ANNALS OF THE NEW YORK ACADEMY OF SCIENCES

Volume 928

EDITORIAL STAFF

Executive Editor
BARBARA M. GOLDMAN

Managing Editor
JUSTINE CULLINAN

Associate Editor
TRUMBULL ROGERS

The New York Academy of Sciences
2 East 63rd Street
New York, New York 10021

THE NEW YORK ACADEMY OF SCIENCES
(Founded in 1817)

BOARD OF GOVERNORS, September 2000 – September 2001

BILL GREEN, *Chairman of the Board*
TORSTEN WIESEL, *Vice Chairman of the Board*
RODNEY W. NICHOLS, *President and CEO* [ex officio]

Honorary Life Governors
WILLIAM T. GOLDEN   JOSHUA LEDERBERG

JOHN T. MORGAN, *Treasurer*

Governors

ELEANOR BAUM   D. ALLAN BROMLEY   KAREN BURKE
     LAWRENCE B. BUTTENWIESER   PRAVEEN CHAUDHARI
JOHN H. GIBBONS   MICHAEL GOLDEN   RONALD L. GRAHAM
ROBERT G. LAHITA   JACQUELINE LEO   WILLIAM J. McDONOUGH
JOHN F. NIBLACK   SANDRA PANEM   RICHARD RAVITCH
RICHARD A. RIFKIND   SARA LEE SCHUPF   JAMES H. SIMONS

HELENE L. KAPLAN, *Counsel* [ex officio]   PETER H. KOHN, *V.P. & Secretary* [ex officio]

HEALTHY AGING FOR FUNCTIONAL LONGEVITY
MOLECULAR AND CELLULAR INTERACTIONS IN SENESCENCE

ANNALS OF THE NEW YORK ACADEMY OF SCIENCES
Volume 928

HEALTHY AGING FOR FUNCTIONAL LONGEVITY
MOLECULAR AND CELLULAR INTERACTIONS IN SENESCENCE

Edited by Sang Chul Park, Eun Seong Hwang, Hyun-Sook Kim, and Woong-Yang Park

The New York Academy of Sciences
New York, New York
2001

Copyright © 2001 by the New York Academy of Sciences. All rights reserved. Under the provisions of the United States Copyright Act of 1976, individual readers of the Annals are permitted to make fair use of the material in them for teaching or research. Permission is granted to quote from the Annals provided that the customary acknowledgment is made of the source. Material in the Annals may be republished only by permission of the Academy. Address inquiries to the Permissions Department (editorial@nyas.org) at the New York Academy of Sciences.

Copying fees: For each copy of an article made beyond the free copying permitted under Section 107 or 108 of the 1976 Copyright Act, a fee should be paid through the Copyright Clearance Center, Inc., 222 Rosewood Drive, Danvers, MA 01923 (www.copyright.com).

∞ The paper used in this publication meets the minimum requirements of the American National Standard for Information Sciences—Permanence of Paper for Printed Library Materials, ANSI Z39.48-1984.

Library of Congress Cataloging-in-Publication Data

Healthy aging for functional longevity : molecular and cellular interactions in senescence / edited by Sang Chul Park ... [et al.].
    p. cm. — (Annals of the New York Academy of Sciences ; v. 928)
"This volume is the result of a conference entitled Healthy aging for functional longevity: molecular and cellular interactions in senescence held by the International Association of Biomedical Gerontology on February 21–s24, 2000 in Kyongju, South Korea."
    Includes bibliographical references and index.
    ISBN 1-57331-285-1 (cloth : alk. paper) — ISBN 1-57331-286-X (pbk. : alk. paper)
    1. Aging—Molecular aspects—Congresses. 2. Longevity —Congresses. I. Park, Sang Chul. II. Last, International Association of Biomedical Gerontology. III. Series.

Q11.N5 vol. 928
[QP86]
500 s—dc21
[612.6'8]
                                                  2001018674

GYAT / PCP
Printed in the United States of America
ISBN 1-57331-285-1 (cloth)
ISBN 1-57331-286-X (paper)
ISSN 0077-8923

ANNALS OF THE NEW YORK ACADEMY OF SCIENCES
Volume 928
April 2001

HEALTHY AGING FOR FUNCTIONAL LONGEVITY
MOLECULAR AND CELLULAR INTERACTIONS IN SENESCENCE

Editors
SANG CHUL PARK, EUN SEONG HWANG, HYUN-SOOK KIM,
AND WOONG-YANG PARK

Conference Organizers
HYON E. CHOY, WOONG-YANG PARK, BOK GHEE HAN,
IN KWON CHUNG, CHEOL HO KIM, EUN SUNG HWANG, IN KYUNG LIM,
HYUN SOOK KIM, AND HAE YOUNG CHUNG

Advisory Board
BYUNG PAL YU, DENHAM HARMAN, KENICHI KITANI,
MOHSEN MEYDANI, AND IMRE ZS. NAGY

This volume is the result of a conference entitled **Healthy Aging for Functional Longevity: Molecular and Cellular Interactions in Senescence** held by the International Association of BioMedical Gerontology during February 2000, in Kyongju, South Korea.

CONTENTS

Preface. *By* SANG CHUL PARK xi

Part I. Main Theme of Current Aging Research

Aging: Overview. *By* DENHAM HARMAN 1

Protein Oxidation in Aging and Age-Related Diseases. *By* EARL R. STADTMAN . 22

Stress Resistance by Caloric Restriction for Longevity. *By* BYUNG P. YU AND
  HAE YOUNG CHUNG 39

Part II. Biomedical Changes Associated with Aging

Protein Glycation: Creation of Catalytic Sites for Free Radical Generation.
  By MOON B. YIM, HYUNG-SOON YIM, CHEOLJU LEE, SA-OUK KANG,
  AND P. BOON CHOCK 48

Implications of Protein Degradation in Aging. *By* SATARO GOTO, RYOYA TAKAHASHI, ATSUSHI KUMIYAMA, ZSOLT RADAK, TOSHIAKI HAYASHI, MASAKI TAKENOUCHI, AND RYOICHI ABE 54

Transglutaminase-Mediated Crosslinking of Specific Core Histone Subunits and Cellular Senescence. *By* JAE HONG KIM, HYON E CHOY, KANG HOON NAM, AND SANG CHUL PARK 65

Proteome and Proteomics for the Research on Protein Alterations in Aging. *By* TOSIFUSA TODA 71

Attenuation of EGF Signaling in Senescent Cells by Caveolin. *By* WOONG-YANG PARK, KYUNG-A CHO, JEONG-SOO PARK, DEOK-IN KIM, AND SANG CHUL PARK 79

Part III. Genomic Instability in Aging

BRCA1 Gene Sequence Variation in Centenarians. *By* JAN VIJG, THOMAS PERLS, CLAUDIO FRANCESCHI, AND NATHALIE J. VAN ORSOUW 85

Increases of Mitochondrial Mass and Mitochondrial Genome in Association with Enhanced Oxidative Stress in Human Cells Harboring 4,977 BP-Deleted Mitochondrial DNA. *By* YAU-HUEI WEI, CHENG-FENG LEE, HSIN-CHEN LEE, YI-SHING MA, CHIA-WEN WANG, CHING-YOU LU, AND CHENG-YOONG PANG 97

DNA Polymerase-β May Be the Main Player for Defective DNA Repair in Aging Rat Neurons. *By* KALLURI SUBBA RAO, V.V. ANNAPURNA, AND N.S. RAJI 113

Premature Aging and Predisposition to Cancers Caused by Mutations in RecQ Family Helicases. *By* YASUHIRO FURUICHI 121

Health Span and Life Span in Transgenic Mice with Modulated DNA Repair. *By* CHRISTI A. WALTER, ZI-QIANG ZHOU, DIWI MANGUINO, YUJI IKENO, ROBERT REDDICK, JAMES NELSON, GABRIEL INTANO, DAMON C. HERBERT, C. ALEX MCMAHAN, AND MARTHA HANES 132

Part IV. Cellular Maintenance and Stress Response

Inhibition Mechanisms of Bioflavonoids Extracted from the Bark of *Pinus maritima* on the Expression of Proinflammatory Cytokines. *By* KYUNG-JOO CHO, CHANG-HYUN YUN, LESTER PACKER, AND AN-SIK CHUNG 141

Gene Expression and Regulation in the Extended Longevity Phenotypes of *Drosophila*. *By* ROBERT ARKING 157

Impairment of Learning and Memory in Rats Caused by Oxidative Stress and Aging, and Changes in Antioxidative Defense Systems. *By* KOJI FUKUI, KOJI ONODERA, TADASHI SHINKAI, SHOZO SUZUKI, AND SHIRO URANO 168

Translocational Inefficiency of Intracellular Proteins in Senescence of Human Diploid Fibroblasts. *By* IN KYOUNG LIM, KWANG WON HONG, IN HAE KWAK, GYESOON YOON, AND SANG CHUL PARK 176

Oxidative Stress and Neurodegeneration in Prion Diseases. *By* JAE-IL KIM, SEUNG-IL CHOI, NAM-HO KIM, JAE-KWANG JIN, EUN-KYOUNG CHOI, RICHARD I. CARP, AND YONG-SUN KIM 182

On the True Role of Oxygen Free Radicals in the Living State, Aging, and Degenerative Disorders. *By* IMRE ZS.-NAGY 187

Cellular and Molecular Pathogenic Mechanisms of Insulin-Dependent Diabetes Mellitus. *By* JI-WON YOON AND HEE-SOOK JUN 200

Part V. Practical Approach for Functional Longevity

Capacity for Recovery and Possible Mechanisms in Immobilization Atrophy of Young and Old Animals. *By* N. ZARZHEVSKY, O. MENASHE, E. CARMELI, H. STEIN, AND A.Z. REZNICK 212

Nutrition Interventions in Aging and Age-Associated Disease. *By* MOHSEN MEYDANI 226

Exercise at Old Age: Does It Increase or Alleviate Oxidative Stress? *By* LI LI JI 236

Do Antioxidant Strategies Work against Aging and Age-associated Disorders? Propargylamines: A Possible Antioxidant Strategy. *By* KENICHI KITANI, CHIYOKO MINAMI, TAKAKO YAMAMOTO, WAKAKO MARUYAMA, SETSUKO KANAI, GWEN O. IVY, AND MARIA-CRISTINA CARRILLO 248

Antioxidant and Immunostimulating Activities of the Fruiting Bodies of *Paecilomyces japonica*, a New Type of *Cordyceps* sp. *By* KUK HYUN SHIN, SOON SUNG LIM, SANG HYUN LEE, YEON SIL LEE, AND SAE YUN CHO 261

A New Function of Green Tea: Prevention of Lifestyle-related Diseases. *By* NAOKO SUEOKA, MASAMI SUGANUMA, EISABURO SUEOKA, SACHIKO OKABE, SATORU MATSUYAMA, KAZUE IMAI, KEI NAKACHI, AND HIROTA FUJIKI 274

Anti-aging and Health-promoting Constituents Derived from Traditional Oriental Herbal Remedies: Information Retrieval Using the TradiMed 2000 DB. *By* IL-MOO CHANG 281

Part VI. Calorie Restriction and Longevity

Caloric Restriction in Primates. *By* M. A. LANE, A. BLACK, A. HANDY, E.M. TILMONT, D. K. INGRAM, AND G. S. ROTH 287

Calorie Restriction Enhances the Expression of Key Metabolic Enzymes Associated with Protein Renewal during Aging. *By* STEPHEN R. SPINDLER 296

Caloric Restriction in Primates and Relevance to Humans. *By* GEORGE S. ROTH, DONALD K. INGRAM, AND MARK A. LANE 305

Aging and Caloric Restriction in Nonhuman Primates: Behavioral and *in Vivo* Brain Imaging Studies. *By* DONALD K. INGRAM, SVETLANA CHEFER, JOHN MATOCHIK, TAMMY D. MOSCRIP, JAMES WEED, GEORGE S. ROTH, EDYTHE D. LONDON, AND MARK A. LANE 316

The Inflammation Hypothesis of Aging: Molecular Modulation by Calorie Restriction. *By* HAE YOUNG CHUNG, HYON JEEN KIM, JUNG WON KIM, AND BYUNG PAL YU 327

Panel Discussion: Perspectives in Aging Research in the New Millennium. *By* SANG CHUL PARK, CHAIR 336

Part VII. Poster Papers

A Thermolabile Variant of Methylenetetrahydrofolate Reductase Is a Determinant of Hyperhomocyst(e)inemia in the Elderly. *By* JUN-HYUN YOO .. 344

Age-related Increase in the Expression of Heat-Shock Protein Genes in the Tissues of Unstressed Rats. *By* RYOYA TAKAHASHI AND SATARO GOTO 345

Amyloid-β-Peptide 25-35 Fragment Modulates the Expression of the Mitochondrial Cytochrome Oxidase Gene. *By* BOK-GHEE HAN, EUN HYE HAN, JEUNG YEUB AHN, AND JUNGSOON PARK 346

Analysis of the Cell Distribution of Endogenous Murine Leukemia Virus in the Brains of SAMR1 and SAMP8 Mice. *By* BYUNG-HOON JEONG, JAE-KWANG JIN, EUN-KYOUNG CHOI, H.C. MEEKER, CHRISTINE A. KOZAK, RICHARD I CARP, AND YONG-SUN KIM 347

Analysis of Traditional Korean Food Patterns According to the Healthy Longevity Diet Based on the Database of Favorite Korean Foods. *By* MEE-SOOK LEE, MEE-KYUNG WOO, CHUNG-SHIL KWAK, SE-IN OH, AND SANG-CHUL PARK 348

Analysis of Proteins in Aged Rat Kidney: The Effect of Calorie Restriction. *By* HYON-JEEN KIM, HYEON-YOUNG JEONG, BYUNG-PAL YU, SATARO GOTO, AND HAE-YOUNG CHUNG 349

Analysis of Redox Status in Serum during Aging. *By* JUNG-WON KIM, JAE-KYUNG NO, BYUNG-PAL YU, AND HAE-YOUNG CHUNG 350

Animal Model for Alzheimer's Disease by *PS2* Gene Transfer. *By* DAE-YOUN HWANG, KAP-RYONG CHAE, TAE-SURK KANG, DONG-HWAN SHIN, IN-SURK JANG, JIN-HEE HWANG, YEON-JU KIM, JOON-YONG CHO, BUM-JIN KIM, YONG-KYU KIM, AND JUNG-SIK CHO 351

Changes in Growth Factor-induced Signal Transduction during the Aging Process of Human Primary Fibroblasts. *By* EUI-JU YEO AND CHANG-MO KANG 352

Contribution of Cyclooxygenase to Age-related Oxidative Stress. *By* HYON-JEEN KIM, BYUNG-PAL YU, MI-AE YU, KYU-WON KIM, JAE-SUK WOO, AND HAE-YOUNG CHUNG 353

Control of Mitochondrial Redox Balance by the Mitochondrial $NADP^+$-dependent Isocitrate Dehydrogenase. *By* TAE-LIN HUH, SEUNG-HEE JO, MI-KYUNG SOHN, SU-MIN LEE, IN-HWANG SONG, HO-JIN KOH, YONG-OU KIM, AND JEEN-WOO PARK 354

The Pro- and Antioxidant Role of Glutathione in Selenite-induced Oxidative Stress and Apoptosis. *By* HAN-MING SHEN, CHENG-FENG YANG, JIN LIU, AND CHOON-NAM ONG 355

Effects of Aging on Aldosterone Secretion in Rat Zona Glomerulosa Cells. *By* MEI-MEI KAU, JIANN-JONG CHEN, AND PAULUS S. WANG 356

Evidence for Differential Structure and Function of Hsp70 Family Members, Mot-1 and Mot-2, in Control of Cellular Senescence. *By* YOUJI MITSUI, RENU WADHWA, SYUICHI TAKANO, AND SUNIL C. KAUL 357

Expression of Growth-Related Genes in the Tissues of Aged Rat Brain. *By* DEOK-KYU AN, SEON-GIL DO, JUN-GYO SUH, JAE-BONG PARK, AND JAE-YONG LEE 358

Expression of Peroxiredoxin in the Skin and Change of Peroxiredoxin by Ultraviolet B Irradiation: A Possible Antioxidant Role against Oxidative Stress in the Skin. *By* SEUNG-CHUL LEE, JUNG EUN LEE, JEE-BUM LEE, YOUNG PIO KIM, AND HO ZOON CHAE 359

Genetic Polymorphism of Presenilin-1 Gene and Apolipoprotein E in Korean Elderly with Dementia. *By* JUNG-EUN PARK AND KYUNG-HEA CHO 361

Impact of Growth Hormone Suppression in the Aging Process and Preliminary Longevity Analysis. *By* ISAO SHIMOKAWA, YOSHIKAZU HIGAMI, KURUMI YANAGIHARA-OUTA, KENJI TANAKA, TOMOSHI TUCHIYA, TAKAHITO KONDO AND SHINJI GOTO 362

Increased Expression of Calsenilin in the Brains of Scrapie-infected Mice. *By* JIN-KYU CHOI, HYUN-PIL LEE, EUN-KYOUNG CHOI, JAE-KWANG JIN, HYOUNG-GON LEE, WILMA WASCO, JOSEPH D. BUXBAUM, RICHARD I. CARP, AND YONG-SUN KIM 363

Induction of Cellular Senescence in Cervical Cancer Cells by Inhibition of HPV Oncogene Expression. *By* CHAN JAE LEE AND EUN SEONG HWANG 364

Induction of Senescence-like Phenotype by an Alkylating Agent, Methyl Methanesulfonante, in Human Diploid Fibroblast. *By* YOUSIN SUH, DEOK-IN KIM, JEONG-SOO PARK, WOONG-YANG PARK, AND SANG CHUL PARK 365

Investigation on Natural Peroxynitrite Scavengers. *By* JI-SUNG YOON, BYUNG-PAL YU, AND HAE-YOUNG CHUNG. 366

Involvement of Caspases in Cell Death Induced by Selenium Compounds in HL-60 Cells. *By* UHEE JUNG, TAE-HO KIM, AND AN-SIK CHUNG 367

Lowered 8-Hydroxyguanine Glycosylase Activity in Senescence-accelerated Mice due to a Single-base Mutation. *By* JEONG-YUN CHOI, HUN-SIK KIM, DONG-WOOK LEE, AND MYUNG-HEE CHUNG 368

Melatonin-related Compounds Have High Free Radical Scavenging Activity. *By* RYUNG YANG, HAE-YOUNG CHUNG, DONG-BUM SHIN, TAE-YEON CHO, AND SEUNG-HYUN YANG 369

Metabolic Modulation of Cellular Redox Potential Can Improve Cardiac Recovery from Ischemia-Reperfusion Injury. *By* HEUN-SOO KANG, JONG-WAN PARK, YANG-SOOK CHUN, MYUNG-SUK KIM, AND SANG CHUL PARK 370

New Directions in Communicating Better Nutrition to Older Adults. *By* GEORGIA SUE GULDAN AND WENDY WAI-HING HUI 371

Nitric Oxide Is Implicated in Apoptotic Cell Death Induced by H_2O_2 in C6 Cells. *By* YOUNG IL LEE, JUNGSOON PARK, YOUNG HEE LEE, AND BOK-GHEE HAN 372

Overexpression of Calsenilin in Sporadic Alzheimer's Disease Brain. *By* JAE KWANG JIN, JIN KYU CHOI, JAE IL KIM, HYOUNG GON LEE, WILMA WASCO, JOSEPH D. BUXBAUM, RICHARD I. CARP, YONG-SUN KIM, AND EUN KYOUNG CHOI 373

Oxidative Stress Associated Antioxidant Enzyme and Neuroendocrine Markers in Dementia. *By* HEUI OG KIM, HYE WON SEO, JUNG EUN PARK, KYUNG HEA CHO, AND IN SUNG KIM 374

p38 Mitogen-activated Protein Kinase Is Involved in H_2O_2-induced Phospholipase D Activation in Vascular Smooth Muscle Cells. *By* EUNG-GOOK KIM, EUN-YOUNG SHIN, DO SIK MIN, BYOUNG-HEE PARK, KYUNG-SUN SHIN, MIN-SOO HYUN, JI-CHEOL SHIN, HEE-YUL AHN, ROGER J. DAVIS, AND SEUNG-RYUL KIM.......................... 376

Photoaging in Asian Skin: New Grading System and the Influence of Environmental Factors. *By* JIN HO CHUNG, SEONG HUN LEE, CHOON SHIK YOON, AND HEE CHUL EUN.......................... 377

Plasma Concentrations of an Endogenous Nitric Oxide Synthase Inhibitor, N^G,N^G-Dimethylarginine: A Novel Risk Factor for Cerebral Infarction in the Elderly. *By* JUN-HYUN YOO AND SUNG-CHANG LEE............. 378

Protection of Mitochondria Permeability Transition by Dihydroxybenzaldehyde against Hydroxyl Radicals. *By* HAE YOUNG CHUNG, HYON JEEN KIM, YOUNG HWAN YANG, WON CHUL CHOI, HYE JIN PARK, JAE SUE CHOI, CHANG MO KANG, AND SANG CHUL PARK.................... 379

Risk Factors for Total Mortality in Centenarians in Aichi Prefecture, Japan. *By* KIYOKO YAGYU, SHOGO KIKUCHI, AND HISASHI TAUCHI............. 380

The Activation Mechanisms of NF-κB and Inflammatory Enzymes during Aging. *By* HYUN JOO KWON, HYON JEEN KIM, MIN JU KANG, RYOYA TAKAHASHI, SATARO GOTO, BYUNG PAL YU, AND HAE YOUNG CHUNG 381

Vitamin and Mineral Supplement Use among Independent-living Korean and American Older Adults. *By* SEUNG-YOUN HONG..................... 382

Vitamin D and Estrogen Receptor Gene Polymorphism and Their Interaction Associated with Bone Mineral Density in Korean Postmenopausal Women. *By* IN SOON KWON, TAIWOO YOO, BYUNG JOO PARK, HEUNG SIK KANG, CHANG MO KANG, IN KYU KIM, SANG HOON BAE, HYUN CHAN CHO, HAENG SHIN LEE, AND CHO-IL KIM.......................... 384

Vitamin-E Dose-Associated Alterations in Mouse Immune Function. *By* HYUN-SOOK KIM, JI-HYE LEE, AND YOU-SOOK LEE................. 385

INDEX OF CONTRIBUTORS.. 387

Financial assistance was received from:

- **FEDERATION OF KOREAN GERONTOLOGICAL SOCIETIES**
- **KOREA SCIENCE & ENGINEERING FOUNDATION**
- **KOREA RESEARCH FOUNDATION**
- **KOREA RESEARCH FOUNDATION FOR HEALTH SCIENCE**
- **SEOUL NATIONAL UNIVERSITY**

> The New York Academy of Sciences believes it has a responsibility to provide an open forum for discussion of scientific questions. The positions taken by the participants in the reported conferences are their own and not necessarily those of the Academy. The Academy has no intent to influence legislation by providing such forums.

Preface

SANG CHUL PARK
Seoul National Universitsy College of Medicine, 28, Yongon-Dong, Chongno-Ku, Seoul 110-799, Korea

The term "functional longevity" is nowadays used to emphasize the biological significance of the elderly. Population epidemiology indicates the inevitable increase in the number of elderly, which makes the future welfare of mankind uncertain. Therefore, improvement in the functional capacity and efficiency of the lives of the elderly is becoming more important than ever before.

The 8th Congress of the International Association of Biomedical Gerontology, titled "Healthy Aging for Functional Longevity: Molecular and Cellular Interactions in Senescence," was held at the Hyundai Hotel in Kyungju, one of Korea's most historic cities, from February 21 to 24, 2000. As the main theme of the congress implies, the organizing committee invited the world's most eminent scientists from not only the fields of basic biomedical gerontology, but also those working with practical and clinical applications.

The basic biomedical changes associated with aging are presented and discussed in Part I, especially such topics of protein modification as oxidation, glycation, and cross-linking in the course of aging. The novel approach of proteomics for protein alteration is also introduced, and signaling attenuation in the senescent cells is explained in terms of receptor-mediated endocytosis.

Part II presents an in-depth exploration of genomic instability in aging. In addition, the difference in genomic stability between aging and cancer, mitochondrial defects in aging, the problem of DNA repair, and the premature aging mechanism are also illustrated.

In Part III, cellular maintenance and the stress response of the senescent cells are presented. Also included is a general discussion of neurodegeneration, prion diseases, diabetic complication, the impact of the oxygen free radical, and dysregulation of the signal transduction system.

Part IV introduces practical approaches for functional longevity, such as nutritional intervention, problems with exercise, and data on drug and herbal medicine. These practical methods were reevaluated, and many ideas for improved efficacy were suggested.

The mechanism of calorie restriction and longevity as regards its effect in primates, potential molecular mechanisms, and calorie restriction mimetics, among other related topics, is discussed in Part V.

Finally, there was a panel on perspectives in aging research of the new millennium. Many new ideas and visions were suggested in this forum, with a possible system of collaboration.

Throughout the conference, most of the participants were keenly interested in the development of an international and interdisciplinary program for aging research, because aging of the organism is not the simple summation of the senescence of each molecule or each cell, but truly the result of the interactive integration of biological, environmental, and social effects on the organism. Moreover, in regard to the welfare of mankind, the importance of the elderly not only in biological life but also in social relations was emphasized. Up to now, however, serious and significant achievement in biomedical gerontology is still waiting to be realized, and it is only through such achievement that the dream of true functional longevity will be accomplished.

Aging: Overview

DENHAM HARMAN

Department of Medicine, University of Nebraska College of Medicine, Omaha, Nebraska 68198-4635, USA

ABSTRACT: Aging is a universal process that began with the origination of life about 3.5 billion years ago. Accumulation of the diverse deleterious changes produced by aging throughout the cells and tissues progressively impairs function and can eventually cause death. Aging changes can be attributed to development, genetic defects, the environment, disease, and an inborn process—the aging process. The chance of death at a given age serves as a measure of the average number of aging changes accumulated by persons of that age, that is, of physiologic age, and the rate of change of this measure as the rate of aging. Chances for death are decreased by improvements in general living conditions. As a result, during the past two millennia average life expectancy at birth (ALE-B), determined by the chances for death, of humans has risen from 30 years, in ancient Rome, to almost 80 years today in the developed countries. Chances for death in the developed countries are now near limiting values and ALE-Bs are approaching plateau values that are 6–9 years less than the potential maximum of about 85 years. Chances for death are now largely determined by the inherent aging process after age 28. Only 1.1% of female cohorts in Sweden die before this age; the remainder die off at an exponentially increasing rate with advancing age. The inherent aging process limits ALE-B to around 85 years, and the maximum life span (MLS) to about 122 years. Past efforts to increase ALE-B did not require an understanding of aging. Such knowledge will be necessary in the future to significantly increase ALE-B and MLS, and to satisfactorily ameliorate the medical, economic, and social problems associated with advancing age. The many theories advanced to account for aging should be used, to the extent it is feasible, to help with these important practical problems, including applications of the free radical theory of aging. Past measures evolved by societies to ensure adequate care for older individuals are rapidly becoming inadequate because of changes in life style, the growing percentage of older people, declining fertility rates, and the diminishing size of the work forces to provide for the elderly. Measures are being advanced to help with this problem. Prospects are bright for further increases in the span of functional life and improvements in the lives of the elderly.

KEYWORDS: Aging; Evolution; Mitochondria; Free radical reactions; Retirement and care of the elderly

INTRODUCTION

Aging and evolution began with the apparent spontaneous origination of life about 3.5 billion years ago.[1] Aging is the accumulation of more or less random di-

Address for correspondence: Denham Harman, Department of Medicine, University of Nebraska College of Medicine, Omaha, Nebraska 68198-4635. Voice: 402-559-4416.
dharman@unmc.edu

verse changes with time. Some changes[2,3] are inheritable, whereas the majority increase the chance of disease and death with advancing age. Together these aging changes ensure evolution. This paper is largely limited to a discussion of aging in mammals, and in particular, to humans.

The rate of accumulation of aging changes under optimal living conditions limits average life expectancy at birth (ALE-B) to about 85 years[4-6] and the maximum life span (MLS) to around 122 years.[7] These limits have been slowly approached over the past 2000 years, owing to gradual improvements in living conditions, for example, nutrition, housing, and medical care. ALE-B, a rough measure of the span of healthy, productive life, has increased from about 30 years in ancient Rome[8] to almost 80 years today in the developed countries.[9] The MLS has apparently remained unchanged.

The accumulation of aging changes throughout the cells and tissues concomitantly progressively lower the ability to cope with work and the stresses and strains of life.[10,11] During recorded history societies continued to develop measures to help minimize the decrements of age. These measures are now under severe strain in many countries,[12] owing in part to the increasing numbers of older persons associated with increasing ALE-Bs.

Future efforts to significantly increase the span of healthy productive life, that is, the functional life span, and to ameliorate problems associated with disproportionate increases in the percentages of older persons in the populations, will require a greater understanding of aging. The purpose of this paper is to contribute to the above goal.

DISCUSSION

Aging

Definition

Aging is the accumulation of diverse deleterious changes in the cells and tissues with advancing age that increase the risk of disease and death.[2,3,9] Aging changes can be attributed to developmental and genetic defects, the environment, disease processes, and an inherent process, referred to as the aging process. The chance of death of an individual of a given age in a population—readily available from vital statistics data—serves as a measure of (1) the average number of adverse changes, that is, aging changes, accumulated by persons of that age, and (2) physiologic age, that is, "true age," in contrast to chronological age. The chances for death in a population determine the ALE-B. ALE-B is a rough measure of the span of healthy, productive life, that is, the functional life span.

Effect of Improved Living Conditions on Aging

Conventional means (CM) of increasing the ALE-B of a population by decreasing the chances for death through improvements in general living conditions—for example, improved nutrition, housing, and medical care—are becoming increasingly futile.[7,9] This is illustrated in FIGURE 1 by the curves of the logarithm of the chance of death versus age for Swedish females for various periods from 1751 to 1992;[13,14] a

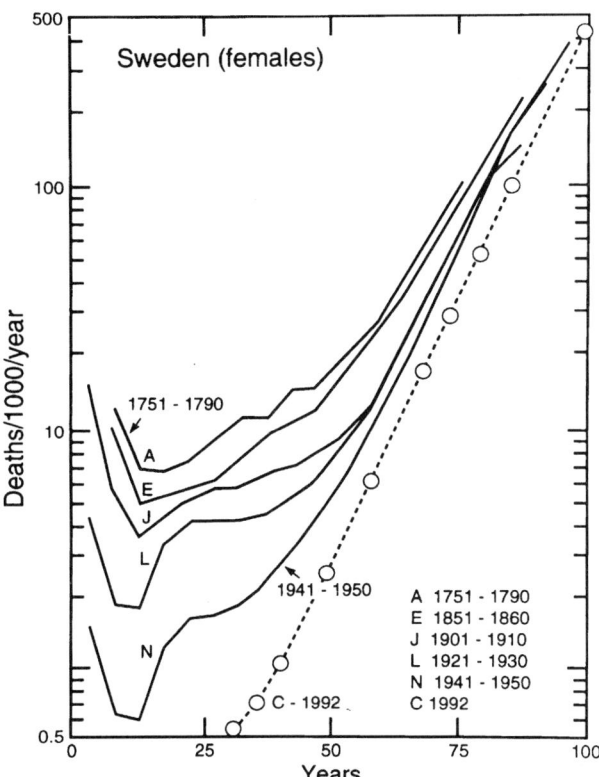

FIGURE 1. Age-specific death rates of Swedish females in various periods from 1751 to 1950 (adapted from H.R. Jones[13]) and for 1992.[14]

straight line represents exponential increases with age. The chances for death in the developed countries are now near limiting values, and ALE-Bs approach plateau values of around 76 years for males and 82 years for females.[7,9]

Thus, as living conditions in a population approach the optimum, and premature deaths the minimum, the logarithmic curve of the chance of death versus age shifts towards a limit determined by the sum of (1) the irreducible contributions to the chance of death by aging changes that can be prevented to varying degrees by CM, for example, those due to the environment and disease, and (2) contributions that can be influenced little, if at all, by CM, that is, those due to the innate aging process. The now-near limiting chances for death rise almost exponentially after about age 28. Only 1–2% of a cohort die before this age.[14]

The Aging Process

The inherent aging process is the major risk factor for disease and death in the developed countries after age 28.[7] It limits ALE-B to about 85 years[4-6] and the MLS to around 122 years.[7] Aging rates are low early in life but rapidly increase with age,

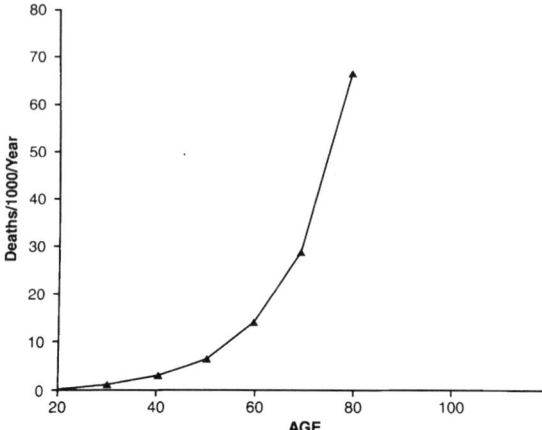

FIGURE 2. The chance of dying in 1985 as a function of age for the total population of the United States.[7]

illustrated in FIGURE 2 by a plot of the chances for death in 1985 for the United States population as a function of age.[7] The innate aging process is caused by chemical reactions that arise in the course of normal metabolism that, collectively, produce aging changes that exponentially increase the chance of death with advancing age even under optimal living conditions.

Theories of Aging: Free Radical Theory

Many theories[7,9] have been advanced to account for the inherent aging process. No theory is generally accepted. The free radical theory of aging (FRTA)[9,15,16] shows promise; the subsequent discussion is based on the assumption that it is correct. The FRTA, and the simultaneous discovery of the important, ubiquitous involvement of free radicals in endogenous metabolic reactions, was proposed in 1954.[15,16] The theory arose from a consideration of aging phenomena from the premise that a single common process, modifiable by genetic and environmental factors, was responsible for the aging and death of all living things.

The FRTA postulates that the common aging process is the initiation of free radical reactions (FRRs). These reactions, however initiated, could be responsible for the progressive deterioration of biological systems over time due to their innate ability to produce random change. The theory was extended in 1972[17,18] with the suggestions that most FRRs were initiated by the mitochondria at an increasing rate with age, and that the life span is determined by the rate of free radical damage to the mitochondria. Collectively, the FRRs initiated by the mitochondria constitute the inherent aging process.

Free Radical Reactions

Free radical reactions can be divided into three stages:[19] initiation, propagation, and termination (FIG. 3). The amount of a compound involved in a free radical reac-

Initiation

$$RH + O_2 \xrightarrow{Cu} R\bullet + HO_2\bullet$$

Propagation

$$R\bullet + O_2 \longrightarrow RO_2\bullet$$
$$RO_2\bullet + RH \longrightarrow R\bullet + ROOH$$

Termination

$$R\bullet + R\bullet \longrightarrow R:R$$

FIGURE 3. Free radical reactions: reaction of O_2 with organic compounds.[19]

tion that is converted to products per unit of time depends on the rate of initiation and the number of times the propagation phase is repeated before termination, that is, the chain length.

Major sources of FRRs today in mammals include the respiratory chain, phagocytosis, prostaglandin synthesis, the cytochrome P-450 system, nonenzymatic reactions of O_2, and ionizing radiation. Defenses that have evolved to minimize free radical–induced damage include antioxidants (e.g., tocopherols and carotenes), heme-containing peroxidases (e.g., catalase), glutathione peroxidase, superoxide dismutases, and DNA repair mechanisms.

Importance of FRRs in Biological Systems

FRRs are ubiquitous in living systems. A reasonable explanation for the presence of this class of chemical reactions is provided by studies on the origin and evolution of life;[1,20] these are summarized in TABLE 1. Life apparently originated spontaneously about 3.5 billion years ago from amino acids, nucleotides, and other basic chemicals of living things produced from the simple, reduced components of the

TABLE 1. Overview of the origin and evolution of life

Years Ago	Main Events
3.5 Billion	Basic chemicals of life formed by free radical reactions, largely initiated by ionizing radiation from the sun. Life begins, excision and recombinational repair processes evolve.
	Ferredoxin appears: RH or $H_2S + CO_2 \to (h\alpha) \to CH$
2.6 Billion	Blue-green algae appear.
	$2H_2O \to (h\alpha) \to 4H + O_2$
1.3 Billion	Atmospheric O_2 reaches 1% of present value. Anaerobic prokaryotes disappear. Eukaryotes become dominate cells. Eukaryotes plus blue-green algae $\to$ the green leaf plants. Eukaryotes plus a prokaryote able to reduce O_2 to $H_2O \to$ animal kingdom. Emergence of multicellular organisms and plants. Meiosis evolves.
500 Million	Atmospheric O_2 reaches 10% of present value. Ozone screen allows emergence of life from the sea.
65 Million	Primates appear.
5 Million	Humans appear.

primitive oxygen-free atmosphere by free radical reactions, initiated mainly by ionizing radiation from the sun.

A picture emerges from the growing knowledge of the role of FRRs in biological systems that naturally follows from their chemical nature. It would appear that life originated as a result of FRRs, selected FRRs to play major metabolic roles, and used them to provide for aging, mutation, and death, thereby assuring evolution. Further, life span evolved in parallel with the ability of organisms to cope with damaging free radical reactions. In short, the origin and evolution of life may be due to free radical reactions and, in particular, to their ability to induce random change. If so, it is remarkable that life with its beautiful order owes its origin to, and is sustained by, a class of chemical reactions whose outstanding characteristic is their unruly nature.

The aging process may be simply the sum of the deleterious FRRs going on continuously throughout the cells and tissues. The process may never have changed; in the beginning the reactions were apparently largely initiated by UV radiation from the sun, and to a lesser extent by volcanic activity; and now they arise from enzymatic and nonenzymatic free radical reactions.

Application of the Free Radical Theory of Aging

The FRTA suggests that measures to decrease the chain lengths of FRRs and/or their rates of initiation can decrease aging changes, even under optimal living conditions, and in turn the rate of aging and of disease pathogenesis. Many studies now support this possibility.[9,16,21–24]

The above studies also indicate that CM increase ALE-B by decreasing the rate of accumulation of aging changes associated with suboptimal living conditions. For example, (1) better nutrition provides more compounds to decrease free radical damage; (2) housing improvements may decrease the amount of food metabolized—and thus free radical production, needed to maintain body temperature; (3) in the case of disease, free radicals are widely involved,[16,21,22] so that measures to improve prevention and treatment would be expected to have beneficial effects on life span; and (4) tissue injury causes free radical formation; thus better accident prevention measures should reduce the accumulation of aging changes.

Increasing Inhibition of Free Radical Reactions

Measures that decrease chain lengths of FRRs include the following: (1) antioxidant enzymes (i.e., superoxide dismutase (SOD), catalase, glutathione peroxidase, and SOD mimics); (2) spin traps; and (3) chain-breaking compounds (i.e., such synthetic compounds as butylated hydroxytoluene (BHT), butylated hydroxyanisole (BHA), 2-mercaptoethylamine (2-MEA), ethoxyquin, 21-aminosteroids, and 2-methylaminochromans (lazaroids); and natural compounds as α-tocopherol, ascorbic acid, β-carotene, melatonin, and α-lipoic acid).

Antioxidant enzymes. Studies with short- and long-lived strains of *Neurospora crassa*,[25] *Drosophila melanogaster*,[26] and *Caenorhabditis elegans*,[27] have shown that activities of antioxidant enzymes are higher in the longer-lived strains. Overexpression in *Drosophila* of both SOD and catalase, which acting in tandem provide the primary enzymatic antioxidant defenses in *Drosophila*, extended the life span by as much as one third.[28]

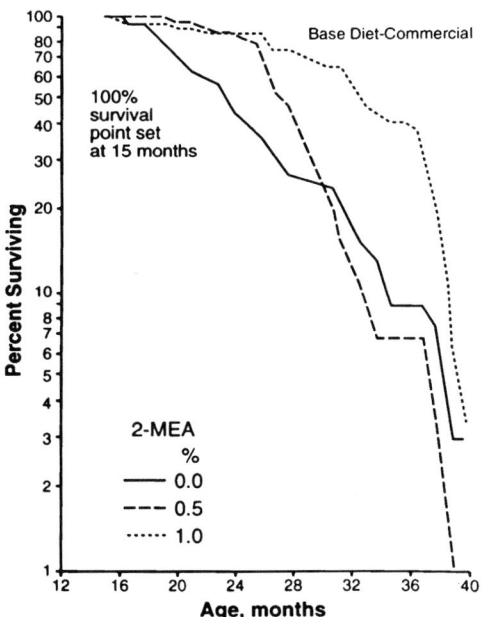

FIGURE 4. Effect of adding 0.5 and 1.0 wt % of 2-MEA to the diet, starting shortly after weaning, on the life span of male LAF_1 mice.[29]

Chain breaking compounds.

- *Dietary antioxidants, from weaning throughout life.* Antioxidants reduce free radical reaction damage by decreasing chain lengths.[19] Most animal studies directed to increasing the life span have used dietary antioxidant supplements to augment the natural defenses against FRR damage. For example, addition of 1% by weight of 2-mercaptoethylamine hydrochloride (2-MEA) to the diet of male LAF mice (FIG. 4), started shortly after weaning, increased ALE-B by 30%;[29] the MLS was increased little, if at all. When 0.5% of ethoxyquin was added to the diet of male and female C3H mice, the increase in ALE-B was 20% for both groups with no change in the MLS.[30] Thus, antioxidant supplements in mice—living under conditions of good animal care, that is, production of free radical reaction–induced aging changes secondary to suboptimal living conditions is small—increased the percentage of older animals in the studies and decreased the senescence periods,[29,30] as there was little, if any, effect on the MLS. The latter is true because the exponentially increasing production of aging changes with age by the inherent aging process progressively nullify the beneficial effects of the antioxidants, keeping increases in maximum life span minimal.

- *Exposure to antioxidants during early life.* FRRs may also produce significant life-shortening changes during the short period of high mitotic and metabolic rate of early life. These reactions, aside from those associated with the envi-

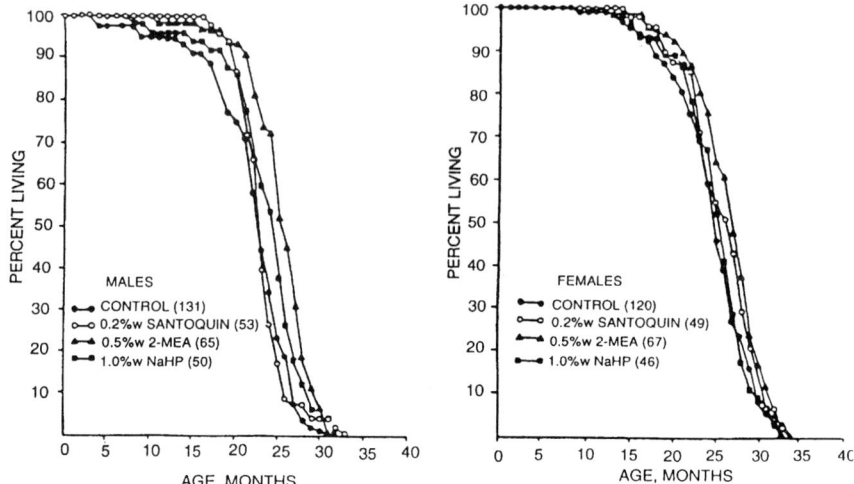

FIGURE 5. Effect of adding antioxidants to the maternal diet on the life spans of their offspring.[35]

ronment, apparently first arise with the onset of mitochondrial function and the associated formation of superoxide radicals in the course of normal metabolism. This occurs on gestational day 10 in the rat.[31] There are at least two other sources of FRRs in early life: (1) steroid estrogens, elevated in pregnancy,[32] can be converted to catechol estrogens that serve as a source of superoxide radicals via the quinone/hydroquinone redox system,[33] and (2) sporadic episodes of transient increases in superoxide radicals, secondary to ischemia-reperfusion injury, due to uteroplacental hypoperfusion.[31,34] The above possibility was assessed twice. In the second experiment[35] groups of female Swiss mice were maintained on a semisynthetic diet, with and without an added antioxidant supplement (0.2 wt % ethoxyquin, 0.5 wt % 2-MEA, or 1.0 wt % sodium hypophosphite), from one month before mating until the offspring were weaned. The male and female offspring were separated and placed on a pelleted commercial diet (no added antioxidants). Survival curves were obtained. Addition of 2-MEA, the most effective of the compounds evaluated, to the maternal diet increased the ALE-B of male offspring by 15% and of females by 8% (FIG. 5). The results of both experiments were similar. The second study confirmed the unexpected results of the first one—the percentage increase in life span was greater for male offspring than for female offspring. The antioxidants had no apparent adverse effects on the pregnancies. The above increases in offspring life spans are attributed to decreases by the 2-MEA in free radical–induced nonspecific aging changes and life-shortening mutations. The lesser effect observed in females may have been largely due to a normally higher level of protection of female embryos from free radical damage during a short period, about 48 hours in the mouse, just prior to the random inactivation of one of the two functioning X chromosomes in the late blastocyst stage of development. The X chromosome codes for glucose-6-phosphate dehydrogenase, a key enzyme in the production of NADPH; NADPH acts to maintain glutathione in the reduced state. Also contributing to the gender difference in longevity are the lower body stores of iron in females prior to the menopause secondary to iron loss during menstruation.[36]

- *Association of disease with age.* The adverse effects of FRRs after conception provide a plausible explanation for the association of disease with age.[23] The ubiquitous FRRs would be expected to produce deleterious changes that accumulate progressively with age. The nature and locations of the changes are influenced by genetic and environmental factors. Those that are more or less common to all persons determine the "normal" sequential alterations with time. Superimposed on this common pattern of change are patterns that differ from individual to individual owing to genetic and environmental differences that modulate FRR damage, for example, defective Cu/Zn SOD in Lou Gehrig disease[37] and probable higher rates of formation of superoxide radicals in the vessel walls in essential hypertension.[38] The superimposed patterns of change may become progressively more discernable with time, and some may eventually be recognized as diseases, at ages influenced by genetic and environmental risk factors. In agreement with the preceding: (1) FRRs have been implicated in the pathogenesis of a growing number of disorders—the free radical diseases[23,24] (i.e., atherosclerosis, cancer, Alzheimer disease, Parkinson disease, essential hypertension, cataracts, Fanconi anemia, Bloom syndrome, amyloidosis, diabetes mellitus, Laennec cirrhosis, and amyotrophic lateral sclerosis), and (2) accumulating recent data demonstrate that many diseases of adulthood that shorten life[39,40]—for example, breast and prostate cancer, coronary heart disease, hypertension, and diabetes mellitus—have their origins in events of early life.[39,40] This is also probably true for Alzheimer disease.[39]

- *Decreasing the incidence of free radical diseases.* Although the exact etiologies of the free radical diseases are not known, the probability of developing any one of them should be decreased by lowering levels of the more or less random FRRs by any of the following means: (1) during early development, enhance antioxidant content of maternal diets, reduce catechol estrogens, and increase efforts to lower episodes of uteroplacental ischemia; (2) food restriction; (3) minimization of exposure to ionizing radiation; (4) increasing antioxidant intake (dietary and/or supplements); and (5) in the case of a specific disease, decreasing environmental risk factors, for example, cholesterol in atherosclerosis and carcinogens in cancer. In some instances it may be necessary to "target" the inhibitor(s) in order to achieve effective inhibitor concentrations. Thus, the blood pressure of spontaneously hypertensive rats is not lowered by intravenously injected Cu/Zn SOD, but it is lowered when the enzyme is coupled with a basic peptide to form HB-SOD.[38] Unlike SOD, HB-SOD undergoes transendothelial transport and localizes within arterial walls.

- *Failure to increase the maximum life span.* The general failure of antioxidants to increase maximum life span is attributed to[9,39] (1) depression of mitochondrial function by the compounds at concentrations below those needed to slow free radical damage to the mitochondria (that is, as the dietary concentration of an antioxidant is increased it significantly impairs mitochondrial function before it slows mitochondrial aging)—2-mercaptoethanol[41] and two pyridine compounds[42,43] may be exceptions, and/or (2) progressive increases in the initiation of free radical reactions with age by the mitochondria eventually nullify the beneficial effects of the added antioxidant.

Decreasing FRR Initiation Rates

Measures to reduce FRR initiation rates, and thus increase life span, can be divided into two categories: those that produce increases in ALE-B but have little, if any, effect on MLS, and those that produce increases in both ALE-B and MLS. The following measures fit into the first category.

Measures That Increase ALE-B.

- *Minimize intake of dietary componnents prone to increase inintiation rates.* For example, copper, iron, and manganese, polyunsaturated lipids, and easily peroxidized amino acids. Thus, increasing the the dietary content of easily peroxidized amino acids might increase FRR damage and thereby decrease life expectancy. In agreement, when 1 wt % of either histidine or lysine was added to a semisynthetic diet containing 20 wt % of casein as the sole source of protein, average life expectancy was decreased by 5 and 6%, respectively.[44] Conversely, replacing casein by a soybean protein containing a lesser amount of easily oxidized amino acids increased life expectancy by 13 percent.

- *Cruciferous vegetables.* Cruciferous vegetables[9] contain compounds that induce enzymes that catalyze the two-electron reduction of dietary quinones to hydroquinones, thereby decreasing the likelihood that the compounds would undergo one electron reduction to the semiquinone radical. These can react spontaneously with O_2 to form the superoxide radical and regenerate the quinones, thus resulting in oxidative stress by redox cycling.

- *Phlebotomy and chelation.* The life span may be increased further by measures such as phlebotomy[36,45] and chelation.[46–48] These minimize accumulation in the body of metals capable of initiating adverse free radical reactions, for example, iron, copper, and manganese, as well as of such heavy metals as lead, mercury, and cadmium that can impair activities of sulfur and selenium-containing enzymes.

- *Peroxisomal activity.* Peroxisomes[49,50] are organelles that have large complements of flavin oxidases and catalase. Normally a small amount of the H_2O_2 formed by the oxidases escapes catalase action and diffuses from the organelle. This peroxisomal-derived H_2O_2 can be increased, for example, by peroxisomal proliferators such as clofibrate and high fat diets. Thus, minimizing peroxisomal proliferator activity should have a beneficial effect on life span.

Measures That Increase both ALE-B and MLS. The rate of mitochondrial superoxide radical formation is the major determinant of the life span. The major source of endogenous free radical reactions are superoxide radicals arising from the mitochondrial respiratory chain in the course of normal metabolism. The rate of mitochondrial superoxide radical formation increases with age.[17,22,51–58] This makes it progressively more difficult, and eventually impossible, to prevent free radical damage to the body by dietary means, including the use of dietary supplements. Decreases in caloric intake are associated with (a) decreases in O_2 utilization and in superoxide radical formation, and (b) increases in life span. Comparing birds and mammals of similar metabolic rates, the much longer life spans of the birds is related to a lower rate of formation of superoxide radicals by the mitochondria.[59,60] This also occurs in two closely related rodent species.[61] Life spans of different mammalian species[53] are related to the rates of mitochondrial superoxide radical formation. The frequency of the mitochondrial genotype, Mt5178A, in Japan is higher in centenarians than in healthy blood donors.[62] The high frequency of this genotype in the Japanese population (45%) may be related to the fact that the Japanese are the longest lived of the the world's populations. As expected, because mitochondria are of maternal origin, siblings of centenarians live longer than the normal life span.[63] In accord with the foregoing, oxidative stress has been reported to be less in healthy centenarians than in younger individuals.[64]

The following measures can/may decrease mitochondrial superoxide formation without lowering ATP production below a level compatible with normal life. These are followed by a further comment on decreasing damage during the early period of life.

• *Caloric restriction.* Decreases in caloric intake are associated with proportionate decreases in O_2 utilization. Over 90% of the O_2 consumed by mammals is used by mitochondria; of this, a small fraction is diverted to form superoxide radicals, causing a corresponding decrease in ATP production. Thus, food restriction decreases both superoxide radical formation and ATP production. The former decreases the aging rate,[9,21,22] thereby increasing life span, whereas the latter decreases energy input, resulting in adapted metabolic changes in an effort to sustain body maintenance and function. The foregoing provides the most parsimonious explanation of the numerous changes[65] found in caloric restriction studies.

In accordance with the above possibility, decreasing the daily caloric intake of rats by 40%, while maintaining essential nutrients,[66] decreased body weight by 40% and increased average life span by 40% and maximum life span by 49 percent. The metabolic rate, that is, the caloric consumption per day per unit of body weight, was the same for the two dietary groups because the percentage decrease in the restricted group, in caloric intake per day and in body weight, was equal. This study demonstrated that caloric restriction slows production of aging changes by the inherent aging process: the slope of the curve of the log of the chance of death versus age for restricted animals is less than that of the controls.[9,21] A similar study has been initiated with primates.[67]

Caloric restriction can almost certainly increase the MLS of humans. However, the increase associated with a tolerable level of restriction would undoubtedly be small. The goal for humans is to significantly increase our healthy life span while living a normal life. Efforts to achieve this goal should also include some acceptable degree of caloric restriction.

Compounds that compete with O_2 for access to "electron-rich areas" of the mitochondria.

• *Spin traps.* Spin traps commonly used in biological systems are nitrones ($\rightarrow$N $\rightarrow$ O) or nitroso (>N = O) compounds.[68] They react with free radicals to form relatively stable nitroxides (>N − O•) that are readily reduced to hydroxylamines (>N − OH). Although spin traps are antioxidants, in a biological system their antioxidant activity seems small in comparison to the apparent ability of the nitroxide derivatives, at least that of *N-tert*-butyl-*"*-phenylnitrone (PBN), to inhibit initiation of FRRs. PBN gradually enhanced performance of old gerbils[69,70] in a radial-arm maze test (a measure of memory) to near that of young gerbils, over a two-week period of twice a day intraperitoneal injections of 32 mg/kg PBN (the threshold dose for protection against ischemia/reperfusion brain injury).[69] This was accompanied by increases in the brain of the ratio of unoxidized to oxidized protein and of the activities of glutamine synthetase and neutral protease. After injections were stopped these measures returned slowly over two weeks to the original values. The above results are those to be expected if PBN had disproportionately lowered the FRR level in old gerbils to near that of the young. This would have increased activities of both neutral protease and glutamine synthetase. The protease would have increased the turnover rate of oxidized proteins,[71,72] changing the ratio of normal protein to oxidized protein towards that of the young and improving maze performance. Assuming the foregoing is correct, it was in part a consequence of the free radical scavenging effect of PBN. However, most likely the major action of PBN was to decrease the initiation rate of adverse FRRs. This could probably be accomplished by the joint action of the following: (a) Addition of a free radical, for example, superoxide radical, to PBN followed by association of the resulting nitroxide with a mitochondrial respiratory chain,[73] where, in competition with O_2 for electrons, a hydroxylamine is formed instead of a superoxide radical. The hydroxylamine could then diffuse away from the mitochondria and be readily converted back to the nitroxide by reacting with a free radical, for example, a hydroxyl radical, thus resulting in cyclic oxidation of the respiratory chain. In essence, the spin trap in a cyclic fashion causes the removal of a free radical while preventing formation of a new one. (b) Decrease formation of the hydroxyl radical by helping to maintain cellular iron in the ferric state;[74,75] (c) the nitroxide serving as a superoxide dismutase mimic; and (d) depressing hydroxyl radical formation inside Cu/Zn SOD.[74] In accordance with the above discussion:

(i) C57BL male mice at 24.5 months of age were divided into two groups of 50 each.[76] The experimental group received 0.25 mg/mL of PBN in their drinking water. The mean life spans for the control and treated groups were 29.0 and 30.1 months, respectively, whereas the corresponding maximum life spans (last survivors) were 31.7 and 33.3 months.

(ii) Eleven 24-month-old male Sprague-Dawley rats were started on daily ip injections of 32 mg/kg of PBN for the 9.5-month study period; the 12 controls of the same age were similarly injected with 0.9% saline solution.[77] The average life span of the controls was 28 months, whereas that of the experimental group was 30. At the end of the study period, 36% (4 rats) of the PBN group was alive, but only 8% (1 rat) of the controls was alive. PBN improved cognitive performance in several tasks associated with decreased oxidative brain damage.

(iii) Daily intraperitoneal injection of senescence-accelerated mice (SAM-P8)—mice that seem to age at a higher than normal rate—with 30 mg/kg of PBN increased both average and maximum life spans.[78] This study suggests that the increased FRR levels in SAM-P8 mice[79] are caused by higher than normal rates of mitochondrial formation of superoxide radical.

- *Nitroxides and hydroxylamines.* In view of the above discussion, these two classes of compounds should act like nitrones and nitroso compounds.

Blocking agents. Compounds that can associate with the electron-rich areas of the mitochondrial respiratory chain, but not react significantly with it or elsewhere, may block access of O_2 to these areas to some extent and thus decrease superoxide radical formation. A search for such substances may be productive.

- The "free radical sponge,"[80] buckyball—for example, fullerene (C_{60}), or some of its derivatives—may have the foregoing properties. These empty ball-like compounds show promise as neuroprotective agents.[81]

- The antiviral agent, amantadine,[82] may also be useful. This soluble, stable 10-carbon amine prevents cellular entry of a virus,[83] possibly by coating the virus. This compound is excreted unchanged in the urine.

Compounds that may decrease loss of mtDNA function with age.

- *Coenzyme Q_{10}.* This compound is an essential component of the electron transport chain and serves also as an important antioxidant in both mitochondria and lipid membranes. Levels of coenzyme Q_{10} in both animals and humans decrease with age. Dietary supplementation of rats with coenzyme Q_{10} significantly increased mitochondrial content of the compound.[84] The decline in the level of this substance with age hinders the transfer of electrons from complexes I and II to complex III.[85] This increases the electron density of complexes I and II, resulting in a higher rate of formation of superoxide radical. Thus coenzyme Q supplementation should both decrease the block and the oxidative damage to the mitochondria. Apparently very few long-term studies have been made with coenzyme Q_{10}. A lifelong study of mice and rats supplemented with coenzyme Q_{10} found no increase in life span, and no shortening;[86] further studies are indicated.

- *R-"-Lipoic acid.* This form of the disulfide lipoic acid is the naturally occurring enantiomer in mammalian cells. It is a coenzyme for the mitochondrial dehydrogenases for pyruvate and α-ketoglutarate.[87] Supplementation of the diet of rats with (R)-α-lipoic acid "significantly attenuates the age-related increase in hepatocellular oxidant production as well as lipid peroxidation."[88] Supplementation also increased the cellular levels of glutathione and ascorbic in old rats to be like those of the young. Further, "feeding acetyl-L-carnitine (ALCAR) in combination with lipoic acid effectively increases mitochondrial metabolism without an increase in oxidative stress," which was observed with using ALCAR alone.[89] Thus, (R)-α-lipoic acid may serve, at least in part, to decrease mitochondrial superoxide radical formation.

- *Glutathione.* Increases in oxidative damage to mtDNA with age are associated with decreases in mitochondrial glutathione (GSH) content.[90,91] The changes are reversed with oral antioxidants—for example, thiazolidine carboxylate (TC)[90] and a *Ginkgo biloba* extract (EGb 761).[91] Other measures directed to increasing mitochondrial GSH[92] include providing GSH esters, and precursors of substrates for GSH synthetase and γ-glutamylcysteine synthetase. The MLS[93] of *Drosophila melanogaster* was increased about 18% when maintained on a diet supplemented with either sodium or magnesium thiazolidine carboxylate.
- *Aminoethylcysteine ketimine decarboxylated dimer.* This compound[94] may slow mitochondrial superoxide radical formation by inhibiting oxidation of mitochondrial components at concentrations that do not inhibit function of complex I.
- 2-Mercaptoethanol[41] and two pyridine compounds[42,43] have been reported to increase the MLS (see above). If these studies can be reproduced they should prompt evaluation of other antioxidants.

Genetic change. Birds have high metabolic rates compared to comparable sized mammals and yet have relatively long life spans. This is attributed to a genetically determined diversion of a smaller fraction of the oxygen they use to superoxide radicals than do mammals.[59,60] Likewise,[61] and apparently for the same reason, the white-footed mouse (*Peromyscus leucopus*) lives longer than the common mouse (*Mus musculus*).

Efforts to determine the cause(s), such as more detailed knowledge of the structure of the complexes[95] of these differences in O_2 diversion to superoxide radicals, may result in measures to decrease the diversion in humans. These efforts may be helped by studies of neuroleptics; these compounds may alter mitochondrial gene expression.[96,97]

The short life span of SAM-P8 mice, discussed above, is probably also caused by a mutation(s) that increased mitochondrial superoxide formation. Recently it has been demonstrated that a single targeted mutation of the mouse $p66^{shc}$ gene[98] induces resistance to oxidative stress and increases life span by about 30% without apparent negative side effects.[98] A reasonable possibility is that mutation of the $p66^{shc}$ gene decreases the fraction of O_2 diverted to superoxide radicals by the mitochondria (see above).

Rate of Mitochondrial Superoxide Radical Formation

Decreasing Ill Effects of Early Life

Accumulating data implicates abnormal changes in early life that predispose to diseases of adulthood that shorten life.[39,40] Measures to ameliorate these changes have been briefly discussed above. In addition, efforts to minimize the rise[99,100] in estrogen levels in pregnancy, for example, by a low fat diet,[101] may also increase the life span of offspring.

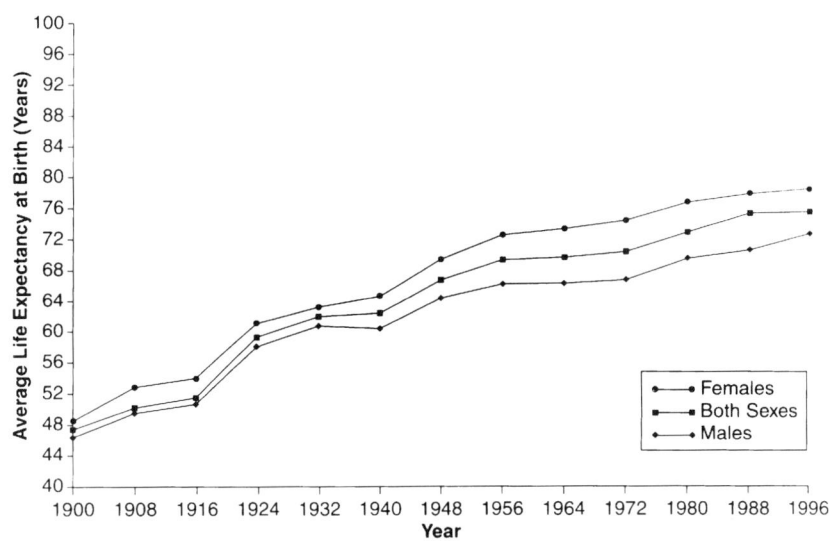

FIGURE 6. Average life expectancy at birth: United States, 1900–1996.[102]

Satisfactorily Accommodating Disproportionate Increases in the Numbers of Older Persons in the Populations

Increases in longevity by continued improvements in CM[102] (FIG. 6) are accompanied by progressive increases in the percentages of older people in the population[10] (FIG. 7), illustrated by data for the United States for 1900–1996. Thus, in the United States the ALE-B rose from 69.7 years in 1960 to 75.4 years in 1990.[102] The 38.7% increase in the total population during this 30-year period was accompanied by an 86.7% increase in the 65+ group (the elderly), and the 85+ group (the oldest old) grew by 225.2%.[10,103] Such disproportionate increases in the numbers of older members, particularly of the oldest old, of many populations are now beginning to (1) severely stress the measures that societies have evolved to help make the lives of older individuals worth living,[12,104–106] and (2) stimulate efforts to cope.

It is in the self-interest of all individuals in a society that it have acceptable, sustainable measures that satisfactorily ameliorate the medical, economic, and social problems of the elderly. Because everyone eventually benefits, everyone should contribute. These measures must recognize that each individual has different abilities, opportunities, and interests, while each individual must accept the responsibility for his/her life and those of their children. These responsibilities include efforts to ensure "successful aging"[104] and to put their children on a course to do likewise.

A sustainable, and probable acceptable, measure in many societies would mandate each individual to save and invest for retirement throughout their working life. This is akin to the present successful plans[107] in England, Australia, and Chile. Life

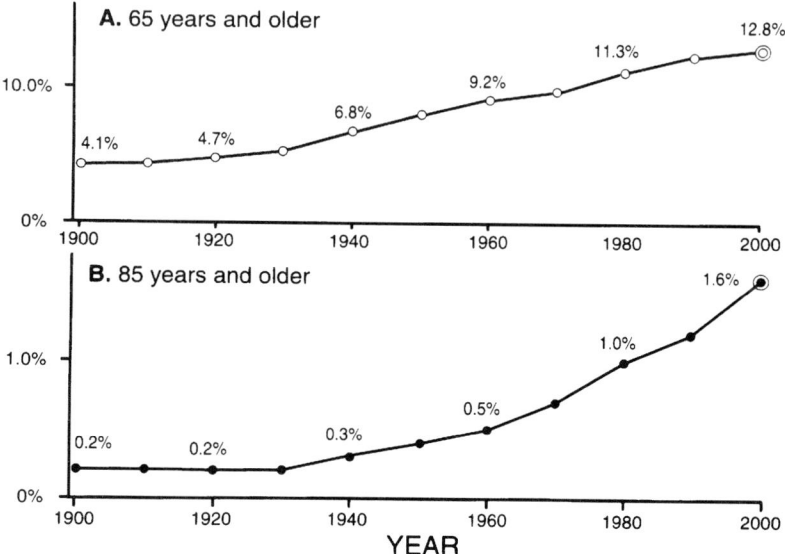

FIGURE 7. Percentage of the population of the United States from 1900 to 2000[7] that are (A) aged 65 and older, and (B) aged 85 and older.

is not perfect. Society must continue to make provisions for those who are unable or unwilling, for whatever reason, to take care of themselves. When necessary, society should provide a means-tested safety net. Humankind has the ability to both extend human life and to make the extensions worthwhile.

COMMENT

Future efforts to increase ALE-B will be largely confined to slowing the inherent aging process because attempts to do so by CM are now almost futile. Some measures that may significantly increase the MLS and/or the ALE-B without lowering ATP below acceptable levels are suggested above. More will be available in the future from the growing biomedical gerontology data base, for example, the recent study mentioned above with the $p66^{shc}$ gene,[98] and the synthesis of a nonpeptidyl mimic of superoxide dismutase with therapeutic activity in rats.[108] Although the measures evolved by societies to make the latter part of life worthwhile are now under increasing stress, efforts are already under way to replace them by ones that are acceptable and sustainable.

REFERENCES

1. HARMAN, D. 1981. The aging process. Proc. Natl. Acad. Sci. USA **78:** 7124–7128.
2. KOHN, R.R. 1985. Aging and age-related diseases: Normal processes. *In* Relation Between Normal Aging and Disease. H.A. Johnson, Ed.: 1–44. Raven Press. New York.

3. UPTON, A.C. 1977. Pathology. *In* The Biology of Aging. C.E. Finch & L. Hayflick, Eds.: 513–535. Van Nostrand. New York.
4. WOODHALL, B. & S. JOBLON. 1957. Prospects for future increases in average longevity. Geriatrics **12**: 586–591.
5. FRIES, J.F. 1988. Aging, natural death, and the compression of morbidity. N. Engl. J. Med. **303**: 130–135.
6. OLSHANSKY, S.J., B.A. CARNES & C. CASSEL. 1990. In search of Methuselah: estimating the upper limits to human longevity. Science **250**: 634–640.
7. HARMAN, D. 1998. Aging: Phenomena and theories. Ann. N.Y. Acad. Sci. **854**: 1–7.
8. DUBLIN, L.I., A.J. LOTKA & M. SPIEGLEMAN. 1949. The life table as a record of progress to the end of the nineteenth century. *In* Length of Life. 26–43. Ronald Press. New York.
9. HARMAN, D. 1994. Aging: prospects for further increases in the functional life span. Age **17**: 119–146.
10. F.B. HOBBS & B.L. DAMON. 1996. Bureau of the Census. Current population reports, Special Studies, P23–190, Sixty-five plus in the United States. U.S. Government Printing Office. Washington, D.C.
11. KRAMAROW, E., H. LENTZNER, R. ROOKS, J. WEEKS & S. SAYDAH. 1999. Health and Aging Chartbook. Health, United States. Hyattsville, Maryland: National Center for Health Statistics.
12. PETERSON, P.G. 1999. Gray Dawn. Times Books, a division of Random House. New York.
13. JONES, H.R. 1955. The relation of human health to age, place and time. *In* Handbook of Aging and the Individual. J.E. Birren, Ed: 333–363. Chicago University Press. Chicago, IL.
14. SVERIGES OFFICIELLA STATISTIK. 1993. Befolknings-forandringar. Livslangstabeller, 1951–1993. Statistiska centralbyran: 114–115. Stockholm, Sweden.
15. HARMAN, D. 1956. Aging: a theory based on free radical and radiation chemistry. J. Gerontol. **11**: 298–300.
16. HARMAN, D. 1992. Free radical theory of aging: history. *In* Free Radicals and Aging. I. Emerit & B. Chance, Eds. 1–10. Birkhauser. Basel, Switzerland.
17. HARMAN, D. 1972. The biologic clock: the mitochondria? J. Am. Geriatr. Soc. **20**: 145–147.
18. HARMAN, D. 1983. Free radical theory of aging: consequences of mitochondrial aging. Age **6**: 86–94.
19. NONHEBEL, D.C. & J.C. WALTON. 1974. Free Radical Chemistry. University Press. Cambridge, MA.
20. DAY, W. 1979. Genesis on Planet Earth. House of Talos. East Lansing, MI.
21. HARMAN, D. 1993. Free radical involvement in aging: pathophysiology and therapeutic implications. Drugs & Aging **3**: 60–80.
22. HARMAN, D. 1986. Free radical theory of aging: role of free radicals in the origination and evolution of life, aging, and diseases processes. *In* Free Radicals, Aging, and Degenerative Diseases. J.E. Johnson, Jr., R. Walford, D. Harman & J. Miquel, Eds.: 3–49. Alan R. Liss. New York.
23. HARMAN, D. 1984. Free radical theory of aging: the "free radical" diseases. Age **7**: 111–131.
24. HALLIWELL, B. & J.M.C. GUTTERIDGE. 1989. Free Radicals in Biology and Medicine, 2nd edit. Clarendon Press. Oxford, England.
25. MUNKERS, K.D., R.S. RANA & E. GOLDSTEIN. 1984. Genetically determined conidial longevity is positively correlated with superoxide dismutase, catalase, glutathione peroxidase, cytochrome c peroxidase, and ascorbate free radical reductase activities in *Neurospora crassa*. Mech. Ageing Dev. **24**: 83–100.
26. DWYER, D., A. BERRIOS & R. ARKING. 1989. Extended longevity and enhanced antioxidant defenses in *Drosophila*. Gerontology **29**: 186a.
27. JOHNSON, T.E. & G.J. LITHGOW. 1992. The search for the genetic basis of aging: the identification of gerontogenes in the nematode *Caenorhabditis elegans*. J. Am. Geriatr. Soc. **48**: 936–945.
28. ORR, W.C. & R.S. SOHALL. 1994. Extension of life-span by overexpression of superoxide dismutase and catalase in *Drosophila melanogaster*. Science **263**: 1128–1130.

29. HARMAN, D. 1968. Free radical theory of aging: effect of free radical inhibitors on the mortality rate of male LAF$_1$ mice. J. Gerontol. **23:** 476–482.
30. COMFORT, A. 1971. Effect of ethoxyquin on the longevity of C3H mice. Nature **229:** 254–255.
31. FANTERL, A.G., R.E. PERSON, R.W. TUMBIC, T.-D. NGUYEN & B. MACKLER. 1995. Studies of mitochondria in oxidative embryo toxicity. Teratology **52:** 190–195.
32. MCFADYEN, I.R., H.G.J. WORTH, D.J. WRIGHT & S.S. NOTTA. 1982. High oestrogen excretion in pregnancy. Br. J. Obstet. Gynaecol. **87:** 81–86.
33. LIEHR, J.G. 1990. Genotoxic effects of estrogens. Mutat. Res. **238:** 269–276.
34. IWASA, H., T. AONO & K. FUKUZAWA. 1990. Protective effect of vitamin E on fetal distress induced by ischemia of the uteroplacental system in pregnant rats. Free Radic. Biol. Med. **8:** 393–400.
35. HARMAN, D. & D.E. EDDY. 1979. Free radical theory of aging: beneficial effect of adding antioxidants to the maternal mouse diet on life span of offspring: possible explanation of the sex difference in longevity. Age **2:** 109–122.
36. SULLIVAN, J.L. 1981. Iron and the sex difference in longevity. Lancet **1:** 1293–1294.
37. ROSEN, D.R., T. SIDDIQUE, D. PATTERSON et al. 1993. Mutations in Cu/Zn superoxide dismutase gene are associated with familial amyotrophic lateral sclerosis. Nature **362:** 59–62.
38. NAKAZONO, K., N. WATANABE, K. MATSUNO, J. SASKI, T. SATO & M. INOUE. 1991. Does superoxide underlie the pathogenesis of hypertension? Proc. Natl. Acad. Sci. USA **88:** 10045–10049.
39. HARMAN, D. 1999. Aging: minimizing free radical damage. J. Anti-Aging Med. **2:** 15–36.
40. CURHAN, G.C., W.C. WILLETT, E.R. RIMM et al. 1996. Birth weight and adult hypertension, diabetes mellitus, and obesity in US men. Circulation **94:** 3246–3250.
41. HEIDRICK, M.L., L.C. HENDRICKS & D.E. COOK. 1984. Effect of dietary 2-mercaptoethanol on the life span, immune system, tumor incidence, and lipid peroxidation damage in spleen lymphocytes of aging BC3F$_1$ mice. Mech. Ageing Dev. **27:** 341–358.
42. EMANUEL, N.M. 1976. Free radicals and the action of inhibitors of radical processes under pathological states and aging in living organisms and man. Q. Rev. Biophys. **9:** 283–308.
43. EMANUEL, N.M., G. DUBURS, L.K. OBUKHOV et al. 1981. Drug for prophylaxis of aging and prolongation of lifetime. Chem. Abstr. **94:** 9632a.
44. HARMAN, D. 1978. Free radical theory of aging: nutritional implications. Age **1:** 145–152.
45. CASIE, G., M. BIGNAMINI & P. DE NICOLA. 1983. Does blood donation prolong life expectancy? Vox Sang. **45:** 398–399.
46. EDITORIAL. 1985. Metal chelation therapy, oxygen radicals, and human disease. Lancet **1:** 143–145.
47. OLSZEWER, E., F.C. SABBAG & J.P. CARTER. 1990. A pilot double-blind study of sodium-magnesium EDTA in peripheral vascular disease. J. Natl. Med. Assoc. **82:** 173–177.
48. DEUCHER, G.O. 1992. Antioxidant therapy in the aging process. In Free Radicals and Aging. I. Emerit & B. Chance, Eds.: 428–437. Birkhauser. Basel, Switzerland.
49. MASTERS, C. & D. CRANE. 1995. The Peroxisome: A Vital Organelle. Press Syndicate, University of Cambridge. Cambridge.
50. GIBSON, G. & B. LAKE. 1993. Peroxisomes: Biology and Importance in Toxicology and Medicine. Taylor & Francis. London.
51. CHANCE, B., H. SIES & A. BOVERIS. 1979. Hydroperoxide metabolism in mammalian organs. Physiol. Rev. **59:** 527–605.
52. NOHL, H. & D. HEGNER. 1978. Do mitochondria produce oxygen radicals *in vivo*? Eur. J. Biochem. **82:** 863–867.
53. KU, H-H., U.T. BRUNK & R.S. SOHAL. 1993. Relationship between mitochondrial superoxide and hydrogen peroxide production and longevity of mammalian species. Free Radic. Biol. Med. **15:** 621–627.
54. BANDY, B. & A.J. DAVISON. 1990. Mitochondrial mutations may increase oxidative stress: implications for carcinogenesis and aging? Free Radic. Biol. Med. **8:** 523–539.

55. SOHAL, R.S. & B.H. SOHAL. 1991. Hydrogen peroxide release by mitochondria increases during aging. Mech. Ageing Dev. **57:** 187–202.
56. FLEMING, J.E., J. MIQUEL, S.F. COTTRELL, L.S. YENGOYAN & A.C. ECONOMOS. 1982. Is cell aging caused by respiratory-dependent injury to the mitochondrial genome? Gerontology **28:** 44–53.
57. MIQUEL, J., A.C. ECONOMOS, J. FLEMING & J.E. JOHNSON, JR. 1988. Mitochondrial role in cell aging. Exp. Gerontol. **15:** 575–591.
58. SOHAL, R.S., H-H. KU, S. AGARWAL, M.J. FORSTER & H. LAL. 1994. Oxidative damage, mitochondrial oxidant generation and antioxidant defenses during aging and in response to food restriction in the mouse. Mech. Ageing Dev. **74:** 121–133.
59. KU, H-H. & R.S. SOHAL. 1993. Comparison of mitochondrial pro-oxidant generation and anti-oxidant defenses between rat and pigeon: possible basis of variation in longevity and metabolic potential. Mech. Ageing Dev. **72:** 67–76.
60. BARJA, G., S. CADENAS, C. ROJAS, R. PEREZ-CAMPO & M. LOPEZ-TORRES. 1994. Low mitochondrial free radical production per unit O_2 consumption can explain the simultaneous presence of high longevity and high aerobic metabolic rate in birds. Free Radic. Res. **21:** 317–328.
61. SOHAL, R.S., H-H. KU & S. AGARWAL. 1993. Biochemical correlates of longevity in two closely related rodent species. Biochem. Biophys. Res. Commun. **196:** 7–11.
62. TANAKA, M., J-S. GONG, J. ZHANG, M. YONEDA & K. YAGI. 1998. Mitochondrial genotype associated with longevity. Lancet **351:** 185–186.
63. PERIS, T.T., E. BUBRICK, C.C. WAGER, J. VIJG & L. KRUGALYAK. 1998. Siblings of centenarians live longer. Lancet **351:** 1560.
64. PAOLISSO, G., M.R. TAGLIAMONTSE, M.R. ROSARIA, D. MANZELLA, A. GAMBARDELLA & M. VARRICCHIO. 1998. Oxidative stress and advancing age: results in healthy centenarians. J. Am. Geriatr. Soc. **46:** 833–838.
65. SOHAL, R.S. & R. WEINDRUCH. 1996. Oxidative stress, caloric restriction, and aging. Science **273:** 59–63.
66. YU, B.P., E.J. MASORO, E.J. MURATA, H.A. BERTRAND & F.T. LYND. 1982. Life span study of SPF Fischer 344 male rats fed ad libitum or restricted diets: longevity, growth, lean body mass and disease. J. Gerontol. **37:** 130–141.
67. INGRAM, D.K., R.G. CUTLER, R. WEINDRUCH, D.M. RENQUIST, J.J. KNAPKA, M. APRIL, C.T. BELCHER, M.A. CLARK, C.D. HATCHERSON, B.M. MARRIOTT & G.S. ROTH. 1990. Dietary restriction and aging: the initiation of a primate study. J. Gerontol.: Biol. Sci. **45:** B148–B163.
68. JANZEN, E.G. A critical review of spin trapping in biological systems. *In* Free Radicals in Biology. W.A. Pryor, Ed. **4:** 115–154. Academic Press. New York.
69. CARNEY, J.M., P.E. STARKE-REED, C.N. OLIVER, R.W. LANDUM, M.S, CHENG, J.F. WU & R.A. FLOYD. 1991. Reversal of age-related increase in brain protein oxidation, decrease in enzyme activity, and loss in temporal and spatial memory by chronic administration of the spin-trapping compound *N-tert*-butyl-"-phenylnitrone. Proc. Natl. Acad. Sci. USA **88:** 3633–3636.
70. FLOYD, R.A. 1991. Oxidative damage to behavior during aging. Science **254:** 1597.
71. STADTMAN, E.R. 1990. Covalent modification reactions are marking steps in protein turnover. Biochemistry **29:** 6328–6331.
72. STADTMAN, E.R. 1992. Protein oxidation and aging. Science **257:** 1220–1223.
73. QUINTANILHA, A.T. & L. PACKER. 1977. Surface localization of sites of reduction of nitroxide spin-labeled molecules in mitochondria. Proc. Natl. Acad. Sci. USA **74:** 570–574.
74. VOEST, E.E., E. VAN FAASSEN & J.J.M. MARX. 1993. An electron paramagnetic resonance study of the antioxidant properties of the nitroxide free radical tempo. Free Radic. Biol. Med. **15:** 589–595.
75. MITCHELL, J.B., A. SAMUNI, M.C. KRISHNA, W.G. DEGRAFF, M.S, AHN, U. SAMURI & A. RUSSO. 1990. Biologically active metal-independent superoxide dismutase mimics. Biochemistry **29:** 2802–2807.
76. SAITO, K., H. YOSHIOKA & R.G. CUTLER. 1998. A spin trap, *N-tert*-butyl-α-phenylnitrone extends the life span of mice. Biosci. Biotechnol. Biochem. **62:** 792–794.

77. SACK, C.A., D.J. SOCCI, B.M. CRANDALL & G.W. ARENDASH. 1996. Antioxidant treatment with phenyl-α-*tert*-butyl nitrone (PBN) improves cognitive performance and survival of aging rats. Neurosci. Lett. **205**: 181–184.
78. EDAMATSU, R., A. MORI & L. PACKER. 1995. The spin-trap *N-tert*-α-butylnitrone prolongs the life span of the senescence accelerated mouse. Biochem. Biophys. Res. Commun. **211**: 847–849.
79. LIU, J. & A. MORI. 1993. Age-associated changes in superoxide dismutase activity, thiobarbituric acid reactivity and reduced glutathione level in the brain and liver in senescence accelerated mice (SAM): a comparison with ddY mice. Mech. Ageing Dev. **71**: 23–30.
80. CULOTTA, E. & D.E. KOSHLAND JR. 1991. Buckyballs: Wide open playing field for chemists. Science **254**: 1706–1709.
81. DUGAN, L.L., D.M. TURETSKY, C. DU, D. LOBNER, M. WHEELER, C.R. ALMLI *et al.* 1997. Carboxyfullerenes as neuroprotective agents. Proc. Natl. Acad. Sci. USA **94**: 9434–9439.
82. VERNIER, V.G., J.B. HARMON, J.M. STUMP, T.E. LYNES, J.P. MARVEL & D.H. SMITH. 1969. The toxicologic and pharmacologic properties of amantadine hydrochloride. Toxicol. Appl. Pharmacol. **15**: 642–665.
83. HOFFMANN, C.E., E.M. NEUMAYER, R.F. HAFF & R.A. GOLDSBY. 1965. Mode of action of the antiviral activity of amantadine in tissue culture. J. Bacteriol. **90**: 623–628.
84. MATTHEWS, R.T., L. YANG, S. BROWNE, M. BAIK & M.F. BEAL. 1998. Coenzyme Q_{10} administration increases brain mitochondrial concentrations and exerts neuroprotective effects. Proc. Natl. Acad. Sci. USA **95**: 8892–8897.
85. FORSMARK-ANDREE, P., C-P. LEE, G. DALLNER & L. ERNSTER. 1994. Lipid peroxidation and changes in the ubiquinone content and the respiratory chain enzymes of submitochondrial particles. Free Radic. Biol. Med. **22**: 391–400.
86. LONNROT, K., P. HOLM, A. LAGERSTEDT, H. HUHTALA & H. ALHO. 1998. The effects of lifelong ubiquinone Q_{10} supplementation on the Q_9 and Q_{10} tissues concentrations and life span of male rats and mice. Biochem. Mol. Biol. Int. **44**: 727–737.
87. BUSTAMANTE, J., J.K. LODGE, L. MARCOCCI, H.J. TRITSCHLER, L. PACKER & B.H. RIHN. 1998. α-Lipoic acid in liver metabolism and disease. Free Radic. Biol. Med. **24**: 1023–1039.
88. HAGEN, T.M., R.T. INGERSOLL, J. LYKKESFELDT, J. LIU, C.M. WEHR, V. VINARSKY, J.C. BARTHOLOMEW & B.N. AMES. 1999. (R)-α-lipoic acid–supplemented old rats have improved mitochondrial function, decreased oxidative damage, and increased metabolic rate. FASEB J. **13**: 411–418.
89. HAGEN, T.M., R.T. INGERSOLL, C.M. WEHR, J. LYKKESFELDT, V. VINARSKY, J.C. BARTHOLOMEW, M-H. SONG & B.N. AMES. 1998. Proc. Natl. Acad. Sci. USA **95**: 9562–9566.
90. GARCIA DE LA ASUNCION, J., A. MILLAN, R. PLA, L. BRUSESGHINI, A. ESTERAS, F.V. PALLARDO, J. SASTRE & J. VINA. 1996. Mitochondrial glutathione oxidation correlates with age-associated oxidative damage to mitochondrial DNA. FASEB J. **10**: 333–338.
91. SASTRE, J., A. MILLAN, J. GARCIA DE LA ASUNCION, R. PLA, G. JUAN, F.V. PALLARDO, E. O'CONNER, J.A. MARTIN, M-T. DROY-LEFAIX & J. VINA. 1998. A *Ginkgo biloba* extract (EGb 761) prevents mitochondrial aging by protecting against oxidative stress. Free Radic. Biol. Med. **24**: 298–304.
92. MEISTER, A. 1994. Glutathione-ascorbic acid antioxidant system in animals. J. Biol. Chem. **269**: 9397–9400.
93. MIQUEL, J. & A.C. ECONOMOS. 1979. Favorable effects of the antioxidants sodium and magnesium thiazolidine carboxylate on the vitality and life span of *Drosophila* and mice. Exp. Gerontol. **14**: 279–285.
94. PECCI, L., M. FONTANA, G. MONTEFOSCHI & D. CAVALLINI. 1994. Aminoethylcysteine ketimine decarboxylated dimer protects submitochondrial particles from lipid peroxidation at a concentration not inhibitory of electron transport. Biochem. Biophys. Res. Commun. **205**: 264–268.
95. FINEL, M., J.M. SKEHEL, S.P.J. ALBRACHT, I.M. FEARNLEY & J.E. WALKER. 1992. Resolution of NADH:ubiquinone oxidoreductase from bovine heart mitochondria into two

subcomplexes, one of which contains the redox centers of the enzyme. Biochemistry **31:** 11425–11434.
96. WHATLEY, S.A., D. CURTI, F.D. GUPTA, I.N. FERRIER, S. JONES, C. TAYLOR & R.M. MARCHBANKS. 1998. Superoxide, neuroleptics and the ubiquinone and cytochrome b5 reductases in brain and lymphocytes from normals and schizophrenic patients. Mol. Psychiatry **3:** 227–237.
97. WHATLEY, S.A., D. CURTI & R.M. MARCHBANKS. 1996. Mitochondrial involvement in schizophrenia and other functional psychoses. Neurochem. Res. **21:** 995–1004.
98. MIGLLACCIO, E., M. GIORGIO, S. MELE, G. PELICCI, P. REBOLDI, P.P. PANDOLFI, L. LANFRANCONE & G. PELICCI. 1999. The p66^{shc} adaptor protein controls oxidative stress response and life span in mammals. Nature **402:** 309–313.
99. TRICHOPOULOS, D. 1990. Hypothesis: does breast cancer originate in utero? Lancet **335:** 939–940.
100. EKBOM, A., C-C. HSIESH, LIPWORTH, H-O. ADAMI & D. TRICHOPOULOS. 1997. Intrauterine environment and breast cancer risk in women: a population-based study. J. Natl. Cancer Inst. **88:** 71–76.
101. HILAKIVI-CLARKE, L., R. CLARKE, I. ONOJAFE, M. RAYGADA, E. CHO & M. LIPPMAN. 1997. A maternal diet high in n-6 polyunsaturated fats alters mammary gland development, puberty onset, and breast cancer risk among female rat offspring. Proc. Natl. Acad. Sci. USA **94:** 9372–9377.
102. PETERS, K.D., K.D. KOCHANEK & S.L. MURPHY. 1998. Deaths: Final Data for 1996. National vital statistics reports: vol. 7 no. 9. Hyattsville, Maryland: National Center for Health Statistics.
103. CAMPION, E.W. 1994. The oldest old. N. Engl. J. Med. **330:** 1819–1820.
104. ROWE, J.W. & R.L. KAHN. 1998. Successful Aging. Pantheon Books. New York.
105. BULLETIN ON AGEING, Nos. 2 and 3. 1999. Division for Social Policy and Development, United Nations Secretariat, Room DC2-1358. Department of Economic and Social Affairs of the United Nations Secretariat. New York.
106. FRIEDLAND, R.B. & L. SUMMER, EDS. 1999. Demography is not Destiny. Gerontology Society of America. Washington, D.C.
107. PETERSON, P. 1999. Gray Dawn. 160–178. Times Books, a division of Random House. New York.
108. DANIELS, S., Z-Q. WANG, J.L. ZWEIER, A. SAMOUILOV, H. MACARTHUR, T.P. MISKO, M.G. CURRIE, S. CUZZOCREA, J.A. SIKORSKI & D.P. RILEY. 1999. A nonpeptidyl mimic of superoxide dismutase with therapeutic activity in rats. Science **286:** 304–306.

Protein Oxidation in Aging and Age-Related Diseases

EARL R. STADTMAN

Laboratory of Biochemistry, National Heart, Lung, and Blood Institute, National Institutes of Health, Bethesda, Maryland 20892-0342, USA

ABSTRACT: Although different theories have been proposed to explain the aging process, it is generally agreed that there is a correlation between aging and the accumulation of oxidatively damaged proteins, lipids, and nucleic acids. Oxidatively modified proteins have been shown to increase as a function of age. Studies reveal an age-related increase in the level of protein carbonyl content, oxidized methionine, protein hydrophobicity, and cross-linked and glycated proteins as well as the accumulation of less active enzymes that are more susceptible to heat inactivation and proteolytic degradation. Factors that decelerate protein oxidation also increase the life span of animals and vice versa. Furthermore, a number of age-related diseases have been shown to be associated with elevated levels of oxidatively modified proteins. The chemistry of reactive oxygen species–mediated protein modification will be discussed. The accumulation of oxidatively modified proteins may reflect deficiencies in one or more parameters of a complex function that maintains a delicate balance between the presence of a multiplicity of prooxidants, antioxidants, and repair, replacement, or elimination of biologically damaged proteins.

KEYWORDS: Oxidatively modified protein; Reactive oxygen species; Amino acid residues; Apoptosis

INTRODUCTION

There is a considerable difference of opinion on the definition of aging. Some believe that aging is the manifestation of a normal process of differentiation that fixes the maximum life span of the species. Others consider aging as the progressive loss of physical and cognitive function over time of survival. Although one definition does not preclude the other, it makes little sense that organisms would select for life span limitation a process of differentiation that involves slow progressive debilitation over time, from middle age to death. In any case, from a biochemical point of view, there is growing support for the free radical theory of aging advanced by Denham Harman in 1956.[1] According to this theory, the changes in biological function with passage of time are due to the accumulation of free radical–provoked cellular damage. In the meantime, this proposition finds support from studies showing that during aging there is a progressive, almost exponential, increase in the accumulation

---

Address for correspondence: Earl R. Stadtman, Laboratory of Biochemistry, National Heart, Lung, and Blood Institute, National Institutes of Health, Building 3, Room 222, 3 Center Drive, MSC-0342, Bethesda, MD 20892-0342. Voice: 301-496-4096; fax: 301-496-0599.
erstadtman@nih.gov

of oxidatively damaged protein, lipids, and nucleic acids. It is the purpose of this report to review some of the evidence showing that aging, by whatever mechanism, is associated with an increase in the level of oxidatively modified protein.

Before considering specific events, it is important to note that the accumulation of oxidatively modified protein is a complex function of a multitude of factors that govern (a) the rates of formation of various kinds of reactive oxygen species (ROS); (b) the levels of antioxidant defenses that guard against ROS-mediated protein damage; (c) the sensitivity of proteins to oxidative attack; and (d) the repair or elimination of damaged proteins. The interplay between these various factors is illustrated in FIGURE 1, which shows that ROS are formed by ionizing radiation, activation of neutrophils and macrophages, oxidase-catalyzed reactions, lipid peroxidation, and glycation/glycoxidation reactions, and are present as pollutants in the atmosphere. However, once they are formed, the ability of these ROS to modify proteins may be prevented by the action of various enzymic and nonenzymic antioxidants that can neutralize their prooxidant capacities. Nevertheless, as will be discussed below, the antioxidant defenses are not normally sufficient to prevent significant oxidative damage to occur. Moreover, depending upon the nature of the modifications, oxidation can lead to forms that are preferentially degraded by several intracellular pro-

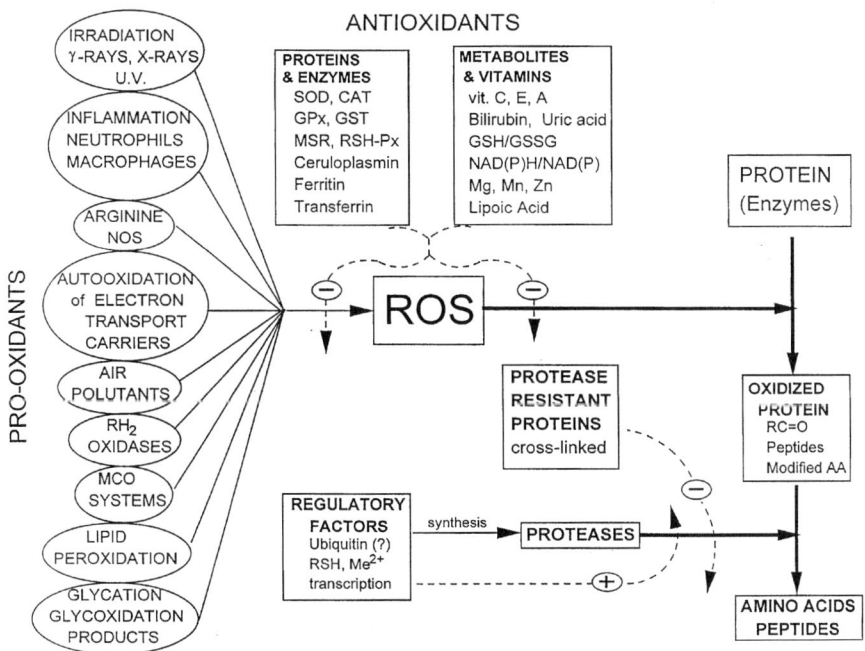

FIGURE 1. Accumulation of oxidized protein reflects balance between prooxidant, antioxidant, and proteolytic activities. MSR, methionine sulfoxide reductase; Gp_x, glutathione peroxidase; CAT, catalase; $RSHP_x$, thiol-specific peroxidase; NOS, nitric oxide synthase; SOD, superoxide dismutase; GST, glutathione transferase.

teases (the 20 S proteosome, calpain, cathepsin B),[2-4] whereas some protein modifications may lead to derivatives that are not only resistant to proteolysis but may inhibit the ability of proteases to degrade other forms of oxidatively modified proteins.[2,5-7] The accumulation of oxidized proteins is therefore dependent not only on the levels of proteases that selectively degrade oxidized proteins, but also on the levels of metabolites and metal ions that activate or inhibit their activities.

Finally, it must be realized that most of the many factors that govern the rates of protein oxidation and degradation of oxidized proteins are of genetic origin. Their concentrations and activities are therefore subject to genetic fidelity, which is also subject to compromise by ROS-mediated DNA damage. There is, in fact, substantial evidence that accumulation of oxidative DNA damage occurs with advancing age.[8-10]

It follows from these considerations that the accumulation of oxidized protein during aging and in age-related diseases could reflect random DNA damage to one or more of the multitude of genes that are implicated in the synthesis of proteins that govern the generation of ROS, the antioxidant defense systems, and the proteolytic activities that degrade oxidized proteins. It also follows that aging in this context is not a single process, rather it is the overall manifestation of the contributions of a myriad of activities. Thus, the accumulation of oxidatively modified protein may be a reliable marker of aging, but the accumulation of oxidized protein in one individual may reflect biological deficiencies in a different set of parameters than are responsible for its accumulation in another individual. For example, the accumulation of oxidized protein in one case might reflect an increase in the rate of ROS formation, whereas accumulation in another could reflect either a loss of antioxidant activity or a loss of proteolytic capacity, or any combination thereof. It follows that, if the free radical theory of aging is valid, then the search for a single common gene, or even several genes, that dictate aging may be disappointing, because genetic deficiencies that underlie the ROS damage in one individual may be very different from those that are responsible for the damage in another. Nevertheless, the identification of genes that underlie alterations in the biosynthesis of ROS, the synthesis and regulation of antioxidant activities, and the biosynthesis and regulation of the proteases that degrade oxidized proteins, together with the identification of genes that define the differentiation process that specifies the life span of the species, will undoubtedly contribute to a better understanding of the aging process.

PROTEIN MODIFICATIONS

Oxidation of Protein Backbone

Much of our knowledge about the mechanisms of free radical–mediated protein modification is derived from the results of studies by Garrison *et al.*,[11,12] Swallow,[13] and Schuessler and Schilling,[14] who subjected aqueous solutions of proteins to ionizing radiation (X rays, gamma rays) in the presence of oxygen under conditions where only HO$^\bullet$ or $O_2^{\bullet-}$, or a mixture of both, were formed. Results of these studies demonstrated that a major pathway, illustrated in FIGURE 2, involves the HO$^\bullet$-dependent abstraction of the alpha-hydrogen atom from any one of the amino acid residues to form a carbon-centered radical derivative (reaction *c*, FIG. 1) that is followed by the addition of O_2 to form an alkyl-peroxyl radical (reaction *d*), which upon reaction

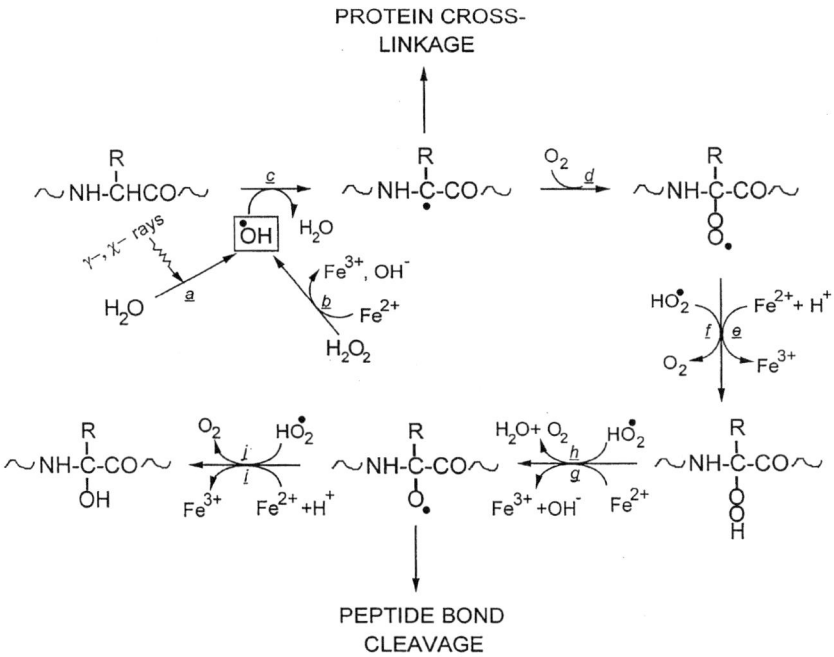

FIGURE 2. Free radical–mediated oxidation of proteins.

with the protonated form of superoxide anion ($HO_2^\bullet$) gives rise to an alkyl peroxide (reaction *f*). Interaction of the peroxide with $HO_2^\bullet$ leads to formation of a protein alkoxyl radical (reaction *h*), which can undergo peptide bond cleavage or react further with $HO_2^\bullet$ to yield a hydroxyl derivative (reaction *j*). Although not shown in FIGURE 2, the proteins alkyl-, peroxyl-, and alkoxyl-radical intermediates may also abstract hydrogen atoms from amino acid residues in the same or a different protein molecule to produce another carbon-centered radical capable of undergoing a similar series of reactions. It is also noteworthy that the same series of reactions can be initiated by $HO^\bullet$ produced in the Fe^{2+}-dependent cleavage of H_2O_2 (reaction *b*, FIG. 2), and that Fe^{2+} can replace $HO_2^\bullet$ in reactions *f*, *h*, and *j*. This underscores the importance of metal-catalyzed oxidation (MCO) reactions in protein modification.

Peptide Bond Cleavage

As indicated in FIGURE 2, alkoxyl derivatives of proteins are also capable of undergoing peptide bond cleavage. As illustrated in FIGURE 3, this cleavage can occur by either of two mechanisms:[12] the diamide pathway (reaction *a*) or the α-amidation pathway (reaction *b*); but peptide bond cleavage can occur also by ROS-mediated oxidation of glutamyl side chains. In this mechanism, oxalic acid is formed and the N-terminal amino acid of one peptide fragment exists as the pyruvyl derivative.[12] Finally, based on the observation that the number of peptides formed during the exposure of proteins to ionizing radiation is approximately equal to the number of prolyl residues present, Schuessler and Schilling[14] proposed that the oxidation of proline residues leads to peptide bond cleavage. Subsequently, Uchida et al.[15] demonstrated that proline residues of collagen are oxidized to 2-pyrrolidone derivatives with concomitant peptide bond cleavage, according to overall reaction 1. They showed further that, upon acid hydrolysis, the 2-pyrrolidone moiety of the N-terminal fragment is converted to 4-aminobutyric acid. The presence of 4-aminobutyric acid in acid hydrolysates of proteins is therefore presumptive evidence for oxidative cleavage by this mechanism.

-Gly-Hypro-Pro-Gly-Hypro-Pro + HO$^•$ →

$$\text{-Gly-Hypro-2-Prolidone + Gly-Hypro-Pro-} \quad (1)$$

Oxidation of Amino Acid Residue Side Chains

All amino acid residues of proteins are potential targets for oxidation by HO$^•$ generated upon exposure to ionizing radiation[11–14] or by high concentrations of hydrogen peroxide and Cu^{2+} or Fe^{2+}.[16,17] However, unambiguous characterization of the products formed has been established in only a few cases. Thus, phenylalanine residues are converted to mono- and dihydroxy derivatives.[12,16,18–20] Tyrosine residues are converted to the 3,4-dihydroxyphenylanine (dopa) derivative,[12,16,19,21–23] which can undergo redox cycling and thereby production of more ROS.[22,24] Tyrosine residues are also converted to nitrotyrosine,[25–30] chlorotyrosine,[29,31] and to tyrosyl radicals that can interact with one another to form dityrosine inter- or intraprotein cross-linked derivatives.[5,16,26] Because myeloperoxidase can catalyze the formation of dityrosine protein derivatives, it has been proposed that the presence of dityrosine might be used to pinpoint targets where phagocytes inflict oxidative damage *in vivo*.[26] Tryptophan residues are oxidized to various hydroxy derivatives—kynurenine, N-formyl-kynurenine, and 3-hydroxy-kynurenine, oxindole, and hydropyrroloindole derivatives.[32–38] Histidine residues are oxidized to 2-oxohistidine, 4-OH-glutamate, asparagine, and aspartate.[37,39,40]

Oxidation of Sulfur-Containing Amino Acids

Cysteine and methionine residues of proteins are by far the most sensitive to oxidation by almost all kinds of ROS.[12,13,41–46] Unlike other amino acid oxidation reactions, however, the primary oxidation products of cysteine residues to form protein disulfides (P^1SSP^2) can be repaired by disulfide exchange reactions carried out by a class of thiol transferases[47] that catalyze reactions between glutathione (GSH) or thioredoxin, $Th(SH)_2$, to regenerate the protein sulfhydryl (PSH) groups and the disulfide derivatives of glutathione (GSSG) or thioredoxin, Th(SS), respectively (reactions 2 and 3):

$$P^1SSP^2 + 2GSH \rightarrow P^1SH + P^2SH + GSSG \quad (2)$$

$$P^1SSP^2 + Th(SH)_2 \rightarrow P^1SH + P^2SH + Th(SS) \quad (3)$$

The disulfide derivatives of glutathione and thioredoxin can both be reduced back to the sulfhydryl forms by specific reductases using NADPH as an electron donor.

In an analogous manner, the oxidation of methionine residues of proteins to methionine sulfoxide can be reversed by the $Th(SH)_2$-dependent reaction catalyzed by methionine sulfoxide reductase (MSR).[48,49] As illustrated below, when the oxidation of methionine (Met) residues to methionine sulfoxide (MetO) by H_2O_2 (reaction 4) is coupled with the regeneration of Met (reaction 5) and the regeneration of $Th(SH)_2$ (reaction 6), the overall reaction is described by reaction 7, that is, by the NADPH-dependent conversion of H_2O_2 to 2 moles of H_2O. It is also evident that the substitution of almost any other form of ROS for H_2O_2 in reaction 4 will lead to the NaDPH-dependent conversion of that ROS to an inactive species. Based on this consideration, it was proposed that the oxidation of methionine residues of proteins might serve as a first line of antioxidant defense against ROS damage:[50]

$$Met + H_2O_2 \rightarrow MetO + H_2O \quad (4)$$

$$MetO + Th(SH)_2 \rightarrow Met + Th(SS) + H_2O \quad (5)$$

$$Th(SS) + NADPH + H^+ \rightarrow Th(SH)_2 + NADP^+ \quad (6)$$

$$\text{Sum: } NADPH + H^+ + H_2O_2 \rightarrow NADP^+ + 2H_2O \quad (7)$$

In an analogous manner, the oxidation of cysteine sulfhydryl groups might in some cases also serve an antioxidant function. The antioxidant function of methionine residue oxidation and reduction was supported by studies with yeast showing that the overexpression of MSR leads to increased resistance to oxidative stress, whereas strains lacking MSR are more sensitive to oxidative stress. Moreover, there was a good correlation between the differences in oxidative stress sensitivities and the intracellular accumulation of both free and protein-bound MetO.[50–52]

Peroxynitrite-Mediated Protein Modification

Although nitric oxide derived from arginine metabolism plays an important role as a second messenger in the regulation of various cellular functions, upon reaction with superoxide anion it is converted to the highly toxic peroxynitrite[3,5,54] (reaction 8), which has been found to nitrosate cysteine sulfhydryl groups,[44,55,56] nitrate tyrosine,[25,27,28,30] and tryptophan[38] residues, and oxidize methionine[28,30] residues of proteins. However, it was subsequently found that peroxynitrite (PN) reacts rapidly with CO_2 to form the $ONOOCO_2^-$ derivative (reaction 9) that is able to nitrate aromatic compounds.[57,62] In fact, at physiological CO_2 concentrations, PN will exist almost entirely as the $ONOOCO_2^-$ derivative:[63]

$$O_2^{\bullet-} + NO^{\bullet} \rightarrow ONOO^- \quad (8)$$

$$ONOO^- + CO_2 \rightarrow ONOOCO_2^- \quad (9)$$

In further studies, it was found that the ability of PN to oxidize methionine residues is almost completely inhibited by physiological concentrations of CO_2, whereas the nitration of tyrosine residues is almost completely dependent upon the presence of CO_2.[62,63] Based on these and other observations not discussed here, it seems established that the toxicity of peroxynitrite is governed by its ability to gen-

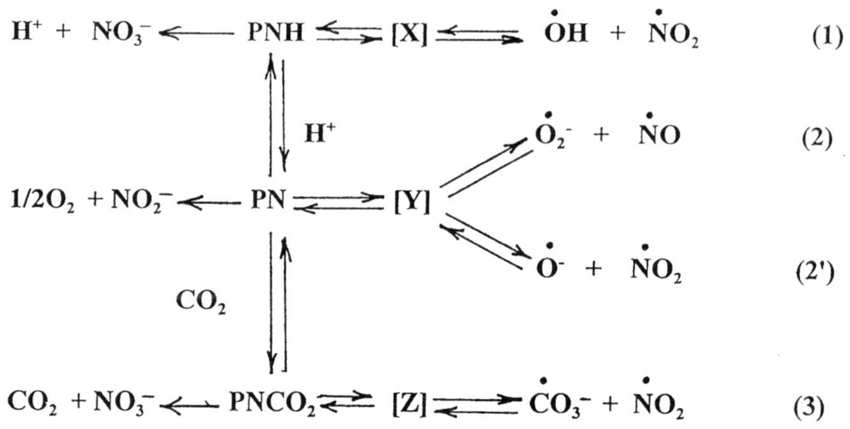

$$H^+ + NO_3^- \longleftarrow PNH \rightleftarrows [X] \rightleftarrows \overset{\bullet}{O}H + \overset{\bullet}{N}O_2 \quad (1)$$

$$\updownarrow H^+$$

$$1/2 O_2 + NO_2^- \longleftarrow PN \rightleftarrows [Y] \diagup \overset{\nearrow \overset{\bullet}{O}_2^- + \overset{\bullet}{N}O \quad (2)}{\searrow \overset{\bullet}{O}^- + \overset{\bullet}{N}O_2 \quad (2')}$$

$$\updownarrow CO_2$$

$$CO_2 + NO_3^- \longleftarrow PNCO_2 \rightleftarrows [Z] \rightleftarrows \overset{\bullet}{C}O_3^- + \overset{\bullet}{N}O_2 \quad (3)$$

FIGURE 3. Reactions of peroxynitrite (PN).

erate various radical species (HO$^\bullet$, O$_2^{\bullet-}$, NO$_2^\bullet$, and CO$_2^{\bullet-}$) by the mechanisms illustrated in FIGURE 3, where X, Y, and Z represent "caged radical pairs," as indicated.[63]

Biological Significance of Tyrosine Nitration

Interconversion of tyrosine residues between phosphorylated and unmodified forms plays an important role in the regulation of many cell signaling pathways, and the interconversion of tyrosine residues of glutamine synthetase between nucleotidylated and unmodified forms is the basis of an elegant mechanism for the regulation of this enzyme by end-product feedback inhibition in *Escherichia coli*. The singular importance of nitration of tyrosine residues in regulatory proteins is highlighted by the demonstration that nitration of the tyrosine residue in regulatory proteins prevents their capacities to be phosphorylated[66] or nucleotidylated.[30,62] Furthermore, nitration of the functional tyrosine residue in glutamine synthetase was shown to mimic the effect of nucleotidylation.[30] It follows that, because the nitration of tyrosine residues of proteins is an irreversible process, it can seriously interfere with one of the most important mechanisms of cellular regulation.

Generation of Carbonyl Derivatives

Lysine, arginine, proline, and threonine residues of proteins are particularly sensitive to metal-catalyzed oxidation, leading in each case to the formation of carbonyl derivatives.[67] As noted above, peptide carbonyl derivatives are also obtained as fragmentation products of peptide bond cleavage reactions. Furthermore, carbonyl derivatives of proteins are also formed by the interaction of protein amino acid side chains (cysteine sulfhydryl groups, histidine imidazole groups, and lysine amino groups) with lipid peroxidation products,[68] including 4-hydroxy-2-nonenal,[69,70] acrolein,[71] and malondialdehyde,[72] and also as a result of glycation/glycoxidation reactions that lead directly to carbonyl adducts[23,73] and indirectly to the formation of

N-carboxymethyl-lysine derivatives[74] that, because of their strong chelating ability,[75] are able to promote the generation of carbonyl groups by metal-catalyzed reactions.[76]

In view of the fact that carbonyl derivatives are formed by many different processes, a number of simple, highly sensitive specific methods for the assay of protein carbonyls have been developed.[77-79] Using these methods, the carbonyl content of proteins has become a widely used marker of ROS-mediated damage during oxidative stress, aging, and in age-related diseases.

Role of Protein Oxidation in Aging

A role of protein oxidation in aging is supported by the results of studies showing that the level of protein carbonyls in cultured human fibroblasts increases almost exponentially as a function of the age of the fibroblast donor,[79] and that similar age-related increases in protein carbonyl content occur in human brain tissue[80,81] and eye lens,[82] as well as in other animal models—namely, in whole body proteins of house flies,[83] rat liver,[84] and gerbil brain.[85] The role of protein oxidation in aging is emphasized also by the results of studies showing that mutations and variations in dietary or environmental factors that lead to an increase in animal life span lead also to a decrease in the level of intracellular protein carbonyl content, and vice versa.[86-91]

Age-related changes in other markers of protein oxidation have also been observed. Thus, the level of oxidized methionine (MetO) in rat liver was found to increase with animal age. This age-related increase in MetO correlated also with an age-related increase in protein surface hydrophobicity.[92] In other studies, it was demonstrated that the H_2O_2-dependent oxidation of methionine residues in glutamine synthetase is associated with a parallel increase in surface hydrophobicity,[49] and suggests that hydrophobicity might also be used as a presumptive marker of protein oxidation in aging.

Age-Related Changes in Enzyme Activities

It has been recognized for decades that aging is associated with the accumulation of altered forms of a number of enzymes.[93] These alterations often lead to the formation of catalytically less active enzymes that are more sensitive to heat inactivation and to proteolytic degradation. In fact, the subsequent finding that these age-related changes could be mimicked by exposure of enzymes to ROS-mediated oxidation provided some of the first experimental support for the propositions (a) that aging may be associated with protein oxidation, and (b) that the age-related accumulation of oxidatively modified proteins might be due to an age-related decrease in the levels or activities of proteases that selectively degrade oxidized proteins. In the meantime, support for both propositions has been obtained.[5,41,79,94-100]

Generation of Protein–Protein Cross-Linkages

Protein oxidation can lead to the formation of several different kinds of protein–protein cross-linked derivatives (for review, see ref. 101), as follows. (a) In the absence of O_2, two different carbon-centered protein radicals formed by HO• abstraction of H atoms (FIG. 1) can react with one another to form –C–C– protein cross-linked products. (b) The oxidation of protein sulfhydryl groups can lead to disulfide

–S–S– cross-linked proteins. (c) The oxidation of tyrosine residues can lead to –Tyr–Tyr– cross-linked derivatives. (d) Michael addition reactions of either cysteine sulfhydryl groups, lysine amino groups, or histidine imidazole groups of proteins with the double bonds of 4-hydroxy-2-nonenal and other α,β-unsaturated aldehydes (e.g., acrolein), formed during the oxidation of polyunsaturated fatty acids, lead to the formation of a protein carbonyl derivative, which upon further reaction with the lysine amino group of the same or a different protein will lead to Schiff-based cross-linked derivatives. (e) Reaction of both aldehyde groups of malondialdehyde (formed in the oxidation of polyunsaturated fatty acids) with lysine amino groups within the same or two different proteins will lead to Schiff-based cross-linked products. (f) The carbonyl groups obtained in the direct oxidation of amino acid side chains of one protein (see above) may react with the lysine amino groups of another protein to form Schiff-based cross-linked products. Of particular significance is the demonstration that, although a protein oxidation reaction may convert proteins to forms that are more susceptible to proteolytic degradation, the oxidized forms of some proteins are not only resistant to proteolytic degradation but they may also inhibit the ability of some proteases to degrade the oxidized forms of other proteins. Thus, protein–protein cross-linked derivatives have been found to resist proteolytic degradation and to inhibit the ability of the 20 S proteosome to degrade the oxidized forms of other proteins.[5–7]

Protein Oxidation and Diseases

Based on various markers, it is well established that the accumulation of oxidized proteins is associated with a number of diseases. Elevated levels of protein carbonyls have been observed in Alzheimer's disease,[102–107] amyotrophic lateral sclerosis,[108] cataractogenesis,[82] systemic amyloidosis,[109] muscular dystrophy,[110] Parkinson's disease,[111] progeria,[79] Werner's syndrome,[79] rheumatoid arthritis,[112] and respiratory distress syndrome.[113] Elevated levels of proteins modified by lipid oxidation products (HNE, malondialdehyde) are associated with Parkinson's disease,[111] iron-induced renal carcinogenesis,[114,115] cardiovascular disease,[116] experimental pancreatitis,[117] dextran sulfate-induced colitis,[118] atherosclerosis,[119] and Alzheimer's disease.[120–123] Elevated levels of protein glycation/glycoxidation end products (AGEs) are associated with diabetes mellitus,[124–126] Alzheimer's disease,[105,127] atherosclerosis,[128] Parkinson's disease,[129] and Down's syndrome.[130] Elevated levels of protein nitrotyrosine damage are associated with atherosclerosis,[131] Alzheimer's disease,[132] lung injury,[133–134] multiple sclerosis,[135] and endotoxemia.[136] However, whether nitrotyrosine formation is due to reactions with the peroxynitrite-CO_2 complex or with one of the other mechanisms of nitration remains to be established.

Apoptosis

There is overwhelming evidence that low levels of ROS serve as key second messengers in the regulation of diverse signal transduction pathways that control a number of very important biological functions, including cell replication and cell death. At first glance, it seems difficult to reconcile this with the fact that ROS-mediated damage to proteins, nucleic acids, and lipids is associated with aging and several age-related diseases. Why would cells choose ROS to regulate their metabolism, when these same ROS are able to cause so much cellular damage? When viewed from a different perspective, this makes good sense. When tissues have reached a normal size as dictated by differentiation processes, cellular replication ceases to take place as a consequence of "cell–cell contact inhibition." Under these conditions, cellular replication occurs only to replace an established cell, including nonfunctional cells that have been damaged by ROS. In view of this consideration, it makes sense that H_2O_2 and other forms of ROS serve as messengers for the regulation of cell signaling pathways. For example, under conditions of oxidative stress, the cells may sense a significant increase in the level of H_2O_2 and, to prepare for the eventuality that further increases could lead to loss of biological function, they take steps to set in place a mechanism to get rid of oxidatively damaged, nonfunctional cells and to replace them with good cells. In this context, it makes sense that H_2O_2 would serve as a second messenger to initiate cell destruction by apoptosis and at the same time to activate the potential for cellular replication so that the bad cell could be replaced by a good one.

If this concept has any merit, then apoptosis is the key to maintenance of high tissue integrity and focuses attention on the need to determine if oxidatively damaged cells are selectively targeted for apoptosis and, if so, to identify those modifications that are recognized by the apoptotic system. It also raises the possibility that the accumulation of oxidative protein damage during aging and in age-related diseases might, in addition to the various mechanisms discussed above, reflect a loss of apoptotic capacity. That is, are the oxidatively modified proteins present mainly in cells that have escaped apoptosis because of insufficient damage or because of age-dependent changes in the apoptotic machinery?

REFERENCES

1. HARMAN, D. 1956. Aging theory based on free radical and radiation chemistry. J. Gerontol. **2:** 298–300.
2. RIVETT, A.J., J.E. ROSEMAN, C.N. OLIVER, R.L. LEVINE & E.R. STADTMAN. 1985. Covalent modification of proteins by mixed-function oxidation: recognition by intracellular proteases. *In* Intracellular Protein Catabolism. E.A. Khairallah, J.S. Bond & J.W.C. Bird, Eds.: 317-328. Alan R. Liss. New York.
3. DAVIES, K.J.A. & S.W. LIN. 1988. Degradation of oxidatively denatured proteins in *Escherichia coli*. Free Radical Biol. Med. **5:** 215–223.
4. DEAN, R.T. 1987. A mechanism for accelerated degradation of intracellular proteins after limited damage by free radicals. FEBS Lett. **220:** 278–282.
5. GIULIVI, C. & K.J. DAVIES. 1993. Dityrosine and tyrosine oxidation products are endogenous markers for the selective proteolysis of oxidatively modified red blood cell hemoglobin by the 19 S proteasome. J. Biol. Chem. **268:** 8752–8759.
6. FRIGUET, B., E.R. STADTMAN & L. SZWEDA. 1994. Modification of glucose-6-phosphate dehydrogenase by 4-hydroxy-2-nonenal. J. Biol. Chem. **269:** 21639–21643.
7. GRUNE, T., T. REINHECKEL, M. JOSHI & K.J.A. DAVIES. 1995. Proteolysis in cultured liver epithelial cells during oxidative stress. J. Biol. Chem. **270:** 2344–2351.
8. AMES, B.N., M.K. SHIGENAGA & T.M. HAGEN. 1993. Oxidants, antioxidants, and the degenerative diseases of aging. Proc. Natl. Acad. Sci. USA **90:** 7915–7922.
9. SHIGENAGA, M.K., T.M. HAGEN & B.N. AMES. 1994. Oxidative damage and mitochondrial decay in aging. Proc. Natl. Acad. Sci. USA **91:** 10771–10778.
10. BECKMAN, J.S. & B.N. AMES. 1998. The free radical theory of aging matures. Physiol. Rev. **78:** 547–581.

11. GARRISON, W.M., M.E. JAYKO & W. BENNET. 1962. Radiation-induced oxidation of proteins in aqueous solution. Radiat. Res. **16:** 487–502.
12. GARRISON, W.M. 1987. Reaction mechanisms in the radiolysis of peptides, polypeptides, and proteins. Chem. Rev. **87:** 381–398.
13. SWALLOW, A.J. 1960. Effect of ionizing radiation on proteins, RCO groups, peptide bond cleavage, inactivation, -SH oxidation. *In* Radiation Chemistry of Organic Compounds. A.J. Swallow, Ed.: 211–224. Pergamon Press. New York.
14. SCHUESSLER, H. & K. SCHILLING. 1984. Oxygen effect in radiolysis of proteins. Part 2. Bovine serum albumin. Int. J. Radiat. Biol. **45:** 267–281.
15. UCHIDA, K., Y. KATO & S. KAWAKISHI. 1990. A novel mechanism for oxidative damage of prolyl peptides induced by hydroxyl radicals. Biochem. Biophys. Res. Commun. **169:** 265–271.
16. HUGGINS, T.G., M.C. WELLS-KNECHT, N.A. DETORIE, J.W. BAYNES & S.R. THORPE. 1993. Formation of *O*-tyrosine and dityrosine in proteins during radiolytic and metal-catalyzed oxidation. J. Biol. Chem. **268:** 12341–12347.
17. NEUZIL, J., J.M. GEBIKI & R. STOCKER. 1993. Radical-induced chain oxidation of proteins and its inhibition by chain-breaking antioxidants. Biochem. J. **293:** 601–606.
18. SOLAR, S. 1985. Reactions of OH with phenylalanine in neutral aqueous solutions. Radiat. Phys. Chem. **26:** 103–108.
19. MASKOS, Z., J.D. RUSH & W.H. KOPPENOL. 1992. The hydroxylation of tryptophan. Arch. Biochem. Biophys. **296:** 514–520.
20. KAUR, H. & B. HALLIWELL. 1994. Aromatic hydroxylation of phenylalanine as an assay for hydroxyl radicals. Measurement of hydroxyl radical formation from ozone and in blood from premature babies using improved HPLC methodology. Anal. Biochem. **220:** 11–15.
21. FLETCHER, G.L. & S. OKADA. 1961. Radiation-induced formation of dihydroxy phenylalanine from tyrosine and tyrosine-containing peptides in aqueous solution. Radiat. Res. **15:** 349–351.
22. SIMPSON, J.A., S.P. GIESEG & R.T. DEAN. 1993. Free radical and enzymatic mechanisms for the generation of protein bound reducing moieties. Biochim. Biophys. Acta **1156:** 190–196.
23. WELLS-KNECHT, M.C., T.G. HUGGINS, G. DYER, S.R. THORPE & J.W. BAYNES. 1993. Oxidized amino acids in lens protein with age. J. Biol. Chem. **268:** 12348–12352.
24. WAITE, J.H. 1995. Precursors of quinone tanning: dopa-containing proteins. Methods Enzymol. **258:** 1–20.
25. BECKMAN, J.S., H. ISCHIROPOULOS, L. ZHU, M. VAN DER WOERD, C. SMITH, J. CHEN, J. HARRISON, J.C. MARTIN & M. TSAI. 1992. Kinetics of superoxide dismutase- and iron-catalyzed nitration of phenolics by peroxynitrite. Arch. Biochem. Biophys. **298:** 438–445.
26. HEINECKE, J.W., W. LI, H.L. DAEHNKE III & J.A. GOLDSTEIN. 1993. Dityrosine, a specific marker of oxidation, is synthesized by the myeloperoxidase-hydrogen peroxide system of human neutrophils and macrophages. J. Biol. Chem. **268:** 4069–4077.
27. VAN DER VLIET, A., J.P. EISERICH, C.A. O'NEILL, B. HALLIWELL & C.E. CROSS. 1994. Tyrosine modification by reactive nitrogen species. A closer look. Arch. Biochem. Biophys. **319:** 341–349.
28. PRYOR, W.A. & G. SQUADRITO. 1995. The chemistry of peroxynitrite: a product from the reaction of nitric oxide with superoxide. Am. J. Physiol. **268:** L699–L722.
29. EISERICH, J.P., C.E. CROSS, A.D. JONES, B. HALLIWELL & A. VAN DER VLIET. 1996. Formation of nitrating and chlorinating species by reaction of nitrite with hypochlorous acid. A novel mechanism for nitric oxide–mediated protein modification. J. Biol. Chem. **271:** 19199–19208.
30. BERLETT, B.S., B. FRIGUET, M.B. YIM, P.B. CHOCK & E.R. STADTMAN. 1996. Peroxynitrite-mediated nitration of tyrosine residues of *Escherichia coli* glutamine synthetase mimic adenylylation: relevance to signal transduction. Proc. Natl. Acad. Sci. USA **93:** 1776–1780.
31. DOMIGAN, N.M., T.S. CHARLTON, M.W. DUNCAN, C.C. WINTERBOURN & A.J. KETTLE. 1995. Chlorination of tyrosyl residues in peptides by myeloperoxidase and human neutrophils. J. Biol. Chem. **270:** 16542–16548.

32. ARMSTRONG, R.C. & A.J. SWALLOW. 1969. Pulse- and gamma-radiolysis of aqueous solutions of tryptophan. Radiat. Res. **41:** 563–579.
33. WINCHESTER, R.V. & K.R. LYNN. 1970. X- and γ-radiolysis of some tryptophan dipeptides. Int. J. Radiat. Biol. **17:** 541–549.
34. KURODA, M., F. SAKIYAMA & K. NARITA. 1975. Oxidation of tryptophan in lysozyme by ozone in aqueous solution. J. Biochem. **78:** 641–651.
35. KNIGHT, K.L. & J.B. MUDD. 1984. The reaction of ozone with glyceraldehyde-3-phosphate dehydrogenase. Arch. Biochem. Biophys. **229:** 259–269.
36. GUPTASARMA, P., D. BALASUBRAMANIAN, S. MATSUGO & I. SAITO. 1992. Hydroxyl radical mediated damage to proteins, with special reference to the crystallins. Biochemistry **31:** 4296–4302.
37. BERLETT, B.S., R.L. LEVINE & E.R. STADTMAN. 1996a. A comparison of the effects of ozone on the modification of amino acid residues in glutamine synthetase and bovine serum albumin. J. Biol. Chem. **271:** 4177–4182.
38. KATO, Y., K. UCHIDA & S. KAWAKISHI. 1992. Oxidative fragmentation of collagen and prolyl peptide by CuII/H_2O_2 conversion of proline residue to 2-pyrrolidone. J. Biol. Chem. **267:** 23646–23651.
39. UCHIDA, K. & S. KAWAKISHI. 1993. 2-Oxohistidine as a novel biological marker for oxidatively modified proteins. FEBS Lett. **332:** 208–210.
40. FARBER, J.M. & R.L. LEVINE. 1986. Sequence of a peptide susceptible to mixed-function oxidation: probable cation binding site in glutamine synthetase. J. Biol. Chem. **261:** 4574–4578.
41. ZHOU, J.Q. & A. GAFNI. 1991. Exposure of rat muscle phosphoglycerate kinase to a nonenzymatic MFO system generates the old form of enzyme. J. Gerontol. **46:** B217–B221.
42. BRODIE, E. & D.J. REED. 1990. Cellular recovery of glyceraldehyde-3-phosphate dehydrogenase activity and thiol status after exposure to hydroperoxide. Arch. Biochem. Biophys. **277:** 228–233.
43. TAKAHASHI, R. & S. GOTO. 1990. Alteration of aminoacyl-tRNA synthetase with age: heat labilization of the enzyme by oxidative damage. Arch. Biochem. Biophys. **277:** 228–233.
44. STAMLER, J.S. 1994. Redox signaling: nitrosylation and related target interactions of nitric oxide. Cell **78:** 931–936.
45. MOHR, S., J.S. STAMLER & B. BRUNE. 1994. Mechanism of covalent modification of glyceraldehyde-3-phosphate dehydrogenase at its active site thiol by nitric oxide, peroxynitrite, and related nitrosating agents. FEBS Lett. **348:** 223–227.
46. MUDD, J.B., R. LEAVITT, A. ONGUN & T.T. MCMANUS. 1969. Reaction of ozone with amino acids and proteins. Atmos. Environ. **3:** 669–682.
47. MANNERVICK, B., I. CARLBURG & K. LARSON. 1989. Glutathione: General review of mechanism of action. *In* Glutathione, Part A. D. Dolphin, R. Paulson & O. Avramovic, Eds.: 476–516. John Wiley & Sons. New York.
48. BROT, N. & H. WEISSBACH. 1983. Biochemistry and physiological role of methionine sulfoxide reductase in proteins. Arch. Biochem. Biophys. **233:** 271–288.
49. MOSKOVITZ, J., M.A. RAHMAN, J. STRASSMAN, S.O. YANCEY, S.R. KUSHNER, N. BROT & H. WEISSBACH. 1995. *Escherichia coli* peptide methionine sulfoxide reductase gene: regulation of expression and role in protecting against oxidative damage. J. Bacteriol. **177:** 502–507.
50. LEVINE, R.L., L. MOSONI, B.S. BERLETT & E.R. STADTMAN. 1996. Methionine residues as endogenous antioxidants in proteins. Proc. Natl. Acad. Sci. USA **93:** 15036–15040.
51. MOSKOVITZ, J., B.S. BERLETT, J.M. POSTON & E.R. STADTMAN. 1997. The yeast peptide-methionine sulfoxide reductase functions as an antioxidant *in vivo*. Proc. Natl. Acad. Sci. USA **94:** 9585–9589.
52. MOSKOVITZ, J., E. FLESCHER, B. BERLETT, J. AZARE, J.M. POSTON & E.R. STADTMAN. 1998. Overexpression of peptide-methionine sulfoxide reductase in *Saccharomyces cerevisiae* and human T cells provides them with high resistance to oxidative stress. Proc. Natl. Acad. Sci. USA **95:** 14071–14075.
53. BECKMAN, J.S., T.W. BECKMAN, J. CHEN, P.A. MARSHALL & S. FREEMAN. 1990. Apparent hydroxyl radical production by peroxynitrite: implications for endothelial injury from nitric oxide and superoxide. Proc. Natl. Acad. Sci. USA **87:** 1620–1624.

54. BECKMAN, J.S., J. CHEN, H. ISCHIROPOULOUS, J.P. CROW & Y.Z. YE. 1994. Oxidative chemistry of peroxynitrite. Methods Enzymol. **233:** 229–239.
55. VINER, R.I., T.D. WILLIAMS & C. SCHONEICH. 1999. Peroxynitrite modification of protein thiols: oxidation, nitrosylation, and S-glutathiolation of functionally important cysteine residue(s) in the sarcoplasmic reticulum Ca-ATPase. Biochemistry **38:** 12408–12415.
56. RUBBO, H., A. DENICOLA & R. RADI. 1994. Peroxynitrite inactivates thiol-containing enzymes of *Trypanosoma cruzi* energetic metabolism and inhibits cell respiration. Arch. Biochem. Biophys. **308:** 96–102.
57. LYMAR, S.V. & J.K. HURST. 1995. Rapid reaction between peroxynitrite ion and carbon dioxide: implications for biological activity. J. Am. Chem. Soc. **117:** 8867–8868.
58. LYMAR, S.V. & J.K. HURST. 1996. Carbon dioxide: physiological catalyst for peroxynitrite-mediated cellular damage or cellular protectant? Chem. Res. Toxicol. **9:** 845–850.
59. LYMAR, S.V., Q. JIANG & J.K. HURST. 1996. Mechanisms of carbon dioxide–catalyzed oxidation of tyrosine by peroxynitrite. Biochemistry **35:** 7855–7861.
60. UPPU, R.M., G.L. SQUADRITO & W.A. PRYOR. 1996. Acceleration of peroxynitrite oxidations by carbon dioxide. Arch. Biochem. Biophys. **327:** 335–343.
61. DENICOLA, A., B.A. FREEMAN, M. TRUJILLO & R. RADI. 1996. Peroxynitrite reaction with carbon dioxide/bicarbonate: kinetics and influence on peroxynitrite-mediated oxidations. Arch. Biochem. Biophys. **333:** 49–58.
62. BERLETT, B.S. & E.R. STADTMAN. 1996. Carbon dioxide stimulates nitration of tyrosine residues and inhibits oxidation of methionine residues in *Escherichia coli* glutamine synthetase by peroxynitrite. FASEB J. **10:** Abstract #585.
63. TIEN, M., B.S. BERLETT, R.L. LEVINE, P.B. CHOCK & E.R. STADTMAN. 1999. Peroxynitrite-mediated modification of proteins at physiological carbon dioxide concentration: pH dependence of carbonyl formation, tyrosine nitration, and methionine oxidation. Proc. Natl. Acad. Sci. USA **96:** 7809–7814.
64. HUNTER, T. 1995. Protein kinases and phosphatases: the Ying and Yang of protein phosphorylation and signaling. Cell **80:** 225–236.
65. STADTMAN, E.R., P.B. CHOCK & S.G. RHEE. 1981. Interconvertible enzyme cycles in cellular regulation. Curr. Top. Cell. Regul. **18:** 79–83.
66. KONG, S.-K., M.B. YIM, E.R. STADTMAN & P.B. CHOCK. 1996. Peroxynitrite disables the tyrosine phosphorylation regulatory mechanism: lymphocyte-specific tyrosine kinase fails to phosphorylate nitrated cdc2(6-20)NH_2 peptide. Proc. Natl. Acad. Sci. USA **93:** 3377–3382.
67. AMICI, A., R.L. LEVINE, L. TSAI & E.R. STADTMAN. 1989. Conversion of amino acid residues in proteins and amino acid homopolymers to carbonyl derivatives by metal-catalyzed reactions. J. Biol. Chem. **264:** 3341–3346.
68. REFSGAARD, H., L. TSAI & E.R. STADTMAN. 2000. Modifications of proteins by polyunsaturated fatty acid peroxidation products. Proc. Natl. Acad. Sci. USA **97:** 611–616.
69. SCHUENSTEIN, E. & H. ESTERBAUER. 1979. Formation and properties of reactive aldehydes. *In* Submolecular Biology of Cancer, CIBA Foundation Series 67, Excerpta Medica: 225–244. Elsevier. Amsterdam, the Netherlands.
70. UCHIDA, K. & E.R. STADTMAN. 1993. Covalent modification of 4-hydroxynonenal to glyceraldehyde-3-phosphate. J. Biol. Chem. **268:** 6388–6393.
71. UCHIDA, K., M. KANEMATSU, Y. MORIMITSU, T. OSAWA, N. NOGUCHI & E. NIKI. 1998. Acrolein is a product of lipid peroxidation reaction. Formation of free acrolein and its conjugate with lysine residues in oxidized low density lipoproteins. J. Biol. Chem. **273:** 16058–16066.
72. BURCHAM, P.C. & Y.T. KUHAN. 1996. Introduction of carbonyl groups into proteins by the lipid peroxidation product, malondialdehyde. Biochem. Biophys. Res. Commun. **220:** 996–1001.
73. CERAMI, A., H. VLASSARA & M. BROWNLEE. 1987. Glucose and aging. Sci. Am. **256:** 90–96.
74. REQUENA, J.R., M.X. FU, M.U. AHMED, A.J. JENKINS, Y.J. LYONS & S.R. THORPE. 1996. Lipoxidation products as biomarkers of oxidative damage to proteins during lipid peroxidation reactions. Nephrol. Dial. Transplant. **11:** 48–53.

75. SAXENA, A.K., P. SAXENA, X. WU, M. OBRENOVICH, M.F. WEISS & V.M. MONNIER. 1999. Protein aging by carboxymethylation of lysines generates sites for divalent metal and redox active copper binding: relevance to diseases of glycoxidative stress. Biochem. Biophys. Res. **260:** 332–338.
76. REQUENA, J.R. & E.R. STADTMAN. 1999. Conversion of lysine to N^ε-carboxymethyl lysine increases susceptibility of proteins to metal-catalyzed oxidation. Biochem. Biophys. Res. Commun. **264:** 207–211.
77. LEVINE, R.L., D. GARLAND, C.N. OLIVER, A. AMICI, I. CLIMENT, A.G. LENZ, B.-W. AHN, S. SHALTIEL & E.R. STADTMAN. 1990. Determination of carbonyl groups in oxidatively modified proteins. Methods Enzymol. **186:** 464–478.
78. LEVINE, R.L., J.A. WILLIAMS, E.R. STADTMAN & E. SCHACTER. 1994. Carbonyl assays for determination of oxidatively modified proteins. Methods Enzymol. **233:** 346–357.
79. OLIVER, C.N., B.-W. AHN, E.J. MOERMAN, S. GOLDSTEIN & E.R. STADTMAN. 1987. Age-related changes in oxidized proteins. J. Biol. Chem. **262:** 5488–5491.
80. SMITH, C.D., J.M. CARNEY, P.E. STARKE-REED, C.N. OLIVER, E.R. STADTMAN & R.A. FLOYD. 1991. Excess brain protein oxidation and enzyme dysfunction in normal and Alzheimer's disease. Proc. Natl. Acad. Sci. USA **88:** 10450–10543.
81. SMITH, C.D., J.M. CARNEY, T. TATSUMO, E.R. STADTMAN, R.A. FLOYD & W.R. MARKESBERY. 1992. Protein oxidation in aging brain. In Aging and Cellular Defense Mechanisms. C. Franceschi, G. Cerpaldi, V.J. Cristofalo & J. Vijg, Eds.: **663:** 110–119. The New York Academy of Sciences. New York.
82. GARLAND, D., P. RUSSELL & J.S. ZIGLER. 1988. The oxidative modification of lens proteins. In Oxygen Radicals in Biology and Medicine. M.G. Simic, K.S. Taylor, J.F. Ward & V. von Sontag, Eds.: 347–353. Plenum. New York.
83. SOHAL, R.S., S. AGARWAL, A. DUBEY & W.C. ORR. 1993. Protein oxidative damage is associated with life expectancy of houseflies. Proc. Natl. Acad. Sci. USA **90:** 7255–7259.
84. STARKE-REED, P.E. & C.N. OLIVER. 1989. Protein oxidation and proteolysis during aging and oxidative stress. Arch. Biochem. Biophys. **275:** 559–567.
85. CARNEY, J.M., P.E. STARKE-REED, C.N. OLIVER, R.W. LANDUM, M.S. CHENG, J.F. WU & R.A. FLOYD. 1991. Reversal of age-related increase in brain protein oxidation, decrease in enzyme activity loss and loss of temporal and spatial memory by chronic administration of the spin-trapping compound N-$tert$-butyl-α-phenylnitrone. Proc. Natl. Acad. Sci. USA **88:** 3633–3636.
86. SOHAL, R.S., H.-H. KU & S. AGARWAL. 1993. Biochemical correlates of longevity in two closely related rodent species. Biochem. Biophys. Res. Commun. **196:** 7–11.
87. SOHAL, R.S., H.-H. KU, S. AGARWAL, M.J. FORSTER & H. LAL. 1994. Mech. Aging & Dis. **79:** 121–133.
88. ISHII, N., M. FUJII, P.S. HARTMAN, M. TSUDA, K. YASUDA, N. SENOO-MATSUDA, S. YANASE, D. AYUSAWA & K. SUZUKI. 1998. A mutation in succinate dehydrogenase cytochrome b causes oxidative stress and ageing in nematodes. Nature **394:** 694-697.
89. LASS, A., B.H. SOHAL, R. WEINDRUCH, M.J. FORSTER & R.S. SOHAL. 1998. Caloric restriction prevents age-associated accrual of oxidative damage to mouse skeletal muscle mitochondria. Free Radical Biol. Med. **25:** 1089–1097.
90. SOHAL, R.S., H.H. KU, S. AGARWAL, M.J. FORSTER & H. LAL. 1994. Oxidative damage, mitochondrial oxidant generation and antioxidant defenses during aging and in response to food restriction in the mouse. Mech. Ageing Dev. **74:** 121–133.
91. AGARWAL, S. & R.S. SOHAL. 1993. Relationship between susceptibility to protein oxidation, aging, and maximum life span potential of different species. Exp. Gerontol. **31:** 365–372.
92. CHAO, C.-C., Y.-S. MA & E.R. STADTMAN. 1997. Modification of protein surface hydrophobicity and methionine oxidation by oxidative stress. Proc. Natl. Acad. Sci. USA **94:** 2969–2974.
93. ROTHSTEIN, M. 1984. Changes in enzymatic proteins during aging. In Molecular Basis of Aging. A.K. Roy & B. Chatterjee, Eds.: 209–232. Academic Press. New York.
94. SZWEDA, L.I. & E.R. STADTMAN. 1992. Iron-catalyzed oxidative modification of glucose-6-phosphate dehydrogenase from Leuconostoc. mesenteroides. J. Biol. Chem. **267:** 3096–3100.

95. RIVETT, A.J. 1986. Regulation of intracellular protein turnover: covalent modification as a mechanism of marking proteins for degradation. Curr. Top. Cell. Regul. **28:** 291–337.
96. FRIGUET, B., L. SZWEDA & E.R. STADTMAN. 1994. Susceptibility of glucose-6-phosphate dehydrogenase modified by 4-hydroxy-2-nonenal and metal-catalyzed oxidation to proteolysis by the multicatalytic protease. Arch. Biochem. Biophys. **311:** 168–173.
97. DEAN, R.T., S. GIESEG & M.J. DAVIES. 1993. Reactive species and their accumulation on radical-damaged proteins. Trends Biochem. Sci. **18:** 437–441.
98. STADTMAN, E.R. 1990. Covalent modification reactions are marking steps in protein turnover. Biochemistry **29:** 6323–6331.
99. STADTMAN, E.R. 1986. Oxidation of proteins by mixed-function oxidation systems: implication in protein turnover, ageing and neutrophil function. Trends Biochem. Sci. **11:** 11–12.
100. STADTMAN, E.R. 1990. Metal ion-catalyzed oxidation of proteins: Biochemical mechanism and biological consequences. Free Radical Biol. Med. **9:** 315–325.
101. STADTMAN, E.R. 1997. Free radical mediated oxidation of proteins. *In* Free Radicals, Oxidative Stress, and Antioxidants. Pathological and Physiological Significance. NATO ASI Series, Series A: Life Sciences, Volume 296. T. Özben, Ed.: 51–65. Plenum Press. New York
102. CARNEY, J.M., C.D. SMITH, A.M. CARNEY & D.A. BUTTERFIELD. 1994. Aging- and oxygen-induced modifications in brain biochemistry and behavior. *In* Aging and Cellular Defense Mechanisms. C. Franceschi, G. Crepaldi, V. J. Cristofalo & J. Vijg, Eds.: **663:** 110–119. The New York Academy of Sciences. New York.
103. HARRIS, M., K. HENSLEY, D.A. BUTTERFIELD, R.A. LEEDLE & J.M. CARNEY. 1995. Direct evidence of oxidative injury produced by Alzheimer's β-amyloid peptide 1-40 in cultured hippocampal neurons. Exp. Neurol. **131:** 193–202.
104. CHAUHAN, A., V.P.S. CHAUHAN, H. BROCKERHOFF & H.M. WISNIEWSKI. 1991. Action of amyloid β-protein on protein kinase C activity. Life Sci. **49:** 1555–1556.
105. SMITH, M.A., S. TANEDA, P.L. RICHEY, S. MIYATA, S.-D. YAN, D. STERN, L.M. SAYRE, V. MONNIER & G. PERRY. 1994. Advanced Maillard reaction end products are associated with Alzheimer's disease pathology. Proc. Natl. Acad. Sci. USA **91:** 5710–5714.
106. SMITH, M.A., M. RUDNICKA-NAWROT, P.L. RICHEY, D. PRAPROTNIK, P. MULVIHILL, C.A. MILLER, C.A. SAYRE & G. PERRY. 1995. Carbonyl-related posttranslational modification of neurofilament protein in neurofibrillary pathology of Alzheimer's disease. J. Neurochem. **64:** 2660–2666.
107. SMITH, M.A., P.L. PERRY, L.M. SAYRE, V.E. ANDERSON, M.F. BEAL & N. KOWAL. 1996. Oxidative damage in Alzheimer's disease. Nature **382:** 120–121.
108. BOWLING, A.C., J.B. SCHULTZ, R.H. BROWN JR. & M.F. BEAL. 1993. Superoxide dismutase activity, oxidative damage, and mitochondrial energy metabolism I familial and sporadic amyotrophic lateral sclerosis. J. Neurochem. **61:** 2322–2325.
109. ANDO, Y., N. NYHLIN, O. SUHR, G. HOLMGREN, K. UCHIDA, M. EL SAHLY, T. YAMASHITA, H. TERASAKI, M. NAKAMURA, M. UCHINO & M. ANDO. 1997. Oxidative stress is found in amyloid deposits in systemic amyloidosis. Biochem. Biophys. Res. Commun. **232:** 497–502.
110. MURPHY, M.E. & J.P. KHERER. 1989. Oxidation state of tissue thiol groups and content of protein carbonyl groups in chickens with inherited muscular dystrophy. Biochem. J. **260:** 359–364.
111. YORITAKA, A., N. HATTORI, A. UCHIDA, M. TANAKA & E.R. STADTMAN. 1996. Immuochemical detection of 4-hydroxy-nonenal protein adducts in Parkinson's disease. Proc. Natl. Acad. Sci. USA **93:** 2696–2701.
112. CHAPMAN, M.L., B.R. RUBIN & R.W. GRACY. 1989. Increased carbonyl content of proteins in synovial fluid from patients with rheumatoid arthritis. J. Rheumatol. **16:** 15–18.
113. GLADSTONE, I.M. & R.L. LEVINE. 1994. Oxidation of proteins in neonatal lungs. Pediatrics **93:** 764–768.
114. TOYOKUNI, S., K. UCHIDA, K. OKAMOTO, Y. HATTORI-NAKAKUKI, H. HIAI & E.R. STADTMAN. 1994. Formation of 4-hydroxy-2-nonenal-modified proteins in the renal proximal tubules of rats treated with a renal carcinogen ferric nitrilotriacetate. Proc. Natl. Acad. Sci. USA **91:** 2616–2620.

115. UCHIDA, K., A. FUKUDA, S. KAWAKISHI, H. HIAI & S. TOYOKUNI. 1995. A renal carcinogen ferric nitriloacetate mediates a temporary accumulation of aldehyde-modified proteins within cytosolic compartments of rat kidney. Arch. Biochem. Biophys. **317:** 405–411.
116. KRSEK-STAPLES, J.A. & R.O. WEBSTER. 1993. Ceroplasmin inhibits carbonyl formation in endogeneous cell proteins. Free Radical Biol. Med. **14:** 115–125.
117. REINHECKEL, T., B. NEDELEV, J. PRAUSE, W. AUGUSTIN, H.U. SCHULZ, H. LIPPERT & W. HALANGK. 1998. Occurrence of oxidatively modified proteins: an early event in experimental acute pancreatitis. Free Radical Biol. Med. **24:** 393–400.
118. BLACKBURN, A.C., W.F. DOE & G.D. BUFFINTON. 1999. Protein carbonyl formation on mucosal proteins *in vitro* and in dextran sulfate-induced colitis. Free Radical Biol. Med. **27:** 262–270.
119. UCHIDA, K., S. TOYOKUNI, K. NISHIKAWA, S. KAWAKISHI, H. ODA, H. HIAI & E.R. STADTMAN. 1994. Michael addition-type 4-hydroxy-2-nonenal adducts in modified low density lipoproteins: markers for atherosclerosis. Biochemistry **33:** 12487–12494.
120. MARK, R.J., M.A. LOVELL, W.R. MARKESBERY, K. UCHIDA & M.P. MATTSON. 1997. A role for 4-hydroxynonenal, an aldehydic product of lipid peroxidation, in disruption of ion homeostasis and neuronal death induced by amyloid beta-peptide. J. Neurochem. **68:** 255–264.
121. MARKESBERY, W.R. & J.M. CARNEY. 1999. Oxidative alterations in Alzheimer's disease. Brain Pathol. **9:** 133–146.
122. SAYRE, L.M., D.A. ZELASKO, P.L. HARRIS, G. PERRY, R.G. SALOMON & M.A. SMITH. 1997. 4-Hydroxynonenal-derived advanced lipid peroxidation end products are increased in Alzheimer's disease. J. Neurochem. **68:** 2092–2097.
123. DYER, D.G., J.A. DUNN, S.R. THORPE, K.E. BAILIE, T.J. LYONS, D.R. MCCANCE & J.W. BAYNES. 1993. Accumulation of Maillard reaction products in skin collagen in diabetes and aging. J. Clin. Invest. **91:** 2463–2469.
124. MAKITA, Z., S. RADOFF, E.J. RAYFIELD, Z. YANG, E. SKOLNIK, V. DELANEY, E.A. FRIEDMAN, A. CERAMI & H. VLASSARA. 1991. Advanced glycosylation end products in patients with diabetic nephropathy. N. Engl. J. Med. **325:** 836–842.
125. BAYNES, J.W. 1991. Perspectives in diabetes. Role of oxidative stress in development of complications in diabetes. Diabetes **40:** 405–411.
126. MATSUMOTO, K., K. IKEDA, S. HORIUCHI, H. ZHAO & E.C. ABRAHAM. 1997. Immunochemical evidence for increased formation of advanced glycation end products and inhibition by aminoguanidine in diabetic rat lenses. Biochem. Biophys. Res. Commun. **241:** 352–354.
127. TAKEDO, A., T. YASUDA, T. MIYATA, K. MIZUNO, M. LI, S. YONEYAMA, K. HORIE, K. MAEDA & G. SOBUE. 1996. Immunohistochemical study of advanced glycation end products in aging and Alzheimer's disease brain. Neurosci. Lett. **211:** 17–20.
128. KUME, S., M. TAKEYA, T. MORI, N. ARAKI, H. SUZUKI, T. KODAMA, Y. MIYAUCHI & K. TAKAHASHI. 1995. Immunohistochemical and ultrastructural detection of advanced glycation end products in atherosclerotic lesions of human aorta with a novel specific monoclonal antibody. Am. J. Pathol. **147:** 654–667.
129. CASTELLANI, R., M.A. SMITH, P.L. RICHEY & G. PERRY. 1996. Glycoxidation and oxidative stress in Parkinson disease and diffuse Lewy body disease. Brain Res. **737:** 195–200.
130. ODETTI, P., G. ANGELINI, D. DAPINO, D. ZACCHEO, S. GARIBALDI, F. DAGNA-BRICARELLI, G. PIOMBO, G. PERRY, M. SMITH, N. TRAVERSO & M. TABATON. 1998. Early glycoxidation damage in brains from Down's syndrome. Biochem. Biophys. Res. Commun. **243:** 849–851.
131. BECKMAN, J.S., Y.Z. YE, P. ANDERSON, J. CHEN, M.A. ACCAVETTI, M.M. TARPEY & C.R. WHITE. 1994. Extensive nitration of protein tyrosines observed in human atherosclerosis detected by immunochemistry. Biol. Chem. Hoppe-Seyler **335:** 81–85.
132. SMITH, M.A., P.L. RICHEY HARRIS, L.M. SAYRE, J.S. BECKMAN & G. PERRY. 1997. Widespread peroxynitrite-mediated damage in Alzheimer's disease. J. Neurosci. **17:** 2653–2657.
133. KOOY, N.W., J.A. ROYALL, Y.Z. YE, D.R. KELLY & J.S. BECKMAN. 1995. Evidence for *in vivo* peroxynitrite production in human acute lung injury. Am. J. Respir. Crit. Care Med. **15:** 1250–1254.

134. HADDAD, I.Y., G. PATAKI, P. HU, C. GALLIANI, J.S. BECKMAN & S. MATALON. 1994. Quantitation of nitrotyrosine levels in lung sections of patients and animals with acute lung injury. J. Clin. Invest. **94:** 2407–2413.
135. BAGASRA, O., F.H. MICHAELS, Y.M. ZHENG, L.E. BOBROSKI, S.V. SPITSIN, Z.F. FU, R. TAWADROS & H.O. KOPROWSKI. 1995. Activation of the inducible form of nitric oxide synthase in the brains of patients with multiple sclerosis. Proc. Natl. Acad. Sci. USA **92:** 2041–12045.
136. SZABO, C., A.L. SALZMAN & H. ISCHIROPOULOS. 1995. Endotoxin triggers the expression of an inducible isoform of nitric oxide synthase and the formation of peroxynitrite in the rat aorta *in vivo*. FEBS Lett. **363:** 235–238.

Stress Resistance by Caloric Restriction for Longevity

BYUNG P. YU[a] AND HAE YOUNG CHUNG[b]

[a]*Department of Molecular Biology, Pusan National University, Pusan, Korea, and Department of Physiology, University of Texas Health Science Center at San Antonio, San Antonio, Texas 78229, USA*

[b]*College of Pharmacy, Pusan National University, Pusan, Korea*

> ABSTRACT: Hardly an aspect of aging is more important than an organism's ability to withstand stress or to resist both internally and externally imposed insults. We know that as organisms loose their ability to resist these insults, aged organisms suffer more than the young. Therefore, a prime strategy for an organism's survival has been the evolutionarily adapted defense systems that guard against insult. For better survivability, an organism's defense system must be maximized to its full effect through well-coordinated networks of diverse biologically responsive elements. Although terms like stress, resistance, and adaptablity have long been used in biology, they remain mechanistically and quantitatively poorly defined. In a gerontological context, stress resistance or susceptibility are often discussed in association with an organism's vulnerability to disease and age-related damage. However, to date, there is no clear molecular delineation of cellular and molecular mechanisms for such complex biological phenomena. The life-prolonging action of caloric restriction (CR) seems to offer an excellent opportunity for investigating the interrelationship between stress and the aging process. As an omnipotent intervention, CR provides a unique opportunity to probe the organism's ability to withstand age-related stress as a survival strategy. In this context, the antiaging action of CR can be viewed as "nutritional stress," because the organism's reduced caloric intake seems to be a stimulatory metabolic response for survivability. Recent gerontologic research has provided sufficient experimental data supporting this antiaging property of CR, of which several pertinent, key examples are discussed below.
>
> KEYWORDS: Caloric restriction; Corticosterone; Oxidative stress; Mitochondria; Hormesis

DESCRIPTION OF STRESS IN AGING

When exposed to a certain stressor, an organism's adaptive response undergoes three interrelated stages: alarm reaction, stage of resistance, and stage of exhaustion, according to Selye's definition.[1] Because stress itself is a most effective factor in eliciting adaptive responses, the organism's innate nature is to use some form of

---

Address for correspondence: Byung P. Yu, Department of Physiology, University of Texas Health Science Center at San Antonio, San Antonio, Texas 78229. Voice: 210-567-4376; fax: 210-567-4410.

bpyu@usa.net

stress for its own benefit.[2] Such a notion is in line with the basic premise of the proposed stress theory of aging[3] and adaptation hypothesis for longevity.[4]

One well-known, exemplified response to stress is the hormonal increase in adrenal corticosterone levels in plasma during aging,[5-7] where increases in these levels appear to be proportional to the degree of stress. Aged animals appear to have a diminished ability to attenuate the increase, causing the aged to have continually elevated plasma levels of corticosterones.[5] These authors suggested that increased levels of corticosterone in aged rats result in hippocampal neuronal cell death, that is, the stage of exhaustion. However, this scenario in the glucocorticoid cascade hypothesis is obviously not applicable in the case of the CR paradigm, because CR results in an increased life span in spite of chronically elevated diurnal levels of serum corticosterone.[6] This apparent contradiction makes the interrelation of glucocorticoid and aging far more complex than one might want to narrowly define it and needs other mechanistic explanations like stress resistance to resolve the disparity in responses (see below for further discussion).

CALORIC RESTRICTION AS A STRESSOR

A hallmark of CR is life span extension.[2] Indeed many researchers have produced an overwhelming body of data establishing CR as the most effective measure in retarding the aging process.[8,9] It should be clear by now that the sole, critical factor responsible for CR's antiaging action is reduced calories, not dietary nutrients, such as reduced lipids or proteins and their components, as they seem to play minor roles in the life-extension action.[9]

Several studies have also shown that CR's life-extending action is not likely brought about by a slowed metabolic rate. When food consumption of animals who had their food restricted was compared with controls, restricted rats had equal or higher caloric intakes when normalized to body weight, suggesting a similar metabolic rate. Thus, it seems reasonable that an adjustment in metabolic rate *per se* may not be the major mechanism of CR's antiaging action.[2,9] It appears, however, that CR animals seem to "reset" their energy utilization machinery geared for a higher efficiency under limited energy resources (see FIG. 1). This interpretation is in line with what is known about increased glucose utilization in CR rats with low insulin levels.[9]

What then is the mechanism that underlies CR's life-extending action? By understanding CR's diverse effects on biological and pathological processes, it is hardly conceivable that any single factor could be responsible for this action. As exemplified in CR's antioxidative strategy, CR mobilizes well-coordinated, multilevel networks of various defenses to maintain homeostatic mechanisms.[10]

EVIDENCE OF STRESS RESISTANCE BY CALORIC RESTRICTION

It is clear that organisms could not have evolved under aerobic conditions without proper defenses against free radicals and oxidants. Because oxidative stress causes an imbalance in the redox state of the cell, an adaptive response to oxidative stress is therefore a critical factor in its survival as shown in CR animals.

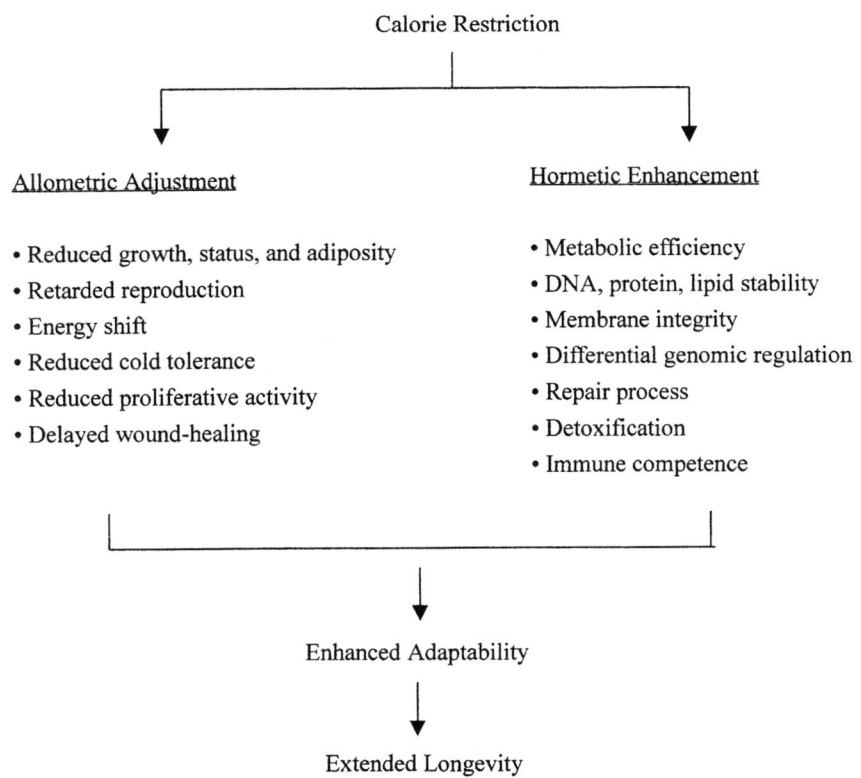

FIGURE 1. Survival strategy by caloric restriction.

TABLE 1. Mean 24-hour plasma-free corticosterone levels (nM)[6]

Age	Ad libitum fed	Caloric restriction
3–7	10.4 ± 3.7	25.4 ± 3.7
9–13	9.9 ± 3.7	22.3 ± 3.7
15–19	17.3 ± 3.7	19.5 ± 3.7
21–25	17.5 ± 4.4	35.0 ± 3.9
27–31	—	54.8 ± 4.7

Frame *et al.* viewed elevated glucocorticoids as the major adaptive response to nutrient stress.[10] Data clearly show that biologically active free corticosterone levels in CR rats are higher than those in ad libitum–fed rats throughout the animals' life spans (TABLE 1).[6] An interesting and more important question, however, is how chronically elevated, deleterious glucocorticoid levels cause no apparent harm to CR animals, and how these animals use it for their own advantage.[10] The answer can, in part, be found in the stabilized neuronal membrane status by CR.[9]

CALORIC RESTRICTION AS A PROTECTOR AGAINST OXIDATIVE STRESS

In addition to CR's ability to resist hormonal stress, accumulated evidence has proven CR to be the most effective modulator of free radical–induced oxidative stress.[3] The oxidative stress hypothesis explains how an organism's ability promotes resistance of oxidative stress.[2,11] One such action is exhibited in the protection of membrane integrity by CR.

Resistance to oxidative stress is especially important to biological membranes because of their essential role for cellular homestasis.[11] As an outstanding membrane protector, CR was shown to reduce age-related oxidative damage by modulating the membrane fatty acid composition. This is an interesting revelation because no such data were previously reported, showing that reduced caloric intake *per se* alters membrane fatty acid composition, although various dietary sources are known to readily change membrane composition.[2] Even more intriguing is the way CR modulates membrane compositional changes by decreasing polyunsaturated fatty acids (PUFA), such as 22:4 and 22:5, which were replaced by increased 18:2 fatty acid to maintain proper membrane fluidity and reduce peroxidizability.[12] As shown in FIGURE 2, CR manipulates the membrane fatty acid components as an adaptive measure against age-related peroxidizability—an efficient and smart strategy to resist oxidative stress. This strategy seems to develop as an adaptive trait through the evolutionary process revealed by the work of Pamplona *et al.*[13] The authors show an inverse relationship between the amount of PUFA with increased peroxidizability and the life spans of rats, pigeons, and humans: the higher the PUFA, the shorter the life span, a similar trend found when comparing ad libitum–fed rats to CR rats.[9] Thus, CR manipulation seems to take an adaptive strategy in protecting the most basic requirement for membrane integrity. Several other examples are given below for further expansion of this point of view.

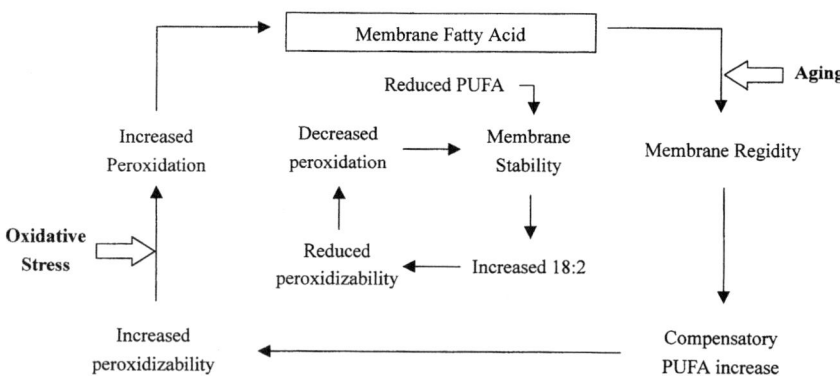

FIGURE 2. Protection of membrane integrity by CR.

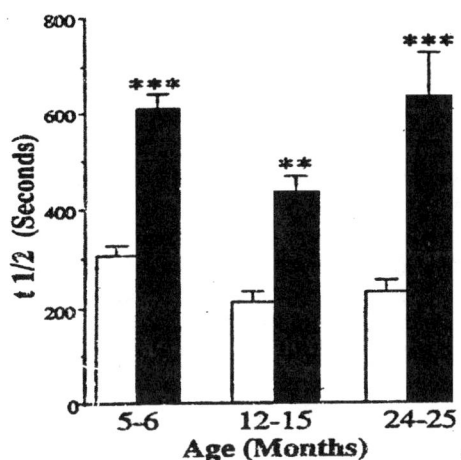

FIGURE 3. Resistance to *t*-butyl hydroperoxide challenge in mitochondria isolated from CR rats. The induction time for permeability transition was much prolonged compared to ad libitum–fed controls. This shows CR's ability to maintain a more stable membrane structure under oxidative stress. □, ad libitum–fed controls; ■, CR rats. (Reproduced with permission from Kristal and Yu.[12])

PROTECTION OF MITOCHONDRIAL MEMBRANE BY CALORIC RESTRICTION

Exposure of mitochondria to various oxidants causes mitochondrial deterioration with concurrent functional loss. One functional change sensitive to oxidant treatment is mitochondrial permeability transition (MPT). Using liver mitochondria isolated from male Fischer 344 rats, 6–24 months of age, our laboratory obtained evidence showing that CR regimens greatly delay the opening of the MPT Ca^{2+} megachannel upon exposure to various oxidants (FIG. 3).[12] CR slowed the opening of the MPT when challenged by *t*-butyl hydroperoxide by approximately 50%, indicating resistance of mitochondria to oxidative stress. The increased resistance to MPT induction was maintained through 24 months of age in CR animals, showing the resilient nature of the membrane of CR animals, as described in the previous section and shown in FIGURE 2.

EFFECT OF CALORIC RESTRICTION ON HEAT SHOCK PROTEIN

In response to stressed conditions, cells take various adaptive measures, activating a wide variety of evolutionarily conserved machinery.[14] The heat shock response is one such mechanism. A characteristic feature of the heat shock response is the rapid stress-induced synthesis of many cytoprotective proteins.[15] Thus, the expression of cytoprotective heat shock proteins (HSPs) was found to be a major endogenous cellular defense mechanism in ischemia/reperfusion damage, inflammation, and aging.

TABLE 2. Reduction of the incidence of tumors following reduction of food intake[20]

Treatment	No. of Rats	Rats Bearing Tumors	Percent
Ad libitum fed	89	43	48
Restriction	77	0	0
Control/radiation	102	91	89
Restriction/radiation	128	29	23

In this regard, the effects of the conserved action of CR on an age-related decline in transcription and the degradation of HSP 70 are noteworthy. Heydari et al. showed that one-half of the hepatic nuclear transcription activity of HSP 70 was lost in aged rats fed ad libitum, compared to the hepatocytes isolated from CR rats.[16] The age-related changes in the degradation of HSP 70, with a half-life of 140 min, were shortened to 60 min in CR rats, restoring the value of the young. These findings are of interest in the sense that CR can provide cytoprotection against heat challenge by activating conserved resources to withstand stress.[15,16]

STRESS RESISTANCE TO CARCINOGENS AND IRRADIATION BY CALORIC RESTRICTION

CR's resistance to various stressors was perhaps best exemplified when animals were subjected to life-threatening toxic agents or radiation, as shown in the 1942 pioneering work of Tannenbaum using mouse skin tumors induced by benzo(a)pyrene. A more recent report by Chou et al. revealed further insights into how CR enhances resistance by inhibiting the interaction of DNA with the potent carcinogenic aflatoxin B (AFB_1).[17] These investigators found that AFB_1-induced hepatic tumors are reduced by more than 50% in CR rats. Moreover, CR reduced AFB_1-DNA adduct formation by as much as 71%, depending on adduct type, compared to control rats. Furthermore, the authors found that *in vitro* nuclear DNA binding of AFB_1 is 37% lower in CR rats than in controls, although exposure to activated AFB_1 was the same for both groups. A similar resistance was shown in a DNA strand break experiment. A more stable double-stranded DNA was maintained following alkaline treatment in CR rats, whereas about a fourfold increase of damaged single-stranded DNA was found in ad libitum–fed rats.[17]

A study by ThyagaRajan et al. showed CR's resistance against hormone-inducible tumorigenesis.[18] They investigated the mechanism by which CR suppresses carcinogen-induced mammary tumors in the rat and whether CR rats can blunt the action of tumor-promoting estrogen and/or prolactin. The results show that when challenged with the tumor-promoting hormones, tumor progression was significantly suppressed by CR, indicating again a strong ability to resist tumor growth even under powerful tumor stimulation by estrogen and prolactin.

An even more remarkable example of CR's ability to resist irradiation is shown in the work of Gross and Dreyfuss, who challenged mice with gamma irradiation to induce tumorigenesis.[19] They not only show a clear-cut tumor suppression by CR (TABLE 2) but also that CR rats had a far better capability of resisting one of the most deleterious forms of stressors.[19]

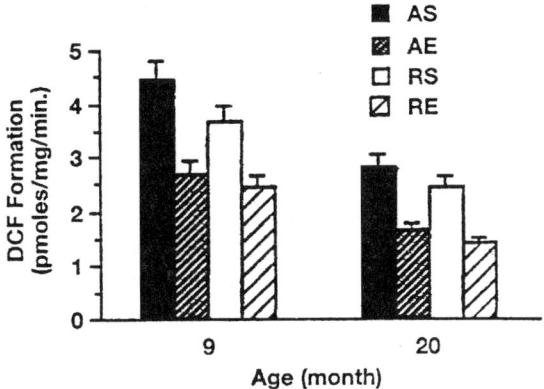

FIGURE 4. Suppression of microsomal production of reactive oxygen species by CR. AS, ad libitum–fed, sedentary; AE, ad libitum–fed, exercising; RS, CR, sedentary; RE, CR, exercising; DCF=2'7'-dichlorodihydrofluorescin. (Reproduced with permission from Kim et al.[20])

CALORIC RESTRICTION AND EXERCISE-INDUCED STRESS

A consequence of the increased metabolic demand that physical exercise presents is increased oxidative stress, as indicated by the increased production of oxidants in mitochondria.[20] However, a recent report shows longer survival spans for exercised CR rats.[20] Exercised CR animals are shown to have an additional extended mean life span of ~10% beyond their nonexercised CR counterparts.[21] An interesting question arises: How can this be possible if exercise promotes oxidative stress? The answer could come from the CR's unique ability to mobilize a series of adaptive defense mechanisms. For example, the free radical generation of microsomes, in contrast to mitochondria, was shown to be significantly suppressed by exercise in CR rats, even at 20 months old (FIG. 4).

Another interesting manipulation by CR is its ability to resist exercise-induced oxidative stress on membrane integrity of exercised CR rats.[11,21] Data show that exercised CR rats, despite having increased mitochondrial oxidant production, can maintain mitochondrial membrane fluidity as good as that of sedentary rats.[21] The mechanisms for such remarkable resistance to stress are likely to be derived from concerted networks of stress-responsive elements, like the lowered membrane peroxidability and antioxidant defenses.

CALORIC RESTRICTION AS A BIOLOGICAL HORMESIS

Numerous studies on CR have established its efficacy as the most effective life-prolonging intervention, extending both average and maximum life spans. Emerging views on extended longevity lead us to believe that CR's resistive action against stress is an evolutionary, adapted measure,[3,4] which is characteristic of a hormetic response (TABLE 3).

TABLE 3. Characteristics of hormesis

Metabolic adaptability
Dose and time-dependent response
Induction by a variety of factors
Evolutionarily conserved genomic adjustment

The concept of hormesis may well offer a biological basis for such a phenomenon by CR.[8] The term *hormesis* by definition describes the beneficial, biological effect at low levels, as seen in reduced caloric intake, which at higher levels would cause deleterious effects.[21] The evidence strongly suggests that an organism's adaptive response to CR was acquired through evolution by its turning on the proper genes essential for a high metabolically efficient state for the survival of the species.[22] The maintenance of homeostasis by an ability to adapt to stress during aging should be the key determinant for extended longevity and a case for the CR paradigm, as depicted in FIGURE 1.

REFERENCES

1. SELYE, H. & B. TUCHWEBER. 1976. Stress in relation to aging and disease. *In* Hypothalamus Pituitary and Aging. A.V. Everitt & J.A. Burgess, Eds: 553–569. Charles C Thomas. Pub. Springfield, MO.
2. YU, B.P. 1994. Modulation of Aging Processes by Dietary Restriction. CRC Press. Boca Raton, FL.
3. PARSON, P.A. 1996. The limit to human longevity: an approach through a stress theory of ageing. Mech. Aging Dev. **87:** 211–218.
4. HOLLIDAY, R. 1989. Problems and paradigms. BioEssays **10:** 125–127.
5. SAPOLSKY, R.M., L.C. KERY & B.S. MCEWEN. 1986. The neuroendocrinology of stress and aging: the glucocorticoid cascade hypothesis. Endocr. Rev. **7:** 284–301.
6. SABATINO, F., E.J. MASORO, C.A. MCMAHAN & R.W. KUHN. 1991. Assessment of the role of the glucocorticoid system in aging process and in the action of food restriction. J. Gerontol. **46:** B171–B179.
7. MERRY, B.J. & A.M. HOLEHAN. 1985. The endocrine response to dietary restriction in the rat. *In* Molecular Biology of Aging. A.D. Woodhead, D. Blackett & A. Hollander, Eds: 117–141. Plenum Press. New York.
8. NEAFSEY, P.J. 1990. Longevity hormesis. A review. Mech. Ageing Dev. **51:** 1–31.
9. KRISTAL, B.S. & B.P. YU. 1994. Aging and its modulation by dietary restriction. *In* Modulation of Aging Processes by Dietary Restriction. B.P. Yu, Ed: 1–36. CRC Press. Boca Raton, FL.
10. FRAME, L.T., R.W. HART & J.E.A. LEAKEY. 1998. Calorie restriction as a mechanism mediating resistance to environmental disease. Environ. Health Perspect. **106:** 313–324.
11. YU, B.P., D.Y. LEE, E.H. HWANG & B.O. LIM. 1999. Calorie restriction: a potent mechanistic solution to the oxygen paradox. *In* The Paradoxes of Longevity. J. M. Robin, B. Forette, C. Franceschi & M. Allard, Eds: 93–102. Springer-Verlag. Berlin.
12. KRISTAL, B.S. & B.P. YU. 1998. Dietary restriction augments protection against induction of the mitochondrial permeability transition. Free Radical Biol. Med. **24:** 269–277.
13. PAMPLONA, R., M. PORTERO-OTIN, D. RIBA, C. RUIZ, J. PRAT, M.I. BELLMUNT & G. BARJA. 1998. Mitochondrial membrane peroxidizability index is inversely related to maximum life span in mammals. J. Lipid Res. **39:** 1989–1994.
14. MAULIK, N. & D.K. DAS. 2000. Redox regulation of ischemic adaptation. *In* Antioxidant and Redox Regulation of Genes. C.K. Sen, H. Sie & P.A. Baeuerle, Eds: 491–516. Academic Press. San Diego, CA.

15. MORIMOTO, R.I. & G. SANTORO. 1998. Stress-inducible response and heat shock proteins: new pharmacologic targets for cytoprotection. Nat. Biotechnol. **16:** 833–836.
16. HEYDARI, A.R., B. WU, R. TAKAHASHI, R. STRONG & A. RICHARDSON. 1993. Expression of heat shock protein 70 is altered by age and diet of the level of transcription. Mol. Cell Biol. **13:** 2909–2918.
17. CHOU, M.W., R.A. PEGRAM, P. GAO & W.T. ALLABEN. 1991. Effects of calorie restriction, aflatoxin B, metabolism and DNA modification in Fischer 344 rats. *In* Biological Effects of Dietary Restriction. L. Fishbein, Ed: 42–54. Springer-Verlag. Berlin.
18. THYAGARAJAN, S., J. MEITES & S.K. QUADRI. 1993. Underfeeding-induced suppression of mammary tumors: counteraction by estrogen and haloperidol. Proc. Soc. Exp. Biol. Med. **203:** 236–242.
19. GROSS, L. & Y. DREYFUSS. 1990. Prevention of spontaneous and radiation-induced tumors in rats by reduction of food intake. Proc. Natl. Acad. Sci. USA **87:** 6795–6797.
20. KIM, J.D., R.J.M. MCCARTER & B.P. YU. 1996. Influence of age, exercise, and dietary restriction on oxidative stress in rats. Aging Clin. Exp. Res. **8:** 123–129.
21. CALABRESE, E.J. & L.A. BALDWIN. 1998. Hormesis as a biological hypothesis. Environ. Health Perspect. **106:** 357–362.
22. LEE, C.K., R.G. KLOPP, R. WEINDRUCH & T.A. PROLLA. 1999. Gene expression profile of aging and its retardation by calorie restriction. Science **285:** 1390–1393.

Protein Glycation

Creation of Catalytic Sites for Free Radical Generation

MOON B. YIM,[a] HYUNG-SOON YIM,[a] CHEOLJU LEE,[b] SA-OUK KANG,[b] AND P. BOON CHOCK[a]

[a]*Laboratory of Biochemistry, NHLBI, National Institutes of Health, Bethesda, Maryland 20892, USA*

[c]*Laboratory of Biophysics, Department of Microbiology, College of Natural Sciences, and the Research Center for Molecular Microbiology, Seoul National University, Seoul 151-742, Republic of Korea*

ABSTRACT: In a glycation reaction, α-dicarbonyl compounds such as deoxyglucosone, methylglyoxal, and glyoxal are more reactive than the parent sugars with respect to their ability to react with amino groups of proteins to form inter- and intramolecular cross-links of proteins, stable end products called advanced Maillard products or advanced end products (AGEs). The AGEs, which are irreversibly formed, accumulate with aging, atherosclerosis, and diabetes mellitus, and are especially associated with long-lived proteins such as collagens, lens crystallins, and nerve proteins. It was suggested that the formation of AGEs not only modifies protein properites but also induces biological damage *in vivo*. In this report, we summarize results obtained from our studies for (1) identifying the structure of the cross-linked radical species formed in the model system—the reaction between α-dicarbonyl methylglyoxal with amino acids, and (2) the reactivity of the radical center of the protein created by the similar reaction. These results indicate that glycation of protein generates active centers for catalyzing one-electron oxidation-reduction reactions. This active center, which exhibits enzyme-like character, is suggested to be the cross-linked Schiff-based radical cation of the protein. It mimics the characteristics of the metal-catalyzed oxidation system. These results together indicate that glycated proteins accumulated *in vivo* provide stable active sites for catalyzing the formation of free redicals.

KEYWORDS: Nonenzymatic glycosylation; Maillard reaction; Methylglyoxal

In a glycation reaction (nonenzymatic glycosylation, Maillard reaction), which produces brown fluorescent compounds, free amino groups of protein react slowly with the carbonyl groups of reducing sugars to yield Schiff base intermediates (FIG. 1) that undergo Amadori rearrangement to stable ketoamine derivatives.[1] These Schiff bases and Amadori products subsequently degrade into alpha-dicarbonyl compounds, such as deoxyglucosone, methylglyoxal, and glyoxal.[2-5] These compounds

Address for correspondence: Moon B. Yim, Laboratory of Biochemistry, NHLBI, National Institutes of Heath, Bethesda, MD 20892. Voice: 301-496-9494; fax 302-496-0599
yimm@nhlbi.nih.gov

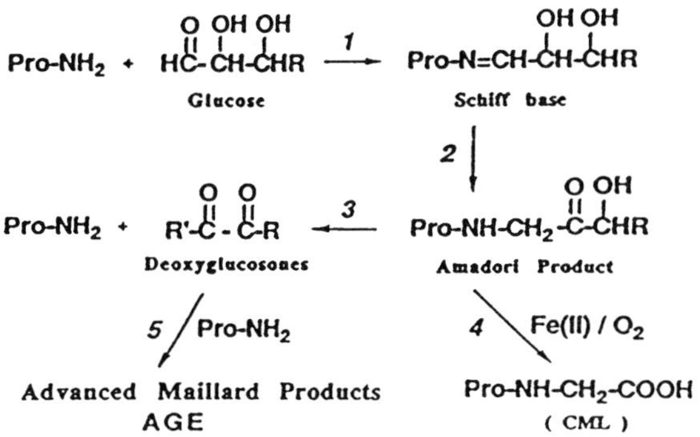

FIGURE 1. A general scheme of the glycation or Maillard reaction. (Reproduced with permission from Yim et al.[26])

are more reactive than the parent sugars with respect to their ability to react with amino groups of proteins to form inter- and intramolecular cross-links of proteins called advanced Maillard products or advanced glycation end products (AGEs). The AGEs, which are irreversibly formed, accumulate with aging, atherosclerosis, and diabetes mellitus and are especially associated with long-lived proteins such as collagens, lens crystallins, and nerve proteins.[5-12] It was suggested that the formation of AGEs not only modifies protein properties but also induces biological damage *in vivo*. For example, AGEs deposited in the arterial wall or glycated tau protein in Alzheimer disease could themselves induce oxidant stress capable of promoting further damage, in hyperglycemic diabetic patients,[13-15] or neuronal dysfunction.[12] Although molecular structures of some AGEs in the heterogeneous products had been identified as pentosidines,[16-19] pyrrole derivatives,[20] pyrazine derivatives,[4] N^ε-carboxyalkyllysine,[21,22] imidazolone compounds,[23] and imidazolium cross-linked species,[5,24,25] it is not known what and how free radicals are generated in the glycation reaction and by glycated proteins.

The formation of α-dicarbonyl compounds seems to be an essential step for the cross-linking reaction (FIG. 1), which leads to the formation of AGEs. In this report, we describe results obtained from our studies for identifying the structure of the cross-linked radical species and their reactivity that may cause deleterious effects *in vivo*.[26,27] For this purpose, we studied a model system consisting of the reaction between three-carbon α-dicarbonyl methylglyoxal and L-alanine, to identify the radical species generated during the glycation reaction.[26] We then studied the oxidation reduction property of glycated protein formed between bovine serum albumin and methylglyoxal.[27]

STRUCTURE OF FREE RADICALS

Although N^ε of lysine residues may be the dominant sites for glycation, alanine was chosen in this study to facilitate EPR analysis because all of ^{15}N- and ^{13}C-substituted alanines are available commercially, and also the electronic structure of the

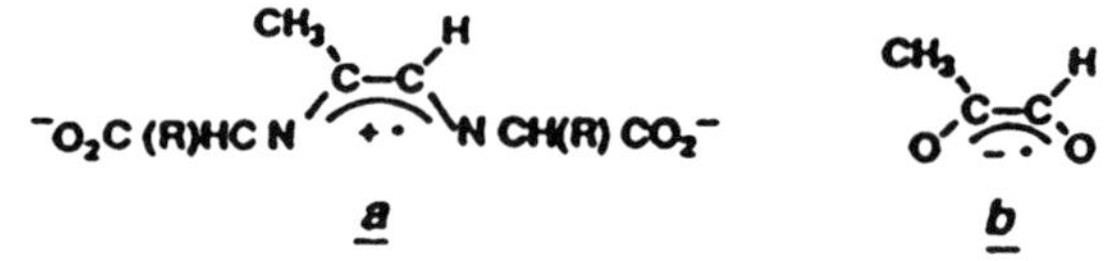

FIGURE 2. Structure of free radicals observed in this reaction and identified by EPR results.

cross-linked radical site is probably similar to that of lysine on the basis of the EPR, absorption, and fluorescence data.[26,27] The reaction between methylglyoxal and L-alanine produced yellow fluorescent products (absorbance maxima, 285 and 334 nm; excitation and emission maxima, 334 and 385 nm, respectively), as formed in some glycated proteins. In addition, we found that three types of free radical species were produced, and their structures were identified using the EPR spectroscopic method.[26] These free radicals are (1) the cross-linked dialkylimine radical cation (FIG. 2a); (2) the methylglyoxal radical anion (FIG. 2b); and (3) the superoxide radical anion generated only in the presence of oxygen molecules. The generation of the cross-linked radical cations and methylglyoxal radical anions does not require transition metal ions or oxygen. The addition of $NaCNBH_3$, which is known to reduce Schiff base selectively, inhibits both the formation of the cation radicals and yellow fluorescent products. These results are summerized in equations 1 and 2.

$$MGDI + MG \rightarrow MGDI^{+\cdot} + MG^{-\cdot} \quad (1)$$

$$MG^{-\cdot} + O_2 \rightarrow MG + O_2^{-\cdot} \quad (2)$$

The dicarbonyl compounds cross-linked free amino groups of protein by forming methylglyoxal dialkylimine (MGDI) Schiff bases, which donate electrons directly to dicarbonyl compounds, resulting in the cross-linked radical cations ($MGDI^{+\cdot}$) and the methylglyoxal radical anions ($MG^{-\cdot}$). Oxygen can accept an electron from an anion to generate a superoxide radical anion, which can initiate damaging chain reactions or cell signaling. The cross-linked radical cations, which have an extensively delocalized unpaired electron, are quite stable. These radical sites in cross-linked proteins will be more persistent and could be a reactive site for putative reducing and oxidizing molecules, which produce free radicals for a long duration. We examined this hypothesis by using methylglyoxal-modified bovine serum albumin (BSA).

GLYCATED PROTEINS

The treatment of BSA with methylglyoxal also produced yellow fluorescent products that exhibited a single broad EPR line at a g value of 2.006.[27] It indicates that glycation of BSA by methylglyoxal also generated a protein-bound, cross-linked free radical (FIG. 3, species D), as observed with alanine, but with much higher stability. Addition of an oxidizing ferricytochrome c to the methylglyoxal-treated BSA (MG-BSA) sample caused a large increase in the amplitude of the EPR signal, which was accompanied by the reduction of ferri- to ferrocytochrome c (FIG. 3, re-

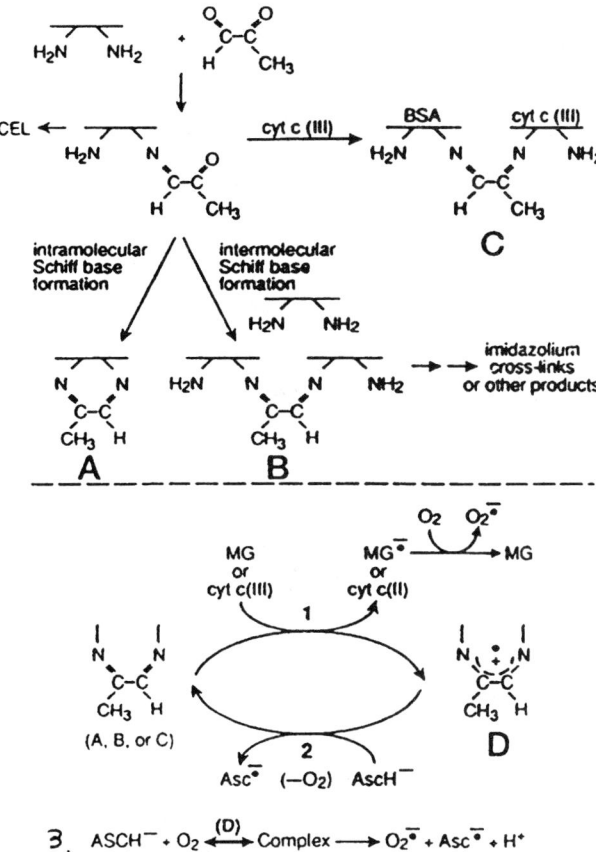

FIGURE 3. Proposed reaction scheme for glycation of protein by methylglyoxal and reaction of glycated protein. CEL, N-(carboxyethyl)lysine. (Reproduced with permission from Lee et al.[27])

action 1). This result indicates that ferricytochrome c receives one electron directly from the cross-linked Schiff bases, such as MGDI (FIG. 3, species A, B, or C), to produce the radical cation of the cross-linked Schiff base MGDI$^{+\cdot}$ (species D). Addition of a reducing ascorbate to MG-BSA quenched the EPR signal, which was also accompanied by the degradation of ascorbate (FIG. 3, reaction 2). Moreover, the oxidation reaction of ascorbate by MG-BSA is catalytic in the presence of oxygen (FIG. 3, reaction 3). Superoxide dismutase, but not catalase, exerts partial inhibition on the degradation of ascorbate in this catalytic reaction. The fact that this inhibition is only partial indicates that O_2, but not $O_2^{-\cdot}$, is directly involved in this catalytic reaction. The partial inhibition, however, suggests that superoxide radical anions are produced during this reaction (FIG. 3, reaction 3), and they play a role in ascorbate degradation, probably via the superoxide-scavenging reaction by ascorbate. Together, these results indicate that MG-BSA behaves as an enzyme, which has the ability to catalyze the oxidation of ascorbate in the presence of oxygen to produce the superoxide radical anion and the semidehydroascorbyl radical. This reaction is initiated by the protein radical cation of MG-BSA.

CREATION OF CATALYTIC SITES

We have shown that the cross-linked Schiff base and its radical cation of proteins produced by glycation behaves as an active site of an enzyme for one-electron oxidation-reduction reactions. This active site has similar characteristics, as observed in the MGDI/MGDI$^{+\cdot}$ pair. Frye et al.[5] have recently detected the methylglyoxal-lysine and glyoxal-lysine cross-links in collagen and lens proteins. The concentration of these cross-links increases with aging and in disease, and in a AGEs-dependent manner. Therefore, the MGDI/MGDI$^{+\cdot}$-type catalytic site of glycated proteins may exert significant effects to their biological environment by generating free radicals for a long duration.

ACKNOWLEDGMENTS

This work was supported, in part, by the International Collaborative Research Program of the National Heart, Lung, and Blood Institute, National Institutes of Health, and by the Korea Science and Engineering Foundation.

REFERENCES

1. REYNOLDS, T.M. 1963. Chemistry of non-enzymatic browning. Adv. Food. Res. **12:** 1–52.
2. KATO, H., D.B. SHIN & F. HAYASE. 1987. 3-Deoxyglucosone cross-links proteins under physiological conditions. Agric. Biol. Chem. **51:** 2009–2011.
3. WELLS-KNECHT, K.J., D.V. ZUZAK, J.E. LITCHFIELD, S.R. THORPE & J.W. BAYNES. 1995. Mechanism of autoxidative glycosylation: identification of glyoxal and arabinose as intermediates in the autoxidative modification of proteins by glucose. Biochemistry **34:** 3702–3709.
4. HAYASHI, T., S. MASE & M. NAMIKI. 1985. Formation of the N,N'-dialkylpyrazine cation radical from glyoxal dialkylimine produced on the reaction of sugar with an amine or amino acid. Agric. Biol. Chem. **49:** 3131–3135.
5. FRYE, E.B., T.P. DEGENHARDT, S.R. THORPE & J.W. BAYNES. 1998. Role of the Maillard reaction in aging of tissue proteins. Advanced glycation end product–dependent increase in imidazolium cross-links in human lens proteins. J. Biol. Chem. **273:** 18714–18719.
6. GORDILLO, E., A. AYALA, J. BAUTISTA & A. MACHADO. 1989. Implication of lysine residues in the loss of enzymatic activity in rat liver 6-phosphogluconate dehydrogenase found in aging. J. Biol. Chem. **264:** 17024–17028.
7. MONNIER, V.M., R.R. KOHN & A. CERAMI. 1984. Accelerated age-related browning of human collagen in diabetes mellitus. Proc. Natl. Acad. Sci. USA **81:** 583–587.
8. ELGAWISH, A., M. GLOMB, M. FREIDLANDER & V.M. MONNIER. 1996. Involvement of hydrogen peroxide in collagen cross-linking by high glucose in vitro and in vivo. J. Biol. Chem. **271:** 12964–12971.
9. MONNIER, V.M. & A. CERAMI. 1981. Nonenzymatic browning in vivo: possible process for aging of long-lived proteins. Science **211:** 491–493.
10. VLASSARA, H., M. BROWNLEE & A. CERAMI. 1983. Excessive nonenzymatic glycosylation of peripheral and central nervous system myelin components in diabetic rats. Diabetes **32:** 670–674.

11. CHOU, S.M., H.S. WANG, A. TANIGUCHI & R. BUCALA. 1998. Advanced glycation endproducts in neurofilament conglomeration of motorneurons in familial and sporadic amyotrophic lateral sclerosis. Mol. Med. **4:** 324–332.
12. YAN, S.D., X. CHEN, A.M. SCHMIDT, J. BRETT, G. GODMAN, Y.S. ZOU, C.W. SCOTT, C. CAPUTO, T. FRAPPIER, M.A. SMITH et al. 1994. Glycated tau protein in Alzheimer disease: a mechanism for induction of oxidant stress. Proc. Nat. Acad. Sci. USA **91:** 7787–7791.
13. BROWNLEE, M., H. VLASSARA & A. CERAMI. 1984. Nonenzymatic glycosylation and pathogenesis of diabetic complications. Ann. Intern. Med. **101:** 527–537.
14. MULLARKEY, C.J., D. EDELSTEIN & M. BROWNLEE. 1990. Free radical generation by early glycation products: a mechanism for accelerated atherogenesis in diabetes. Biochem. Biophys. Res. Commun. **173:** 932–939.
15. SAKURAI, T. & S. TSUCHIYA. 1988. Superoxide production from nonenzymatically glycated protein. FEBS Lett. **236:** 406–410.
16. SELL, D.R. & V.M. MONNIER. 1989. Structure elucidation of a senescence cross-link from human extracellular matrix. Implication of pentoses in the aging process. J. Biol. Chem. **264:** 21597–21602.
17. SELL, D.R. & V.M. MONNIER. 1990. End-stage renal disease and diabetes catalyze the formation of a pentose-derived crosslink from aging human collagen. J. Clin. Invest. **85:** 380–384.
18. GRANDHEE, S.K. & V.M. MONNIER. 1991. Mechanism of formation of the Maillard protein cross-link pentosidine. Glucose, fructose, and ascorbate as pentosidine precursors. J. Biol. Chem. **266:** 11649–11653.
19. DYER, D.G., J.A. BLACKLEDGE, S.R. THORPE & J.W. BAYNES. 1991. Formation of pentosidine during nonenzymatic browning of proteins by glucose. Identification of glucose and other carbohydrates as possible precursors of pentosidine in vivo. J. Biol. Chem. **266:** 11654–11660.
20. MIYATA, S. & V.M. MONNIER. 1992. Immunohistochemical detection of advanced glycosylation end products in diabetic tissues using monoclonal antibody to pyrraline. J. Clin. Invest. **89:** 1102–1112.
21. AHMED, M.U., S.R. THORPE & J.W. BAYNES. 1986. Identification of N-epsilon-carboxymethyllysine as a degradation product of fructoselysine in glycated protein. J. Biol. Chem. **261:** 4889–4894.
22. AHMED, M.U., E. BRINKMANN FRYE, T.P. DEGENHARDT, S.R. THORPE & J.W. BAYNES. 1997. N-epsilon-(carboxyethyl)lysine, a product of the chemical modification of proteins by methylglyoxal, increases with age in human lens proteins. Biochem. J. **324:** 565–570.
23. LO, T.W.C., M.E. WESTWOOD, A.C. MCLELLAN, T. SELWOOD & P.J. THORNALLEY. 1994. Binding and modification of proteins by methylglyoxal under physiological conditions. A kinetic and mechanistic study with N alpha-acetylarginine, N alpha-acetylcysteine, and N alpha-acetyllysine, and bovine serum albumin. J. Biol. Chem. **269:** 32299–32305.
24. WELLS-KNECHT, K.J., E. BRINKMANN, M.C. WELLS-KNECHT, J.E. LITCHFIELD, M.U. AHMED, S. REDDY, D.V. ZYZAK, S.R. THORPE & J.W. BAYNES. 1996. New biomarkers of Maillard reaction damage to proteins. Nephrol. Dial. Transplant. **11**(Suppl. 5): 41–47.
25. NAGARAJ, R.H., I.N. SHIPANOVA & F.M. FAUST. 1996. Protein cross-linking by the Maillard reaction. Isolation, characterization, and in vivo detection of a lysine-lysine cross-link derived from methylglyoxal. J. Biol. Chem. **271:** 19338–19345.
26. YIM, H.-S., S.-O. KANG, Y.-C. HAH, P.B. CHOCK & M.B. YIM. 1995. Free radicals generated during the glycation reaction of amino acids by methylglyoxal. A model study of protein-cross-linked free radicals. J. Biol. Chem. **270:** 28228–28233.
27. LEE, C., M.B. YIM, P.B. CHOCK, H.-S. YIM & S.-O. KANG. 1998. Oxidation-reduction properties of methylglyoxal-modified protein in relation to free radical generation. J. Biol. Chem. **273:** 25272–25278.

Implications of Protein Degradation in Aging

SATARO GOTO,[a] RYOYA TAKAHASHI,[a] ATSUSHI KUMIYAMA,[a]
ZSOLT RADÁK,[b] TOSHIAKI HAYASHI,[a] MASAKI TAKENOUCHI,[a]
AND RYOICHI ABE[a]

[a]*Department of Biochemistry, School of Pharmaceutical Sciences, Toho University, Funabashi, Chiba 274-8510, Japan*

[b]*Laboratory of Exercise Physiology, Hungarian University of Physical Education, Budapest, Hungary*

ABSTRACT: Aging is characterized by accumulation of potentially harmful altered proteins that could lead to gradual deterioration of cellular functions and eventually result in increased probability of death. Metabolic turnover of proteins thus plays an essential role in maintaining the life of an organism. In this article we summarize our current knowledge on age-related changes in protein turnover with special reference to degradation. Increase in half-life of proteins with advancing age is well documented. Qualitative rather than quantitative changes of proteasomes appear to be responsible for this change. Dietary restriction and moderate long-term exercise seem to restore higher proteasome activity and turnover rate of proteins in aged animals.

KEYWORDS: Proteasomes; Hepatocytes; Dietary restriction; Exercise; Ubiquitin

INTRODUCTION

Living organisms have evolved a variety of cellular and molecular mechanisms to cope with endogenous and exogenous stresses potentially harmful to life. Cells, if damaged seriously, are removed by apoptosis or necrosis and the damaged cells are then renewed by replication of remaining intact cells to establish a new steady state in an organism. Nonreplicating cells, such as neurons and cardiac muscle cells, or slowly replicating cells, as hepatocytes, are never or only slowly replaced by cell turnover.

Metabolic turnover of macromolecules, on the other hand, is an alternative means of escaping from the damaging consequences of possibly detrimental internal milieu or external environments. DNA with modified bases or base deletion can be repaired by a variety of repair enzymes,[1] without which death of cells or mutation might result. Peroxidized fatty acid esters in membrane phospholipids may also be repaired.[2] The oxidized phospholipids, if not repaired, can decrease membrane fluidity and/or give rise to various kinds of aldehydes that could modify adjacent proteins,[3] thus deteriorating membrane functions such as signal transduction and membrane transport. Altered protein molecules would be degraded by proteolytic systems, and new intact

---

Address for correspondence: Dr. Sataro Goto, Department of Biochemistry, School of Pharmaceutical Sciences, Toho University, 2-2-1 Miyama, Funabashi, Chiba 274-8510, Japan. Voice: +81-47-472-1531; fax: +81-47-472-1531.

goto@phar.toho-u.ac.jp

molecules would be synthesized instead. Altered proteins do not only lose or lower cellular functions but also often gain toxicity if they accumulate, as in the aggregation of β-amyloid[4] and paired helical filament[5] in Alzheimer disease, α-synuclein in Parkinson's disease,[6] or crystalline in cataract.[7]

Thus, the cellular and metabolic turnovers appear to be among the most fundamental survival strategies of an organism. Aging may therefore be characterized by a decrease in such life-maintenance systems, resulting in increased probability of death. It has been hypothesized that age-related decline of cellular functions is due to accumulation of harmful proteins or proteins with reduced or lost function, extreme cases being the serious age-related diseases mentioned above. We have investigated age-related changes of protein turnover with special reference to degradation and possible means to intervene in the aging process by preventing accumulation of altered proteins.

CHANGE IN DEGRADATION OF CELLULAR PROTEINS WITH AGE

Medvediev and Orgel independently presented an error catastrophe theory of aging that predicts catastrophic deterioration of cellular functions due to exponential increase of altered proteins or nucleic acids by expanding the rate of errors in replication, transcription, and/or translation.[8,9] Although this theory has not gained experimental support so far (see, e.g., Refs. 10–12), an important realization has been advanced that one of the reasons errors do not increase is that error-containing molecules would be largely degraded, thus preventing their accumulation.[13-15] Nevertheless, altered proteins do increase with age.[16,17] Meanwhile, Sharma et al.[18] and Reznick et al.[19] convincingly demonstrated an age-related decrease in the turnover rate of pulse-labeled proteins in nematode and mouse, respectively. In addition, Lavie et al.[20] showed that prematurely terminated puromycinyl peptides are much more slowly degraded in the liver of old mice than in young counterparts. These findings suggested that degradation of normal and abnormal proteins is impaired in old animals.

Hepatocytes in primary culture isolated from young and old rodents provide a good model to investigate protein turnover as a function of age. They can easily be isolated and may be cultivated *in vitro* for the period necessary to study protein turnover without appreciable changes of protein metabolism.[21] Proteins can be introduced into the cultured cells by the osmotic method involving enhanced formation of pinosomes containing the protein to be studied.[22] We have reported that half-lives of proteins introduced into hepatocytes of old mice were extended significantly as compared with those in the cells from young animals (FIG. 1). Chicken lysozymes oxidatively modified *in vitro* were degraded as expected more rapidly than the unmodified counterpart in the cells of both young and old animals, the half-life again being longer in the latter cells (Takahashi *et al.*, in preparation).

Intracellular protein degradation in eukaryotes occurs primarily by one of the two major proteolytic mechanisms, that is, the lysosomal or the proteasomal pathway. The proteasome has been implicated in selective degradation of oxidatively modified proteins[23] and the majority of normal cellular proteins.[24] The degradation of oxidatively modified and unmodified chicken lysozymes introduced into hepatocytes

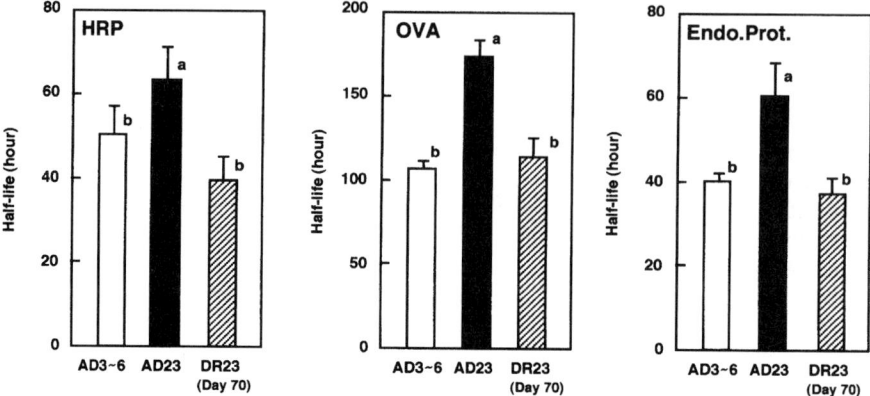

FIGURE 1. Effects of aging and dietary restriction initiated at old age on the half-lives of proteins in hepatocytes from mice (BDF1). HRP: horseradish peroxidase; OVA: ovalbumin; and Endo.Prot.: endogenous proteins. AD3-6: ad libitum–fed, 3~6 months old; AD23: ad libitum–fed, 23 months old; DR23: dietary restricted, 23 months old; mean ± SD. (**a**) Significantly different from AD3-6 ($p < 0.05$); (**b**) significantly different from AD23 ($p < 0.05$).

from both young and old mice was inhibited by a proteasomal inhibitor, Z-leucyl-leucyl-norvalinal, suggesting that the proteasome is responsible for the age-related increase in the half-life of proteins (Kumiyama et al., in preparation).

The proteasome is believed to exist *in vivo* in two different molecular forms, 20S and 26S proteasome, as detected on glycerol gradient centrifugation of cell extracts.[25] The 26S form consists of a 20S core proteasome and two 19S regulatory complexes. Proteins to be degraded by the 26S proteasome are marked with multiple ubiquitin molecules in steps requiring two or three kinds of enzymes. The polyubiquitinated proteins are recognized, deubiquitinated, and perhaps unfolded by a group of subunits called 19S regulatory complex in the 26S proteasome, and then the deubiquitinated proteins are degraded by the catalytic core of the 20S proteasome (FIG. 2). The 20S proteasome consists of two outer rings made up of seven different α-subunits each and two inner rings made up of seven different β-subunits each, some of which contain catalytic domains for peptide bond cleavage. Among at least five peptidase activities in the proteasomes, chymotrypsin-like, trypsin-like, and peptidylglutamyl-peptide hydrolyzing (PGPH) activities are often studied as proteasomal activity. Each of these peptidases catalyzes cleavage of a peptide bond at the carboxyl-terminal side of hydrophobic, basic, and acidic amino acid residues, respectively, giving rise to oligo peptides or amino acids from protein substrates. Inasmuch as the proteasome has been implicated in the degradation of oxidatively modified proteins,[23,26] it was of interest to study age-related changes in them.

Starke-Reed and Oliver[27] were perhaps the first to show that the activity of alkaline protease in the liver of rat (strain not described) declines with age. The major alkaline protease was apparently believed to be an enzyme, later called proteasome. They found a dramatic decline of the activity between 16 and 26 months of age using soluble liver proteins oxidatively modified by metal catalyzed oxidation. This observation was confirmed by Agarwal and Sohal[28] who reported an age-related decline

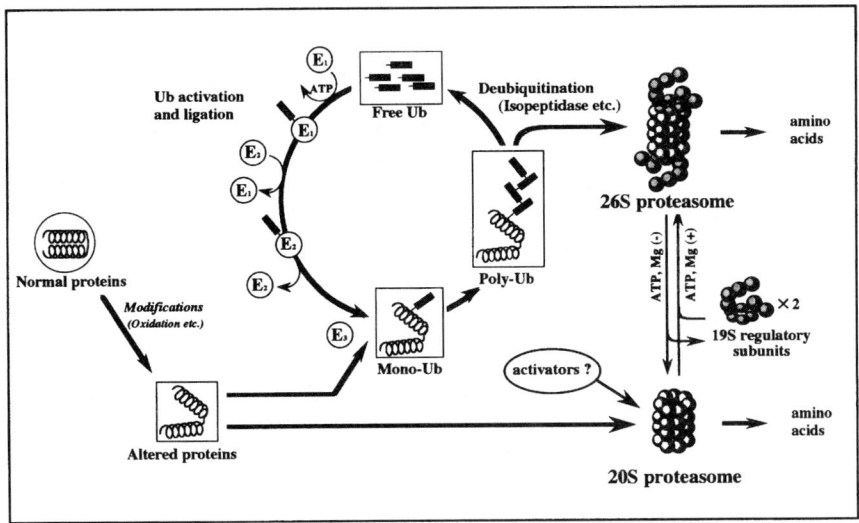

FIGURE 2. 20S and 26S proteasome pathways of altered protein degradation. Ub: ubiquitin.

of alkaline protease activity in the liver of SD rats using X-ray irradiated bovine serum albumin as a substrate. No significant change of the activity, however, was observed in the brain or heart among animals of 3, 13, and 23 months of age. Carney et al.[29] also found significant decrease in alkaline protease activity in the brain of old gerbils. Cao and Cutler[30] critically examined alkaline protease activity in the brain of aging male F344 rats using oxidized glutamine synthetase (GS) or oxidized brain cortex protein as substrate. They found no change of the enzyme with age, making a conclusion that the reported age-dependent change in alkaline protease activity remains to be confirmed. Sahakian et al.[31] also found that the multicatalytic protease activity in liver homogenates of F344 rats at 8, 14, and 26 months of age did not change with age significantly when oxidatively modified bulk liver soluble proteins or oxidatively modified GS were used as substrates. The same group of investigators also reported that specific activity of the PGPH activity in purified multicatalytic proteinase declined by 50% with age when young (8 months old) and old (24 months old) rats were compared.[32] In accordance with the finding of age-related decrease in PGPH activity, Shibatani et al.[33] reported that the activity in F344 rat liver supernatant ($100,000 \times g$) decreased by 40% with age (7 vs. 26 months of age). More recently, Keller et al.[34] described that chymotrypsin-like activity of proteasome decreases with age (3, 12, 24, and 28 months old) in the homogenates of heart, lung, kidney, and liver as well as some portions of the brain of male F344 rats. In all of the investigations cited above, tissue homogenates or the supernatant was used as enzyme sources. It is, therefore, likely that the 20S and 26S proteasome activities together or the 20S proteasome activity alone was measured, depending on what substrate was used and under what assay conditions the activity was determined. This is because the two forms of the proteasome appear to have distinct functions, the 26S form being involved in ATP-dependent degradation of ubiquitinated proteins and the 20S form degrading proteins ATP and ubiquitin independently. The 20S form does not appear to be simply an artificially dissociated form of the 26S proteasome (Ref. 35, see FIG. 2). We therefore studied changes in the two forms of the proteasome with age.

The proteasomal peptidase activities in the liver extracts of young (8- to 10-month-old), middle-aged (15- to 18-month-old), and old (25- to 28-month-old) male F344 rats were studied using fluorogenic peptide substrates for chymotrypsin-like, trypsin-like, and PGPH activities. The $100,000 \times g$ supernatant of the extracts in 5% glycerol was fractionated on glycerol gradient (15–35%) centrifugation to separate 20S and 26S.[36] Glycerol is believed to preserve the physiological state of the proteasomes in cells.[25] The trypsin-like activity in the sum of 20S and 26S fractions decreased significantly by 17% when the level of the old group was compared with that of the young. The chymotrypsin-like activity in the absence of the activator sodium dodecyl sulfate (SDS) declined significantly by 30%, but age-related change was abolished in the presence of SDS under which condition much higher activity was attained. The age-related percentage decrease in the total PGPH activity of 20S and 26S regions in the presence of SDS was most notable, being 60% (old vs. young) (FIG. 3b). Differences between the 20S and 26S forms in age-related changes of the activities were not significant (FIG. 3a), indicating that both ubiquitin-dependent and -independent proteasomal protein degradation are equally impaired in old animals. Remarkably, the relative amount of an α-subunit (C2) of the proteasomes per milligram tissue protein did not decrease appreciably with age, as shown by Western blot analysis.[36] Shibatani et al.[33] also noted that the amount of 20S proteasome did not change with age, as detected by immunoblot analysis of $100,000 \times g$ supernatant

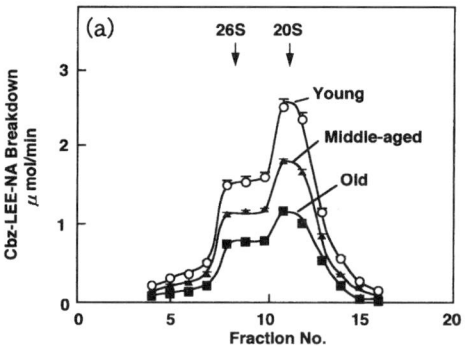
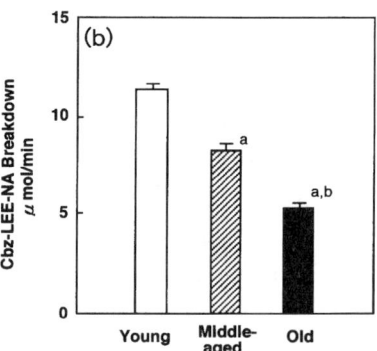

FIGURE 3. Age-related changes in the activity of peptidylglutamyl-peptide hydrolyzing (PDPH) activities of proteasomes (26S and 20S) in the livers of rats (F344). (**a**) Distribution of proteasomal activities on the glycerol gradient centrifugation. (**b**) The PGPH activity in each fraction of the gradient shown in FIG. 3a was totaled for individual animals. Young: 8 to 10 months old; middle-aged: 15 to 18 months old; old: 25 to 28 months old. Values are mean ± SE (n = 6). (a) Significantly different from young ($p < 0.05$); (b) significantly different from middle-aged ($p < 0.05$).[36]

proteins of the liver of male F344 rats 7, 16, and 26 months of age. These findings suggest that the quality rather than quantity of proteasome subunits is decreased with age. It is possible that the proteasomes are themselves modified oxidatively either directly or by aldehydes derived from peroxidized lipids.[31,34] We recently found in male BDF1 mouse liver that although the PGPH activity tended to decrease with age, though not significantly, a significant 50% increase in the amount of the proteasome subunit was found in old animals, again suggesting that the quality of the proteasome decreases with age (Takenouchi et al. in preparation). Thus, an age-related decline in the quality of proteasomes could be at least part of the cause of the accumulation of altered proteins.

Consistent with this hypothesis, ubiquitinated proteins accumulate with age in various tissues, including different regions of the brain of mouse (FIG. 4).[37] It is interesting that proteins that contain errors in translation or that are misfolded during translation were shown to be polyubiquitinated and rapidly degraded by the proteasome, and the ubiquitinated proteins therefore accumulate if the proteasome activity is inhibited.[38] It is possible that the age-associated increase in ubiquitinated proteins is partly a result of abortive translation in addition to being due to well-documented nonphysiological posttranslational modifications. Regarding the accumulation of ubiquitinated proteins, it should be pointed out that their deposition in neurodegenerative disorders, including Alzheimer's and Parkinson's diseases, may be causally related to the deterioration of the ubiquitin/proteasomal system of protein degradation.[39,40]

DIETARY INTERVENTION FOR DECREASED PROTEIN TURNOVER IN AGED ANIMALS

Dietary restriction (DR) or caloric restriction initiated soon after weaning or even in middle age is perhaps the only reliable means of retarding aging in a variety of organisms.[41,42] Because the majority of age-related changes are attenuated by this regimen, it is suggested that general mechanisms that are likely to be the basis of aging might be involved in the beneficial effects of DR. In the present context Ward and his collaborators reported that proteasomal PGPH activity that declines with age in ad libitum fed F344 rats was maintained at higher levels by DR throughout life.[33] Interestingly, the age-related increase rather than decrease in chymotrypsin-like activity was abolished by DR. The significance of this change is unclear. Vittorini et al.[43] reported that proteasomal chymotrypsin-like and trypsin-like activities in the liver extract (23,000 × g supernatant) of SD rats fed every other day decreased significantly from those of ad libitum–fed animals at the age of 2, 24, and 27 months. On the other hand the PGPH activity that declined significantly between 24 and 27 months of age was not affected by the regimen. Thus, available data on the effect of life-long DR on proteasome activity are controversial.

Of particular interest is the mechanism of beneficial effects of DR initiated relatively later in life on the extension of life or a healthy life span because such intervention might provide a biological basis for human application. We have previously shown that DR initiated at old ages and continued for two months in BDF1 mice resulted in significant reduction of altered proteins and half-life of proteins, including

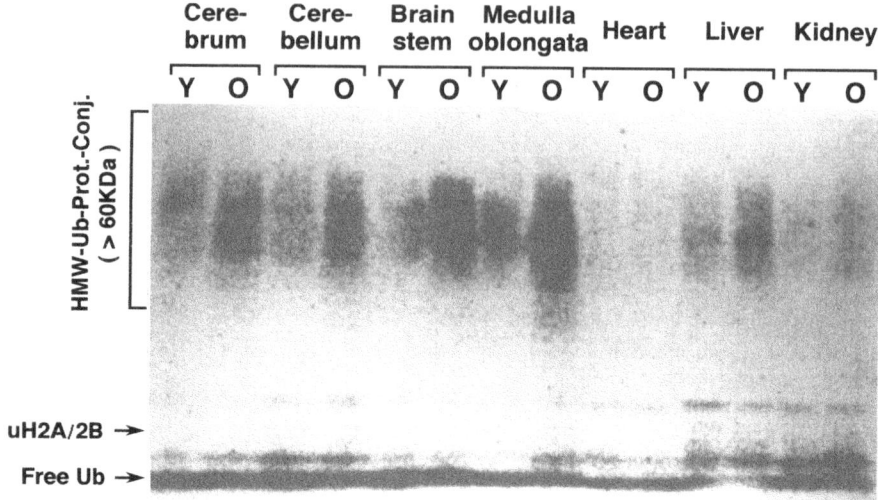

FIGURE 4. Accumulation of high-molecular-weight (HMW) ubiquitin conjugates in BDF1 mouse tissues with age. Y: young (3 to 6 months old); O: old (32 to 36 months old). (Reproduced with permission from Ohtsuka et al.[37])

oxidatively modified ones[44,45] (Takahashi et al., in preparation). These findings, and in view of protein turnover being involved in the general process of life, suggest that an increase in protein turnover by DR late in life may be part of the mechanism of its beneficial effects in prolonging life.

Our more recent results for F344 rat liver suggest that DR by feeding every other day initiated at an old age (26.5 months old) and continued for 3.5 months restored higher PGPH activity, comparable to the level of young animals (10 months old), with no apparent change in the amount of proteasome (Kumiyama et al., in preparation). This finding suggests that proteasome complexes with reduced activity, possibly due to some kind of modification, are replaced by intact ones during DR. It is noted that such "rejuvenization" can be achieved even in the latest half of life (the average life span of male F344 rats being 29 months in our animal facility).

EFFECT OF EXERCISE ON THE PROTEOLYTIC SYSTEM IN AGING ANIMALS

Regular moderate exercise is believed to be beneficial for health, reducing age-related disorders and eventually extending functional life or health span and life span.[46,47] The biochemical basis of this well-documented phenomenon is not, however, well understood.[48] Paradoxically, physical exercise increases the generation of reactive oxygen species that are potentially harmful to proteins and other macromolecules in cells. It is true that a single bout of exercise does indeed damage these mac-

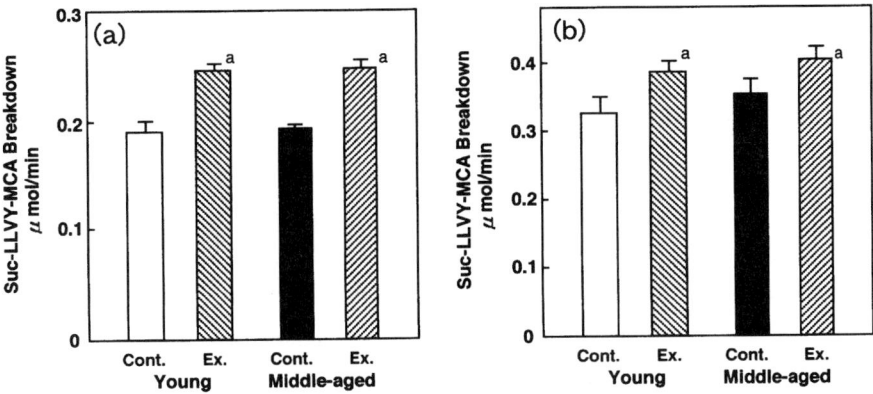

FIGURE 5. Effect of exercise on the activity of chymotrypsin-like activity of proteasomes (26S and 20S) in the (**a**) skeletal muscle and (**b**) brain of rats (Wistar). Cont.: control, Ex.: exercised. Young: 4 weeks old; middle-aged: 14 months old. Values are mean ± SE (n = 6). a: significantly different from the control groups ($p < 0.05$).[52, 53]

romolecules in laboratory rodents.[49–51] This is perhaps not unexpected because sedentary laboratory rodents are probably not prepared for the massive oxidative stress caused by acute exercise. It is, however, conceivable that moderate long-term exercise induces higher protection mechanisms against oxidative damage due to slightly but significantly elevated generation of reactive oxygen species. To test this hypothesis we conducted a moderate swimming exercise of 5 days a week for 9 weeks on young (4-week-old) and middle-aged (14-month-old) male Wistar rats.[52] Although the amount of protein carbonyls in the skeletal muscle was not changed significantly by the exercise, the activities of proteasomal chymotrypsin-like and trypsin-like peptidases increased significantly (FIG. 5a). Remarkably, the same exercise training improved cognitive functions assessed by active and passive avoidance tests of the rats with concomitant decrease in protein carbonyl and increase in proteasomal peptidase activities in the brain (FIG. 5b).[53] It is tempting to speculate that the decrease in protein carbonyls is involved in the improved learning and memory of rats by the exercise, and the enhanced proteasomal activity could have a role in the reduction of these carbonyls. Our findings are in accordance with previous reports on negative correlation between the extent of carbonylation of brain proteins and cognitive function, and the positive correlation between alkaline protease activity of the brain and cognitive function in aging animals.[29,54] It is thus conceivable that, in addition to an increase in the activity of antioxidant enzymes known to occur in the brain as a result of regular physical exercise, upregulation of proteasomes to promote protein turnover may play a significant role in improved cognitive functions by reducing damaged proteins in the brain. It would be interesting to know whether or not improvement of cognitive functions can be attained by moderate regular exercise in older animals, such as those used in our DR experiments described above.

ACKNOWLEDGMENTS

This work was supported by the Research Grant from the Japan Foundation for Aging and Health, the Research Grant of the Japan Society for the Promotion of Science, and a grant from the Hungarian Academy of Sciences Cooperative Science Program to Z. Radák and S. Goto.

REFERENCES

1. LINDAHL, T. & R.D. WOOD. 1999. Quality control by DNA repair. Science **286:** 1897–1905.
2. GIROTTI, A.W. 1998. Lipid hydroperoxide generation, turnover, and effector action in biological systems. J. Lipid Res. **39:** 1529–1542.
3. ESTERBAUER, H., R.J. SCHAUR & H. ZOLLNER. 1991. Chemistry and biochemistry of 4-hydroxynonenal, malonaldehyde and related aldehydes. Free Radic. Biol. Med. **11:** 81–128.
4. COTMAN, C.W., A.J. TENNER & B.J. CUMMINGS. 1996. β-Amyloid converts an acute phase injury response to chronic injury responses. Neurobiol. Aging **17:** 723–731.
5. IQBAL, K., A.C. ALONSO, C.X. GONG et al. 1998. Mechanisms of neurofibrillary degeneration and the formation of neurofibrillary tangles. J. Neural. Transm. **153:** 169–180.
6. MEZEY, E., A. DEHEJIA, G. HARTA et al. 1998. Alpha synuclein in neurodegenerative disorders: murderer or accomplice? Nature Med. **4:** 755–757.
7. OTTONELLO, S., C. FORONI, A. CARTA et al. 2000. Oxidative stress and age-related cataract. Ophthalmologica **214:** 78–85.
8. MEDVEDEV, ZH. A. 1962. Ageing at the molecular level and some speculations concerning maintaining the functioning of systems for replication of specific macromolecules. In Biological Aspects of Ageing. N. Shock, Ed.: 255–266. Colombia University Press. New York.
9. ORGEL, L.E. 1963. The maintenance of the accuracy of protein synthesis and its relevance to ageing. Proc. Natl. Acad. Sci. USA **49:** 517–521.
10. MORI, N., K. HIRUTA, Y. FUNATSU et al. 1983. Codon recognition fidelity of ribosomes at the first and second positions does not decrease during aging. Mech. Ageing Dev. **22:** 1–10.
11. TAKAHASHI, R. & S. GOTO. 1988. Fidelity of aminoacylation by rat liver tyrosyl-tRNA synthetase. Eur. J. Biochem. **178:** 381–386.
12. HOLLIDAY, R. 1996. The current status of the protein error theory of aging. Exp. Gerontol. **31:** 449–452.
13. LEVIS, C.M. 1972. Protein turnover in relation to Orgel's error theory of aging. Mech. Ageing Dev. **1:** 43–47.
14. CALOW, P. 1978. Bidder's hypothesis revisited. Solution to some key problems associated with general molecular theory of ageing. Gerontology **24:** 448–458.
15. MEDVEDEV, ZH. A. 1980. The role of infidelity of transfer of information for the accumulation of age changes in differentiated cells. Mech. Ageing Dev. **14:** 1–14.
16. ROTHSTEIN, M. 1983. Detection of altered proteins. In Altered Proteins and Aging. R.C. Adelman & G.S. Roth, Eds.: 2–8. CRC Press. Boca Raton, FL.
17. GERSHON, D. 1979. Current status of age altered enzymes. Alternative mechanisms. Mech. Ageing Dev. **9:** 189–196.
18. SHARMA, H.K., H.R. PRASANNA, R.S. LANE et al. 1979. The effect of age on enolase turnover in the free-living nematode, *Turbatrix aceti*. Arch. Biochem. Biophys. **194:** 275–282.
19. REZNICK, A.Z., L. LAVIE, H.E. GERSHON et al. 1981. Age-associated accumulation of altered FDP aldolase B in mice. Conditions of detection and determination of aldolase half-life in young and old animals. FEBS Lett. **128:** 221–224.
20. LAVIE, L., A.Z. REZNICK & D. GERSHON. 1982. Decreased protein and puromycinyl-peptide degradation in livers of senescent mice. Biochem J. **202:** 47–51.

21. IKEDA, T., A. ISHIGAMI, K. ANZAI et al. 1992. Changes with donor age in the degradation rate of endogenous proteins of mouse hepatocytes in primary culture. Arch. Gerontol. Geriatr. **15:** 181–188.
22. OKADA, C.Y. & M. RECHSTEINER. 1982. Introduction of macromolecules into cultured mammalian cells by osmotic lysis of pinocytic vesicles. Cell **29:** 33–41.
23. GRUNE, T., T. REINHECKEL & K.J. DAVIES. 1997. Degradation of oxidized proteins in mammalian cells. FASEB J. **11:** 526–534.
24. ROCK, K.L., C. GRAMM, L. ROTHSTEIN et al. 1994. Inhibitors of the proteasome block the degradation of most cell proteins and the generation of peptides presented on MHC class I molecules. Cell **78:** 761–771.
25. TANAKA, K., K. LI & A. ICHIHARA et al. 1986. A high molecular weight protease in the cytosol of rat liver. I. Purification, enzymological properties, and tissue distribution. J. Biol. Chem. **261:** 15197–15203.
26. RIVETT, A.J. 1985. Preferential degradation of the oxidatively modified form of glutamine synthetase by intracellular mammalian proteases. J. Biol. Chem. **260:** 300–305.
27. STARKE-REED, P. & C. OLIVER. 1989. Protein oxidation and proteolysis during aging and oxidative stress. Arch. Biochem. Biophys. **275:** 559–567.
28. AGARWAL, S. & R.S. SOHAL. 1994. Aging and proteolysis of oxidized proteins. Arch. Biochem. Biophys. **309:** 24–28.
29. CARNEY, J.M., P.E. STARKE-REED, C.N. OLIVER et al. 1991. Reversal of age-related increase in brain protein oxidation, decrease in enzyme activity, and loss in temporal and spatial memory by chronic administration of the spin-trapping compound *N-tert*-butyl-alpha-phenylnitrone. Proc. Natl. Acad. Sci. USA **88:** 3633–3636.
30. CAO, G. & R.G. CUTLER. 1995. Protein oxidation and aging. II. Difficulties in measuring alkaline protease activity in tissues using the fluorescamine procedure. Arch. Biochem. Biophys. **320:** 195–201.
31. SAHAKIAN, J.A., L.I. SZWEDA, B. FRIGUET et al. 1995. Aging of the liver: proteolysis of oxidatively modified glutamine synthetase. Arch. Biochem. Biophys. **318:** 411–417.
32. CONCONI, M., L.I. SZWEDA & R.L.I. LEVINE. 1996. Age-related decline of rat liver multicatalytic proteinase activity and protection from oxidative inactivation by heat-shock protein 90. Arch. Biochem. Biophys. **331:** 232–240.
33. SHIBATANI, T., M. NAZIR & F.W. WARD. 1996. Alteration of rat liver 20S proteasome activities by age and food restriction. J. Gerontol. **54A:** B316–B322.
34. KELLER, J.N., K.B. HANNI & W.R. MARKESBERY. 2000. Possible involvement of proteasome inhibition in aging: implications for oxidative stress. Mech. Ageing Dev. **113:** 61–70.
35. COUX, O., K. TANAKA & A.L. GOLDBERG. 1996. Structure and functions of the 20S and 26S proteasomes. Annu. Rev. Biochem. **65:** 801–847.
36. HAYASHI, T. & S. GOTO. 1998. Age-related changes in the 20S and 26S proteasome activities in the liver of male F344 rats. Mech. Ageing Dev. **102:** 55–66.
37. OHTSUKA, H., R. TAKAHASHI & S. GOTO. 1995. Age-related accumulation of high-molecular-weight ubiquitin protein conjugated in mouse brains. J. Gerontol. **50A:** B277–281.
38. SCHUBERT, U., I. ANT, J. GIBBS et al. 2000. Rapid degradation of a large fraction of newly synthesized proteins by proteasomes. Nature **404:** 770–774.
39. ALVES-RODRIGUES, A., L. GREGORI & M.E. FIGUEIREDO-PEREIRA. 1998. Ubiquitin, cellular inclusions and their role in neurodegeneration. Trends Neurosci. **21:** 516–520.
40. ARNOLD, J., S. DAWSON, J. FERGUSSON et al. 1998. Ubiquitin and its role in neurodegeneration. Prog. Brain Res. **117:** 23–34.
41. YU, B.P. 1995. Putative interventions. *In* Handbook of Physiology. Section 11 Aging. E.J. Masoro, Ed.: 613–631. Oxford University Press.
42. WEINDRUCH, R. 1996. Caloric restriction and aging. Sci. Am. **274:** 46–52.
43. VITTORINI, S., C. PARADISO, A. DONATI et al. 1999. The age-related accumulation of protein carbonyl in rat liver correlates with the age-related decline in liver proteolytic activities. J. Gerontol. **54:** B318–323.
44. TAKAHASHI, R. & S. GOTO. 1987. Influence of dietary restriction on the accumulation of heat-labile aminoacyl tRNA synthetase in senescent mice. Arch. Biochem. Biophys. **257:** 200–206.

45. ISHIGAMI, A. & S. GOTO. 1990. Effect of dietary restriction on the degradation of proteins in senescent mouse liver parenchymal cells in culture. Arch. Biochem. Biophys. **283:** 362–366.
46. BLAIR, S.N., H.W. KOHL, C.E. BARLOW et al. 1995. Changes in physical fitness and all-cause mortality. A prospective study of healthy and unhealthy men. J. Am. Med. Assoc. **273:** 1093–1098.
47. SARNA, S., T. SAHI, M. KOSKENVUO et al. 1993. Increased life expectancy of world class male athletes. Med. Sci. Sports Exercise **25:** 237–244.
48. RADÁK, Z. & S. GOTO. 1998. The effects of exercise, aging and caloric restriction on protein oxidation and DNA damage in skeletal muscle. *In* Oxidative Stress in Skeletal Muscle. A.Z. Reznick et al., Eds.: 87–102. Birkhäuser Verlag. Basel/Switzerland.
49. DAVIES, K.J.A., A.T. QUINTANILHA, G.A. BROOKS et al. 1982. Free radicals and tissue damage produced by exercise. Biochem. Biophys. Res. Commun. **107:** 1198–1205.
50. REZNICK, A.Z., E. WITT, M. MATSUMOTO et al. 1992. Vitamin E inhibits protein oxidation in skeletal muscle of resting and exercising rats. Biochem. Biophys. Res. Commun. **189:** 801–806.
51. RADÁK, Z., K. ASANO, A. NAKAMURA et al. 1998. Single bout of exercise increases accumulation of reactive carbonyl derivatives in lung of rats. Pflueger Arch. Eur. J. Physiol. **435:** 439–441.
52. RADÁK, Z., T. KANEKO, S. TAHARA et al. 1999. The effect of exercise training on oxidative damage of lipids, proteins and DNA in rat skeletal muscle: evidence for beneficial outcome. Free Radic. Biol. Med. **27:** 69–74.
53. RADÁK, Z., T. KANEKO, S. TAHARA et al. 2000. Regular exercise improves cognitive function and decreases oxidative damage to proteins in rat brain. 2000. Neurochem. Int. **38:** 17–23.
54. BUTTERFIELD, D.A., B.J. HOWARD, S. YATIN et al. 1997. Free radical oxidation of brain proteins in accelerated senescence and its modulation by *N-tert*-butyl-alpha-phenylnitrone. Proc. Natl. Acad. Sci. USA **94:** 674–678.

Transglutaminase-Mediated Crosslinking of Specific Core Histone Subunits and Cellular Senescence

JAE HONG KIM, HYON E CHOY, KANG HOON NAM, AND SANG CHUL PARK[a]

Department of Biochemistry, Aging and Physical Culture Research Institute, Seoul National University College of Medicine, Seoul, 110-799, Korea

ABSTRACT: We observed that the transglutaminase (tTGase) level and activity increased in aged rats and senescent primary fibroblasts, suggesting that the tTGase-mediated macromolecule crosslinking may play a mechanistic role during aging. Although preliminary, our *in vitro* experiment suggests that the target of tTGase is core histones: H2A:H2B and H3:H4 are specifically crosslinked by tTGase. On the basis of these data, we postulate that the changes of DNA metabolism in association with cellular aging may be ascribed primarily to the crosslinking of core histone subunits. Further speculation awaits substantive data showing increased histone crosslinking in senescent cells and also what crosslinked histones in various DNA metabolisms may imply. At the moment, present data are sufficient to propose that tTGase is a senescence marker and it may be primarily responsible for the phenotypes associated with cellular senescence.

KEYWORDS: Transglutaminase; Macromolecular crosslinking; Histones

INTRODUCTION

Two of the many theories accounting for aging are genetics and environment. The genetic theory explains aging as a genetically programmed process; that is, cells have a certain clock that counts their own age, once proposed as a "mitotic clock." This clock might be certain genes or subcellular structures such as telomore. The environmental theory proposed that the aging is an environmentally modulated process. As an animal grows old, there is an accumulation of repairable and nonrepairable damage caused by various environmental insults, such as free radicals. Accumulation of such damage, according to this theory, leads to aging. There is a "crosslinking theory of aging" that belongs grossly to the category of this environmental theory. The crosslinking theory of aging, originally proposed by Bjorkstein,[1] is that aging process is closely associated with an increase of macromolecular crosslinking. It is generally perceived that macromolecular crosslinking increases as a function of aging, and the crosslinking limits the mechanistic function of various macromolecules that are crosslinked during the aging process. Here, we adopted this crosslinking theory, but extended it beyond what was originally proposed to account

---

[a]Corresponding author. Voice: 82-2-740-8244; fax: 82-2-744-4534.
scpark@plaza.snu.ac.kr

for cellular aging. That is, macromolecular crosslinking may be responsible for the phenotypes associated with senescent cells at the level of DNA metabolism—transcription, replication, etc.

Biological crosslinking reactions can be enzymatically mediated or nonenzymatically activated. Nonenzymatic crosslinking activities are mediated by the Maillard glycation reaction, aldol-aldimine condensation, or the interaction of lipid peroxides, which are random events but reported to increase during the aging process. In contrast, there are enzyme-mediated crosslinking reactions that catalyze the specific crosslinking of macromolecules. Several enzymes, including lysyl oxidase tyrosine peroxidase, sulfhydryl oxidase and transglutaminase, have been shown to crosslink the various macromolecules. We conjectured that if enzyme-mediated crosslinking of macromolecules is implicated in aging, the enzyme catalyzing the crosslinking reaction must increase its activity or protein content as a function of aging. However, in the case of lysyl oxidase, not only the amount but also its products, such as elastin, pyridinoline and glucitolylllysine, decrease with aging. In the case of tyrosine peroxidase and sulfhydryl oxidase, the regulation of redox potential and radical generation is prerequisite for the control of their activity, which again makes it unlikely to be involved in the aging process. On the other hand, transglutaminase (tGase)-mediated crosslinking has already been suggested to play a role in several age-related phenomena such as cataract formation, Alzheimer's disease, Mallory's bodies of the liver, atrophic muscle fiber and senescent keratinocytes.[2–4] Thus, it is most likely that if an enzyme-mediated crosslinking is implicated in aging, it involves transglutaminase.

Transglutaminases are a class of enzymes that catalyze the acyl-transfer reaction in which γ-carboxamide groups of peptide-bound glutamine residues serve as acyl donors, and ε-amino group of peptide-bound lysine residues as acyl acceptors, forming ε (γ-glutamyl)lysine bond between two peptides. Transglutaminases have been found to be widespread in cells and body fluids of a number of mammals including humans. Five different transglutaminases have been discovered in human: transglutaminase K, C, E, P and FactorXIII.[5] In an attempt to understand the role of enzyme-mediated macromolecular crosslinking in aging, we focused on macromolecule crosslinking by tGase (TGase C, tissue TGase, TGase 2) since it is ubiquitously present. We report here that tGase expression increased in aged rats and *in vitro* cultured primary cells; specifically, tGase was capable of crosslinking core histone subunits in the nucleus.

CHANGES OF TRANSGLUTAMINASE ACTIVITIES DURING AGING

We set up an experiment with the rationale that if enzyme-mediated crosslinking is implicated in aging the crosslinking enzyme activity must increase during aging. First, we determined the tGase activity in the liver and brain tissues of Sprague-Dawley rats at various ages—4, 12, 18 and 24 months.

tGase activity increased in both the liver and brain as the animals aged, although more significantly in brain owing to low activity in the 4-month-old rats—approximately 3-fold less than in the liver.[6] The increase of tGase in the liver was determined to be about 2-fold and that in the brain about 7-fold when activity in the 4- and 24-month-old rats was compared. Thus, we could establish a positive correlation between tTGase activity and animal age. Subsequently, we examined the tTGase activity in *in vitro* cultured human diploid primary fibroblast cells. Primary fibroblasts undergo only about 50 to 60 population doublings in culture. The senescent primary fibroblasts show the phenotype of aged cells: enlarged flat cells that could be stained by β-galactosidase, the sole marker of cellular senescence presently available. The tTGase activity remained about the same until passage 42. Thereafter, the tTGase activity increased abruptly. It should be pointed out that from the passage 42 cell growth also begins to slow down and the cell morphology begins to change to that of the senescent cells. tTGase activity at passage 56 was about 7 times of that at passage 20 or 42.

H_2O_2, a free radical generator, has been reported to induce cellular senescence. When the fibroblast cells at passage 42 were treated with H_2O_2, it caused cellular senescence indistinguishable from that of naturally senescent cells. When they were analyzed for tTGase activity, we observed an elevation of the activity (520 cpm × 01^{-3}/mg protein), which is comparable to that of naturally senescent cells (540 cpm × 10^{-3}/mg protein) at passage 56. Thus, tTGase activity increased in the senescent fibroblast cells irrespective of mode of aging, natural or induced. Transglutaminase activity increased in the aged rats and *in vitro* cultured senescent cells, although the rate of increase seems to be somewhat different. In liver and in cultured fibroblasts, the increase was abrupt at the late age, while in brain the increase was gradual. Nevertheless, it seems that tTGase, amongst those enzymes capable of crosslinking macromolecules, may play some role in cellular aging.

tTGase protein level and activity increase during aging both in rat organs and *in vitro* cultured primary human diploid fibroblast (HDF). The tTGase level *in vitro* increased in the senescent cells regardless of method of senescence, either induced or natural. Since HDF *in vitro* should not be subject to the same environmental influence as those cells *in vivo* (e.g., rats), but the level of tTGase was elevated in both cases, it is suggested that tTGase is implicated in intrinsic cellular aging rather than the aging through environmental stress. In contrast, tTGase has been also implicated in apoptosis, on the basis of the observation that overexpression of tTGase in human neuroblastoma cells renders these cells susceptible to death by apoptosis.[7] It should be noted, however, that a typical characteristic of senescent cells is resistance to environmental insults, presumably owing to a selective modification of cytoplasmic membrane components.[8] It is therefore most likely that the apoptosis induced by the overexpression of tTGase is physiological phenomenon not directly associated with that of cellular senescence.

It has been reported that the expression of tTGase is sensitive to the cytosine methylation of the CpG-rich segment of its promoter.[9] Cytosine residues of mammalian genome, especially in the CpG doubles, are known to be methylated. Certain transcription factors such as cAMP-reponsive element (CRE) binding protein (CREB) are sensitive to the cytosine methylation. An inverse correlation between the degree of cytosine methylation and the tTGase promoter activity suggests a possibility that the age-dependent increase in tTGase expression may be ascribed to a selective demethylation of CpG doublets on tTGase promoter.

Most recently it has been reported that about 2% of total genes in mouse change their expression during aging: of this 2%, expression increased in roughly half while it decreased in the other half.[10] In this study, using a high-density oligonucleotide array to define transcriptional response to aging in mouse gastronemius muscle revealed that those genes encoding stress mediator increased but those involved in energy metabolism and biosynthesis decreased their expression. Interestingly, it should be noted that in addition to tTGase many other proteins such as tumor suppressors p53 or cell cycle regulators known to increase during aging were not included in the list. It is certainly possible that the activity rather than the protein level of tTGase increases during aging if it plays a critical regulatory role at the top of cascade leading the aging process. Following this line of thought, the increased tTGase activity must result in significant changes of cellular function.

TARGETS OF TRANSGLUTAMINASE ACTION

tTGase has been considered solely a cytosolic enzyme, although its role has not been fully understood. Interestingly, however, the possibility that transglutaminase may function in nucleus instead of cytosol was recently reported. When neuroblastoma cells were treated with retinoic acid and mitotoxin, which elevate intracellular Ca^{++} concentration, the tTGase translocates from cytoplasm into nucleus. Both tTGase activity and the protein were found localized in nucleus following the elevation of intracellular Ca^{++} concentration. It is not totally unreasonable to consider that tTGase acts in the nucleus since it has been shown repeatedly that DNA metabolism, such as the pattern of transcription, changes through aging, which may be ascribed to the increased nuclear macromolecule crosslinking. What should, then, be the substrate for tTGase in the nucleus? To answer this question, we turned out attention to the most abundant nuclear proteins—notably, the histones. Histone proteins are organized in loose ends with a compact core. The C-termini of core histone subunits are particularly rich in lysine residues, possible acyl acceptors for transglutaminase-mediated crosslinking reaction. To test whether core histone proteins can be substrates of tTGase in nucleus, we set up an *in vitro* experiment using tTGase purified from human erythrocytes using HPLC and linker (H1)-depleted nucleosome core from chicken erythrocytes. FIGURE 1 shows the result of an *in vitro* reaction in which H1-depleted chromatin was incubated in the absence (–) or presence (+) of tTGase. In the absence of tTGase, roughly an equal amount of each of the histone subunits was displayed on 15% denaturing polyacrylamide gel: H3, H2A, H2B, and H4 in order. Note that H1 was completed removed. In the presence of tTGase, two products with molecular weight of approximately 30 kD were formed, which was accompanied by a reduction of substrate core histones. Two product bands were analyzed for composition by Western blot analysis using specific antibodies, and it was found that the upper band consisted of H2A and H2B and the lower band of H3 and H4 (data not shown). It appeared that the crosslinking of histone subunits by tTGase is not random but substrate specific. Although further study is needed, these data demonstrated clearly that core histones could be the substrate for tTGase in nucleus.

Histone subunits have been shown to be crosslinked during the development of starfish (*Asterina pectinifera*) testis.[11] It was reported that nuclei of the testis contains a significant amount of covalently crosslinked histones, p28: Gln^9 of H2B and Lys^5 or Lys^{12} of H4 crosslinked by ε (γ-glutamyl)lysine bond formed presumably by a transglutaminase. It was also noted during embryogenesis of the starfish, especially at the midblastula stage, that p28 was also produced. Since the enzyme capable of breaking the ε (γ-glutamyl)lysine bond has not been found, the fate of crosslinked

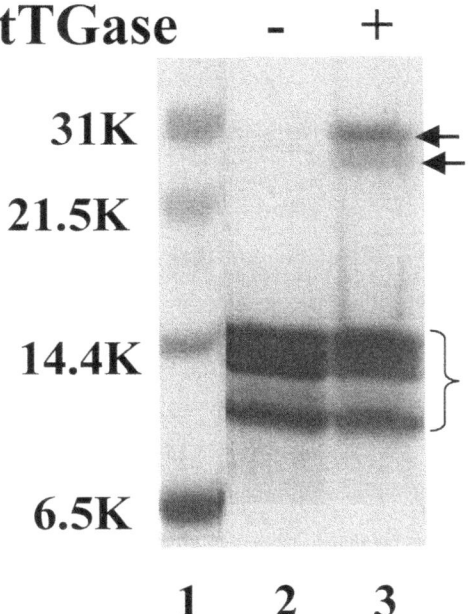

FIGURE 1. Crosslinking of core histone subunit by tTGase. H1-depleted chromatin was incubated at 37°C in the absence (−) or presence (+) of tTGase. The reactants were displayed on 15% SDS-PAGE gel. *Lane 1* shows the protein size maker; *lane 2*, the reactant without tTGase; and *lane 3* shows the reactant with tTGase.

H2B and H4 is a mystery. It is also unclear whether the crosslinked subunits can participate in nucleosome assembly or not. But, we propose that histone crosslinking during aging by tTGase may be responsible for the changes in DNA metabolism such as transcription and replication. It has been reported, that nucleosome arrangements in young and old cells are vastly different.[12] An electron microscopic observation of 10 nm chromatin fiber from human embryonic fibroblast revealed that the nucleosome arrangement from young fibroblasts was compact and extended through out most of chromatin fiber, but that from old fibroblasts was loose and scarce. This difference might be exaggerated, but it points out that chromatin structure may be vastly different between young and old cells, reflected as a differential gene expression between young and old cells. We speculate that histone crosslinking by elevated tTGase may be responsible for the changes in chromatin structure in old cells.

ACKNOWLEDGMENTS

This work has been supported by the grants from the Korea Science and Engineering Foundation and the Korea Research Foundation for Health Science to S.C. Park.

REFERENCES

1. BJORKSTEN, J. 1968. The crosslinking theory of aging. J. Am. Geriatr. Soc. **16:** 408.
2. DUDEK, S.M. & G.V. JOHNSON. 1993. Transglutaminase catalyzes the formation of sodium dodecyl sulfate insoluble, Alz 50-reactive polymers of tau. J. Neurochem. **61:** 1159–1162.
3. KNIGHT, R.L., D. HAND, M. PIACENTINI & M. GRIFFIN. 1993. Characterization of the transglutaminase-mediated large molecular weight polymer from rat liver: its relationship to apoptosis. Eur. J. Cell Biol. **60:** 210–216.
4. PARK, S.C., W.H. KIM, M.C. LEE, et al. 1994. Modulation of transglutaminase expression in rat skeletal muscle by induction of atrophy and endurance training. J. Kor. Med. Sci. **9:** 490–496.
5. HAN, J.A. & S.C. PARK. 1999. Reduction of transglutaminase 2 expression is associated with an induction of drug sensitivity in the PC 14 human lung cancer cell line. J. Cancer Res. Clin. Oncol. **125:** 89–95.
6. PARK, S.C., E.J. YEO, J.A. HAN, et al. 1999. Aging process is accompanied by increase of transglutaminase C. J. Gerontol. (Biol. Sci.) **54A:** B78–B83.
7. MELINO, G., M. ANNICCHIARIO-PETRUZZELLI & L. PIREDDA. 1994. Tissue transglutaminase and apoptosis: sense and antisense transfection studies with human neuroblastoma cells. Mol. Cell Biol. **14:** 6584–6596.
8. PARK, W.Y., J.S. PARK, K.A. CHO, et al. 2000. Upregulation of caveolin attenuates EGF signaling in senescent cells. J. Biol. Chem. In press.
9. LU, S., M. SAYDAK, V. GENTILE, et al. 1995. Isolation and characterization of the human tissue transglutaminase gene promoter. J. Biol. Chem. **270**(17): 9748–9756.
10. LEE, C.K., R.G. KLOPP, R. WEINDRUCH & T.A. PROLLA. 1999. Gere expression profile of aging and its retardation by caloric restriction. Science **285:** 1390–1393.
11. SHIMIZU, T., T. TAKAO, K. HOZUMI, et al. 1997. Structure of a covalently cross-linked form of core histones present in the starfish sperm. Biochemistry **36:** 12071–12079.
12. MOZZHUKHINA, T.G., V.N. CHABANNY, E.L. LEVITSKY & A. LITOSHENKO. 1991. Age-related changes of supranucleosomal structures and DNA-synthesizing properties of rat liver chromatin. Gerontology **37:** 181–186.

Proteome and Proteomics for the Research on Protein Alterations in Aging

TOSIFUSA TODA

Department of Gene Regulation and Protein Function,
Tokyo Metropolitan Institute of Gerontology, Tokyo, Japan

ABSTRACT: Functional decline of tissues in aged animals is a result of cellular aging. Though any process of somatic cell aging basically depends on genomic instructions, phenotypes of aged cells are expressed in a given internal environment of each cell type that was made with translated proteins and post-translationally modified products. Therefore, research on age-dependent protein alterations in each cell type is very important in clarifying mechanisms of aging. The novel term "proteome" is a compound of "prote_in" and "gen_ome_," which means constitutive whole proteins including post-translationally modified products in a cell type. Proteomics is a novel strategy for analyzing proteomes. In proteomics, high resolution two-dimensional electrophoresis is exclusively performed for isolation of proteins followed by mass spectrometry for identification of proteins and determination of modifications. Thus, proteomics is becoming appreciated as a powerful tool to find out proteins responsible for cellular aging, symptoms of senility and geriatric diseases.

KEYWORDS: Proteome; Proteomics; Bioinformatics; Protein alterations; Aging

INTRODUCTION

DNA sequencing projects have been progressing rapidly and are or soon will be complete for many organisms including human.[1,2] Accumulated information about DNA sequences will be helpful for us in understanding mechanisms of cellular differentiation, tissue development and genetic diseases better. It is, however, doubtful that the genomic information alone is enough to clarify complete mechanisms of aging. Only a small part of genomic instructions are transcribed into mRNAs in a specific cell type in a strictly regulated fashion. Many proteins are modified enzymatically and/or non-enzymatically after translation.[3,4] Phenotypes of senescent cells appear through functions of expressed and modified proteins (FIG. 1). Even in premature aging caused by genetic abnormality, the acceleration of aging may come through missing or abnormal function of gene products.

The term "proteome" was invented by Marc Wilkins and Keith Williams at the Macquarie University Center for Analytical Biotechnology in Australia in 1995. In the same way that the genome is the collective name for all the genetic material in the cell of a living organism, the proteome is the term for the complete set of the pro-

---

Address for correspondence: Dr. Tosifusa Toda, Department of Gene Regulation and Protein Function, Tokyo Metropolitan Institute of Gerontology, 35-2 Sakaecho, Itabashi-ku, Tokyo 173-0015, Japan. Voice: +81-3-3964-3241; fax: +81-3-3579-4776.

ttoda@tmig.or.jp

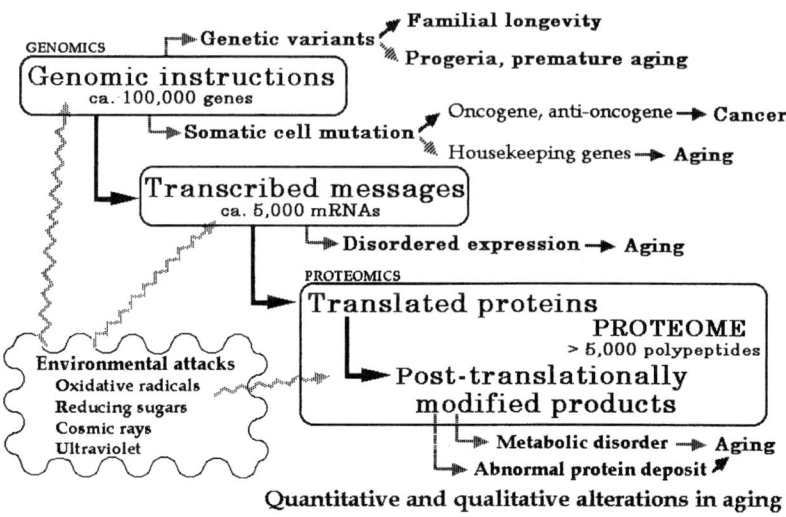

FIGURE 1. Possible causes of aging.

teins produced from the genetic instructions and modified after translation. Proteomics is a combined technique of two-dimensional polyacrylamide gel electrophoresis (2-D PAGE) and mass spectrometry (MS) to separate, quantitate, identify and characterize proteins of interest. The methodology is especially appropriate for research on molecular mechanisms of aging.

GENERAL PROCEDURE FOR PROTEOME ANALYSIS

Proteome analysis is generally carried out in a simple procedure as described in FIGURE 2. So-called Differential Protein Display is accomplished by 2-D PAGE followed by image analysis. Proteins are separated by 2-D PAGE, and proteome profiles are displayed as spots on a gel slab. Quantitative and/or qualitative differences of corresponding spots among gels are analyzed using a computer software system for image processing.[5,6] Subsequently, protein in a spot of interest is digested with an endoproteinase and subjected to MS for protein identification by peptide mass fingerprinting.[7,8] Information of peptide sequence is obtained by secondary MS after collision-induced dissociation (CID)[9,10] or by Edman degradation microsequencing.[11] Post-translational modifications of peptides are detectable as mass shifts in fingerprints by CID-MS/MS analysis. Edman degradation microsequencing is an alternative method for determining peptide sequences of proteins for which mass spectrometry does not work well. In the final step of proteomics, possible functions of a given protein are hypothesized and determined in bioinformatics using an on-line search on internet web sites.

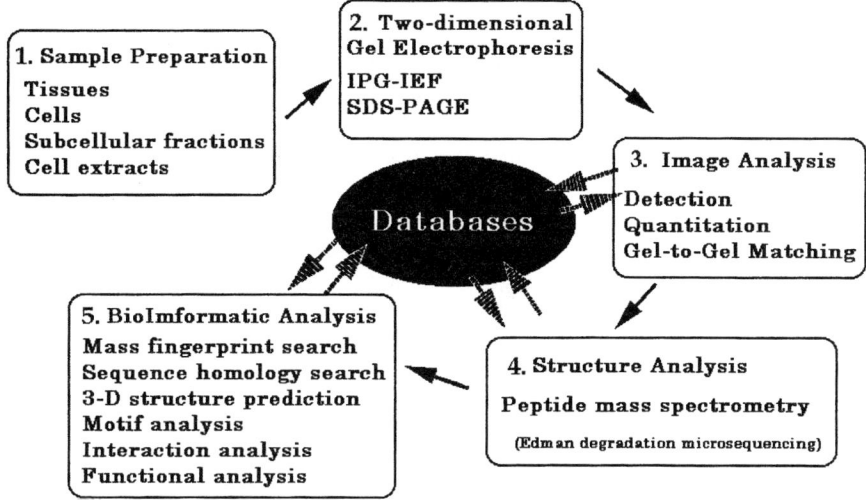

FIGURE 2. General procedure for proteomics.

Sample Preparation

Reproducibility of sample preparation in the procedure for proteome analysis is of critical importance to get reliable data about protein alterations during aging. Protein profiling by 2-D PAGE is readily affected by a sample-to-sample difference in cell population. Therefore, special care should be taken to obtain exactly corresponding tissue preparations from different animals at various ages. This is a reason why cultured cell lines are often used as samples for proteome analysis in research on aging. Isolation of a specific cell type, subcellular fractionation, selective protein extraction and immuno-affinity purification of protein are effective for detecting trace amount of minor components in a given cell type.

Two-Dimensional Gel Electrophoresis

In a general procedure for proteomic analysis, proteins in a sample are separated by an advanced method of two-dimensional polyacrylamide gel electrophoresis (IPG-DALT 2-D PAGE),[12–14] in which isoelectric focusing (IEF) is performed on an immobilized pH-gradient (IPG) first, and followed by SDS polyacrylamide gel electrophoresis (SDS-PAGE). IPG gel strips for various ranges of pH are available in a dry form from Amersham Pharmacia Biotech AB (Uppsala, Sweden) and Bio-Rad Laboratories (Hercules, CA, USA) commercially. To achieve the best reproducibility of protein separation in the first-dimensional IEF, a batch of gel strips, that were prepared at a time, should be used through out a series of experiment. Dry gel strips are storable in a deep freezer under −75°C for several years or more without any deterioration in quality. After reconstitution with a swelling buffer, each gel strip is loaded with a small chip of filter paper absorbing 10–20 μl of 1–3 mg/ml protein solution for analytical scale of differential protein display. A dry strip can be loaded with a maximum of 0.2 ml protein sample by supplementing the swelling buffer with protein if much protein should be treated at a time for mass spectrometry. IPG gel strips with a narrower pH range gives higher first-dimensional resolution to separate more spots in crowded area on a 2-D gel. In our laboratory, two types of Immobiline Drystrip, pH 4–7 and pH 6–11, are generally used for profiling acidic and basic ranges of a proteome separately.

After IEF, the IPG gel strip is incubated in a SDS/iodoacetamide-containing buffer for carbamoylmethylation of sulfhydryl groups of proteins. Details of the incubation condition are described in our home page at <http://proteome.tmig.or.jp/2D/>. The IPG gel strip is fix on a top of gel slab, and followed by SDS-polyacrylamide gel electrophoresis (SDS-PAGE) for separating protein according to their molecular masses.

Detection of Protein Spots

After second-dimensional SDS-PAGE, proteome profiles are visualized by Coomassie staining, silver staining, copper staining, CYPRO Ruby fluorostaining, or autoradiography. Silver staining is often used because it has the highest sensitivity excepting autoradiography; however, optical densities of silver-stained spots are not exactly correlated to absolute quantities of protein in a gel slab. Sensitivity of CYPRO Ruby fluorostaining is almost the same as silver staining, and the fluorescence intensities of stained spots show a better linearity in wide dynamic range of protein concentration, even though an expensive fluoroscanner is required. Coomassie staining is less sensitive, but suitable for detecting spots for MS because the sensitivities of Coomassie staining and MS are comparable and Coomassie-stained proteins are detectable by MS.

Image Analysis

Computerized image analysis is a necessity for differential protein display in gerontology research. Aging is a very complicated process, and many differences are displayed among gels for proteome profiling because more than a few proteins may alter during aging. Subtraction and equilibration of background level of optical density on each gel are very important for reliability in quantitative comparison of corresponding spots among gels. Several types of software are commercially available. PDQuest is the best choice for differential protein display analysis because programs for background subtraction, spot detection, spot matching and spot quantitation are well designed to get reliable data by image comparison. Melanie II software is an alternative choice when a spot of interest should be identified by matching to a corresponding spot on a standard gel image that may be downloaded from an internet web site such as SWISS-2DPAGE.[15]

Peptide Structure Analysis

Protein in a spot at which age-related alteration is detected is easily identified by peptide mass fingerprinting followed by homology search to an internet web site of a peptide sequence database such as MASS-Fit at a UCSF server. For peptide mass fingerprinting, spot protein in a gel slab is digested with endoproteinase directly or after being transferred onto a PVDF membrane. Trypsin is suitable for "in-gel diges-

TABLE 1. Theoretical mass shifts by various post-translational modifications

Functional modifications	
Phosphorylation	+80 D
Acetylation	+42 D
Methylation	+14 D
Disulfide bridging	−2 D
Undesirable modifications	
Deamidatio	+2 D
Ditylosine bridging	−2 D
Methionine sulfoxidation	+16 D
Lysine carboxymathylation	+58 D
Lysine carbonylaton	−2 D

tion." On the other hand, "on-membrane" digestion of protein is often incomplete with trypsin. Lysylendoproteinase (Lys-C) is the best choice for "on-membrane" digestion. Details of digestion condition are described in our homepage. Peptide mass signals for fingerprinting can be obtained by matrix-assisted laser desorption ionization-time of flight MS (MALDI-TOF-MS), electrospray ionization-time of flight MS (ESI-TOF-MS) or electrospray ionization-fourier transform MS (ESI-FT-MS). Identification of protein can be achieved using proteomic tools in Web sites such as SWISS-2DPAGE or UCSF Proteomic Web site.

When no peptide is hit by the query for fingerprinting, internal peptide sequences obtained by collision-induced dissociation (CID) MS/MS analysis or by Edman degradation microsequencing are then used as tags for sequence homology search. Two tandem mass spectrometers are employed in MS/MS. Between the two analyzers (MS1 and MS2) is a collision gas cell. Precursor ions selected by MS1 collide with an inert gas such as helium in the cell and undergo fragmentation. The resulting daughter ions are analyzed by scanning with MS2. The collision process is called collision-induced dissociation. TOF-MS is better than FT-MS for CID-MS/MS analysis, because fragmentation by CID in a cell of FT-MS is inadequate for peptide sequencing.

Post-translational modifications are also detectable by CID-MS/MS[16] if the modification causes a mass shift. Theoretical mass shifts that are caused by typical post-translational modifications are shown in TABLE 1. Phosphorylation, acetylation, methylation and disulfide bridging are known as functional modifications. Besides, peptidyl lysine carboxymethylation is formed by non-enzymatic glycation by attacking with reducing sugars.[17,18] Peptidyl methionine sulfoxidation and peptidyl lysine carbonylation are products of protein oxidation.[19–22] Though the mass shift in peptidyl lysine carbonylation is too small to be detected by MS, dinitrophenylhydrazine (DNPH) derivatization offers enough mass shift for MS analysis (FIG. 3).

Protein-to-protein, protein-to-DNA and protein-to-metabolites interactions are also detected by proteome analysis for ascertaining the physiological meaning of proteins that show significant alterations during aging.

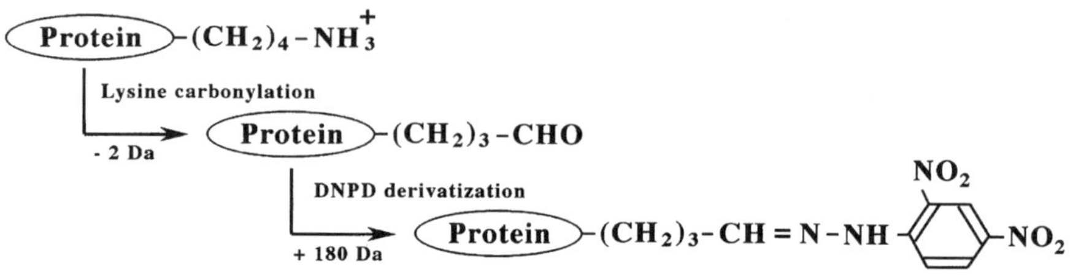

$$\text{Protein}-(CH_2)_4-NH_3^+$$

$$\underset{-2\,Da}{\xrightarrow{\text{Lysine carbonylation}}} \text{Protein}-(CH_2)_3-CHO$$

$$\underset{+180\,Da}{\xrightarrow{\text{DNPD derivatization}}} \text{Protein}-(CH_2)_3-CH=N-NH-\underset{NO_2}{\overset{NO_2}{\bigcirc}}$$

FIGURE 3. Theoretical mass shift in peptidyl lysine carbonylation and DNPH derivatization.

Bioinformatic Analysis

The deposition of sequence information for entire human genomes in databases will be a fruit of the human genome project. Besides, many DNA sequences are expected to be identified as cellular senescence-responsible genomes. However, there will remain many protein sequences for which no biological function has yet been assigned yet. On the other hand, much fragmentary information about protein structures and functions is independently deposited in separate databases on discrete web sites. Construction of an integrated database by linking home pages to each other with HTML tags or by redirecting on a clickable imagemap of proteome database is expected to offer a powerful tool to assign functions to proteins.

A query for protein identification with peptide mass fingerprint data may be successfully answered from a site if the complete sequence of the protein has already been reported to the database. If not, information on peptide sequence obtained by CID-MS/MS or microsequencing may be helpful for searching family proteins or homologous proteins for creating hypotheses about functions. Prediction of three dimensional structures by computer simulation may give us information about protein interactions and functions. Motif analysis is also useful to assign each domain of the protein to a specific group of functions.

CONCLUSION

Many useful databases for bioinformatics have been constructed in the internet. Some of two-dimensional gel protein databases, mass spectrometry databases, peptide sequence databases, DNA sequence databases, EST databases, 3-D structure databases, protein motif databases, and disease databases have already been linked to each other.[23] The new concepts of proteomics and bioinformatics are expected to promote further integration of these databases; and computerized technologies of proteomics and bioinformatics will surely open a new path to approach complex molecular mechanisms of cellular aging.

REFERENCES

1. WHEELAN, S. & W. MAKALOWSKI. 2000. Genome research: the second decade. A report on the XI Cold Spring Harbor Laboratory Meeting on Genome Mapping and Sequencing, May 13–17, 1998, Cold Spring Harbor, NY. Comput. Chem. **24:** 125–127.

2. ABBOTT, A. 1999. A post-genomic challenge: learning to read patterns of protein synthesis. Nature **402**(6763): 715–720.
3. GARNER, B., D.C. SHAW, R.A. LINDNER, et al. 2000. Non-oxidative modification of lens crystallins by kynurenine: a novel post-translational protein modification with possible relevance to ageing and cataract. Biochim. Biophys. Acta **1476**: 265–278.
4. ZHAO, W., P.S. DEVAMANOHARAN & S.D. VARMA. Fructose-mediated damage to lens alpha-crystallin: prevention by pyruvate. Biochim. Biophys. Acta **1500**: 161–168.
5. TODA, T., K. KAJI & N. KIMURA. 1998. TMIG-2DPAGE: a new concept of two-dimensional gel protein database for research on aging. Electrophoresis **19**: 344–348.
6. TODA, T., M. SATOH, M. SUGIMOTO, et al. 1999. A comparative analysis of the proteins between the fibroblasts from Werner's syndrome patients and age-matched normal individuals using two-dimensional gel electrophoresis. Mech. Ageing Dev. **100**:133–143.
7. GRAS, R., M. MULLER, E. GASTEIGER, et al. 1999. Improving protein identification from peptide mass fingerprinting through a parameterized multi-level scoring algorithm and an optimized peak detection. Electrophoresis **20**: 3535–3550.
8. GAY, S., P.A. BINZ, D.F. HOCHSTRASSER & R.D. APPEL. 1999. Modeling peptide mass fingerprinting data using the atomic composition of peptides. Electrophoresis **20**: 3527–3534.
9. HUA, Y. & R.B. COLE. 2000. Electrospray ionization tandem mass spectrometry for structural elucidation of protonated brevetoxins in red tide algae. Anal. Chem. **72**: 376–383.
10. LAPKO, V.N., X.Y. JIANG, D.L. SMITH & P.S. SONG. 1999. Mass spectrometric characterization of oat phytochrome A: isoforms and posttranslational modifications. Protein Sci. **8**: 1032–1044.
11. SINHA, P., G. HUTTER, E. KOTTGEN, et al. 1999. Increased expression of epidermal fatty acid binding protein, cofilin, and 14-3-3-sigma (stratifin) detected by two-dimensional gel electrophoresis, mass spectrometry and microsequencing of drug-resistant human adenocarcinoma of the pancreas. Electrophoresis **20**: 2952–2960.
12. GORG, A., C. OBERMAIER, G. BOGUTH & W. WEISS. 1999. Recent developments in two-dimensional gel electrophoresis with immobilized pH gradients: wide pH gradients up to pH 12, longer separation distances and simplified procedures. Electrophoresis **20**: 712–717.
13. GORG, A. & W. WEISS. 1999. Horizontal SDS-PAGE for IPG-Dalt. Methods Mol. Biol. **112**: 235–244.
14. GORG, A. & W. WEISS. 1999, Analytical IPG-Dalt. Methods Mol. Biol. **112**: 189–195.
15. APPEL, R.D., J.C. SANCHEZ, A. BAIROCH, et al. 1996. The SWISS-2DPAGE database of two-dimensional polyacrylamide gel electrophoresis, its status in 1995. Nucleic Acids. Res. **24**:180–181.
16. WILKINS, M.R., E. GASTEIGER, A.A. GOOLEY, et al. 1999. High-throughput mass spectrometric discovery of protein post-translational modifications. J. Mol. Biol. **289**: 645–657.
17. REQUENA, J.R. & E.R. STADTMAN. 1999. Conversion of lysine to N(epsilon)-(carboxymethyl)lysine increases susceptibility of proteins to metal-catalyzed oxidation. Biochem. Biophys . Res. Commun. **264**: 207–211.
18. JONSSON, A.P., M. CARLQUIST, B. HUSMAN, et al. 1999. Structural analysis of the thyroid hormone receptor ligand binding domain: studies using a quadrupole time-of-flight tandem mass spectrometer. Rapid Commun. Mass Spectrom. **13**: 1782–1791.
19. POCERNICH, C.B., M. LA FONTAINE & D.A. BUTTERFIELD. In-vivo glutathione elevation protects against hydroxyl free radical-induced protein oxidation in rat brain. Neurochem. Int. **36**: 185–191.
20. BUTTERFIELD, D.A., S.M. YATIN & C.D. LINK. 1999. In vitro and in vivo protein oxidation induced by Alzheimer's disease amyloid β-peptide (1–42). Ann. N.Y. Acad. Sci. **893**: 265–268.
21. WINTERBOURN, C.C., I H. BUSS, T.P. CHAN, et al. 2000. Protein carbonyl measurements show evidence of early oxidative stress in critically ill patients. Crit. Care Med. **28**: 143–149.

22. ODETTI, P., S. GARIBALDI, G. NOBERASCO, *et al.*1999. Levels of carbonyl groups in plasma proteins of type 2 diabetes mellitus subjects. Acta. Diabetol. **36:** 179–183.
23. MEWES, H.W., D. FRISHMAN, C. GRUBER, *et al.* 2000. MIPS: a database for genomes and protein sequences. Nucleic Acids Res. **1:** 37–40

Attenuation of EGF Signaling in Senescent Cells by Caveolin

WOONG-YANG PARK, KYUNG-A CHO, JEONG-SOO PARK, DEOK-IN KIM, AND SANG CHUL PARK

*Department of Biochemistry and Molecular Biology,
Seoul National University College of Medicine, Seoul, 110-799, Korea*

ABSTRACT: One of the characteristics of senescent cells is unresponsiveness to external stimuli like EGF. Although they have a normal level of receptors and downstream signaling molecules, EGF cannot induce the activation of Erk kinases and DNA synthesis in senescent cells as much as in young cells. Caveolin proteins directly interact with signaling molecules including EGF receptor and suppress the activation of EGFR upon EGF stimulation. We found that Erk activation after EGF stimulation in senescent human diploid fibroblasts was down-regulated. Those senescent cells showed an increased level of three isoforms of caveolin proteins. This change seems to lie in transcriptional control in senescent cells. We also demonstrated up-regulated caveolin proteins were co-localized with EGFR proteins in detergent-insoluble fractions. From these results, we suggest that the up-regulated expression of caveolin might explain the unresponsiveness of senescent fibroblasts to EGF stimulation.

KEYWORDS: EGF signaling; Caveolin; Erk kinases

INTRODUCTION

Age-related diseases might be due to the improper response to external stimuli,[1,2] which can be seen in *in vitro* human diploid fibroblasts (HDFs). Replicative senescence of HDF has long been used as an *in vitro* model for aging research. Hayflick first reported a phenomena as a replicative senescence in which primary cells do not grow indefinitely.[3] After a finite number of divisions, senescent cells do not grow or respond to growth factors like EGF. However, the mechanisms of signal-attenuation in senescent cells have never yet been fully explained. Senescent cells also showed an attenuated response to toxic stimuli.

EGF SIGNALING IN SENESCENT CELLS

Old rat hepatocytes or senescent human diploid fibroblasts showed an age-dependent decline in DNA synthesis and cell division upon growth-factor stimulation. Reenstra *et al.* reported EGFR phosphorylation and trafficking was affected in

---

Address for correspondence: Dr. Sang Chul Park at Department of Biochemistry, Seoul National University College of Medicine, 28 Yongon-dong, Chongno-gu, Seoul, 110-799, Korea. Voice: 82-2-740-8244; fax: 82-2-744-4534.
scpark@plaza.snu.ac.kr

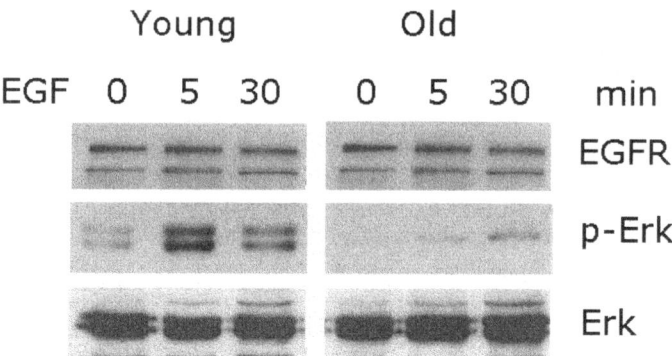

FIGURE 1. Attenuation of EGF signaling in old HDFs. Erk activation by EGF stimulation was attenuated in old human diploid fibroblasts. HDFs were starved of FBS for more than 24 hours and treated with EGF at 100ng/ml for the indicated time. Using young cells at PDL 20–30 and old cells at PDL 55–65, total cell lysates were analyzed by western blot using polyclonal anti-phospho-Erk antibody to detect the activation of Erk-1/2 kinases. Using polyclonal anti-Erk-1/2 and EGFR antibody, the amounts of each sample were normalized.

aged fibroblast.[4] They emphasized the interaction of EGFR and Shc in aged hepatocytes. Liu *et al.*[5] also showed that the overexpression of MKP-1 in old rat hepatocytes mediate the attenuated activation of Erk2. In old rat hepatocyte, basal level of MKP-1 was higher that young control rats although induction was lower in old hepatocyte. More recently the activities of Ras and MEK following EGF stimulation were demonstrated to be significantly lower in aged hepatocytes.[6]

Although we did not check the DNA synthesis directly, we used senescent fibroblasts which are not divide within 2 weeks and showed increased beta-galactosidase activity. We examined the Erk phosphorylation upon EGF stimulation in human diploid fibroblasts with aging (FIG. 1). As previous reports, we clearly demonstrate Erk activation was attenuated in HDFs to EGF stimulation. However, the level of signaling proteins like EGFR and Erk itself were not changed at all. Therefore, the reduced responsiveness of old cells may not be due to the altered protein turnover and post-translational modification. These results suggested that there would be a specific modulation mechanism for the signal attenuation and reduced proliferation of old cells upon EGF stimulation.

CAVEOLIN PROTEINS IN SENESCENT CELLS

General unresponsiveness of old cells to growth signals and even to apoptotic stimuli might require more wide and broad barrier at the level of signal entrance at the senescent cell membranes. Membrane peroxidation by repeated toxic insults through multiple passages in vitro or *in vivo* might modify the membrane rigid and finally might block the efficient firing of signal upon external stimuli. Membranes undergo marked alterations during aging. An age-related increase in free cholesterol is associated with a decrease in the phospholipid content.[7] Together with peroxidation and increased saturated:unsaturated fatty acid ratio, the plasma membranes of old cells decreased fluidity or increased structural order, which might lead to functional alterations. Increased level of cholesterol in the membrane of senescent cells can explain another cause for the membrane rigidity.

We have assumed that caveolin might be a possible culprit for the mechanism of the attenuation of EGF signaling in senescent cells. Caveolin is a major structural component of caveolae, which is a vesicular organelle and present mostly in fully differentiated cells like adipocyte and endothelial cells. In this structure, caveolin, an integral membrane protein, works as a scaffolding protein. Interaction of caveolin with various signaling molecules including heterotrimeric G-proteins, eNOS, c-Src and EGFR can suppress their enzymatic activity by holding these proteins in an inactive conformation.[8] In particular, the cytoplasmic membrane proximal region, residues 82–101, mediates the interaction with those signaling proteins.[9] The amino acid residues between 889–979 of EGFR binds to caveolin-1 *in vitro* and the peptides containing these residues of EGFR and caveolin modified the autophosphorylation activity of EGFR. Interestingly, Palmer *et al.* showed that Shc binding to EGFR was suppressed in old rat hepatocytes,[10] suggesting the age-related attenuation of EGF signaling cascade. The overexpression of caveolin can be the cause of the inhibition of EGF signaling in old HDF cells. The direct interaction between EGFR and caveolin-1 in senescent fibroblasts may result in functional inhibition of EGFR.[11,12]

In our experiment we found that the expression level of caveolin-1 was increased in aging HDF (FIG. 2). The up-regulation of caveolin-1 protein was regulated at the transcription level. We also examine whether the EGFR from old HDF could be co-localized to caveolae fractions as described previously (FIG. 3). The overexpression of caveolin-1 in caveolae-deficient cells can form structurally competent caveolae. We found that senescent cells had an increased number of caveolae structures in

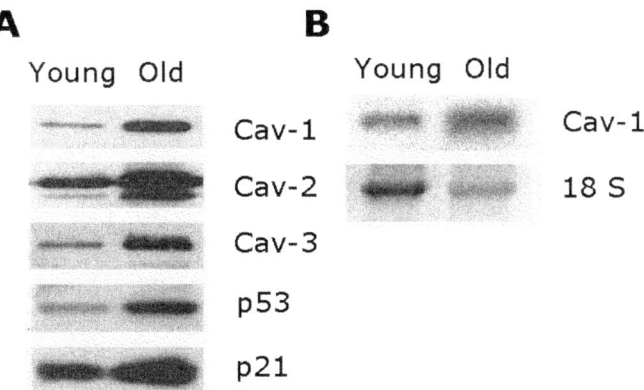

FIGURE 2. Overexpression of caveolin-1 in old HDF. (A) Total cell lysates from young, middle and old-passage HDFs or IMR-90 cells were analyzed by western blot with anti-caveolin antibodies. Along with other proteins like p53 and p21, all of three isoforms of caveolin was increased in western blot analysis. (B) Total RNAs from each HDFs were also analyzed by northern blot and mRNA for caveolin-1 was increased in old HDFs.

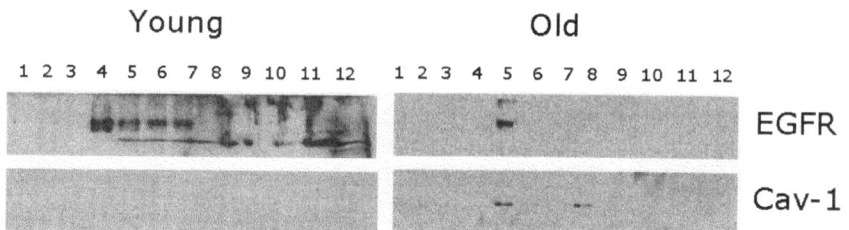

FIGURE 3. Co-localization of caveolin-1 and EGFR in caveolae fractions. Young and old fibroblasts were fractionated by sucrose-density gradient to isolate caveolae fractions. Each fraction was separated by SDS-PAGE and probed with anti-caveolin-1 and anti-EGFR antibodies in western blot.

electron microscopic analysis. Moreover, caveolin-1 in senescent cells can directly interact with EGFR as reported previously in NIH3T3 cells.

Caveolin-2, a homologue of caveolin-1,[13] is expressed ubiquitously in most cell types, supposedly forming a hetero-oligomer in basolaterally localized caveolae. Although the overexpression of caveolin-2 itself was not sufficient to form functional caveolae structures,[14] we found that the expression of caveolin-2 in senescent HDF was also increased with aging. The role of caveolin-2 is not well defined, but we suggest that caveolin-2 might potentiate caveolae formation in aged cells or might regulate the signaling in a different way.

Although the expression of caveolin-3 is restricted to striated muscle cells,[15] heterologous expression of caveolin-3 in old human fibroblasts was detected in senescent HDF (FIG. 2). We also found the overexpression of caveolin proteins in old rat tissues including brain and spleen, in which caveolin is not present normally.[11]

THE ROLE OF CAVEOLIN IN SENESCENT CELLS

Caveolin-1 expression correlates inversely with the level of oncogenic transformation in NIH3T3 cells, indicating the strong relation of caveolin in caveolae with regulation of normal cell proliferation. Moreover, caveolin-1 re-expression inhibits tumor growth in culture.[9] Caveolin levels in skeletal muscle increased in aged rats compared to young rats.[16] Furthermore, the up-regulation of caveolin with aging or high fat feeding might be associated with the insulin resistance.

Caveolin-1 and -2 show the ubiquitous expression while caveolin-3 distributes only in striated muscles. Although the function of caveolin-2 is not properly defined so far, concerted role of caveolin hetero-oligomer might explain the role in old tissues or fibroblasts. Moreover overexpression of caveolin-2 was consistent in every tissues we examined. The expression pattern of caveolin proteins in various tissues from old rat would suggest a possible meaning in age-related diseases. Recently the role of caveolin in different physiological and pathological phenomena has been proposed.

THE REGULATION OF CAVEOLIN EXPRESSION IN SENESCENT CELLS

There are three different regulation mechanism for caveolin transcription; p53-dependent regulation, CpG methylation in the upstream region of caveolin genes, and through the sterol-response element in the promoter region. The increased level of caveolin required the presence of p53 in cell cycle-dependent regulation.[17] However, in EJ-p53 cells, the overexpression of p53 for 7 days did not induced the up-regulation of caveolin proteins.[11] Although caveolin-2 was slight increased, caveolin-1 and –3 was not detected at all. Because genes encoding human caveolin-1 and -2 are localized to the fragile site (FRA7G) that is frequently deleted in human cancers,[18] there might be deletion or other types of mutation along the caveolin genes in EJ-p53 cells

Discrete elements for promoters of caveolin genes are not yet fully determined. Methylation of a CpG island in the promoter region of the caveolin-1 gene in human breast cancer cell lines was reported by Engelman *et al.*[19] Alteration of methylation and chromatin structures with aging might induce the expression of caveolin proteins. Gradual changes of chromatin structures seem to be rather important for caveolin expression. It is possible that cholesterol might trigger the induction of caveolin proteins, which aid the trafficking of cholesterol to plasma membranes. If this is so, then, caveolin expression and accompanied caveolae formation may be secondary phenomena. Nevertheless resulting caveolae regulate the signaling through membrane, which confers old cells resistance to external stimuli.

According to the genetic hypothesis on aging, gerontogenes might regulate actively the aging process. For example, fused young and senescent fibroblasts were unable to divide actively like young cells.[20] This result suggests that senescence appears to be a dominant process,[21] supporting the genetic hypothesis of aging. Cellular senescence is a kind of phenotype like differentiation or apoptosis. Expression of gerontogene or other age-related genes might actively drive some types of cells into senescence. A certain population of cells in aged organisms should redistribute their functional populations for overall activity. During the development, a process like apoptosis will select unwanted cells. After the full development, we propose that the selection mechanisms might be working through apoptosis and senescence as well. If not, aged cells will function improperly and finally accumulate the errors into cancers. In this case, concerted overexpression of caveolin in some types of old cells will help the selection procedures.

ACKNOWLEDGMENTS

This work was supported by the Seoul National University Research Fund (to W.-Y. Park), and by Ministry of Health and Welfare, Korea (HMP-98-MS-001 to W.-Y. Park) and by KOSEF (1999-2-208-001-5 to S.-C. Park).

REFERENCES

1. SESHADRI, T. & J. CAMPISI. 1990. Science **247**: 205–209.
2. RIABOWOL, K., J. SCHIFF & M.Z. GILMAN. 1992. Proc. Natl. Acad. Sci. USA **89**: 157–161.

3. HAYFLICK, L. & P.S. MOOREHEAD. 1961. Exp. Cell Res. **25:** 585–621.
4. REENSTRA, W.R., M. YAAR & B.A. GILCHREST. 1996. Exp. Cell Res. **227:** 252–255.
5. LIU, Y., M. GOROSPE, C. YANG & N.J. HOLBROOK. 1995. J. Biol. Chem. **270:** 8377–8380.
6. HUTTER, D., Y. YO, W. CHEN, et al. 2000. J. Gerontol. **55:** B125–134.
7. WANG, J. & K. WALSH. 1996. Science **273:** 359–361.
8. OKAMOTO, T., A. SCHLEGEL, P.E. SCHERER & M.P. LISANTI. 1998. J. Biol. Chem. **273:** 5419–5422.
9. GALBIATI, F., D. VOLONTE, J.A. ENGELMAN, et al. 1998. EMBO J. **17:** 6633–6648.
10. PALMER, H.J., C.T. TUZON & K.E. PAULSON. 1999. J. Biol. Chem. **274:** 11424–11430.
11. PARK, W.Y., J.S. PARK, K.A. CHO, et al. 2000. J. Biol. Chem. **275:** 20847–20852.
12. COUET, J., M. SARGIACOMO & M.P. LISANTI. 1997. J. Biol. Chem. **272:** 30429–30438.
13. SCHERER, P.E., T. OKAMOTO, M. CHUN, et al. 1996. Proc. Natl. Acad. Sci. USA **93:** 131–135.
14. LI, S., F. GALBIATI, D. VOLONTE, et al. 1998. FEBS Lett. **434:** 127–134.
15. TANG, Z., P.E. SCHERER, T. OKAMOTO, et al. 1996. J. Biol. Chem. **271:** 2255–2261.
16. MUNOZ, P., S. MORA, L. SEVILLA, et al. 1996. J. Biol. Chem. **271:** 8133–8139.
17. LEE, S.W., C.L. REIMER, P. OH, et al. 1998. Oncogene **16:** 1391–1397.
18. ENGELMAN, J.A., C. CHU, A. LIN, et al. 1998. FEBS Lett. **428:** 205–211.
19. ENGELMAN, J.A., A.H. BERG, R.Y. LEWIS, et al. 1999. J. Biol. Chem. **274:** 35630–35638.
20. LI, S., K.S. SONG & M.P. LISANTI. 1996. J. Biol. Chem. **271:** 568–573.
21. FIELDING, C.J., A. BIST & P.E. FIELDING. 1997. Proc. Natl. Acad. Sci. USA **94:** 3753–3758.

BRCA1 Gene Sequence Variation in Centenarians

JAN VIJG,[a,b] THOMAS PERLS,[c] CLAUDIO FRANCESCHI,[d] AND NATHALIE J. VAN ORSOUW[b]

[a]*University of Texas Health Science Center, San Antonio, Texas 78245, USA*

[b]*Cancer Therapy and Research Center, San Antonio, Texas 78229, USA*

[c]*Gerontology Division, Beth Israel Deaconess Medical Center, Boston, Massachusetts 02215, USA*

[d]*Department of Gerontological Research, Italian National Research Center on Aging (INRCA), Ancona, Italy*

ABSTRACT: With the ample gene sequence information that has become available with the human genome project virtually completed, it has become possible to identify functional gene variants and their frequencies in elderly populations with different aging-related characteristics. Such a genetic epidemiological approach could lead to new insights with respect to the basic mechanisms of aging and longevity as well as the identification of new targets to prevent or retard some of the late-age adverse effects. Using our recently developed two-dimensional gene scanning (TDGS) technology platform we demonstrate the feasibility of this approach by screening two different populations of centenarians for polymorphic variation in the *BRCA1* breast cancer susceptibility gene, one of the many genes involved in genome maintenance. The initial results obtained with this approach suggest differences in *BRCA1* genotype frequencies between the centenarian populations and controls.

KEYWORDS: 2-D gene scanning; *BRCA1*; Centenarians; Allelic variants; Genome instability

The success of the human genome project combined with new technologies of genetic analysis have greatly facilitated the identification of genes with inherited mutations that predispose to various age-related disorders, including specific cancers. Such genes are often involved in genome stability pathways, to maintain DNA integrity. Examples are the DNA mismatch repair genes, *MLH1* and *MSH2*, heritable mutations in which predispose to colon cancer,[1] and the breast cancer susceptibility genes *BRCA1* and *BRCA2*.[2,3] It is assumed that increased genomic instability and mutation accumulation is causally related to the increased risk of cancer observed in individuals with heritable defects in these genes.

Address for correspondence: Dr. Jan Vijg, University of Texas Health Science Center, Texas Research Park, South Texas Centers for Biology in Medicine, 15355 Lambda Drive, San Antonio, TX 78245. Voice: 210-562-5027; fax: 210-562-5028.

vijg@uthscsa.edu

In a more general sense, genomic instability in organs and tissues has been considered as a major cause of aging. In this respect, increased mutation accumulation could lead to tissue atrophy and neoplasms, as well as increased loss of cellular function.[4–6] This process could be driven by oxygen free radicals and other sources of spontaneous DNA damage, although unambiguous evidence for such a causal relationship is still lacking.[7,8] Oxidative stress is known to induce genome rearrangement mutations, such as large deletions, inversions or translocations.[9,10] These types of mutation have been demonstrated to accumulate during aging in various tissues of normal mice.[11] In this respect, it has been speculated that, in addition to causing cell death and cell transformation, a relatively small number of such large mutations could destabilize the genome, leading to dysregulation of normal patterns of gene expression.[6]

Ultimately, the quality of genome stability systems determines the rate and spectrum of mutation accumulation during aging. In this respect, evidence is accumulating that defects in those systems that control the frequency of large DNA rearrangement mutations are associated with symptoms of accelerated senescence, in both mice and humans. This is the case for mice with defects in double-strand break repair genes, which can be expected to greatly accelerate the rate of illegitimate recombinations. Recent evidence indicates that mice with inactivated genes involved in non-homologous end joining, i.e., *Ku86*, prematurely exhibit symptoms of age-related degeneration in various tissues, including liver, skin and bone.[12] Disruption of the mouse *Ercc1* gene, which is involved in both nucleotide excision repair and a mitotic recombination pathway, also shows symptoms of accelerated senescence, including premature replicative senescence of Ercc1-mutant cells.[13] Premature replicative senescence, which could be an important marker for *in vivo* aging,[14] has also been observed for murine cells deficient for other genes involved in recombinational repair and non-homologous end joining, including *Atm*, *Brca2*, *Ku70* and DNA ligase IV.[12] Cellular proliferation defects have also been observed in murine *Brca1* mutant cells and a mammary-specific conditional *Brca1* knock-out mouse model revealed genetic instability and tumorigenesis in combination with growth inhibition *in vivo*.[15]

The possible role of genomic instability in aging is further exemplified by recent work investigating telomere maintenance in the preservation of tissue functioning during aging. In a study of third generation telomerase-deficient mice, shortened life span was found to be accompanied by reduced capacity to respond to stresses such as wound healing, hematopoietic ablation and by an increased incidence of spontaneous malignancies.[16] The results of these studies underscore that in proliferative organs the early initiation of genetic instability due to telomere erosion can greatly accelerate age-related loss of cell viability and increase tumor formation.

An important body of evidence that large genomic mutations are causally related to the degenerative aspects of the aging process has been derived from human syndromes of accelerated aging, such as Werner syndrome. Werner syndrome, which is caused by a heritable mutation in a human homologue of the bacterial *RecQ* gene, termed *WRN* in humans,[17] is characterized by the accelerated occurrence of certain aspects of the senescent phenotype, including cancer.[18] The *WRN* gene encodes both a helicase and an exonuclease[19] and is thought to play a role in suppressing genomic instability.[20] Indeed, cultured somatic cells from patients with Werner syndrome dis-

TABLE 1. Genome stability pathways that control large rearrangements and aging

Genome stability pathway	Genes	Null mice	Symptoms of accelerated senescence		Human syndrome
			In vitro	In vivo	
DSB-repair	KU70, KU86, DNA-PKcs SIR2/3/4	Ku70, Ku86 PKcs, SCID	Yes	Yes	
	RAD51		Yes	Yes	
	BRCA1/2	Brca1/2			Hereditary breast cancer
			Yes	Yes	
	ERCC1	Ercc1			
Recombination suppression	RECQ1-5	Wrn, Blm			Werner, Bloom, Rothmund Thomson
Telomere maintenance	mTR, hTERT TERF1/2 TNKS TIN2	mTR	Yes	Yes	
Cell cycle check-point activity	ATM TP53	Atm Tp53	Yes		Ataxia telangiectasia Li-Fraumeni

play an increased rate of somatic mutations and a variety of cytogenetic abnormalities, such as deletions and translocations.[21] This high level of genomic instability could be the cause of the severe limitation of *in vitro* life span demonstrated in Werner cells.[18] Also other so-called progeroid syndromes, such as ataxia telangiectasia and Bloom syndrome show increased genomic instability.[18]

TABLE 1 summarizes the pathways and some of the genes thus far identified that are involved in the suppression of large genomic mutations. As discussed above, defects in many of these genes have been found associated with accelerated senescence, but not always and not to the same extent. This is expected, since even if aging would be totally based on genomic instability it would be highly unlikely that complete inactivation of any gene in any of these pathways would closely mimic the normal aging process. Instead, one would expect combinations of subtle allelic variants of these genes to determine the aging phenotype. It is possible to test this by creating mouse models with a variety of knock-in variants of the relevant genome stability genes. However, an alternative and reasonable approach would be to compare frequencies of the various alleles of loci involved in genome maintenance and repair and more specifically the pathways listed in TABLE 1 in different human populations with characteristic aging-related phenotypes. Such phenotypes could include extremely short or extremely long life, extreme susceptibility or extreme resistance to organ-specific age-related loss of function and extreme susceptibility or extreme resistance to age-related disease. One would expect that at least some of those allelic variants that give rise to amino acid changes, has functional consequences in terms of the level of proficiency at which genome maintenance operates. At present, it is

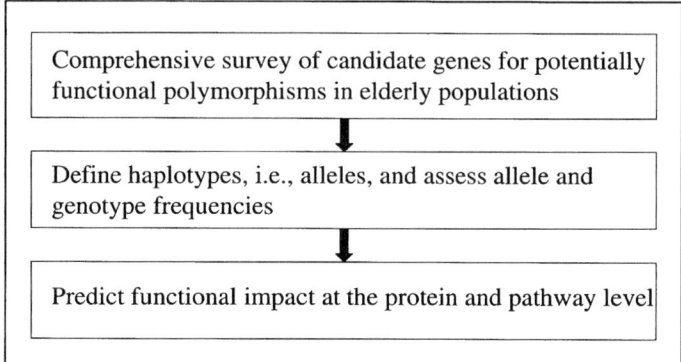

FIGURE 1. Flow chart of the sequential steps in gene-based asssociation studies.

not possible to accurately predict functionality directly from variations in the gene coding sequences. However, statistically significant variations among populations with well-defined aging-related characteristics could provide a good starting point for subsequent functional studies. This approach is schematically depicted in FIGURE 1.

Thus far, association studies have been based on single polymorphisms in candidate genes. The best known example in this respect is the observed lower frequency of the *APOE4* variant in centenarians,[22] a higher frequency of which had previously been found associated with sporadic Alzheimer's disease.[23] However, any positive result could be due to an effect of the polymorphism on the function of the candidate gene or it could be due to some other gene variant that is in linkage disequilibrium with the marker locus. It has recently been shown that the distances over which linkage disequilibrium acts are small, i.e., typically less than 3 kb,[24] although these data have recently been challenged.[25] Nevertheless, unless all polymorphic variation in a large number of candidate genes is detected, this type of studies is unlikely to yield significant results in most cases.

With the rapid emergence of complete sequence information for all human genes it is theoretically possible to scrutinize all genes or families of genes suspected to be involved in a complex phenotype for all possible polymorphic variation in a group of subjects as compared to a control group. Individual differences in complex phenotypes, of which familial aggregation or twin studies suggest a genetic component, could be due to common variants of genes controlling one or more functional pathways thought to play a role in the phenotype. In a recent study, Cargill *et al.*[26] systematically surveyed the coding regions of 106 genes relevant to cardiovascular disease, endocrinology and neuropsychiatry for all possible variants in a sample of mixed ethnic groups. For this purpose, they used a combination of oligonucleotide chip array hybridization and DHPLC (HPLC of DNA fragments in a temperature gradient). In these 106 genes a total of 560 single nucleotide polymorphisms were discovered.

To identify potentially functional SNPs involved in blood pressure homeostasis and hypertension Halushka *et al.*[27] used the same technology to assay 75 candidate genes in a sample of 74 ethnically heterogeneous individuals with a range of hypertension phenotype diversity. A total of 387 SNPs were detected in gene coding sequences, 54% of which were predicted to lead to altered protein.

Thus, it is possible to find an informative set of common gene-based SNPs with direct functional relevance to a complex phenotype. There are two potential limitations to this approach. The first involves the relatively small number of genes that have been completely identified in terms of structure and function. Although virtually all human genes are now available as ESTs, only a limited number has been defined by a complete cDNA sequence and functional pathway. Indeed, for only very few genes a complete genomic sequence including 3′UTR, promoter and intronic flanking regions is readily available. With the genome program drawing to a close the next few years it is reasonable to expect that most of these gaps will be filled fairly soon and that complete sequence information and pathway assignments will become available.

A second potential limitation to screen directly for functional polymorphic variants involved in a complex trait involves the technology to screen multiple genes in large numbers of individuals for all possible sequence variation, which is still in its infancy. Most technology in this respect is limited by the need to PCR amplify each individual target sequence for mutational scanning. Moreover, the most advanced methods, such as the DNA chip method used in the two studies described above, involve relatively expensive technology that has not been completely validated (a significant number of variants are missed). A cost-effective method developed in our laboratory is based on extensive multiplex PCR to obtain the target fragments, which are subsequently analyzed on two-dimensional denaturing gradient gels for all possible sequence variants.[28,29]

TWO-DIMENSIONAL GENE SCANNING

The most reliable way of detecting DNA sequence alterations in genes is nucleotide sequencing, the gold standard in mutation detection. Sequencing is PCR-based with preparation of template on an exon-by-exon basis. This is expensive and labor-intensive, even in the semi-automated setting. Other mutation scanning techniques, e.g., single strand conformation polymorphism analysis, trade off accuracy for relative throughput. Many novel methods with the potential of both a high throughput and a high accuracy remain immature and unproven in practice. Moreover, virtually all methods rely on PCR amplification to obtain the target sequences.[30]

A most accurate method for detecting DNA sequence variants is denaturing gradient gel electrophoresis (DGGE). DGGE allows for the separation of DNA fragments differing by as little as one base pair, on the basis of differences in their melting temperature.[31] A given DNA fragment comprises one or more domains, each representing a stretch of between about 50 and 500 base pairs with equal melting temperature (the temperature at which each base pair has a 50% probability of being in either the helical or the denatured state). Therefore, when a double-stranded DNA fragment migrates, parallel to the gradient of denaturants (urea/formamide or temperature), the lowest melting domain will denature first and, because of branching of the DNA strands, the fragment will be retarded in the gel. The melting temperature of a domain is dependent on the base composition of the fragment (G-C base pairs have a higher melting temperature than A-T base pairs) and the stacking interactions of the bases. Therefore, DNA sequence variations will be reflected by the positions in the gel where the fragments are halted.

The sensitivity of DGGE in detecting mutations can be increased dramatically by introducing so-called GC-clamps, i.e., a stretch of 30 to 50 G and C bases, to the target DNA fragments.[32] A convenient way of attaching a GC-clamp to the target fragment is by making it part of one of the primers.[33] Without GC-clamping, a DNA fragment consisting of one melting domain will become completely single stranded upon denaturation and runs off the gel. By adding a GC-clamp, a single high melting domain is artificially created at one end of the target fragment. This will prevent complete melting and ensures that the fragment halts at the melting temperature of the target sequence. However, when the target DNA fragment consists of multiple melting domains, only mutations in the lowest melting domain are readily detected. To facilitate detection of all possible mutations, it is imperative that the target fragment represents only one melting domain. Fortunately, since the addition of a GC-clamp allows for stacking interactions with neighboring bases, the entire target fragment will often behave as one melting domain. However, this is not always the case, and in practice, the target fragment needs to be "designed", e.g., through the strategic positioning of PCR primers to achieve the ideal single melting domain.

The sensitivity of DGGE for detecting variants is further enhanced by the introduction of a heteroduplexing step using one round of denaturation/renaturation, usually at the end of PCR amplification of the target fragment. In this manner, a heterozygous mutation is revealed as four different double-stranded fragments: two homoduplex molecules (one homoduplex wild type and one homoduplex mutant) and two heteroduplex molecules (each comprising one wild type and one mutant strand). The less stable mismatched heteroduplex molecules will melt earlier than the two homoduplex molecules.

Although DGGE has the crucial advantage of having close to 100% sensitivity in detecting mutations,[34,35] it has typically been applied in a serial fashion, e.g., on an exon by exon basis, for analyzing large genes. With the introduction of two-dimensional gene scanning (TDGS) we have transformed the method from the existing serial to a parallel system. The first step in TDGS is a large-scale multiplex PCR. Initial pre-amplification of multiple exons by long-distance PCR has been demonstrated to provide suitable template for a highly specific multiplex PCR. Indeed, the over-representation of the exon-containing genomic fragments, relative to the genomic environment, permits multiplex groups of as many as 24 fragments.[36]

A successful implementation of extensive multiplex PCR amplification in DGGE-based gene mutational scanning tests requires a high-resolution separation system. An example of such a system is the original two-dimensional DGGE format[31] in which fragments are first separated according to size and, subsequently, further sorted as a function of their melting temperature. Although high resolution may also be obtained by using one-dimensional denaturing gradient gels, the 2-D system allows characterization of each fragment on the basis of its xy-coordinates (size and melting temperature). In practice, by using the 2-D system, it is possible to completely visualize all fragments corresponding to an entire gene or multiple genes for a particular DNA sample and immediately recognize each exon and variants therein (schematically depicted for the *BRCA1* gene in FIG. 2). Different sequence

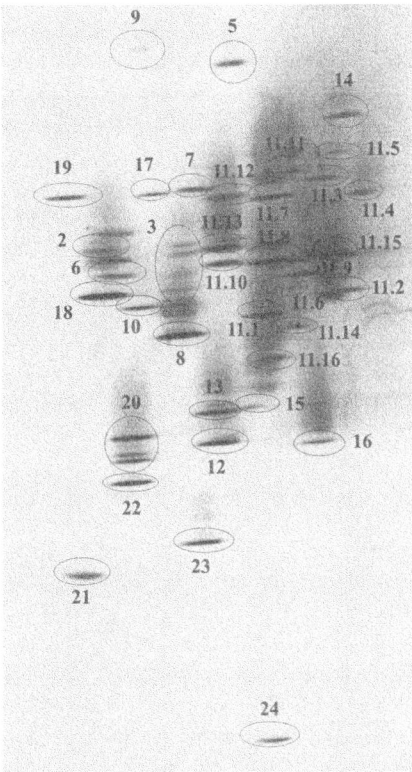

FIGURE 2. Empirical two-dimensional gene scanning pattern of the gene *BRCA1*. All coding exons were amplified from genomic DNA obtained from blood of a normal individual. The sample was found to contain polymorphisms in exons 3 and 20. (Modified after van Orsouw *et al.*[29])

variants in the same exon can be distinguished on the basis of their unique 4-spot patterns.[29] A potential hindrance to the widespread application of this system to multiple, novel genes involves the difficulties in the design of PCR primers generating single-domain fragments which can be resolved under one set of electrophoretic conditions. In order to minimize the time needed to optimize TDGS tests with respect to PCR conditions, melting behavior and distribution of fragments in the 2-D gel, a computerized test design has been developed.[37]

An automated system for 2-D DNA electrophoresis has been developed.[38] This system has a modest throughput of only 4 2-D gels per day. However, with one technician who can easily operate up to three of these systems a total of 140,000 bp of genomic DNA can be comprehensively analyzed per day for all possible sequence variants. The system is presently modified to increase the throughput per instrument to about 500,000 bp per day.

To test the general applicability and usefulness of TDGS in generating complete spectra of sequence variation in large genes or in multiple genes, we screened centenarian and control populations, on a pilot scale, for functional variants of *BRCA1*.

TABLE 2. Polymorphisms defining haplotypes[a]

Type	Exon 11						Exon16
	1186	2196	2731	3232	3238	3667	4956
a	A	G	C	A	G	A	A
b	A	G	T	G	G	G	G
c	A	A	T	G	G	G	G
d	A	G	T	A	G	A	A
e	A	G	C	A	A	A	A
f	G	G	C	A	G	A	A

[a]Out of 256 possible haplotypes.

COMMON *BRCA1* GENE VARIANTS AND SUSCEPTIBILITY TO BREAST CANCER IN CENTENARIANS

BRCA1 is the first human familial breast cancer susceptibility gene cloned.[2] As mentioned above and summarized in TABLE 1, *BRCA1* is a tumor suppressor gene likely to be involved in DNA recombinational repair.[39] A large number of distinct heritable mutations in *BRCA1* have been described, most of which result in a truncated *BRCA1* protein.[40] Heritable mutations in *BRCA1* confer an over 90% life time risk of breast cancer. In view of the large size of the gene (24 exons, comprising 5592 bp of coding DNA) large-scale gene sequence comparisons in population-based studies have not been performed. However, the data available suggest that the frequency of highly penetrant *BRCA1* mutations in the normal population is between 1 in 500 and 1 in 2000 individuals.[41] The lack of cost-efficient re-sequencing technology has also constrained population studies on common polymorphisms in *BRCA1*, which could confer more modest individual risk. In principle, such common variants could explain a far larger part of breast cancer cases.

As mentioned above, one of the benefits of parallel screening by TDGS is that each pattern reveals all homo- and heterozygous variants in the entire gene. The effect of association studies on functional gene variants will now be much more valuable than the study of single polymorphisms in candidate genes, as has been done so far. So far, a total of 7 polymorphic sites in 6 TDGS fragments in *BRCA1* have been identified that give rise to an amino acid change. Owing to strong linkage disequilibrium, these 7 polymorphic sites generate only 6 different haplotypes, i.e., alleles (A–F; TABLE 2). The frequencies of these alleles were compared between groups of centenarians and controls. Centenarians were selected for this study because breast cancer is extremely rare in such individuals of highly advanced age. Hence, it is possible that optimal sequence variants of this gene contribute to this extreme resistancy, possibly as a consequence of its increased proficiency in the process of recombinational repair. Two different centenarian populations were studied, i.e., one population consisted of 102 centenarians from the New England area[42] and one population consisted of 84 centenarians from Italy.[43] The control population consisted of 97 individuals from Italy. All three populations were mainly white.

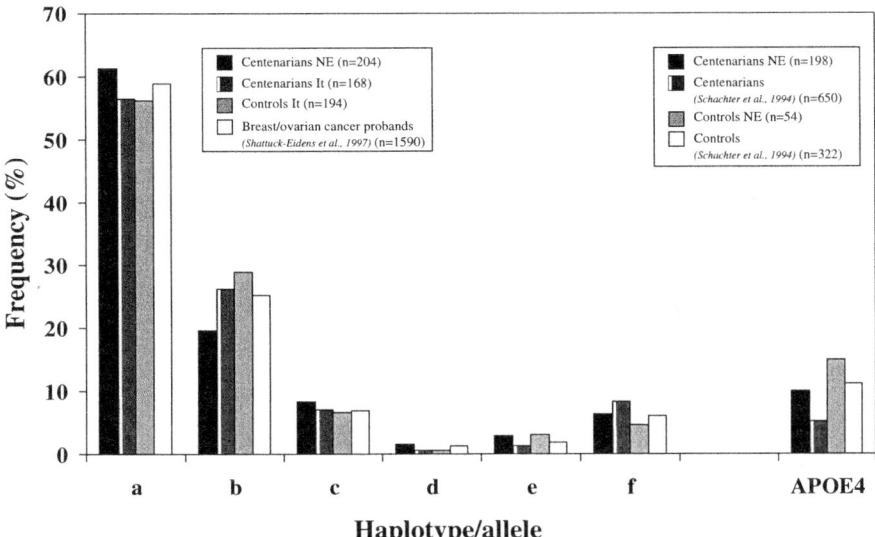

FIGURE 3. *BRCA1* allele frequencies in two different centenarian populations and one control population (NE = New England; IT = Italy). The allele frequency of *APOE4* has been determined in the same populations as a control and was compared with the results of Schächter *et al.*[22]

Results so far obtained indicate that there are no significant differences in *BRCA1* allele (haplotype) frequencies among the three populations (FIG. 3). This also applied to the *APOE4* variant that was included as a positive control. However, in keeping with earlier studies the frequency of the *APOE4* variant was lower in the centenarians as compared to controls (FIG. 3). Comparison to previously published results obtained from 795 breast- and/or ovarian cancer probands sampled from the US and Europe[40] confirmed that at the allele frequency level only minor differences are observed.

Although allele frequencies might give an early indication of possible association of the population-specific effect of the different haplotypes and disease, actual association should be carried out using the frequencies of allele combinations (i.e., genotype frequencies). As shown in FIGURE 4, the *BRCA1* genotype a+a showed to be more frequent in both centenarian groups compared to the control group ($p = 0.1473$), whereas genotype "a+b" was less frequent ($p = 0.0526$). In this case, the A4+A4 *APOE* genotype was not found for any of the 99 New England centenarians and scored 2 times for the 27 control individuals in which this was analyzed (FIG. 4).

The high number of genotypes and the low frequency of some of the alleles require the analysis of large numbers of samples. Only when the sample repository is sufficiently high, reliable conclusions can be drawn regarding the frequencies of all genotypes including some of the rare ones. In this respect, especially haplotype "f" is of interest because of the presence of Arg356 instead of Gln356. There is evidence

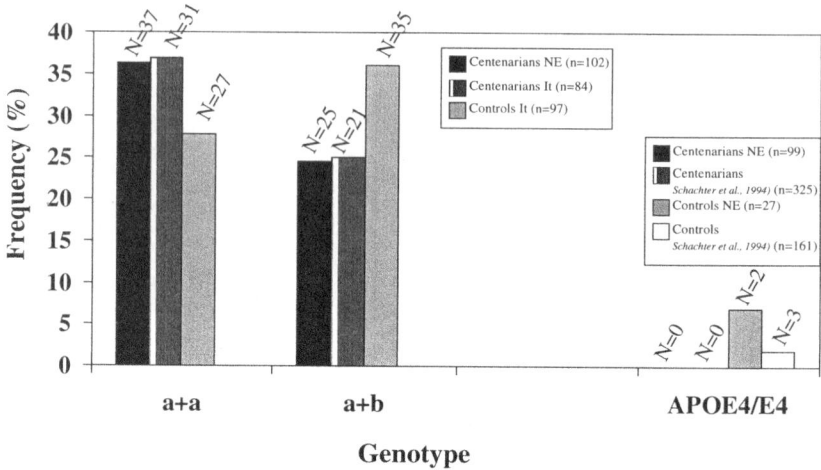

FIGURE 4. Genotype frequency of two of the most frequent *BRCA1* allele combinations in the two centenarian populations and the control population. The *APOE4/E4* frequency has been included as control and compared with Schächter et al.[22] as in FIGURE 3.

that Arg356 homozygosity is less frequent in breast cancer patients than in controls[44] indicating that it may be protective against breast cancer. Although in our present study the frequency of allele f with the Arg356 present was found to be slightly higher in centenarians, the number of individuals analyzed is still too low to draw any definite conclusions.

SUMMARY

One way to test possible causal relationships between various functional pathways and the aging process is to comparatively analyze polymorphic variation in genes participating in these pathways in elderly populations with different aging-related characteristics. The results of the Human Genome Project now make it feasible to identify most if not all genes involved in the candidate pathways that drive the aging process or confer longevity. For this purpose, efficient genotyping methods are needed that allow the comprehensive sequence analysis of multiple genes at the population level. Using our recently developed two-dimensional gene scanning (TDGS) technology platform we demonstrated the feasibility of this approach by screening two different populations of centenarians for polymorphic variation in the *BRCA1* breast cancer susceptibility gene. The results indicate that using this technology relatively large numbers of individuals, i.e., hundreds, can be screened in a relatively short time for all possible sequence variants of this very large gene. Although the number of individuals analyzed is still insufficient to draw definite conclusions, a clear trend towards a difference in genotype frequency involving two of the most common alleles became apparent. Based on these results we conclude that rather than studying individual polymorphisms in groups of elderly with different aging-related characteristics, it should be feasible to analyze multiple genes participating in functional pathways that are possibly involved in aging and longevity for differences in the frequency of potentially functional alleles.

REFERENCES

1. FISHEL, R., M.K. LESCOE, M.R.S. RAO, et al. 1993. The human mutator gene homolog MSH2 and its association with hereditary nonpolyposis colon cancer. Cell **75:** 1027–1038.
2. MIKI, Y., J. SWENSEN, D. SHATTUCK-EIDENS, et al 1994. A strong candidate for the breast and ovarian cancer susceptibility gene BRCA1. Science **266:** 66–71.
3. WOOSTER, R., G. BIGNELL, J. LANCASTER, et al. 1995. Identification of the breast cancer susceptibility BRCA2. Nature **378:** 789–792.
4. FAILLA, G. 1958. The aging process and carcinogenesis. Ann. N.Y. Acad. Sci. **71:** 1124–1135.
5. SZILARD, L. 1959. On the nature of the aging process. Proc. Natl. Acad. Sci. USA **45:** 35–45.
6. VIJG, J. 2000. Somatic mutations and aging: a re-evaluation. Mutation Res. **447:** 117–135.
7. MARTIN, G.M., S.N. AUSTAD & T.E. JOHNSON. 1996. Genetic analysis of ageing: role of oxidative age and environmental stresses. Nature Genet. **13:** 25–34.
8. COLLINS, A.R. 1999. Oxidative DNA damage, antioxidants, and cancer. BioEssays **21:** 238–246.
9. HSIE, A.W., L. RECIO, D.S. KATZ, et al. 1986. Evidence for reactive oxygen species including mutations in mammalian cells. Proc. Natl. Acad. Sci. USA **83:** 9616–9620.
10. GILLE, J.J.P., C.G.M. VAN BERKEL & H. JOENJE. 1994. Mutagenicity of metabolic oxygen radicals in mammalian cell cultures. Carcinogenesis **15:** 2695–2699.
11. DOLLÉ, M.E.T., H. GIESE, C.L. HOPKINS, et al. 1997. Rapid accumulation of genome rearrangements in liver but not in brain of old mice. Nature Genet. **17:** 431–434.
12. VOGEL, H., D.S. LIM, G. KARSENTY, et al. 1999. Deletion of Ku86 causes early onset of senescence in mice. Proc. Natl. Acad. Sci. USA **96:** 10770–10775.
13. WEEDA, G., I. DONKER, J. DE WIT, et al. 1997. Disruption of mouse ERCC1 results in a novel repair syndrome with growth failure, nuclear abnormalities and senescence. Curr. Biol. **7:** 427–439.
14. CAMPISI, J. 1996. Replicative senescence: an old lives' tale? Cell **84:** 497-500.
15. XU, X., K.-U. WAGNER, D. LARSON, et al. 1999. Conditional mutation of Brca1 in mammary epithelial cells results in blunted ductal morphogenesis and tumour formation. Nature Genet. **22:** 37–43.
16. RUDOLPH, K.L., S. CHANG, H.W. LEE, et al. 1999. Longevity, stress response, and cancer in aging telomerase-deficient mice. Cell **96:** 701–712.
17. YU, C-E., J. OSHIMA, Y.-H. FU, et al. 1996. Positional cloning of the Werner's syndrome gene. Science **272:** 258–262.
18. TURKER, M.S. & G.M. MARTIN. 1999. Genetics of human disease, longevity and aging. In Principles of Geriatric Medicine and Gerontology, 4th edit. W.R. Hazzard, J.P. Blass, W.H. Ettinger, Jr., et al., Eds.: 21–44. McGraw-Hill Book Co.
19. HUANG S., B. LI, M.D. GRAY, et al. 1998. The premature ageing syndrome protein, WRN, is a 3'→5' exonuclease. Nature Genet. **20:** 114–116.
20. YAMAGATA, K., J. KATO, A. SHIMAMOTO, et al. 1998. Bloom's and Werner's syndrome genes suppress hyperrecombination in yeast sgs1 mutant: implication for genomic instability in human diseases. Proc. Natl. Acad. Sci. USA **95:** 8733–8738.
21. FUKUCHI, K., G.M. MARTIN & R.J. MONNAT, JR. 1989. Mutator phenotype of Werner syndrome is characterized by extensive deletions. Proc. Natl. Acad. Sci. USA **86:** 5893–5897.
22. SCHÄCHTER, F., L. FAURE-DELANEF, F. GUÉNOT, et al. 1994. Genetic associations with human longevity at the APOE and ACE loci. Nature Genet. **6:** 29–32.

23. CORDER, E.H., A.M. SAUNDERS, W.J. STRITTMATTER, et al. 1993. Gene dose of apolipoprotein E type 4 allele and the risk of Alzheimer's disease in late onset families. Science **261:** 921–923.
24. KRUGLYAK, L. 1999. Prospects for whole-genome linkage disequilibrium mapping of common disease genes. Nature Genet **22:** 139–144
25. COLLINS, A., C. LONJOU & N.E. MORTON. 1999. Genetic epidemiology of single-nucleotide polymorphisms. Proc. Natl. Acad. Sci. USA **96:** 15173–15177.
26. CARGILL, M., D. ALTSHULER, J. IRELAND, et al. 1999. Characterization of single-nucleotide polymorphisms in coding regions of human genes. Nature Genet. **22:** 231–238.
27. HALUSHKA, M.K., J.-B. FAN, K. BENTLEY, et al. 1999. Patterns of single-nucleotide polymorphisms in candidate genes for blood-pressure homeostasis. Nature Genet. **22:** 239–247.
28. VAN ORSOUW, N.J., D. LI, P. VAN DER VLIES, et al. 1996. Mutational scanning of large genes by extensive PCR multiplexing and two-dimensional electrophoresis: application to the RB1 gene. Hum. Mol. Genet. **5:** 755–761.
29. VAN ORSOUW, N.J., R.K. DHANDA, Y. ELHAJI, et al. 1999. A highly accurate, low cost test for BRCA1 mutations. J. Med. Genet. **36:** 747–753.
30. ENG, C. & J. VIJG. 1997. Genetic testing: the problems and the promise. Nature Biotechnol. **15:** 422–426.
31. FISCHER, S.G. & L.S. LERMAN. 1979. Length-independent separation of DNA restriction fragments in two-dimensional electrophoresis. Cell **16:** 191–200.
32. MYERS, R.M., S.G. FISCHER, L.S. LERMAN & T. MANIATIS. 1985. Nearly all single base substitutions in DNA fragments joined to a GC-clamp can be detected by denaturing gradient gel electrophoresis. Nucleic Acids Res. **13:** 3131–3145.
33. SHEFFIELD, V.C., D.R. COX, L.S. LERMAN & R.M. MYERS. 1989. Attachment of a 40-base-pair G + C-rich sequence (GC-clamp) to genomic DNA fragments by the polymerase chain reaction results in improved detection of single-base changes. Proc. Natl. Acad. Sci. USA **86:** 232–236.
34. GULDBERG, P., K.F. HENRIKSEN & F. GUTTLER. 1993. Molecular analysis of phenyketonuria in Denmark: 99% of the mutations detected by denaturing gradient gel electrophoresis. Genomics **17:** 141–146.
35. MOYRET, C., C. THEILLET, P.L. PUIG, et al. 1994. Relative efficiency of denaturing gradient gel electrophoresis and single strand conformation polymorphism in the detction of mutations in exons 5 to 8 of the p53 gene. Oncogene **9:** 1739–1743.
36. LI, D. & J. VIJG. 1996. Multiplex co-amplification of 24 retinoblastoma gene exons after pre-amplification by long-distance PCR. Nucleic Acids Res. **24:** 538–539.
37. VAN ORSOUW, N.J., R.K. DHANDA, R.D. RINES, et al. 1998. Rapid design of denaturing gradient-based two-dimensional electrophoretic gene mutational scanning tests. Nucleic Acids Res. **26:** 2398–2406.
38. DHANDA, R.K., W. SMITH, C.B. SCOTT, et al. 1998. A simple system for automated two-dimensional electrophoresis: applications to genetic testing. Genet. Testing **2:** 67–70.
39. VENKITARAMAN, A.R. 1999. Breast cancer genes and DNA repair. Science **286:** 1100–1102.
40. SHATTUCK-EIDENS, D., A. OLIPHANT, M. MCCLURE, et al. 1997. BRCA1 sequence analysis in women at high risk for susceptibility mutations. Risk factor analysis and implications for genetic testing. JAMA **278:** 1242–1250.
41. FORD, D., D.F. EASTON & J. PETO. 1995. Estimates of the gene frequency of BRCA1 and its contribution to breast and ovarian cancer incidence. Am. J. Hum. Genet. **57:** 1457–1462.
42. PERLS, T.T., K. BOCHEN, M. FREEMAN, et al. 1999. Validity of reported age and prevalence of centenarians in a New England sample. Age Ageing **28:** 193–197.
43. DE BENEDICTIS, G., E. FALCONE, G. ROSE, et al. 1997. DNA multiallelic systems reveal gene/longevity associations not detected by diallelic systems. The APOB locus. Human Genet. **99:** 312–318.
44. DUNNING, A.M., M. CHIANO, N.R. SMITH, et al. 1997. Common BRCA1 variants and susceptibility to breast and ovarian cancer in the general population. Hum. Mol. Genet. **6:** 285–289.

Increases of Mitochondrial Mass and Mitochondrial Genome in Association with Enhanced Oxidative Stress in Human Cells Harboring 4,977 BP-Deleted Mitochondrial DNA

YAU-HUEI WEI, CHENG-FENG LEE, HSIN-CHEN LEE, YI-SHING MA, CHIA-WEN WANG, CHING-YOU LU, AND CHENG-YOONG PANG

Department of Biochemistry and Center for Cellular and Molecular Biology, National Yang-Ming University, Taipei 112, Taiwan

ABSTRACT: In order to investigate the effect of aging- and disease-associated deletion of mtDNA on cellular functions, we used cytoplasm fusion to construct a series of the cybrids harboring varying proportions of mtDNA with 4,977 bp deletion from skin fibroblasts of a patient with chronic progressive external ophthalmoplegia. The cybrids were grown in the Dulbecco's modified Eagle medium supplemented with 5% fetal bovine serum, 100 μg/ml pyruvate and 50 μg/ml uridine. The population doubling time was longer for the cybrids containing higher proportions of 4,977 bp-deleted mtDNA. In addition, we found that the respiratory function was decreased with the increase of mtDNA with 4,977 bp deletion in the cybrids. Since impairment of the respiratory system of mitochondria increases the electron leak of the respiratory chain, we further determined the oxidative stress in these cybrids. The results showed that the specific contents of 8-hydroxy 2'-deoxyguanosine and lipid peroxides of the cybrids harboring > 65% of the 4,977 bp-deleted mtDNA were significantly increased as compared with those of the cybrids containing undetectable mutant mtDNA. On the other hand, we found that the mitochondrial mass and the relative content of the mitochondrial genome in the cybrids harboring 4,977 bp-deleted mtDNA were higher than those of the cybrids containing only wild type mtDNA. The relative content of mtDNA was increased 17% and 30%, respectively, in the cybrids harboring 17% and 56% of mtDNA with 4,977 bp deletion. Moreover, both mitochondrial mass and mtDNA content were concurrently increased by treatment of the cybrids with 180 μM of hydrogen peroxide. Taken these findings together, we conclude that increase of mitochondrial mass and mtDNA are the molecular events associated with enhanced oxidative stress in human cells with impaired respiratory function caused by mtDNA deletion.

KEYWORDS: Oxidative stress; mitochondrial DNA; copy number; mitochondrial mass

Address for correspondence: Professor Yau-Huei Wei, Department of Biochemistry, School of Life Science, National Yang-Ming University, Taipei 112, Taiwan. Voice: 886-2-28267118; fax: 886-2-28264843.

joeman@mailsrv.ym.edu.tw

INTRODUCTION

It has been established that a number of neuromuscular diseases are associated with or caused by mitochondrial DNA (mtDNA) mutations.[1–7] Among them, large-scale deletions are frequently seen in the affected tissues of the patients with mitochondrial myopathies such as chronic progressive external ophthalmoplegia (CPEO) and Kearns-Sayre syndrome.[1,6–8] Abundant evidence have been accumulated to suggest that mtDNA deletions affect the expression of genes in the mitochondrial genome,[9–12] which in turn elicit defects in the respiratory chain. It has been established that impairment of electron transport chain increases the production of the reactive oxygen species (ROS) and free radicals in the mitochondria.[13–15] Thus, the tissues or cultured cells containing mutant mtDNA(s) may be exposed to higher oxidative stress due to defects of the electron transport system. Moreover, some of the patients with mitochondrial diseases have been reported to exhibit premature aging[16] and their clinical symptoms are frequently worsened with time.[17–19] This age-dependent progression of the disease is, in some way, similar to the natural course of some neurodegenerative diseases.[20,21] Recently, we found that oxidative stress and oxidative damage of mitochondria are enhanced in the tissues of old humans that contained mtDNA mutations.[22–24] In the past few years, increase of reactive oxygen species (ROS) and oxidative stress has been shown to stimulate the expression of early growth-related genes such as c-fos and c-jun.[25] Hydrogen peroxide (H_2O_2) has been reported to play a role in the communication between mitochondria and the nucleus in mammalian cells.[26,27] These observations have led us to hypothesize that mitochondrial genome and mitochondrial mass are subject to change in response to enhanced oxidative stress in human cells harboring mtDNA deletions. To test this hypothesis, we used the cytoplasmic transfer technique[28,29] to construct a series of the cybrids harboring different proportions mtDNA with 4,977 bp deletion by fusing enucleated fibroblasts from a CPEO patient with a mtDNA-less human osteosarcoma cell line (termed ρ^0 cells). We then examined the electron transport activities and growth kinetics of the cybrids that harbor different proportions of the mutant mtDNA. The intracellular contents of 8-hydroxy 2′-deoxyguanosine (8-OHdG) and lipid peroxides of the cybrids were determined to assess the oxidative stress of the cybrids. On the other hand, we determined by flow cytometry the mitochondrial mass and measured by slot blot hybridization the relative content of mtDNA in the cybrids treated with and without H_2O_2. The results showed that the cybrids harboring 4,977 bp-deleted mtDNA had higher amounts of mitochondrial genome and mitochondrial mass, which were further increased by oxidative stress elicited by the treatment with sublethal concentrations of H_2O_2.

MATERIALS AND METHODS

Cell Culture

Primary cultures of skin fibroblasts were established from the skin biopsy of a patient with CPEO syndrome and were maintained in the Dulbecco's modified Eagle Medium (DMEM) supplemented with 5% fetal bovine serum (FBS), 100 µg/ml pyruvate and 50 µg/ml uridine.[30] A mtDNA-less human cell line (ρ^0 cells) was established by long-term treatment of the osteosarcoma 143B TK⁻ cells with 50 ng/ml ethidium bromide.[28] A series of the cybrids were then constructed by fusion of the ρ^0 cells with the skin fibroblasts of a CPEO patient, which had been enucleated by treatment with 10 μg/ml of cytochalasin B according to the condition described by King and Attardi.[29] The cybrids were selected in a medium containing 100 μg/ml of 5-bromo 2′-deoxyuridine and were grown in DMEM supplemented with 5% FBS, 100 μg/ml pyruvate and 50 μg/ml uridine and incubated at 37°C in humidfied 5% CO_2/95% air. For oxidative stress treatment, the cybrids were added with H_2O_2 at a final concentration of 180 μM and were then cultured at different periods of time.

Quantification of mtDNA Deletion

Total cellular DNA was prepared from each of the cybrids by the method developed in this laboratory.[31] The proportions of mtDNA with 4,977 bp deletion in the cybrids were quantified by Southern hybridization. An aliquot of 5 μg total DNA of each of the cybrids was linearized by digestion with *Bam*HI (Boehringer Mannheim Co., Mannheim, Germany), and the digested DNA was electrophoresed at 50 V for 17.5 h in a 0.8% agarose gel. DNA bands in the gel were denatured and transferred onto an Hybond N⁺ nylon membrane (Amersham Inc., Buckinghamshire, England), and hybridized with an α-[³²P]dCTP-labeled human D-loop mtDNA probe (spanning np 16455-1462 of the L-strand) at 65°C for 2 h in a rapid hybridization buffer. The filter was first washed with 2x SSC and 0.1% SDS for 20 min at 37°C, and then successively washed with 1x SSC and 0.1% SDS for 15 min at 45°C, 0.5x SSC and 0.1% SDS for 15 min at 50°C, and 0.1x SSC and 0.1% SDS for 15 min at 65°C. The washed filter was wrapped with a Saran Wrap and subjected to autoradiography.

Determination of the Relative Content of mtDNA

The relative content of the cybrid was determined by slot blot using the α-[³²P]dCTP-labeled human D-loop mtDNA encompassing np 16455-1462 of the L-strand as the probe. About 1 μg DNA was denatured in 0.4 N NaOH and 10 mM EDTA at 100°C for 10 min and then transferred onto a piece of Hybond-N⁺ nylon membrane. Hybridization and washing were done essentially according to the conditions described above except that a probe for the 28S rRNA gene was also included to determine the amount of nuclear DNA in each sample. The intensities of the DNA bands representing the mitochondrial genome and nuclear DNA (28S rRNA gene) on the blot were measured on a Phosphorimager.

Cell Viability Assay

Usually, an aliquot of 1×10^4 cybrid cells were seeded on a 12-well culture plate and were grown at 37°C for 36 h to confluency. The cells were washed with the assay medium and then treated with 180 μM of H_2O_2. After treatment for different periods of time, the culture medium was aspirated and stored at 4°C. The remaining cells in the well were disintegrated with a lysis buffer (81.3 mM Tris-HCl, pH 7.2, 203.3 mM NaCl, and 0.5% Triton X-100) at room temperature for 20 min. The activities of lactate dehydrogenase (LDH) in the culture medium and cell lysate were then determined spectrophotometrically by monitoring the decrease of the absorbance of

NADH at 340 nm.[32] The viability of the cells was calculated as the ratio between the LDH activity of the cell lysate and total LDH activity.

Determination of Mitochondrial Mass

The fluorescent dye 10-n-nonyl-acridine orange (NAO; Molecular Probes, Eugene, OR), which binds specifically to cardiolipin at the inner mitochondrial membrane independently of membrane potential ($\Delta\Psi_m$), was used to monitor the mitochondrial mass.[33] Cells were trypsinized and resuspended in 0.5 ml of PBS containing 10 μM of NAO or MitoTracker Green FM (Molecular Probes), which is preferentially accumulated in mitochondria regardless of mitochondrial membrane potential.[34] After incubation for 10 min at 25°C in the dark, cells were immediately transferred to a tube on ice for flow cytometric analysis.

Flow Cytometric Analysis

A FACScan flow cytometer (Becton Dickinson, Bedford, MA) equipped with a 488-nm argon laser system was used for the flow cytometric analysis.[34] Forward and side scatters were used to establish size gates and exclude cellular debris from the analysis. The excitation wavelength was set at 488 nm and the observation wavelength of 530 nm was chosen for green fluorescence and 585 nm for red fluorescence, and the intensities of emitted fluorescence were collected on FL1 and FL2 channels, respectively. In each measurement, a total of 20,000 cells were analyzed. Data were collected and analyzed using the Cell Quest software (Becton Dickinson). Relative change in the mean fluorescence intensity was calculated as the ratio between mean fluorescence intensity in the channel of the treated cells and that of the control cells.

Assay of the Respiratory Functions of the Cybrids

The cybrids were washed twice with 0.25 M sucrose containing 20 mM HEPES (pH 7.2), and 10 mM $MgCl_2$ and pelletted by centrifugation at $500 \times g$ for 5 min at 4°C before use. The pellet of packed cells was then suspended in a small volume of the same medium and stored on ice. Oxygen consumption rate was measured with a Clark electrode in a water-jacketed chamber (Gilson Medical Electronics, Inc., Middleton, WI). The assay medium consisted of air-saturated 0.25 M sucrose, 20 mM HEPES (pH 7.2), 5 mM potassium phosphate, 10 mM $MgCl_2$, and 500 nmol ADP (respiration medium). An aliquot of 50–100 μl of the cell suspension was added to 1.5 ml of the respiration medium and oxygen consumption rates were measured with glutamate-malate, succinate, and tetramethylphenylenediamine (TMPD)-ascorbate, respectively, as the respiratory substrate.[35] The data are expressed in nanogram-atoms of oxygen per minute per 10^7 cells based on the results of three measurements.

Determination of Lipid Peroxides by HPLC

The content of lipid peroxides in the cybrid was measured as malondialdehyde (MDA) according to the method described by Wong *et al.*[36] About 2.0×10^6 cybrid cells were homogenized in 0.5 ml of 0.44 M phosphoric acid plus 0.05 ml of 0.2% butylated hydroxytoluene (BHT) on ice. The homogenate was transferred to a 1.5 ml

Eppendorf vial, to which was added 0.17 ml of 42 mM thiobarbituric acid (TBA) solution, and the final volume was adjusted to 1.2 ml with distilled water. The vial was capped and boiled at 95°C for 1 h and then immediately cooled in icewater bath. An aliquot of 0.25 ml of each boiled sample was pipetted into a new vial and was then neutralized with 0.25 ml of 1 N NaOH in methanol. The neutralized solution was centrifuged at $9,500 \times g$ for 5 min to remove the denatured proteins. An aliquot of 25 µl of the supernatant was injected into a C_{18} column (5-µm particle, 4.6×200 mm, Waters Associates). Before injection of the samples, the column was pre-equilibrated in stepwise manner by 80%, 50%, and 40% (v/v) methanol each for 30 min and then eluted with a mobile phase consisting of methanol and 50 mM potassium phosphate buffer (pH 6.8; 4:6, v/v). The flow rate of the mobile phase was 1.0 ml/min, and the fluorescence of the effluent was monitored for 10 min with a fluorescence detector (excitation wavelength, 525 nm; emission wavelength, 550 nm). The area under the fluorescence peak of the MDA-$(TBA)_2$ adduct was determined by an integrator and the lipid peroxide content of each sample was calculated from a calibration curve constructed by using 1,1,3,3-tetraethoxypropane as standard.

Assay of 8-OHdG Content in the Cybrids

The specific content of 8-OHdG was determined by the method of Shigenaga *et al.*[37] Usually, 5×10^5 cells were trypsinized from a 100 mm culture dish and were suspended in ice cold phosphate-buffered saline (PBS) containing 0.1 mM deferoxamine mesylate (DFAM). After centrifugation, cell pellet was lysed in 1.5 ml of the TE buffer (10 mM Tris-HCl, 1 mM EDTA, pH 8.0) containing 2 mM BHT in ethanol, 100 µg/ml RNase A, and 0.5% SDS. The lysate was incubated at 37°C for 1 h. Proteinase K was added to a final concentration of 100 µg/ml and the lysate was incubated at 56°C overnight. After addition of NaCl to the final concentration of 150 mM, the lysate was extracted each with an equal volume of phenol, phenol/chloroform/isoamyl alcohol (25:24:1) and chloroform/isoamyl alcohol (24:1), respectively. The total DNA was precipitated by adding 1/10 volume of 3 M sodium acetate (pH 5.0) and 2.5 volumes of ice cold 95% ethanol. The precipitated DNA was centrifuged at $10,000 \times g$ for 15 min at 4°C and the DNA pellet was washed with 70% ethanol (v/v), and dried by flushing with a stream of argon. An aliquot of 25 µg DNA was dissolved in 200 µl of 20 mM sodium acetate/1 mM DFAM. The DNA was denatured at 98°C for 10 min and then chilled on ice immediately. To the solution was added 25 µl (20 units) of DNase I (Boehringer Mannheim Co., Mannheim, Germany) and 25 µl of $MgCl_2$ (final concentration 10 mM) and incubated at 37°C for 30 min with gentle shaking. About 38 µl of 0.25 M sodium acetate (pH 5.4), 3 µl of 0.1 M $ZnSO_4$, and 9 µl (2 units) of nuclease P1 were sequentially added and mixed thoroughly, and incubated at 37°C for 1 h. The resulting mixture was adjusted to pH 8.0 by adding 20 µl of 1 M Tris-HCl buffer (pH 8.5) and hydrolyzed to the corresponding nucleosides on incubation with 6 units of calf intestine alkaline phosphatase (Boehringer Mannheim Co., Mannheim, Germany) for 30 min at 37°C. After digestion, the mixture was extracted with 5 ml of acetone and the nucleosides in the acetone layer were vacuum dried and dissolved in 100 µl of 10 mM Tris-HCl (pH 7.4). The nucleoside solution was filtered through an 0.22-µm filter paper (Millipore, Bedford, MA) and stored at −20°C waiting for HPLC analysis. The amount of 8-OHdG in the total DNA was measured by a reverse-phase C_{18} column (4.6 ×

250 mm, Waters Associates, Milford, MA) on an HP 1050 LC system (Hewlett Packard, Palo Alto, CA) according to the conditions described by Lee et al.[38] The amount of deoxyguanosine (dG) was calculated from the peak area of dG recorded through an UV monitor. The amount of 8-OHdG in the sample is expressed in percentile relative to the amount of total dG.

Protein Determination

The cell lysate was suspended in 0.1 N NaOH and 1% deoxycholate and kept for the determination of protein concentration by a modified Lowry method.[39]

RESULTS

Genotyping of the Cybrids

After construction and subcloning of the cybrids, we determined the relative proportion of mtDNA with 4,977 bp deletion in each of the cybrids by Southern hybrid

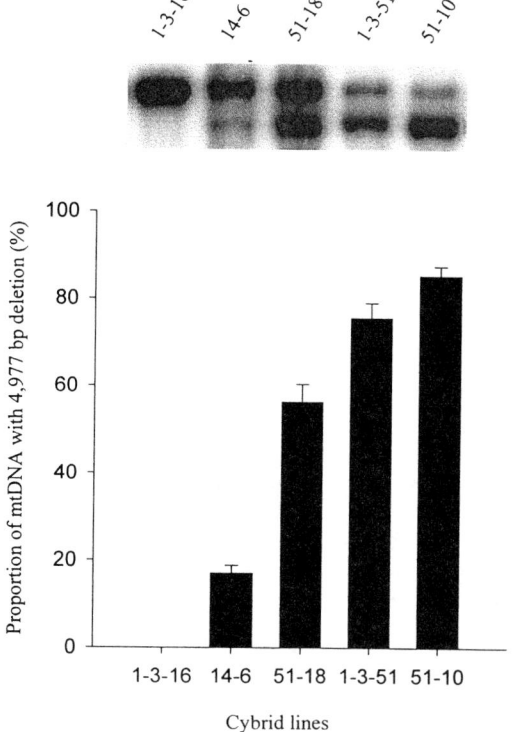

FIGURE 1. Quantification of the proportions of 4,977 bp-deleted mtDNA in the cybrids by using Southern blot analysis. About 5 μg of total DNA of each of the cybrids was hybridized with α-[^{32}P]dCTP-labeled human mtDNA probe (D-loop region), and then quantified by a Phosphorimager as detailed in MATERIALS AND METHODS.

TABLE 1. Summary of the genotype and stress response of the cybrids harboring different proportions of 4,977 bp-deleted mtDNA

	Cybrids				
Feature	1-3-16	14-6	51-18	1-3-51	51-10
Proportion of 4,977 bp-deleted mtDNA (%)	Undetectable	17.1±1.7	56.3±4.1	75.6±3.5	85.4±2.2
Relative amount of mtDNA copy number (%)	100.0	117.3±6.9	129.9±12.5	98.8±11.1	89.7±14.2
Viability (%)					
$-H_2O_2$	92.7±0.4	88.0±0.7	84.5±0.6	80.4±0.5	75.3±1.9
$+H_2O_2$ (180 μM)	72.3±1.3	69.1±1.3	67.3±0.5	61.1±0.4	49.1±0.5
Doubling time (h)					
$-H_2O_2$	15.6±0.9	16.7±0.4	17.1±2.1	19.5±0.2	20.8±0.8
$+H_2O_2$ (180 μM)	19.9±0.7	21.6±0.9	22.9±0.0	30.7±4.1	32.3±4.1
Relative amount of mitochondrial mass (%)					
$-H_2O_2$	NA	100.0±7.9	129.2±10.1	143.9±5.9	205.2±7.8
$+H_2O_2$ (180 μM)	NA	182.8±19.2	226.8±15.7	252.2±3.0	283.3±13.5

NA: Not available.

ization using a probe of D-loop region of human mtDNA. FIGURE 1 shows the proportions of 4,977 bp-deleted mtDNA in the five stable cybrid clones used in this study. One of the clones (designated as 1-3-16) was found to contain undetectable 4,977 bp-deleted mtDNA, which was used as the control cybrid.

Growth Kinetics of the Cybrids Harboring Mutant mtDNAs

The cybrids containing the 4,977 bp-deleted mtDNA were found to grow more slowly than the cybrid harboring only wild-type mtDNA in the presence or absence of H_2O_2. The growth of the cybrid was retarded by the 4,977 bp-deleted mtDNA in a dose-dependent manner (FIG. 2A). The growth of each of the cybrid was further retarded by the treatment with 180 μM of H_2O_2 (FIG. 2B). The population doubling time was 19.5 h for the cybrids containing 75% mtDNA with 4,977 bp deletion, and that was 15.6 h for the control cybrid when grown in the DMEM supplemented with 5% FBS, 100 μg/ml pyruvate, and 50 μg/ml uridine (TABLE 1).

Defective Respiratory Functions of the Cybrids Harboring Mutant mtDNA

The respiratory function of the cybrids harboring 4,977 bp-deleted mtDNA was found to decrease with the increase of the mutant mtDNA. The oxygen consumption rate of the cybrids containing > 65% of 4,977 bp-deleted mtDNA were significantly lower than that of the control cybrids and parental 143B cells (FIG. 3).

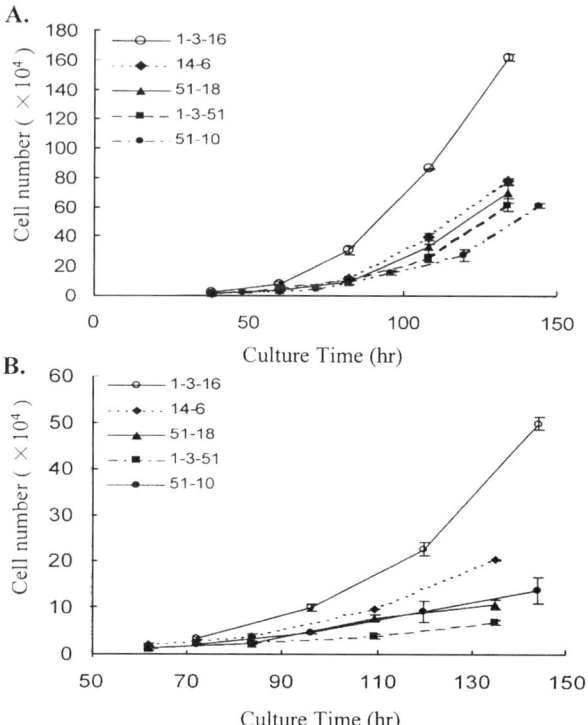

FIGURE 2. Growth kinetics of the cybrids harboring different proportions of 4,977 bp-deleted mtDNA. The five cybrid clones were cultured in the 5% FBS-supplemented DMEM (with 100 μg/ml pyruvate and 50 μg/ml uridine) in the absence (**A**) and presence (**B**) of 180 μM H_2O_2, which was added 36 h after seeding of the cells. The cell number was counted for each of the cybrids at the indicated periods of time.

Oxidative Damage in the Cybrids Harboring 4,977 bp-Deleted mtDNA

As indicated by the level of MDA in the cell lysate, the content of lipid peroxides of the cybrid was elevated in a dose-dependent manner with the proportion of the 4,977 bp-deleted mtDNA. FIGURE 4 shows that the average specific MDA content of the cybrid with deleted mtDNA was higher than that of the cybrid with undetectable mutant mtDNA. Moreover, we observed that the content of 8-OHdG in the cybrid was increased with the increase of the proportion of mtDNA with 4,977 bp deletion (FIG. 5).

Relative Content of mtDNA in the Cybrids Harboring 4,977 bp-Deleted mtDNA

The relative content of mtDNA was found to increase significantly in the cybrids containing <60% of 4,977 bp-deleted mtDNA (TABLE 1). However, as the proportion of the 4,977 bp-deleted mtDNA reached >70%, the relative content of mtDNA was found to be slightly decreased.

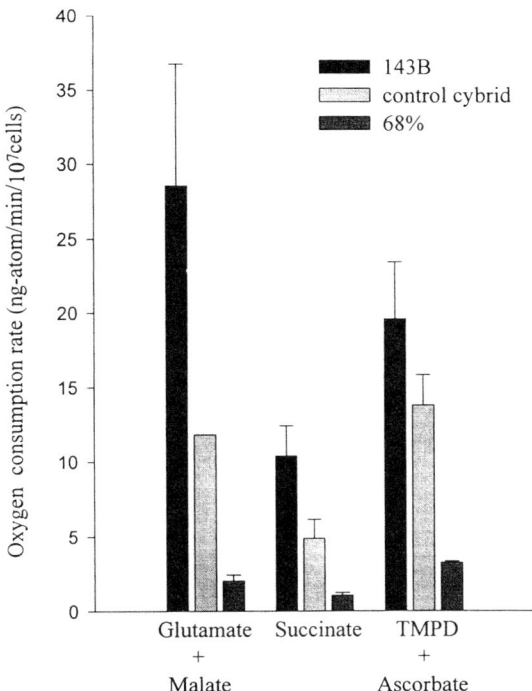

FIGURE 3. Effect of the 4,977 bp deletion of mtDNA on the oxygen consumption rate of the cybrid. The proportion of the 4,977 bp-deleted mtDNA in the cybrid was determined by Southern hybridzation as described in MATERIALS AND METHODS. The respiration rates of the cybrids supported by 5 mM glutamate and 5 mM malate, 5 mM succinate, and 0.2 mM TMPD + 1 mM ascorbate were determined, respectively, in a Gilson 5/6 Oxygraph.

Mitochondrial Mass of the Cybrids Harboring 4,977 bp-Deleted mtDNA

By NAO staining of the mitochondrial membrane, we observed that the mitochondrial mass of the cybrid was increased with the proportion of 4,977 bp-deleted mtDNA (FIG. 6 and TABLE 1).

Response of the Cybrids to Oxidative Stress Treatment

After treatment with 180 μM of H_2O_2 for 48 h, the cell viability was decreased to about 80% for all the cybrids (TABLE 1). In an attempt to determine whether H_2O_2 induces a change of the mitochondrial mass of the cell, we measured the fluorescence intensity of the cybrid after staining with NAO. The results showed that the NAO fluorescence intensities of the treated cybrids were significantly increased (from ca. 40% to 80%) as compared to that of the untreated cybrid (FIG. 7). We observed similar increase in the relative intensity of another fluorescent dye MitoTracker Green FM (data not shown). These results indicate that the oxidative stress induced by H_2O_2 can lead to a further increase of mitochondrial mass in the cybrids harboring 4,977 bp-deleted mtDNA.

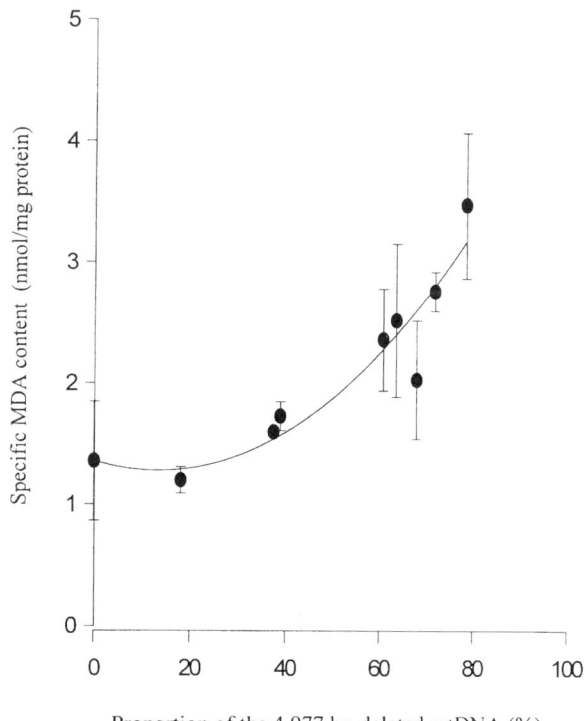

FIGURE 4. Specific MDA contents of the cybrids harboring different proportions of the 4,977 bp-deleted mtDNA. Total lipid peroxides were extracted and specific MDA content of the cybrid was determined by an HPLC system as described in MATERIALS AND METHODS. Each data point represents the mean ± S.D. of the results obtained from 4 determinations.

DISCUSSION

Large-scale deletions of mtDNA have been reported to be associated with about 60% of the patients with the KSS and CPEO syndromes.[8,19] However, it has remained unclear as to how these mtDNA mutations are involved in the pathogenesis of mitochondrial myopathies and encephalomyopathies. It was demonstrated that mtDNA deletions can be caused or driven by defects in nuclear DNA.[40] In order to eliminate possible contributions of the nuclear genotype on the deleterious effect of a mtDNA mutation, the cybrids have been established to provide a system to study the consequence of the mtDNA mutation.[28,29] In addition, the cybrids derived from the same patient that contained varying amounts of a mtDNA mutation can be used to study the quantitative relationship between mtDNA genotype and cell phenotype.[30] The proportion of the mutant mtDNA in each of the cybrids is dictated by the mtDNA genotype of the fibroblast with which the ρ^o cell is fused. Thus, one can usu-

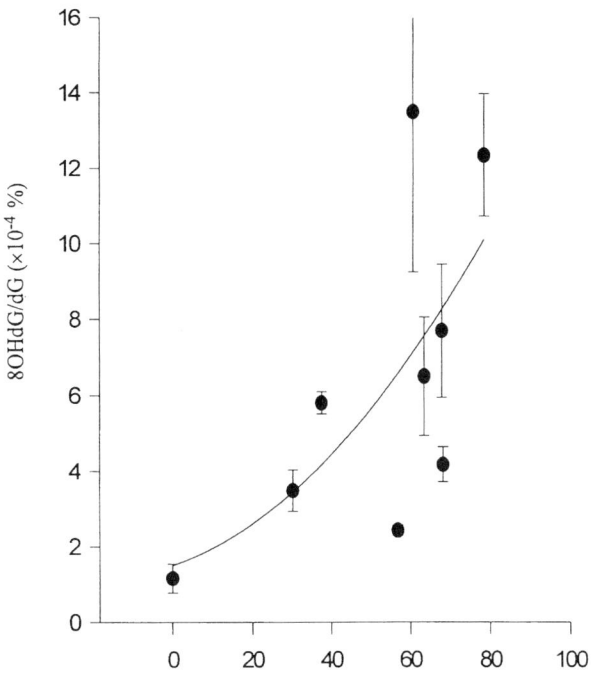

FIGURE 5. The 8-OHdG/dG ratio of the cybrids harboring different proportions of the 4,977 bp-deleted mtDNA. Total DNA was extracted and 8-OHdG/dG ratio was then determined by the HPLC-ECD and HPLC-UV system using a reverse phase C_{18} column as detailed in MATERIALS AND METHODS. Each data point represents the mean ± S.D. of the results obtained from 3 determinations.

ally obtain a series of cybrids harboring widely varied levels of the mutated mtDNA (FIG. 1).

In this study, we found that the proportion of the 4,977 bp-deleted mtDNA was quite stable after two-month of subcloning of the original cybrids. By use of these stable cybrids, the respiratory function was found to decrease with the increase of the proportion of the 4,977 bp-deleted mtDNA (FIG. 3). These results strongly indicate an energy deficit in the cybrids harboring the deleted mtDNA, which are consistent with the previous findings that the bioenergetic function is decreased in the cybrids containing mutant mtDNA.[9–11,30] Since the cybrids harboring the 4,977 bp-deleted mtDNA are defective in mitochondrial respiratory function, an alteration in the intracellular NADH/NAD$^+$ ratio is expected. This may lead to an increase of proton and electron leak through the mitochondrial inner membranes as a result of inefficient NADH oxidation and incomplete reduction of oxygen by the mitochondria.[41] An immediate consequence of the electron leak from the impaired respiratory enzyme system is the increase of the partial reduction of molecular oxygen to form superoxide anions and other ROS in mitochondria.[24,42] Indeed, it has been established

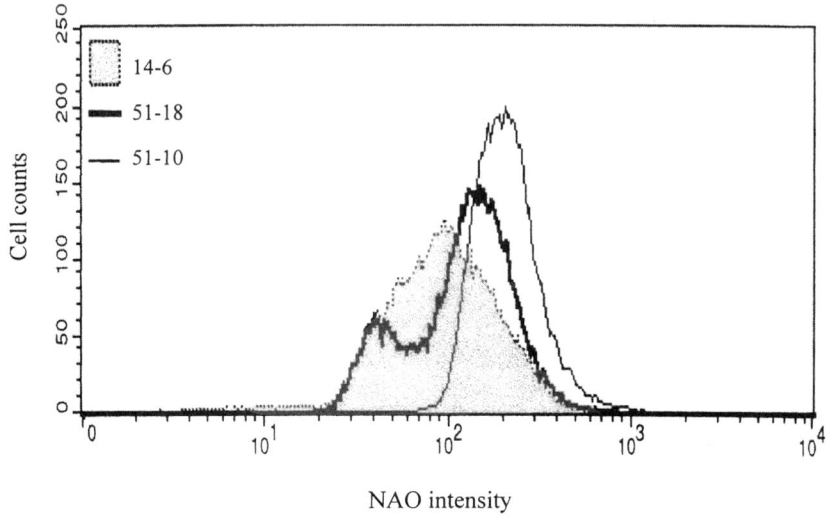

FIGURE 6. Determination of mitochondrial mass in the cybrids harboring different proportions of 4,977 bp-deleted mtDNA by using flow cytometry. Three cybrids clones 14-6 (17.1% mutant), 51-18 (56.3% mutant), and 51-10 (85.4% mutant) were respectively stained with the fluorescent dye NAO and subjected to analysis on a FACScan flow cytometer as described in MATERIALS AND METHODS.

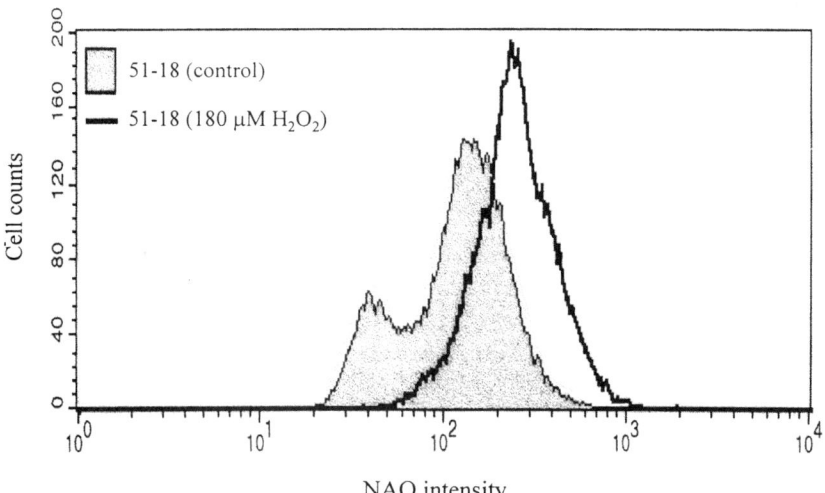

FIGURE 7. Hydrogen peroxide-induced increase of mitochondrial mass in the cybrids harboring 4,977 bp-deleted mtDNA. The cybrid clone 51-18 (containing 56.3% mutant mtDNA) was stained with NAO after treatment with 180 μM H_2O_2 for 48 h. The NAO intensity of the treated cells was increased as determined by the FACScan flow cytometer with the conditions described in MATERIALS AND METHODS.

that impaired respiratory chain function in drug-treated cells or aged human and animal tissues results in the production of higher levels of superoxide anions and/or hydrogen peroxide.[22,26,43–45]

In the past few years, we have proposed that the oxidative stress and oxidative damage in mitochondria and the whole cell are enhanced by mtDNA mutation in a dose-dependent manner.[12,23,24] In this study, we also measured the contents of lipid peroxides and 8-OHdG in the cybrids and found that the levels of 8-OHdG and lipid peroxides in the cybrids containing high proportions of the 4,977 bp-deleted mtDNA were higher than the levels in the control cybrid (FIGS. 4 and 5). These results clearly indicate that the cybrids containing the mtDNA deletion are subject to higher oxidative stress and are afflicted by more severe oxidative damage.

On the other hand, we found that the cybrids harboring high proportions of the 4,977 bp-deleted mtDNA contained higher amounts of mitochondria (FIG. 6). Using slot blot analysis, we found that the mtDNA content was higher in the cybrids harboring low to medium levels of 4,977 bp-deleted mtDNA. By contrast, the cybrids containing high levels (> 70%) of 4,977 bp-deleted mtDNA had slightly lower contents of the mitochondrial genome (TABLE 1). We believe that the increase of mtDNA and mitochondria is one of the molecular events gearing the cells up to cope with the mild to medium stress. However, when the cells are overwhelmed by high oxidative stress, such kind of compensatory mechanism is no longer effective due to the impairment of replication of mtDNA and biogenesis of mitochondria. This is consistent with our earlier finding that the relative content of mtDNA in the lung tissues of light smokers was significantly higher than that of non-smokers and that the lung tissues of heavy smokers contained lower copy number of mtDNA.[46] These observations suggest that mtDNA was amplified in the cybrids with mild oxidative stress but declined in the cybrids with high oxidative stress and profound oxidative damage (see TABLE 1). This notion was supported by our further demonstration that mitochondrial mass was increased by oxidative stress elicited by 180 µM of H_2O_2 in a cybrid with 56% of the 4,977 bp-deleted mtDNA (FIG. 7). In line with these observations, we found that the relative mtDNA content in the primary culture of skin fibroblasts of a patient with CPEO syndrome was about 10% higher than that of skin fibroblasts from healthy subjects.

Taken together, the data obtained in this and previous studies[34] suggest that increase of mitochondrial mass and mtDNA is one of the molecular events associated with enhanced oxidative stress in human cells with impaired respiratory function caused by mtDNA deletion. This may also explain, at least in part, the well-documented but largely unexplained pathological manifestation of overproliferation of abnormal mitochondria in the ragged-red fibers in the muscle of patients with mitochondrial myopathy and encephalomyopathies.[47] The molecular mechanism underlying the increase in the number of mitochondria and mtDNA in human cells with defective respiratory function warrants further investigation.

ACKNOWLEDGMENTS

This work was supported by a grant (NSC89-2316-B010-012) from the National Science Council, Republic of China. The authors are grateful to the assistance of Dr. Edward K. Wang in the procurement of the skin biopsies of the patient used in this study. One of the authors, Yau-Huei Wei, would like to express his sincere appreciation of the generous support of the National Science Council and National Health Research Institutes of the Republic of China in the course of this study.

REFERENCES

1. HOLT, I., A.E. HARDING & J.A. MORGAN-HUGHES. 1988. Deletions of muscle mitochondrial DNA in patients with mitochondrial myopathies. Nature **331:** 717–719.
2. WALLACE, D.C., G. SINGH, M.T. LOTT, et al. 1988. Mitochondrial DNA mutation associated with Leber's hereditary optic neuropathy. Science **242:** 1427–1430.
3. GOTO, Y., I. NONAKA & S. HORAI. 1990. A mutation in the tRNA$^{Leu(UUR)}$ gene associated with the MELAS subgroup of mitochondrial encephalomyopathies. Nature **348:** 651–653.
4. SHOFFNER, J.M., M.T. LOTT, A.M.S. LEZZA, et al. 1990. Myoclonic epilepsy and ragged-red fiber disease (MERRF) is associated with a mitochondrial DNA tRNA^{Lys} mutation. Cell **61:** 931–937.
5. HOLT, I.J., A.E. HARDING, R.K.H. PETY & J.A. MORGAN-HUGHES. 1990. A new mitochondrial disease associated with mitochondrial DNA heteroplasmy. Am. J. Hum. Genet. **46:** 428–433.
6. WALLACE, D.C. 1992. Diseases of the mitochondrial DNA. Annu. Rev. Biochem. **61:** 1175–1212.
7. LARSSON, N.-G. & D.A. CLAYTON. 1995. Molecular genetic aspects of human mitochondrial disorders. Annu. Rev. Genet. **29:** 151–178.
8. WANG, E.K., K.P. KAO, R.H. HSIEH, et al. 1998. Large-scale mitochondrial DNA deletions in patients with CPEO syndrome in Taiwan. J. Biochem. Mol. Biol. Biophys. **1:** 165–170.
9. HAYASHI, J.-I., S. OHTA, A. KIKUCHI, et al. 1991. Introduction of disease-related DNA deletions into HeLa cells lacking mitochondrial DNA results in mitochondrial dysfunction. Proc. Natl. Acad. Sci. USA **88:** 10614–10618.
10. CHOMYN, A., G. MEOLA, N. BRESOLIN, et al. 1991. In vitro genetic transfer of protein synthesis and respiration defects to mitochondrial DNA-less cells with myopathy-patient mitochondria. Mol. Cell. Biol. **11:** 2236–2244.
11. KING, M P., Y. KOGA, M. DAVIDSON & E. A. SCHON. 1992. Defects in mitochondrial proteins and respiratory chain activity segregate with the tRNA$^{Leu(UUR)}$ mutation associated with mitochondrial myopathy, encephalopathy, lactic acidosis, and stroke-like episodes. Mol. Cell. Biol. **12:** 480–490.
12. WEI, Y.H., C.Y. LU, H.C. LEE, et al. 1998. Oxidative damage and mutation to mitochondrial DNA and age-dependent decline of mitochondrial respiratory function. Ann. N.Y. Acad. Sci. **854:** 155–170.
13. TURRENS, F., A. ALEXANDRE & A.L. LEHNINGER. 1985. Ubisemiquinone is the electron donor for superoxide formation by Complex III of heart mitochondria. Arch. Biochem. Biophys. **237:** 408–414.
14. NOHL, H. & W. JORDAN. 1986. The mitochondrial site of superoxide formation. Biochem. Biophys. Res. Commun. **138:** 533–539.
15. ESPOSITO, L.A., S. MELOV, A. PANOV, et al. 1999. Mitochondrial disease in mouse results in increased oxidative stress. Proc. Natl. Acad. Sci. USA **96:** 4820–4825.
16. KATSUMATA, K., M. HAYAKAWA, M. TANAKA, et al. 1994. Fragmentation of human heart mitochondrial DNA associated with premature aging. Biochem. Biophys. Res. Commun. **202:** 102–110.
17. LARSON, N.-G., E. HOLME, B. KRISTIANSSON, et al. 1990. Progressive increase of the mutated mitochondrial DNA fraction in Kearns-Sayre syndrome. Pediatr. Res. **28:** 131–136.
18. FEIGENBAUM, A., D. CHITAYAT, B. ROBINSON, et al. 1996. The expanding clinical phenotype of the tRNA$^{Leu(UUR)}$ A→G mutation at np 3243 of mitochondrial DNA: Diabetes embryopathy associated with mitochondrial cytopathy. Am. J. Med. Genet. **62:** 404–409.

19. PANG, C.Y., C.C. HUANG, M.Y. YEN, et al. 1999. Molecular epidemiologic study of mitochondrial DNA mutations in patients with mitochondrial diseases in Taiwan. J. Formosan Med. Assoc. **98:** 326–334.
20. SAHASHI, K., M. TANAKA, M. TASHIRO, et al. 1992. Increased mitochondrial DNA deletions in the skeletal muscle of myotonic dystrophy. Gerontology **38:** 18–29.
21. BEAL, M.F., B.T. HYMAN & W. KOROSHETZ. 1993. Do defects in mitochondrial energy metabolism underlie the pathology of neurodegenerative diseases? TINS **16:** 125–131.
22. YEN, T.C., K.L. KING, H.C. LEE, et al. 1994. Age-dependent increase of mitochondrial DNA deletions together with lipid peroxides and superoxide dismutase in human liver mitochondria. Free Radic. Biol. Med. **16:** 207–214.
23. WEI, Y.H., S.H. KAO & H.C. LEE. 1996. Simultaneous increase of mitochondrial DNA deletions and lipid peroxidation in human aging. Ann. N.Y. Acad. Sci. **786:** 24–43.
24. WEI, Y.H. 1998. Oxidative stress and mitochondrial DNA mutations in human aging. Proc. Soc. Exp. Biol. Med. **217:** 53–63.
25. BURDON, R.H. 1995. Superoxide and hydrogen peroxide in relation to mammalian cell proliferation. Free Radic. Biol. Med. **18:** 775–794.
26. SUZUKI, H., T. KUMAGAI, A. GOTO & T. SUGIRA. 1998. Increase in intracellular hydrogen peroxide and upregulation of a nuclear respiratory gene evoked by impairment of mitochondrial electron transfer in human cells. Biochem. Biophys. Res. Commun. **249:** 542–545.
27. LEE, H.C. & Y.H. WEI. 2000. Mitochondrial role in life and death of the cell. J. Biomed. Sci. **7:** 2–15.
28. KING, M.P. & G. ATTARDI. 1988. Injection of mitochondria into human cells leads to a rapid replacement of the endogenous mitochondrial DNA. Cell **52:** 811–819.
29. KING, M.P. & G. ATTARDI. 1989. Human cells lacking mtDNA repopulation with exogenous mitochondria by complementation. Science **246:** 500–503.
30. PORTEOUS, W.K., A.M. JAMES, P.W. SHEARD, et al. 1998. Bioenergetic consequences of accumulating the common 4977-bp mitochondrial DNA deletion. Eur. J. Biochem. **257:** 192–201.
31. FANG, W., C.C. HUANG, N.S. CHU, et al. 1994. Myoclonic epilepsy with ragged-red fibers (MERRF) disease: report of a Chinese family with mitochondrial DNA point mutation in tRNA^{Lys} gene. Muscle & Nerve **17:** 52–57.
32. VASSAULT, A. 1983. Lactate dehydrogenase. In Methods of Enzymatic Analysis, 3rd edit. H.U. Bergmeyer, Ed. :118–126. Verlag Chemie GmbH. Weinheim.
33. PETIT, J.M., A. MAFTAH, M.H. RATINAUD & R. JULIEN. 1992. 10-n-nonyl acridine orange interacts with cardiolipin and allows the quantification of this phospholipid in isolated mitochondria. Eur. J. Biochem. **209:** 267–273.
34. LEE, H C., P.H. YIN, C.Y. LU, et al. 2000. Increase of mitochondria and mitochondrial DNA in response to oxidative stress in human cells. Biochem. J. **348:** 425–432.
35. WEI, Y.H., W.H. DING & R.D. WEI. 1984. Biochemical effects of PR toxin on rat liver mitochondrial respiration and oxidative phosphorylation. Arch. Biochem. Biophys. **230:** 400–411.
36. WONG, S.H.Y., J.A. KNIGHT, S.M. HOPFER, et al. 1987. Lipoperoxides in plasma as measured by liquid-chromatographic separation of malondialdehyde-thiobarbituric acid adduct. Clin. Chem. **33:** 214–220.
37. SHIGENAGA, M.K., E.N. ABOUJAOUDE, Q. CHEN & B.N. AMES. 1994. Assays of oxidative DNA damage biomarker 8-oxo-2′-deoxyguanosine and 8-oxoguanine in nuclear DNA and biological fluids by high-performance liquid chromatography with electrochemical detection. Methods Enzymol. **234:** 16–33.
38. LEE, H.C., M.L.R. LIM, C.Y. LU, et al. 1999. Concurrent increase of oxidative DNA damage and lipid peroxidation together with mitochondrial DNA mutation in human lung tissues during aging—smoking enhances oxidative stress on the aged tissues. Arch. Biochem. Biophys. **362:** 309–316
39. LOWRY, O.H., N. ROSEBROUGH, A.L. FARR & R.J. RANDALL. 1951. Protein measurement with the Folin phenol reagent. J. Biol. Chem. **193:** 265–275.

40. ZEVIANI, M., N. BRESOLIN, C. GELLERA, *et al.* 1990. Nucleus-driven multiple large-scale deletions of the human mitochondrial genome: a new autosomal dominant disease. Am. J. Hum. Genet. **47:** 904–914.
41. GIULIVI, C., A. BOVERIS & E. CADENAS. 1995. Hydroxyl radical generation during mitochondrial electron transfer and the formation of 8-hydroxydeoxyguanosine in mitochondrial DNA. Arch. Biochem. Biophys. **316:** 909–916.
42. DE GREY, A.D.N.J. 1998. A mechanism proposed to explain the rise in oxidative stress during aging. J. Anti-Aging Med. **1:** 53–66.
43. SOHAL, R.S. 1993. Aging, cytochrome oxidase activity, and hydrogen peroxide release by mitochondria. Free Radic. Biol. Med. **14:** 583–588.
44. MUSCARI, C., M. FRASCARO, C. GUARNERI & C. CALDARERA. 1990. Mitochondrial function and superoxide generation from submitochondrial particles of aged rat hearts. Biochim. Biophys. Acta **1015:** 200–204.
45. KU, H.H., U.T. BRUNK & R.S. SOHAL. 1993. Relationship between mitochondrial superoxide and hydrogen peroxide production and longevity of mammalian species. Free Radic. Biol. Med. **15:** 621–627.
46. LEE, H.C., C.Y. LU, H.J. FAHN & Y.H. WEI. 1998. Aging- and smoking-associated alteration in the relative content of mitochondrial DNA in human lung. FEBS Lett. **441:** 292–296.
47. DIMAURO, S., E.A. SCHON & L.P. ROWLAND. 1995. Mitochondrial encephalo-myopathies. In Merrit's Textbook of Neurology, 9th edit. L.P. Rowland, Ed.: 618–620. Williams & Wilkins. Philadelphia, PA.

DNA Polymerase-β May Be the Main Player for Defective DNA Repair in Aging Rat Neurons

KALLURI SUBBA RAO, V.V. ANNAPURNA, AND N.S. RAJI

Department of Biochemistry, School of Life Sciences, University of Hyderabad, Hyderabad—500046, India

ABSTRACT: A close relationship between the DNA repair potential of various organisms and their rate of aging has been long suspected. We have been looking into the steps of the DNA repair process in isolated neurons from rats of different ages. Unscheduled DNA synthesis (UDS) was low in aging neurons, and also the response of these cells to raise their DNA repair capacity against a mutagenic challenge was poor. Attempts to identify the possible defective locus in the overall DNA repair pathways indicated that the step involving DNA polymerase may be defective. The activity of DNA polymerase-β, the most predominant DNA polymerase in neurons that is generally considered to be a short-patch repair enzyme, shows a significant decrease in aging neurons. Northern and Southern blotting and immunotitration experiments suggest that there may be an accumulation of inactive β polymerase molecules in the aging rat brain. Most recent preliminary studies reveal significant 3′-5′ exonuclease activity in rat neurons at all ages. However, extension of a primer in a synthetic oligo duplex, either with a mismatch or correct base pair at the 3′ end of the primer, was low in neurons of any age and was very poor (almost undetectable) in older ones. Supplementation of neuronal extracts with pure polymerase enzyme revealed that only polymerase β, but not polymerase α, was able to increase the primer extension activity significantly in old neurons. These findings are taken to indicate an age-dependent decline in the DNA repair capacity of neurons and that DNA polymerase β is a key player in the DNA repair mechanisms of nerve cells.

KEYWORDS: Neurons; Aging; DNA repairs; DNA polymerase β

The inevitability and universality of aging have generated many theories to explain the mechanisms behind this process.[1–5] Many of the hypotheses regarding aging have focused on DNA as a critical molecular target, and theories that seek to explain the process of aging at the genetic level have naturally attracted attention. One such theory is the "DNA damage and repair" theory, which in essence proposes that accumulation of DNA damage and/or decreased DNA repair capacity may be a major

---

Address for correspondence: Prof. Kalluri Subba Rao, Department of Biochemistry, School of Life Sciences, University of Hyderabad, Hyderabad—500046, India. Voice: +91-40-3010451/256; fax: +91-40-3010120/145/451.
ksrsl@uohyd.ernet.in

contributor to the process of aging.[6–12] Several knockout mice that lack a specific DNA repair activity have been generated in the last few years. These mice show, among other things, defective embryogenesis, extreme sensitivity to DNA-damaging agents, premature senescence, and elevated cancer incidence.[11,13] Thus, it has become valid to assume that DNA repair efficiency has a deterministic role in the onset and the rate of the aging process in a given organism.

Mammalian cells have multiple mechanisms, involving many proteins and steps,[14] for repairing damaged DNA. A major category of the repair process is nucleotide and base excision repair (NER and BER, respectively) including mismatch repair. Essentially, the process involves (a) recognition of the damaged site, (b) excision of a portion of the DNA strand harboring the damage, (c) resynthesis of the excised portion by an appropriate DNA polymerase using the other strand as a template, and (d) ligation of the last nucleotide gap through the action of DNA ligase. Although both NER and BER pathways actually converge to become a common pathway, there is a major difference between the two pathways in the length of the nucleotide patch removed and resynthesized. The patch size is much longer in NER, whereas in BER it is usually one nucleotide long—although it can be up to six nucleotides—and is referred to as short-patch repair. Several studies indicate that the polymerase participating in BER is pol β (DNA polymerase β) with an associated activity to remove the deoxyribose-5′ phosphate.[14,15]

Information regarding the specific DNA repair steps in brain cells is scanty, although a number of putative DNA repair enzyme activities have been found in this tissue.[8,16] It is the purpose of this article to briefly present the evidence that has accumulated in our laboratory during the past few years to show that unscheduled DNA synthesis (UDS) decreases in rat brain cells during old age and one of the likely reasons for this is the accumulation of inactive molecules of pol β.

The overall DNA repair capacity, as measured by *in vitro* incorporation of [^{3}H]thymidine into the DNA of isolated neuronal cells in rat brain, was studied as a function of age. Spontaneous UDS in adult and old neurons was low compared to the levels in young neurons. Furthermore, the response of aging neurons, in contrast to that of young and adult neurons or of lymphocytes of any age, to a mutagenic challenge like ultraviolet light (254 nm) is limited.[17] Subsequently, work with isolated nuclei from the cerebral cortex of rats of different ages (young, 10 days postnatal; adult, 6 months; and old, more than 2 years) gave similar results.[18] To begin with, DNA repair activity was inhibited following UV irradiation (60 J/m^2). However, this initial inhibition was overcome with time (2 hours), and the repair activity increased considerably in the nuclei from young brain but not in the nuclei isolated from adult and old brains.

Because DNA repair is a complex, multistep process, it was important to identify which step(s) is most affected in aging brain. Irrespective of the type of repair pathway that is in operation, one major and crucial step is the resynthesis of the excised portion of the damaged strand, which restores the original predamage nucleotide sequence. This step is catalyzed by a DNA polymerase. Mammalian cells possess five different DNA polymerases, the α, β, γ, δ, and ε; although pol γ is mitochondrial, the other four are located essentially in the nucleus. Considering the post-mitotic nature of brain cells, base excision repair (which removes modified and abasic sites) would be of considerable importance. Polymerase β is the main enzyme involved in this

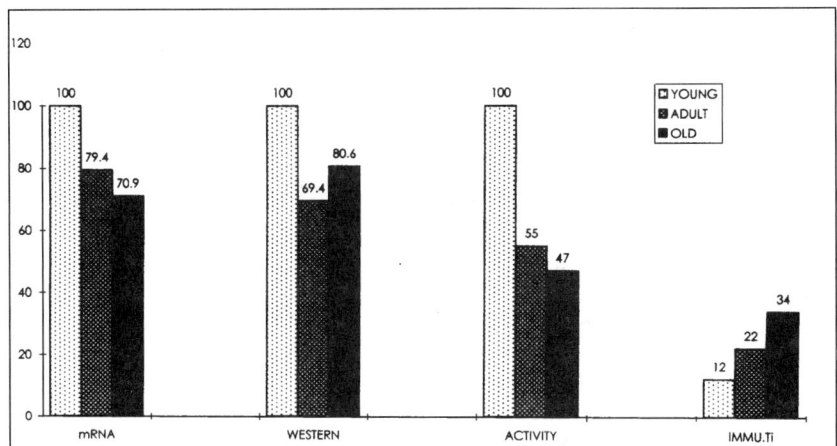

FIGURE 1. Assessment of "active" levels of DNA polymerase b in aging rat brain through different strategies, viz., Northern blotting, Western blotting, activity gel assay, and immunotitration. In the case of immunotitration, the values denote microliters of antiserum required for inhibiting the activity by 50%. An equal amount of activity is taken at all ages. In other cases, the values represent percent of the "young" activity. (From Rao et al.[24] Reproduced with permission. For more details about these studies please refer to Rao et al.[23])

pathway, particularly when a single base replacement is required. In some situations where the patch size is longer (2–10 nucleotides) both pol β and δ or ε, along with some accessory factors like proliferating cell nuclear antigen (PCNA), are implicated.[19]

As early as in 1979, Waser and co-workers found that in adult cortical neurons more than 99% of the DNA polymerase activity was attributable to pol β.[20] They concluded that pol β is the repair enzyme in neurons. All our subsequent and more detailed studies involving the usage of various inhibitors, template-primers, monoclonal antibody to pol α (DNA polymerase α), PCNA, and DMSO (dimethyl sulfoxide) to distinguish different DNA polymerase activities also substantiated the assumption that pol β is the major enzyme in brain cells at all ages.[21,22]

A systematic study to assess the levels of pol β was undertaken. Through Northern and Western blotting, it was found that mRNA and immunologically competent molecules of pol β are reduced by 30% and 20%, respectively, in old rat brain in comparison with young. However, activity gel assay (measuring the pol β activity on the gel itself after the separation of the proteins) and immunotitration with polyclonal antibody revealed a more than 50% reduction in the activity in old brain.[23] All these results are summarized in FIGURE 1. It can be seen that to achieve a 50% reduction from a given amount of activity from old brain extracts, about three times the amount of antiserum is required compared to young brain extracts. These data are taken to indicate accumulation of catalytically inactive molecules of pol β in rat brain with age.

The consequences of accumulation of such "inactive" pol β molecules in aging neurons is examined by using a deoxy oligo duplex as a model template primer. A

14-mer was hybridized with 21–mer, and the nucleotide sequences of the oligos used are shown below.

(1) 5'-c g c g a t c g g t a g c **G**-3' (14-mer)
(2) 3'-g c g c t a g c c a t c g **C** g t t a c c g-5' (21-mer-C)
(3) 3'-g c g c t a g c c a t c g **T** g t t a c c g-5' (21-mer-T)
(4) 3'-g c g c t a g c c a t c g **G** g t t a c c g-5' (21-mer-G)
(5) 3'-g c g c t a g c c a t c g **A** g t t a c c g-5' (21-mer-A)

Out of four 21-mers, one of them has the correct complementary base at the 14th position from 3' end, whereas the other three 21-mers have the three mismatches at that position.

Before the hybridization with any of the 21-mers, the 14–mer was 5'-kinased using γ-^{32}P-ATP and T_4-polynucleotide kinase. The hybridized oligoduplex template primer was used as a substrate for measuring the 3'–5' exonuclease (proofreading) as well as the primer extension activity (referred to as exo extension activities) by the neuronal extracts prepared from young, adult, and old rat brains. The results of a typical experiment are shown in FIGURE 2. As can be seen, neuronal extracts of all ages were able to excise the primer to shorter lengths with good efficiency, pointing to the presence of 3'–5' exonuclease activity in neurons of all ages. However, significant extension of the primer could be seen only with young extracts (lanes 5–8) and there was an age-dependent decrease in this activity (compare the activity in lanes 5–8 to that in 13–16). In fact with old extracts, the activity was barely detectable (lanes 21–24). The extension of the primer was most efficient in case of correctly matched primer (G–C), and with mismatches extension was low. In the absence of dNTPS, no extension was seen.

When the above-mentioned oligoduplexes (unlabeled) were incubated under standard DNA-polymerase conditions with one of the dNTPs being labeled (α-^{32}P-dCTP), detectable template-dependent polymerase activity was seen (TABLE 1). Once again, the activity was less in the case of mismatched duplexes, and overall extension activity was lower in old neurons. From the above two experiments, it was

TABLE 1. Extension of primer under standard DNA-polymerase assay conditions

Base pair at primer 3' end	Age		
	Young	Adult	Old
G-T	37.0	24.2*	22.5*
	±13.1	±6.8	±17.7
G-A	27.3	21.5	9.3*,**
	±11.3	±8.6	±6.5
G-G	25.2	18.4	6.8*,**
	±14.6	±8.0	±5.5
G-C	51.3	33.6*	26.0*,**
	±34.3	±15.6	±9.1

NOTE: The results are the average ± standard deviation of 12 independent experiments. The activities are expressed as femtomoles of radioactive deoxy nucleotide incorporated into the acid-insoluble fraction. The volume of neuronal extracts was adjusted so that in all cases the protein was 10 µg.

*These values are significantly lower than those of the corresponding young group and ** these of the corresponding adult group, at a p value < 0.01.

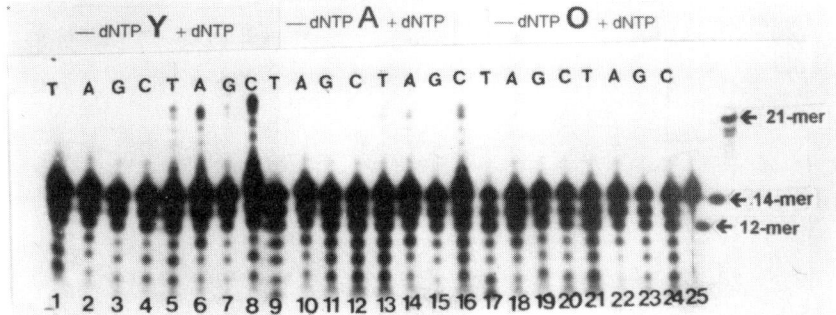

FIGURE 2. Exo-extension activities of neuronal extracts with correctly matched and mismatched oligo duplex template primers. Neuronal cells from rat brain cortex of different ages were isolated as per the previously described procedure.[25] The final preparation of neuronal cells was suspended in extraction medium consisting of 20 mM Tris pH 7.5, 0.1 mM dithiothreitol, 1 mM EGTA, 10% glycerol, 0.5% CHAPS, 0.1 mM PMSF (just before use), 5 mM β-mercaptoethanol, 1 mM $MgCl_2$, 1 µg/ml leupeptin and 1 µg/ml pepstatin A (both just before use), and 0.5 M KCl and sonicated three times for 5 sec with the setting at 5 in a Brasnon sonifier. The suspension was centrifuged at $100,000 \times g$ for 1 hour in a Beckman ultracentrifuge, and the clear supernatant was used as the source for both 3′–5′ exonuclease and DNA polymerase. For the assay, two nanograms (in 1 µl) of the hybridized oligo duplex (14-mer, 21-mer), either with the correct match (G-C) or with mismatches (G-A, G-G, and G-T) was incubated for 20 min at 37°C with the appropriate volume of neuronal extract in a total reaction mixture of 20 µl consisting of 20 mM HEPES, pH 7.5, 1 mM $MgCl_2$, 0.1 mM DTT, 0.1 mg/ml bovine serum albumin, 2% glycerol, and 20 µM of all four dNTPS. The reaction was stopped by adding 1 µl of 0.5 M EDTA, and then the volume was brought up to 100 µl with water. The whole sample was passed through a spin column. The collected sample was dried and resuspended in 5 µl of loading buffer and denatured just before performing the electrophoresis followed by autoradiography. The reaction was carried out both in the presence and absence of dNTPS. At each age, young (Y, 10 days postnatal), adult (A, 6 months), and old (O, more than 2 years), the first four tubes do not contain dNTPS, and the next four contain dNTPS (20 µM). In all the tubes, the protein in neuronal extract was normalized to 10 µg by adjusting the volume. Similarly, equal volumes of the post-reaction reaction mixtures were loaded onto the sequencing gel. Lane 25v is does not contain neuronal extract. Standard 21, 14, and 12 mers are shown.

concluded that the primer extension activity is significantly decreased with age in neurons.

Because the primer extension is essentially a DNA polymerase–catalyzed reaction and because pol β is the most predominant enzyme in the brain, the above exo-extension assay experiments were repeated with the exogenously added pure rat liver pol β or pure calf thymus pol α. First, results with pol α are shown in FIGURE 3. No significant improvement is seen in the primer extension activity with age, and the general pattern of results seen in FIGURE 2 persisted. However, when pol β was supplemented in the extracts, there was a significant improvement in the primer elongation activity at all ages and that too even in the case of mismatched duplexes (FIG. 4). From these experiments, and from our earlier observation on the accumulation of inactive pol β molecules in aging brain,[23] we are inclined to postulate that pol β has a key role in maintaining the genomic stability in brain and this function is compromised with age.

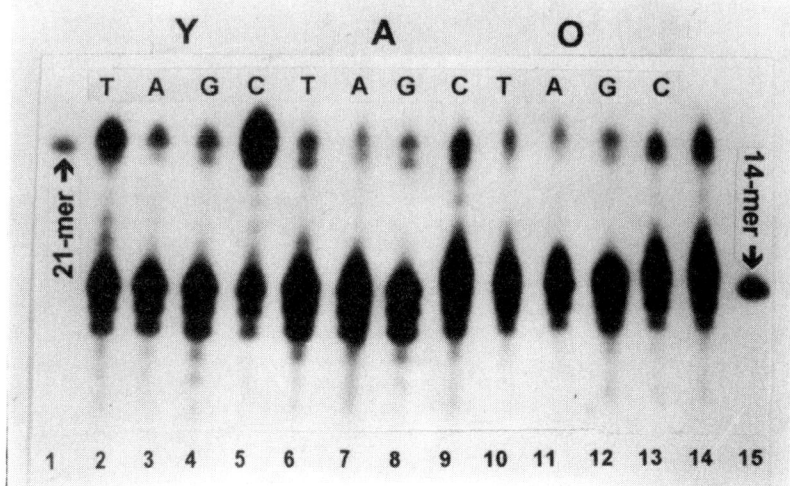

FIGURE 3. Exo-extension activity when rat neuronal extracts (young, Y; adult, A; old, O) were supplemented with 0.25 units (1 unit is equivalent to incorporation of 1 nanomole of total nucleotides into activated DNA in 1 hour at 37°C) of pure calf thymus DNA polymerase α. Other details are the same as in FIGURE 2.

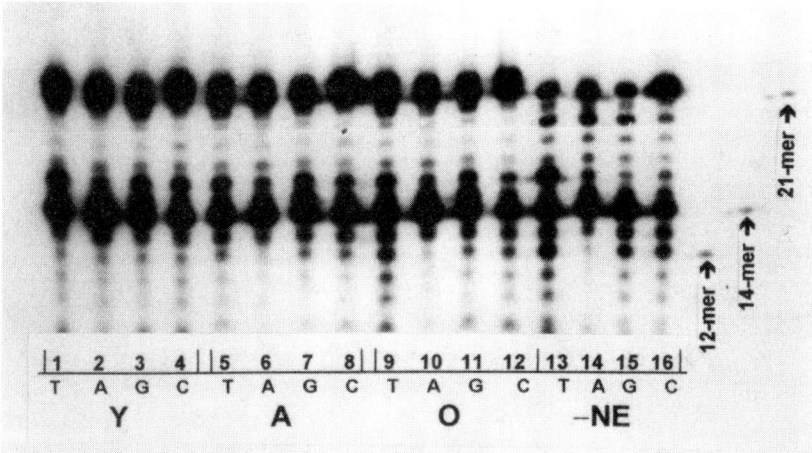

FIGURE 4. Exo-extension activity of rat neuronal extracts supplemented with 2.5 units of rat liver recombinant DNA polymerase β. Lanes 13–16, only DNA polymerase β with no neuronal extracts.

ACKNOWLEDGMENTS

We wish to thank Dr. Akio Matsukage, presently at the Department of Applied Biological Science, Science University of Tokyo, Noda, Chiba, 278-8510, Japan, and Dr. Fred Perrino, Department of Biochemistry, Wake Forest University,

Winston-Salem, NC 27159, USA, for generous gifts of pure DNA polymerase β and calf thymus DNA polymerase α, respectively. Some of the work presented here was supported by the Council of Scientific and Industrial Research, New Delhi, and DST.

REFERENCES

1. WARNER, H.R., R.N. BUTLER, R.L. SPROTT & E.L. SCHNEIDER. 1987. Modern Biological Theories of Aging. Raven Press. New York.
2. RAO, K.S. & L.A. LOEB. 1992. DNA damage and repair in brain: relationship to aging. Mutat. Res. **275**: 317–329.
3. KANUNGO, M.S. 1994. Genes and Aging. Cambridge University Press. New York.
4. SHARMA, R. 1994. Theories of aging. In Physiological Basis of Aging and Geriatrics. P.S. Timiras, Ed.: 37–46. CRC Press. Boca Raton, FL.
5. HARMAN, D. 1998. Aging: phenomena and theories. Ann. N.Y. Acad. Sci. **854**: 1–7.
6. HART, R.W. & R.B. SETLOW. 1974. Correlation between deoxyribonucleic acid excision repair and life span in a number of mammalian species. Proc. Natl. Acad. Sci. USA **71**: 2169–2173.
7. GENSLER, H.L. & H. BERNSTEIN. 1981. DNA damage as the primary cause of aging. Q. Rev. Biol. **56**: 279–303.
8. RAO, K.S. 1997. DNA damage and DNA repair in ageing brain. Indian J. Med. Res. **106**: 423–437.
9. WEI, Q., G.M. MATANOSKI, R.M.A. FARMER, et al. 1993. DNA repair and aging in basal cell carcinoma: a molecular epidemiology study. Proc. Natl. Acad. USA **90**: 1614–1618.
10. CORTOPOSSI, G.A. & E. WANG. 1996. There is substantial agreement among interspecies estimates of DNA repair activity. Mech. Ageing Dev. **91**: 211–218.
11. WILSON, D.M. III & L.H. THOMPSON. 1997. Life without DNA repair. Proc. Natl. Acad. Sci. USA **94**: 12754–12757.
12. RAO, K.S. 1998. Nonapoptotic DNA fragmentation: a molecular pointer of aging. Curr. Sci. **74**: 874–901.
13. FRIEDBERG, E.C. & L.B. MEIRA. 1999. Database of mouse strains carrying targeted mutations in genes affecting cellular responses to DNA damage: version 3. Mutat. Res. **433**: 69–87.
14. WOOD, R.D. 1996. DNA repair in eukaryotes. Ann. Rev. Biochem. **65**: 135–167.
15. WILSON, S.H. 1998. Mammalian base excision repair and DNA polymerase beta. Mutat. Res. **407**: 203–215.
16. MARIETTA, C., F. PALOMBO, P. GALLINARI, et al. 1998. Expression of long-patch and short-patch DNA mismatch repair proteins in the embryonic and adult mammalian brain. Brain Res. Mol. Res. **53**: 317–320.
17. SUBRAHMANYAM, K. & K.S. RAO. 1991. Ultraviolet light induced unscheduled DNA synthesis in isolated neurons of rat brain of different ages. Mech. Ageing Dev. **57**: 283–291.
18. VENUGOPAL, J. & K.S. RAO. 1993. DNA repair/synthesis and RNA synthesis in isolated rat cerebral cortex nuclei: effect of age and UV irradiation. Biochem. Arch. **9**: 341–348.
19. WOOD, R.D. & M.K.K. SHIVJI. 1997. Which DNA polymerases are used for DNA repair in eukaryotes? Carcinogenesis **18**: 605–610.
20. WASER, J., U. HUBSCHER., C.C. KUENZLE & S. SPADARI. 1979. DNA polymerase β from brain neurons is repair enzyme. Eur. J. Biochem. **97**: 361–368.
21. SUBRAMANYAM, K. & K.S. RAO. 1998. On the type of DNA polymerase activity in neuronal, astroglial and oligodendroglial cell fractions from young, adult and old rat brains. Biochem. Int. **16**: 1111–1118.
22. PRAPURNA, D.R. & K.S. RAO. 1997. DNA polymerases δ and ε in developing and aging brain. Int. J. Dev. Neurosci. **15**: 67–73.
23. RAO, K.S., D. VINAYKUMAR, M.S. BHASKAR & G. SRIPAD. 1994. On the "active" molecules of DNA-polymerase β in aging rat brain. Biochem. Mol. Biol. Int. **32**: 287–294.

24. RAO, K.S., M.S. BHASKAR & D. VINAYKUMAR. 1996. Molecular markers of brain aging. *In* Perspectives in Neuroscience Research. C.K. Tan, E.A. Ling & C.B.C. Tan, Eds.: 153–166. Singapore Neuroscience Association. Singapore.
25. USHA RANI, B., N.I. SING, A. RAY & K.S. RAO. 1993. Procedure for isolation of neuron and astrocyte enriched fractions from chick brain of different ages. J. Neurosci. Res. **10:** 101–105.

Premature Aging and Predisposition to Cancers Caused by Mutations in RecQ Family Helicases

YASUHIRO FURUICHI

AGENE Research Institute, Kamakura, 247-0063, Japan

ABSTRACT: DNA helicases, because they unwind duplex DNA, have important roles in cellular DNA events such as replication, recombination, repair, and transcription. Multiple DNA helicase families with seven consensus motifs have been found, and members within each helicase family also share sequence homologies between motifs. The RecQ helicase family includes helicases that have extensive amino acid sequence homologies to the *E. coli* DNA helicase RecQ, which has been implicated in double-strand break repair and suppression of illegitimate recombination. To date, five RecQ helicase species exist in humans, but their exact biological functions remain unknown. In this paper, on the basis of five years of work, I overview the updated molecular biology of five human RecQ helicases; genetic diseases such as Werner's, Bloom's, and Rothmund-Thomson's syndromes caused by helicase mutations; the associated premature aging phenotype; and an increased risk of neoplasms. I also describe a hypothesis of "tissue-specific genomic instability" that accounts for the pathology behind multisymptomatic RecQ helicase syndromes.

KEYWORDS: Werner syndrome; Bloom syndrome; Rothmond-Thomas syndrome; Genomic instability

INTRODUCTION

The human RecQ DNA helicase gene family has five members, RecQ1 (referred to also as RecQL), BLM, WRN, RecQ4, and RecQ5, located on human chromosomes 12p12, 15q26.1, 8p12-11.2, 8q24.3, and 17q25.2-25.3, respectively. Mutations in BLM, WRN, and RecQ4 cause Bloom's syndrome (BS), Werner's syndrome (WS), and Rothmund-Thomson's syndrome (RTS), respectively; these are genetic disorders that increase the rate of generation of genomic instability in the patient's cells, resulting in predisposition to cancer and premature aging (TABLE 1).

RecQ-type helicases from other organisms are from yeasts: Sgs1 of *Saccharomyces cerevisiae* and rqh1+ of *Schizosaccharomyces pombe*. Like *E. coli*, these unicellular organisms contain a single species of RecQ-type helicase. Sgs1 exists in the nucleolus when the cells are young and migrates to the nucleoplasm as the cells senesce and the nucleolus fragments.[1] Mutation of the *Sgs1* gene suppresses the slow-

---

Address for correspondence: Yasuhiro Furuichi, Ph.D., Director, AGENE Research Institute, 200 Kajiwara, Kamakura, 247-0063, Japan. Voice: +81-467-46-9590; fax: +81-467-48-6595.

furuichi@agene.co.jp

TABLE 1. RecQ helicases and genetic diseases

	RecQ1	BLM	WRN	RTS	RecQ5
Homozygous deficiency	Unknown	Bloom syndrome	Werner syndrome	Rothmund-Thomson syndrome	Unknown
Chromosomal location	12p12	15q26.1	8p12-11.2	8q24.3	17q25.2-25.3
Portein (aa)	649	1417	1432	1208	991
Chromosomal	—	Not reported	Yes	Yes	—
Sister chromatid exchange	—	×10 elevated	No	Normal or slightly increased	—
Intracelluar location	Nuclear	Nuclear	Nuclear	Nuclear	Nuclear

growth phenotype of the mutant yeast cell that has a mutation in the topoisomerase 3 gene and causes missegregation of the chromosome during meiosis and mitosis. Biochemically, Sgs1 binds to topoisomerase 2 and topoisomerase 3. The *rqh1+* gene of *S. pombe* was cloned by complementation of the UV sensitivity of the *rqh1-h2* mutant, and the *rqh1−* cells arrested by hydroxyurea at the S phase are unrecoverable because of a high recombination rate.

STRUCTURE AND BIOCHEMICAL NATURE OF HUMAN RECQ HELICASES

All five human RecQ helicase genes have been cloned, and the predicted structure indicates that they contain a consensus helicase domain in the middle of the polypeptides (FIG. 1). Biochemical analyses showed that RecQ1, WRN, and BLM helicases

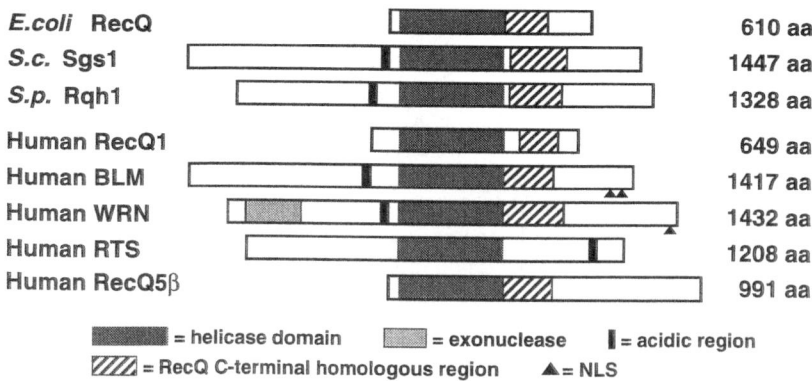

FIGURE 1. Schematic representation of RecQ helicases.

contain DNA-unwinding and ATPase activities. Extended studies on the purified WRN helicase that was expressed in insect cells by a baculovirus system showed that it has RNA/DNA heteroduplex unwinding activity in addition to DNA-unwinding activity, implicating its involvement in transcription.[2] Exonuclease activity was recently found in the NH_2-terminal region of WRN helicase. Some studies on the directionality of the exonuclease, including Gray et al.,[3] proposed that a helicase-independent $3' \rightarrow 5'$ exonuclease exists, but our data[4] clearly indicate that WRN exonuclease has the $5' \rightarrow 3'$ directionality and, most importantly, its activity is dependent on the DNA- or RNA/DNA-unwinding activity of helicase. Controversies between these findings remain to be clarified.

All five RecQ helicases, including the recently identified RecQ5β helicase,[5] migrate to the nucleus. Nuclear localization signals (NLS) composed of basic amino acid arrays have been identified consistently in WRN,[6,7] BLM,[8] and RecQ5β,[5] although the NLS of RecQ1 and RTS helicases have not been determined. We showed that WRN helicase mainly locates in the nucleoplasm of growing cells,[9] but can also exist in the nucleolus depending on the cell conditions. RecQ5 helicase was the last helicase found among the human RecQ helicase family and was considered to be as small as RecQ1 helicase. However, differential splicing of the *RecQ5* gene forms at least three RecQ5 helicase isomers; and one of the three isomers, referred to as RecQ5β, has a larger molecular size.[5] Thus, two size classes of the RecQ helicase family exist: large helicases, BLM, WRN, RTS, and RecQ5β in the nucleus containing 1417, 1432, 1208, and 933 amino acids (aa), respectively, and small helicases, RecQ1 and RecQ5 containing 649 aa and 410 aa, respectively, that exist in both the cytoplasm and nucleus.

Our previous phylogenetic study[10] on the sequence of the helicase domain indicated that the product of the *RecQ5* (and *RecQ5β*) gene is evolutionarily close to the small helicase RecQ1, which is characterized as a human progenitor of the RecQ family helicases, but has no known relation to human disease. Except for the recent RecQ5β helicase, extended studies were performed mostly on large helicases whose mutations cause the disease phenotypes in humans.

WERNER'S SYNDROME, BLOOM'S SYNDROME, AND ROTHMUND-THOMSON'S SYNDROME

Three recessive genetic diseases, WS, BS, and RTS, occur by mutation in WRN, BLM, and RTS helicases, respectively. The clinical phenotypes of these diseases are distinct, but to some extent overlap. Patients have a short stature, a premature aging phenotype, and a high risk of having neoplasms because of chromosomal instability. Some characteristic features of these diseases are briefly described.

Werner's syndrome: The first clinical report of WS[11] was made in 1904 by Otto Werner, an ophthalmologist in Kiel, Germany. Patients with WS show an increased rate of genomic instability: cells show a variegated translocation mosaicism and large deletions in the genomic DNA. Patients have a short stature, juvenile cataracts, atrophy of the skin, graying and loss of hair, early hypogonadism, diabetes mellitus, arteriosclerosis, osteoporosis, and rare tumors.[12] The life span of patients is 46 ± 11.6 years, due mainly to death caused by malignant tumor or cardiovascular infarctions. In 1996, the gene responsible for WS was identified by positional cloning.[13]

Bloom's syndrome: The first clinical report of BS was made in 1966 by David Bloom,[14] a dermatologist in New York City. BS patients have a short stature, skin disorders including hyperpigmentation, immunodeficiency, telangiectasia, male infertility, and various malignant neoplasias. Cells show a high rate of homologous chromosome recombination (sister chromatid exchanges).[15] The gene responsible for WS was identified in 1995.[16]

Rothmund-Thomson's syndrome: In 1868, the German ophthalmologist August Rothmund reported a poikiloderma associated with a high incidence of juvenile cataracts that occurred in 10 young, related patients of his from an isolated Bavarian village.[17] In 1936, the British dermatologist Sidney Thomson reported similar patients with poikiloderma, two of whom had bony abnormalities.[18] The two sets of cases with overlapping clinical features are known as the Rothmund-Thomson syndrome; some debate on the explanation of broadened symptoms has persisted, and the clinical signs among patients has been recognized. The report by Rothmund might conceivably have influenced the later study on WS by Werner. Patients with RTS have growth deficiency, photosensitivity with poikilodermatous skin changes, early graying and hair loss, cataracts, and a predisposition to malignancy, especially osteogenic sarcomas.[19] No consistent cellular abnormality has been identified to facilitate diagnosis, although in several patients acquired clonal chromosomal abnormalities have been observed. The gene responsible for a subset of RTS patients, referred to here as RecQL4 or RTS, was identified in 1999.[20]

IMPAIRED NUCLEAR TRANSPORT OF WRN HELICASES IN CELLS OF WERNER'S SYNDROME PATIENTS

We and others analyzed mutations of Werner helicase genes using DNA samples obtained from over 100 patients.[21,22] These studies showed that mutations occur all over the helicase molecule and generate most, if not all, of the incomplete and truncated polypeptides that lack an NLS in the COOH terminus. Our subsequent cytochemical studies using recombinant fusion proteins showed that the mutated WRN helicase occurring in patient cells is unable to migrate to the nucleus due to the absence of COOH-terminal NLS.[6] This finding provided a new theory clearly explaining why Werner patients show a set of similar symptoms no matter what mutations they carry in their *WRN* helicase genes. The same theory also accounts for clinical phenotypes shared by most patients with BS, because mutations on the Bloom helicase gene are spread throughout the entire molecule of Bloom helicase, whose NLS exists in the COOH terminus.[8,9] Whether RTS also has the same pathologic makeup causing its homologous clinical symptoms among patients remains to be studied.

MUTATIONS IN THE RTS (RECQL4) GENE RESPONSIBLE FOR ROTHMUND-THOMSON'S SYNDROME

RTS is the most recently identified disease in the category of helicase diseases caused by mutation of a gene in the human RecQ helicase family. The number of RTS patients whose gene mutation on the *RTS* helicase gene (originally referred to as RecQL4[10]) was confirmed is still as few as six with an appearance rate of only about

TABLE 2. Mutations on RecQL4 gene in RTS patients

Patient	Mutation		Exon	Consequence	Origin
RTS-B, C (L9552914-J)	1650 del 7 C 2269 T	(mut-1) (mut-2)	10 14	Frameshift Nonsense	Mexican
RTS-E (AG05013)	2492 del 2 3′ splice site, ag→at	(mut-3) (mut-4)	15 13	Frameshift Frameshift	European
RTS-H (B1865425-K)	1573 del 1 3′ splice site, ag→aa	(mut-5) (mut-6)	9 8	Frameshift Altered splicing	European
RTS-M	3′ splice site, ag→aa 3′ splice site, ag→ac	(mut-6) (mut-7)	8 15	Altered splicing Altered splicing	European

40%, perhaps due to the broadened symptoms used for clinical diagnosis. Because the gene responsible for RTS has now been identified at least for a subset of patients, not only will diagnosis at the molecular level be facilitated for patients with the RTS mutation, but also further studies to find other genes involved in non-RecQ4-mediated RTS will be aided. TABLE 2 summarizes the mutations found in RTS patients.

EXPRESSION OF RECQ HELICASES IN NORMAL HUMAN TISSUES

The levels of expression of five RecQ helicase genes in human organs were examined by multiple-tissue Northern blot analysis (FIG. 2). The *RecQ1* gene is highly expressed in all the tissues examined.[10] The *WRN* gene is expressed highly in the pancreas, testis, and ovary. The *BLM* gene is highly expressed in the thymus and testis but not in the ovary, in contrast with *WRN* gene expression. The *RTS* gene is highly expressed in the thymus, testis, and placenta and is moderately expressed in the heart, brain, small intestine, and colon. The *RecQ5β* gene is expressed rather ubiquitously with noticeably high expression in the testis.[5] Thus, the large, disease-causing helicase genes of the RecQ family demonstrate tissue-specific expression.

TISSUE-SPECIFIC GENOMIC INSTABILITY IN PATIENTS

Tissues that express WRN, BLM, or RTS helicases highly correlate with the tissues involved in the representative clinical symptoms of WS, BS, or RTS patients. For example, BS patients have male sterility, but not female sterility, correlating with the high-level expression of the *BLM* gene in the testis and with no expression in the ovary.[15] High expression of the *BLM* gene in the thymus may thus correlate with immunodeficiency associated with BS patients, not with WS patients because no or only a very low expression of the *WRN* gene is found in the thymus. By contrast, high expressions of the *WRN* gene in the pancreas, testis, and ovary directly correlate well with the tissues involved in diabetes mellitus and early hypogonadism in both males

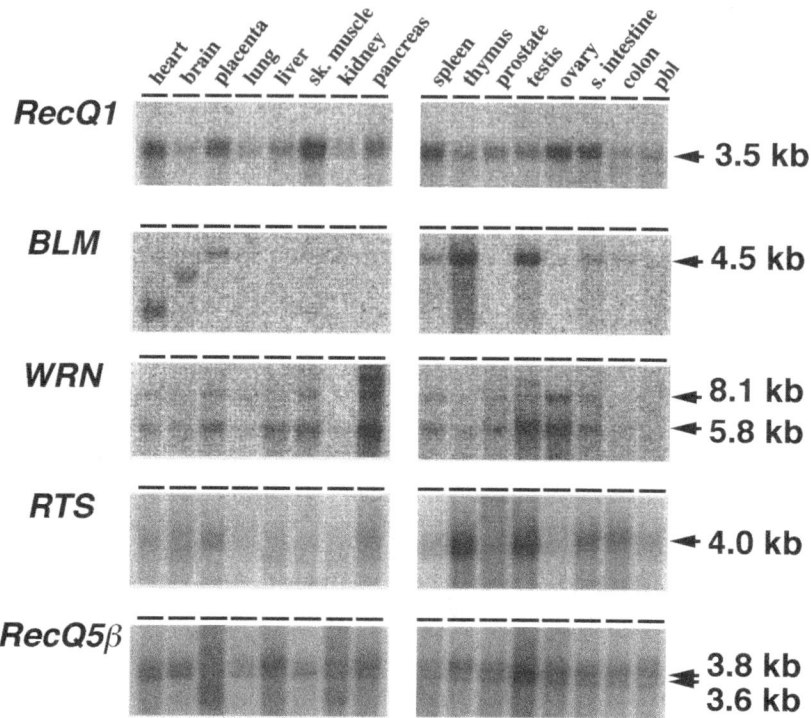

FIGURE 2. Multiple-tissue Northern analysis to compare the expression of RecQ helicase genes in normal human tissues. MTM blot (Clontech) was prepared with 2 μg of poly(A)+ per lane as previously described.[10]

and females, symptoms characteristic of WS. Thus, the distinct clinical symptoms of each disease appear to result from genomic instability due to defective helicases in specified tissues in which a high expression of particular helicases is needed in normal persons. This "tissue-specific genomic instability" hypothesis solves an enigma in the pathology and accounts for complications of multisymptomatic RecQ helicase syndromes.

EACH RECQ HELICASE HAS A SPECIFIC ROLE

Each helicase may have a specific role(s) in the function of differentiated cells in various organs. For example, although *WRN* and *BLM* helicase genes are coexpressed in skin fibroblasts, mutation in the *WRN* helicase gene results in WRN-specific defective phenotypes, such as large deletions associated with the chromosomal instability and a short population-doubling capability characteristic of fibroblasts from WS patients, indicating that the BLM helicase is unable to complement the function of WRN helicase. Also, both *BLM* and *RTS* helicase genes are highly expressed in the thymus, and mutation of the *BLM* helicase gene in BS patients results in immunodeficiency that is not apparently complemented by the RTS helicase, although studies are needed to confirm whether the RTS and BLM helicases are coexpressed in the same cells of the thymus.

Nonetheless, accumulated data suggest that each RecQ helicase is apparently involved in different biological tasks, although the major biochemical function of each RecQ helicase is unwinding duplex DNA: an exception is that WRN helicase can unwind RNA/DNA heteroduplex in addition to DNA/DNA homoduplex and has exonuclease activity as an integral component.[4] Perhaps the biological role of each RecQ helicase is specified by a protein–protein interaction with other nuclear proteins. Further studies are needed to clarify what kind of nuclear proteins cooperate with which kind of RecQ helicases and in which cellular events RecQ helicases are involved. In this regard, DNA replication, repairs, solving the entangled DNA or DNA/RNA structures, and post-replicative chromatid segregation are the candidate events. So far, data are limited except that WRN helicase binds to RPA, p53, topoisomerase I, and PCNA, whereas BLM helicase binds to PCNA and RecQ5β interacts with topoisomerases 3α and 3β.[5]

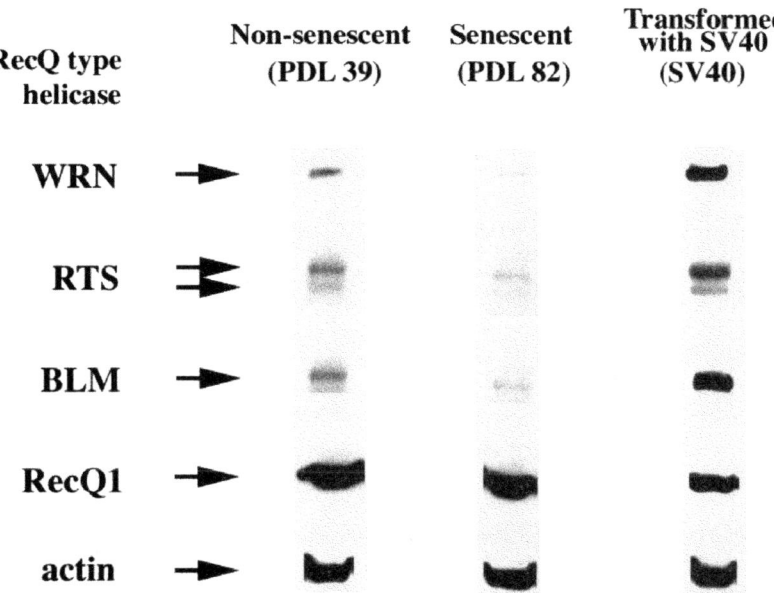

FIGURE 3. Downregulation of WRN, BLM, and RTS helicases in the senescent cells and upregulation of SV40-transformed cells. Proteins extracted from human lung fibroblast TIG-3 cells (60 µg) were analyzed for the expression of five RecQ helicases by immunoblotting using monoclonal antibodies. Bands corresponding to individual helicases were cut out from the stained filters and the intensities compared. For a strict comparison, each helicase band is normalized beforehand with cellular actins present in the extracted proteins. Nonsenescent: cells after culturing of 39 PDL (population doubling); senescent: cells after culturing 82 PDL; transformed with SV40: cells were transformed by SV40 virus as previously described.[9]

WRN, BLM, AND RTS HELICASES ARE DOWNREGULATED IN SENESCENT CELLS

To understand the regulation of gene expression, we previously analyzed the promotor of the *WRN* helicase gene.[23] The promotor region of the *WRN* gene has multiple SP1 elements characteristic of a housekeeping gene. Our subsequent promotor activity assay with luciferase indicated that *WRN* gene transcription is downregulated by tumor suppressor protein p53, whereas it is upregulated, even though marginally, by another tumor suppressor factor, Rb. Because the protein level of p53 increases cellular aging, our findings are consistent with a prediction that *WRN* genes, and perhaps expression of other human RecQ helicase genes, are gradually downregulated along with cell senescence.[23] To prove this hypothesis, we prepared monoclonal antibodies specific to each RecQ helicase and measured the expression kinetics of helicase proteins by immunoblot analysis. The amounts of WRN, BLM, and RST helicases decreased in the senescent fibroblast cells, while the amount of RecQ1 remained unchanged (FIG. 3). These data imply that the activities of large RecQ helicases deteriorate in normal aging, perhaps resulting in increased genomic instability within senescent cells. Patients with WS, BS, and RTS have essentially reduced helicase activities, which means a high incidence of genomic instability from the beginning of their lives.

KNOCKOUT MICE AND OTHER GENE-TARGETED MODEL ORGANISMS

How do these RecQ helicases function in human embryos where cells proliferate rapidly? In an attempt to produce a model animal to address this question, we cloned the mouse *WRN* homologue gene[24] and established the gene-targeted knockout mice (Ichikawa *et al.*, manuscript in preparation). Unfortunately, as we and two other groups noticed, the knockout mice show no marked phenotype of WS. Moreover, they live the same life span as wild mice and were competent in generating baby mice, suggesting that the *WRN* gene is not important for maintaining genomic integrity in mice. To clarify the biological function of WRN and BLM helicases, we used *S. cerevisiae* cells as an alternative model organism. To this end, we replaced the yeast *Sgs1* helicase gene by either *WRN* or *BLM* genes, and the phenotypes of the gene-replaced cells were analyzed.[25] The *Sgs1*$^-$ yeast cells showed increased homologous and nonhomologous recombination rates. Insertion of the human *WRN* or *BLM* gene in the place of the *Sgs1* gene in the right orientation suppressed the increased recombination rates of mutant yeast cells, suggesting that WRN and BLM helicases act similarly as the suppressor of illegitimate recombination in human cells. Also, accelerated aging observed in yeast cells without *Sgs1* was complemented by the human *BLM* gene.[26] These findings support the theory that RecQ helicases prevent apparent aging by suppressing illegitimate hyper-recombination and by eventually maintaining genomic integrity. Other surrogate systems, such as chicken DT-40 cells that show a hyperrecombination,[27] are currently being tested for the effect of human RecQ helicases on the recombination rate.

WRN, BLM, RTS, AND RECQ1 HELICASES ARE UPREGULATED IN RAPIDLY PROLIFERATING TRANSFORMED OR TUMOR CELLS

Strong upregulation occurs in WRN, BLM, and RTS helicases in human B lymphoblastoid cells (LCLs) transformed with Epstein-Barr virus (EBV) and in human fibroblasts infected with SV-40 virus or transformed by the T-antigen gene of SV-40[9] (see also, Kawabe et al.[33]). In particular, upregulation of WRN expression is proven to be T-antigen-dependent because the temperaturesensitive T antigen failed to stimulate WRN expression under a nonpermissive temperature, although it stimulated expression at a permissive temperature. Besides transforming proteins from viruses, a tumor-promoting agent, phorbol myristic acetate (PMA), which stimulates the growth of B cells, exerts a similar stimulatory effect on LCLs by inducing WRN, BLM, RTS, and RecQ1 helicase in vitro[28] (see also, Kawabe et al.[33]). Here, the effect of PMA on the onset of stimulation of individual helicases is differential: *WRN* expression is induced shortly after adding PMA (within 5 hr), whereas *BLM* and *RTS* expressions are slower and are induced after 16 hours. Thus, *WRN* gene expression is stimulated particularly at a very early stage (within 5 hr) of cell commitment to proliferation and may mean that WRN helicase acts mainly in prereplication events and BLM acts in postreplication events, although both are involved in genomic maintenance.

Most tumor cell lines showed increased (approx. 20–50-fold of normal skin fibroblasts) levels of WRN helicase.[9] A similar trend also occurs with BLM and RTS helicases, but the levels of upregulation are variable depending on the tumor cell lines. These findings clearly indicate that RecQ helicases are needed for rapidly growing tumor cell lines, and the difference in the levels of upregulation is perhaps influenced by intrinsic genetic backgrounds of individual tumor clones.

A UNIQUE DOWNREGULATION OF mRNAs AND HELICASE PROTEINS IN PATIENT CELLS: A SUPREME DIAGNOSIS BY IMMUNOBLOTTING

Earlier, we found a severe downregulation of defective WRN mRNA in cultured fibroblasts and LCLs from WS patients and from apparently normal heterozygotes.[28] An early mRNA degradation mediated by a termination codon, reviewed by Maquat,[29] seems to occur in cells of WS and heterozygotic carriers. We confirmed this observation consistently at the protein level by immunoblotting using monoclonal antibodies to WRN and RTS helicases. This observation was used to diagnose WS[30] and RTS[31] by detecting WRN and RTS helicase proteins, respectively, in EBV-transformed B cells from patients or patients suspected of having these diseases. In our laboratory this diagnostic method is run parallel with DNA analysis, and the data consistently confirm the data from DNA analysis. Because immunoblot analysis has been showing unequivocal results, that is, the undoubted presence or absence of helicase proteins in the given B-cell samples, we refer to the immunoblot analysis as a supreme diagnosis. For immunoblot diagnosis, peripheral B cells obtained from patients suspected of having the diseases are transformed by EBV and cultured for several weeks. The rapidly growing B cells are then analyzed for helicase(s), which are assessed.[32] In our experience, DNA analysis sometimes fails to detect the mutation(s) in DNA because of new mutations in difficult regions, for example, in highly GC-rich areas or in introns, but immunoblot analysis is exempted from these problems and never fails. Nevertheless, immunoblot analysis only detects nonsense mutations. Missense mutations have not been found in WS and RTS patients so far.

CONCLUSIONS

Human RecQ helicases are involved in maintaining the integrity of the genome by suppressing illegitimate recombination or by repair of local DNA structural damage. Deterioration or loss of RecQ helicase activity associated with aging or genetic diseases results in genomic instability in tissues and organs where certain RecQ helicases are needed to correct aberrant DNA during proliferation. Such genomic instability, if not corrected, would cause increased apoptotic cell death that results in deterioration of tissues and organs, the phenotypes of aging. Genomic instability would increase the risk of having neoplasms, however, irrespective of benign or malignant phenotypes. Those neoplasms are produced if either a checkpoint system or apoptosis is not functioning appropriately. Malignant tumor cells would then be selected from the mixed population of neoplasms by acquiring phenotypes permitting rapid cell growth and a strong capability to maintain the genome, such as high copy numbers of RecQ helicases, which we observed in various tumor cell lines. Further studies are needed to discover effective measures to control genomic instability and to manage the formation of malignant tumors.

ACKNOWLEDGMENTS

I thank Dr. Makoto Goto at the Tokyo Metropolitan Otsuka Hospital and researchers in the AGENE Research Institute for friendly and efficient cooperation in pursuing this research project over five years. This work was supported by the Drug Organization (The Organization for Drug ADR Relief, R & D Promotion and Product Review, supervised by the Ministry of Health and Welfare of Japanese Government).

REFERENCES

1. SINCLAIR, D.A., K. MILLIS & L. GUARENTE. 1997. Accelerated aging and nucleolar fragmentation in yeast *sgs1* mutants. Science **277:** 1313–1316.
2. SUZUKI, N., A. SHIMAMOTO, O. IMAMURA, *et al.* 1997. DNA helicase activity in Werner's syndrome gene product synthesized in a baculovirus system. Nucleic Acids Res. **25:** 2973–2978.
3. GRAY, M.D., J.C. SHEN, A.S. KAMATH-LOEB, *et al.* 1997. The Werner syndrome protein is a DNA helicase. Nature Genet. **17:** 100–103.
4. SUZUKI, N., M. SHIRATORI, M. GOTO & Y. FURUICHI. 1999. Werner syndrome helicase contains a 5′ → 3′ exonuclease activity that digests DNA and RNA strands in DNA/DNA and RNA/DNA duplexes dependent on unwinding. Nucleic Acids Res. **27:** 2361–2368.
5. SHIMAMOTO, A., K. NISHIKAWA, S. KITAO & Y. FURUICHI. 2000. Human RecQ5β, large isomer of RecQ5 DNA helicase, localizes in the nucleoplasm and interacts with topoisomerases 3α and 3β. Nucleic Acids Res. **28:** 1647–1655.
6. MATSUMOTO, T., A. SHIMAMOTO, M. GOTO & Y. FURUICHI. 1997. Impaired nuclear localization of defective DNA helicases in Werner's syndrome. Nature Genet. **16:** 335–336.
7. MATSUMOTO, T., O. IMAMURA, M. GOTO & Y. FURUICHI. 1998. Characterization of the nuclear localization signal in the DNA helicase involved in Werner's syndrome. Int. J. Mol. Med. **1:** 71–76.

8. KANEKO, H., K.O. ORII, E. MATSUI, et al. 1997. BLM (the causative gene of Bloom syndrome) protein translocation into the nucleus by a nuclear localization signal. Biochem. Biophys. Res. Commun. **240:** 348–353.
9. SHIRATORI, M., S. SAKAMOTO, N. SUZUKI, et al. 1999. Detection by epitope-defined monoclonal antibodies of Werner DNA helicases in the nucleoplasm and their upregulation by cell transformation and immortalization. J. Cell Biol. **144:** 1–9.
10. KITAO S., I. OHSUGI, K. ICHIKAWA, et al. 1998. Cloning of two new human helicase genes of the RecQ family: biological significance of multiple species in higher eukaryotes. Genomics **54:** 443–452.
11. WERNER, O. 1904. Doctoral dissertation, Kiel University, Schmidt and Klauning Kiel.
12. GOTO, M., R.W. MILLER, Y. ISHIKAWA & H. SUGANO. 1996. Excess of rare cancers in Werner's syndrome (adult progeria). Cancer Epidemiol. Biomakers Prev. **5:** 239–246.
13. YU, C.E., J. OSHIMA, Y.H. FU, et al. 1996. Positional cloning of the Werner's syndrome gene. Science **272:** 258–262.
14. BLOOM, D. et al. 1966. The syndrome of congenital telangiectatic erythema and stunted growth. J. Pediatr. **68:** 103–113.
15. GERMAN, J. 1993. Bloom syndrome: a mendelian prototype of somatic mutational disease. Medicine (Baltimore) **72:** 393–406.
16. ELLIS, N.A., J. GRODEN, T.Z. YE, et al. The Bloom's syndrome gene product is homologous to RecQ helicases. 1995. Cell **83:** 655–666.
17. ROTHMUND, A. 1868. Uber cataracten in verbindung mit einer eigenthumlichen hautdegeneration. Arch. Klin. Exp. Ophthal. **4:** 159–182.
18. THOMSON, M.S. 1936. Poikiloderma congenitale. Br. J. Dermatol. **48:** 221–234.
19. LINDOR, N.M., E.M.G. DEVRIES, V.V. MICHELS, et al. 1996. Rothmund-Thomson syndrome in siblings: evidence for acquired in vivo mosaicism. Clin. Genet. **49:** 124–129.
20. KITAO, S., A. SHIMAMOTO, M. GOTO, et al. 1999. Mutations in RECQL4 cause a subset of cases of Rothmund-Thomson syndrome. Nature Genet. **22:** 82–84.
21. MATSUMOTO, T., O. IMAMURA, Y. YAMABE, et al. 1997. Mutation and haplotype analyses of the Werner's syndrome gene based on its genomic structure: genetic epidemiology in the Japanese population. Hum. Genet. **100:** 123–130.
22. OSHIMA, J., C.E. YU, C. PIUSSAN, et al. 1996. Homozygous and compound heterozygous mutations at the Werner syndrome locus. Hum. Mol. Genet. **5:** 1909–1913.
23. YAMABE, Y., A. SHIMAMOTO, M. GOTO, et al. 1998. Sp1-mediated transcription of the Werner helicase gene is modulated by Rb and p53. Mol. Cell. Biol. **18:** 6191–6200.
24. IMAMURA, O., K. ICHIKAWA, Y. YAMABE, et al. 1997. Cloning of a mouse homologue of the human Werner syndrome gene and assignment to 8A4 by fluorescence in situ hybridization. Genomics **41:** 298–300.
25. YAMAGATA, K., J. KATO, A. SHIMAMOTO, et al. 1998. Proc. Natl. Acad. Sci. USA **95:** 8733–8738.
26. SEOK-JIN, H., K. TATEBAYASHI, I. OHSUGI, et al. Bloom's syndrome gene suppresses premature ageing caused by Sgs1 deficiency in yeast. 1999. Genes Cells **4:** 619–625.
27. BUERSTEDD, J.M. & S. TAKEDA. 1991. Increased ratio of targeted to random integration after transfection of chicken B cell lines. Cell **67:** 179–188.
28. YAMABE, Y., M. SUGIMOTO, M. SATOH, et al. 1997. Down-regulation of the defective transcripts of the Werner's syndrome gene in the cells of patients. Biochem. Biophys. Res. Commun. **236:** 151–154.
29. MAQUAT, L.E. 1995. When cells stop making sense: effect of non-sense codons on RNA metabolism in vertebrate cells. RNA **1:** 453–465.
30. GOTO, M., Y. YAMABE, M. SHIRATORI, et al. 1999. Immunological diagnosis of Werner syndrome by down-regulated and truncated gene products. Hum. Genet. **105:** 301–307.
31. KITAO, S., N. LINDOR, M. SHIRATORI, et al. 1999. Rothmund-Thomson syndrome responsible gene, RECQL4: genomic structure and products. Genomics **61:** 268–276.
32. TAHARA, H., Y. TOKUTAKE, S. MAEDA, et al. 1997. Abnormal telomere dynamics of β-lymphoblastoid cell strains from Werner's syndrome patients transformed by Epstein-Barr virus. Oncogene **15:** 1911–1920.
33. KAWABE, T., N. TSUYAMA, S. KITAO, et al. 2000. Differential regulation of human RecQ family helicases in cell transformation and cell cycle. Oncogene **19:** 4764–4772.

Health Span and Life Span in Transgenic Mice with Modulated DNA Repair

CHRISTI A. WALTER,[a,e] ZI-QIANG ZHOU,[a] DIWI MANGUINO,[a]
YUJI IKENO,[b] ROBERT REDDICK,[c] JAMES NELSON,[b] GABRIEL INTANO,[a]
DAMON C. HERBERT,[a] C. ALEX MCMAHAN,[c] AND MARTHA HANES[d]

[a]*Department of Cellular and Structural Biology,* [b]*Department of Physiology,*
[c]*Department of Pathology,* [d]*Department of Laboratory Animal Resources, The University of Texas Health Science Center at San Antonio, 7703 Floyd Curl Drive, San Antonio, Texas 78229-3900, USA*

[f]*South Texas Veterans Health Care System, Audie L. Murphy Hospital, San Antonio, Texas 78284, USA*

ABSTRACT: One way to better understand the contribution of DNA repair, DNA damage, and mutagenesis in aging would be to enhance DNA repair activity, lower DNA damage, and lower mutagenesis. Because the repair protein O^6-methylguanine–DNA methyltransferase (MGMT) acts alone and stoichiometrically, the human MGMT (hMGMT) cDNA was selected to test the feasibility of enhancing DNA repair activity in transgenic mice. MGMT activity is largely responsible for ameliorating the deleterious effects of O^6-methylguanine (O^6mG) lesions in DNA in a direct reversal mechanism. A transgene was constructed consisting of a portion of the human transferrin (TF) promoter and hMGMT cDNA such that hMGMT is expressed in transgenic mouse brain and liver. Expression of hMGMT was associated with a significant reduction in the occurrence of an age-related hepatocellular carcinoma in male mice at 15 months of age. Longitudinal and cross-sectional studies were initiated to determine whether the reduced incidence of hepatocellular carcinoma would impact median or maximum life span. The cross-sectional study performed on 15-month-old male animals confirmed the reduced occurrence of spontaneous hepatocellular carcinoma. At 30 months of age, however, the occurrence of hepatocellular carcinoma in at least one transgenic line was similar to that for nontransgenic animals. The longitudinal study is ongoing; however, at present no significant differences in life span have been detected. Tissues expressing the MGMT transgene also displayed greater resistance to alkylation-induced tumor formation. These results suggest that transgenes can be used to direct enhanced DNA repair gene expression and that enhanced expression can protect animals from certain spontaneous and induced tumors.

KEYWORDS: Transgenic mice; Alkylation damage; Aging; Hepatocellular carcinoma; MGMT

Address for correspondence: Christi A. Walter, Department of Cellular and Structural Biology, The University of Texas Health Science Center at San Antonio, Mail Code 7762, 7703 Floyd Curl Drive, San Antonio, TX 78229-3900. Voice: 210-567-3832; fax: 210-567-3803.
walter@uthscscsa.edu

INTRODUCTION

An age-related decline in genomic integrity has been proposed to be a fundamental mechanism in the aging process.[1-4] The somatic mutation theory of aging encompasses the tenant that accumulation of mutations with time results in the inactivation of genes, decreased protein function, and ultimately cell death. The DNA damage theory of aging embraces the concept that accumulated DNA damage increasingly interferes with DNA replication and transcription, which in turn impairs the ability of cells to perform their functions, thereby leading to aging. More recently it has become accepted that only a certain amount of DNA damage is tolerated before cells commit themselves to a pathway of cell death. These two theories of aging, which are based on genomic integrity, are not mutually exclusive and are difficult to study independently of each other. Some of the data that support the role of genetic integrity in aging are discussed briefly below.

Genetic integrity at the level of the chromosome was among the earliest observations demonstrating a decreased integrity with increased age. For example, chromosomal aberrations have been shown to increase in preparations from mouse liver[5] and mouse kidney cells[6] with older age. The majority of studies involving humans have been performed with peripheral blood cells and have also revealed increases in chromosomal aberrations with increased donor age.[7-13] Thus, there are data linking increased age with increased chromosome aberrations.

Genetic integrity has also been assessed at the level of individual genes, and increases in mutation frequencies have been observed with increased age. The *Hprt* gene can be scored for mutations using selective media and is commonly used for assessing mutation frequencies in humans and other mammals. Several studies have reported an increase in mutation frequency in the *Hprt* gene with increased age in various cell types, but principally in peripheral blood lymphocytes.[12,14-18]

Genomic integrity has been shown to be compromised in male and female germ cells as well. For example, in humans there are clear correlations between increased maternal age and pregnancies with chromosomal abnormalities.[19] In addition, some autosomal dominant disorders display a higher *de novo* germline mutation frequency with increased paternal age. New mutations giving rise to achondroplasia, Marfan's syndrome, and Apert's syndrome are associated with increased paternal age.[20]

More recently, transgenic mouse models have been developed that facilitate assessing mutation frequency for the transgene in any tissue and at any age. Two transgenic models have been developed that utilize shuttle vectors so that individual copies of the transgene can be isolated after being in the mouse and grown as single colonies in appropriate *E. coli* strains. Mutant transgenes are identified by plating the *E. coli* onto agarose with a chromogenic substrate or a selective agent. Both models use a component of the bacterial *lac* operon. Important information about mutation frequency and mutation spectra are being generated with these models. It has been shown in the *lacI* mouse model that the mutation frequency increases approximately fourfold in DNA obtained from spleen as the animals age from birth to 24 months.[21] Similarly, the mutation frequency increases for the *lacZ* transgene in DNA obtained from liver.[22] Nevertheless, the mutation frequency was not observed to increase with age for the *lacZ* gene in DNA obtained from brain.[22] A paternal age effect on mutation frequency in the *lacI* gene has been observed such that a 10-fold increase was noted between 60-day-old mice and 28-month-old mice.[23] Although the data from transgenic mice largely support the theory of decreased genomic integrity with aging, it also appears that changes in genomic integrity may not occur in all tissues as an animal ages.

Dietary restriction is the one experimental intervention known to increase maximal life span in several species.[24] The increase in longevity is associated with a decrease in oxidative DNA damage[25,26] and mutations in the *Hprt* gene.[18] The association between extended life span and reduced DNA damage and mutation supports the somatic mutation and DNA damage theories of aging.

Data also exist that do not support the contribution of decreased genetic integrity to aging. For example, a recent analysis of the effect of dietary restriction on mutation frequency in the *lacI* transgenic mouse model found no significant difference between *ad libitum* and dietary-restricted animals at 6 and 12 months of age.[27] Notably, a 12-month-old mouse has not even begun to approach the median life span. Thus, it is not clear that a conclusion can be made about the effect of dietary restriction on the accumulation of mutations over a lifetime. Furthermore, most DNA repair deficiency syndromes are not associated with premature aging, with the exception of an increased susceptibility to carcinogenesis.

ASSESSING THE IMPACT OF ELEVATED DNA REPAIR ON AGING

The data concerning genetic integrity with old age are largely correlative. This, in combination with the variable results regarding genetic integrity with old age, has contributed to vacillations in enthusiasm for the theories involving genetic integrity in aging. One way to assess the contribution of genetic integrity to aging more directly would be to alter the levels of spontaneous DNA damage and mutation and determine the resulting impact on aging. The levels of DNA damage and mutation are in part a reflection of DNA repair activity. Thus, one potential way of altering spontaneous DNA damage and mutation levels would be to alter DNA repair activity. DNA repair could be reduced or enhanced to achieve altered levels of damage and mutation. We have chosen to try to enhance DNA repair because reductions in DNA repair seem more likely to result in substantial increases in pathology and anomalies that would render the assessment of aging more difficult. Furthermore, enhanced DNA repair might mimic the reduction in DNA damage and mutation observed in conjunction with dietary restriction and have an impact on life span, one quantitative measure of aging.

Most DNA repair mechanisms involve multiple proteins, and it is not presently known which steps are limiting in the pathways. Nevertheless, a few repair processes are performed by single proteins and as such would be more readily amenable to manipulation in a transgenic mouse system. O^6-methylguanine–DNA methyltransferase (MGMT) is a DNA repair protein that removes alkyl lesions at the O^6 position of guanine. It was selected to test the feasibility of overexpressing a DNA repair protein that would then have a biological impact using transgenic mouse technology. MGMT was chosen because (1) it acts in solo, (2) it directly reverses O^6-alkylguanine DNA lesions, (3) it acts stoichiometrically, (4) its activity has been well characterized in mammals, and (5) the lesion it repairs is highly mutagenic and carcinogenic.

The transgene consists of a portion of the human transferrin (TF) promoter, which has been shown to direct robust expression of various genes in brain and liver of transgenic mice.[28–30] The hMGMT cDNA was placed downstream of the promoter and was followed by an SV40 polyadenylation signal.[30] Transgenic mice were generated in two different strains of mice, C57BL/6J and C3HeB/FeJ.[30] The hMGMT transgene was shown to be expressed in brain and liver as expected from previous studies.[30,31] One line in the C3HeB/FeJ strain, however, fortuitously expressed the transgene in lung, and the transcript was slightly larger than expected based on the construction of the transgene[31] and from the transcript size in the seven other lines for which expression was assessed.

Immunohistochemistry was performed with monoclonal antibodies specific for hMGMT to determine which cell types in the various tissues were actually expressing the transgene. The hMGMT protein was detected in hepatocytes in liver, cells that are probably glial cells in brain, and cells in lung that are likely pulmonary interstitial macrophages. The unexpected expression in lung was probably the result of the transgene integrating into a locus that is normally expressed in pulmonary interstitial macrophages. In all cases, the hMGMT protein was found principally in the nucleus. Western blot analysis revealed the protein was the appropriate size in all expressing tissues.[30]

Because the spontaneous level of O^6-methylguanine (O^6mG) is so low it would be difficult to quantitatively measure a decrease of the lesion in DNA, we performed *in vitro* DNA repair assays using a substrate that is recognized and repaired by MGMT. A significant increase in MGMT activity was observed for tissues expressing the transgene.[30,31] Next, our transgenic animals were crossed with *lacI* transgenic mice, and the mutation frequencies in TF/MGMT double transgenic mice compared to single *lacI* transgenic mice with DNA obtained from liver of young adult male animals. No significant differences were found in the spontaneous mutation frequencies;[31] however, this is probably due to the fact that spontaneous O^6mG lesions occur so infrequently that they do not contribute substantially to mutation frequencies.

Male TF/MGMT transgenic mice were then treated with a direct-acting alkylating agent to determine whether the carcinogenic effects of induced O^6mG lesions were reduced in tissues expressing the transgene compared to C3HeB/FeJ control mice. The alkylating agent selected was methylnitrosourea (MNU) because its tumorigenic activity is well established and because it generates O^6mG lesions. Mice were treated monthly with MNU by tail vein injection beginning at 3 months of age until 175 mg/kg body weight had been delivered through a total of seven injections. The animals were euthanized when moribund or at 15 months of age.

A summary of the nonhepatic tumors resulting from MNU treatment is shown in TABLE 1. A significant difference was observed in the prevalence of bronchioloalveolar carcinoma between the untreated control C3HeB/FeJ mice and LC22I animals treated with MNU compared to MNU-treated C3HeB/FeJ and LC26I mice. A difference approaching significance ($p = 0.058$) was detected for gastric squamous cell carcinoma in animals treated with MNU compared with untreated control mice. Increases were also observed for small intestine adenocarcinoma and lymphosarcoma, although these were not significantly different from untreated controls. These data demonstrate that the MNU delivered was an effective carcinogenic agent.

TABLE 1. Prevalence of various tumors among MNU-treated male mice and control male mice

Tumor	Mouse line			
	C3HeB/FeJ	C3HeB/FeJ + MNU	LC22I + MNU	LC26I + MNU
Gastric squamous cell carcinoma	0	41	29	30
Small intestine adenoma	10	24	19	17
Bronchioloalveolar carcinoma[a]	0	18	0	33
Lymphosarcoma	0	12	14	15
Total number of animals[b]	10	17	21	46

NOTE: Prevalence is expressed as the percent animals bearing the tumor.
[a]Denotes a tumor type for which a significant difference in prevalence was detected.
[b]Total number of animals equals tumor-bearing and tumor free.

TABLE 2. Prevalence of hepatocellular carcinoma in MNU-treated mice compared to untreated control mice

	C3HeB/FeJ	C3HeB/FeJ + MNU	LC22I + MNU	LC26I + MNU
Hepatocellular carcinoma	60	12	0	11
Total number of animals[a]	10	17	21	46

NOTE: Prevalence is expressed as percent of animals displaying the tumor.
[a]Total number of animals equals tumor-bearing plus tumor-free animals.

TABLE 3. Prevalence of spontaneous hepatocellular carcinoma

	C3HeB/FeJ	LC22I	LC26I	LC28I
Hepatocellular carcinoma	60	19	18	13
Total number of animals[a]	10	31	22	16

NOTE: Prevalence is expressed as the percent of animals bearing the tumor.
[a]Total number of animals equals tumor-bearing plus tumor-free animals.

One unexpected result was the reduction in hepatocellular carcinoma observed in male MNU-treated mice compared to control animals (TABLE 2). Without MNU treatment the prevalence of hepatocellular carcinoma was 60% in untreated C3HeB/FeJ male mice; however, C3HeB/FeJ, LC22I, and LC26I mice treated with MNU displayed a hepatocellular carcinoma prevalence of ≤12% ($p = 0.001$). Another surprising result was the observed reduction in spontaneous hepatocellular carcinoma in each of three independent transgenic lines (TABLE 3). Because MGMT activity is relatively high in liver in nontransgenic mice and the spontaneous occurrence of O^6mG is low, we expected that there was sufficient MGMT activity to counteract spontaneous O^6mG lesions in liver and did not consider that alkylation damage might contribute to spontaneous hepatocellular carcinoma. Indeed, the level of

TABLE 4. Prevalence of hepatocellular carcinoma in 15–16- and 28–31-month-old mice

Line	15–16 months old	Total No. animals[a]	28–31 months old	Total No. animals
Nontransgenic	50%	10	56%	16
LC22I	10%	10	58%	12
LC26I	30%	10	In progress	12

NOTE: Prevalence is expressed as the percent of tumor-bearing animals.
[a]Total number of animals is the number of tumor-bearing and tumor-free animals.

TABLE 5. Proportion of animals with probable cause of death due to hepatocellular carcinoma in longitudinal life span study

	Nontransgenic	LC22I	LC26I
Hepatocellular carcinoma	13 (35%)	16 (46%)	16 (52%)
Total number of animals	37	35	31

O^6mG in liver of C3HeB mice is not different from that in a nonsusceptible strain such as C57BL/6.[32,33] There are several possible explanations for the reduced spontaneous hepatocellular carcinoma in male C3HeB/FeJ mice. First, alkylation damage is not adequately repaired and does contribute to tumorigenesis in this strain. Second, accessibility to O^6mG lesions may be limited, and overexpression of MGMT corrects the limitation through mass action. Third, hMGMT may have a greater effective repair activity than murine MGMT. Fourth, MGMT may have as yet undetermined substrates or additional activities. Fifth, the TF promoter may compete for transcription factors, which in turn impacts the expression of genes involved in increased susceptibility to hepatocellular carcinoma. Sixth, the immune system may have been altered such that removal of transformed liver cells is improved. Regardless of the mechanism, a larger fraction of male animals remain free of hepatocellular carcinoma for an extended time when MGMT is overexpressed, thereby improving the health span of the animals.

The reduced occurrence of a normally high-frequency tumor presented the opportunity to test whether life span would be correspondingly affected. Accordingly, a longitudinal life span study was initiated, and an adjunct cross-sectional study was begun, both exclusively using male animals. The first cross-sectional study was performed on 15-month-old animals and supported the previous finding of reduced hepatocellular carcinoma at this age (TABLE 4). Notably, the prevalence of hepatocellular carcinoma was similar among transgenic and control mice approximately 30 months old (TABLE 4), thereby indicating that the protection from hepatocellular carcinoma afforded to the transgenic mice was not sustained. The longitudinal study is still in progress, but the current Kaplan-Meier estimate of the survival curve is shown in FIGURE 1. No significant differences in survival curves have been detected at this time. Furthermore, the preliminary results suggest that the prevalence of hepatocellular carcinoma is not reduced in the transgenic mice at the end of their natural lives (TABLE 5).

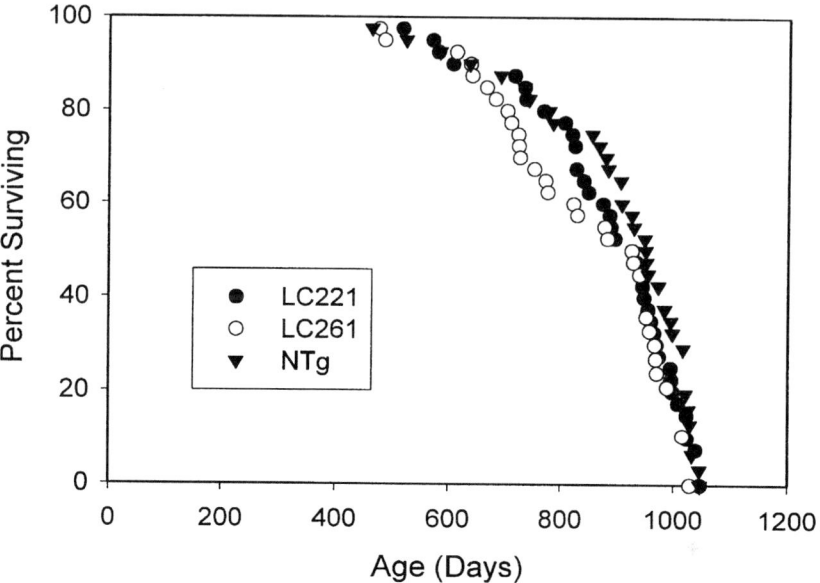

FIGURE 1. Survival curves for two transgenic C3HeB/FeJ transgenic lines and nontransgenic littermates. No significant differences have been observed between any of the mouse lines. LC22I and LC26I refer to two independent transgenic lines. NTg refers to nontransgenic littermates.

SUMMARY

Transgenic mice in the C3HeB inbred strain have been generated that have elevated expression of MGMT in brain and liver, and in lung of one line. The protein is of an appropriate size and is predominantly localized in nuclei of expressing cells. Expression of the transgene correlates with a reduced prevalence of MNU-induced tumors in liver in two independent lines and in lung of one line that fortuitously expresses in this tissue. Spontaneous hepatocellular carcinoma was reduced in three independent lines expressing the transgene in liver at 15 months of age; however, the reduced tumor prevalence was not observed at 30 months of age. Furthermore, a substantial number of transgenic and nontransgenic animals in the longitudinal study appear to die from the hepatocellular carcinoma. No significant impact on life span has been observed in conjunction with delayed onset of hepatocellular carcinoma.

ACKNOWLEDGMENTS

It is a pleasure to thank Kim Hildreth, Traci Reddick, Vivan Diaz, and Jay Cox for outstanding technical assistance. This publication was made possible by Grants ES05798 from the National Institute of Environmental Health Sciences, NIH, AG13560 from the National Institute of Aging, NIH, and AG13319 from the National Institute of Aging, NIH for the Nathan Shock Center for Excellence in Basic Biology of Aging at The University of Texas Health Science Center at San Antonio. The contents of this manuscript are solely the responsibility of the authors and do not necessarily represent the official views of the NIEHS, NIA, or VAHCS.

REFERENCES

1. FAILLA, G. 1958. The aging process and carcinogensis. Ann. N.Y. Acad. Sci. **71:** 1124–1135.
2. SZILARD, L. 1959. On the nature of the aging process. Proc. Natl. Acad. Sci. USA **45:** 30–45.
3. HARMON, D. 1962. Role of free radicals in mutation, cancer, aging and maintenance of life. Rad. Res. **16:** 753–763.
4. ALEXANDER, P. 1967. The role of DNA lesions in processes leading to aging in mice. Symp. Soc. Exp. Biol. **21:** 29–50.
5. STEVENSON, K.G. & H.J. CURTIS. 1961. Chromosomal aberrations in irradiated and nitrogen mustard treated mice. Radiat. Res. **15:** 744–784.
6. MARTIN, G.M., A.C. SMITH, D.J. KETTERER, et al. 1985. Increased chromosomal aberrations in first metaphases of cells isolated from the kidneys of aged mice. Isr. J. Med. **21:** 296–301.
7. DUTKOWSKI, R.T., R. LESH, L. STAIANO-COICO, et al. 1985. Increased chromosomal instability in lymphocytes from elderly humans. Mut. Res. **149:** 505–512.
8. PRIEUR, M., A. ACHKAR, A. AURIAS, et al. 1988. Acquired chromosome rearrangements in human lymphocytes: effect of aging. Hum. Genet. **79:** 147–150.
9. PINCHERIRA, J., C. GALLO, M. BRAVO, et al. 1993. G2 repair and aging: influence of donor age on chromosomal aberrations in human lymphocytes. Mut. Res. **295:** 55–62.
10. GANGULY, B.B. 1993. Cell division, chromosomal damage and micronucleus formation in peripheral lymphocytes of healthy donors: related to donor's age. Mut. Res. **295:** 135–148.
11. TUCKER, J.D., D.A. LEE, M.J. RAMSEY, et al. 1994. On the frequency of chromosome exchanges in a control population measured by chromosome painting. Mut. Res. **313:** 193–202.
12. KING, C.M., E.S. GILLESPIE, P.G. MCKENNA & Y.A. BARNETT. 1994. An investigation of mutation as a function of age in humans. Mut. Res. **316:** 79–90.
13. GUTTENBACH, M., B. KORSCHORZ, U. BERNTHALER, et al. 1995. Sex chromosome loss and aging: in situ hybridization studies on human interphase nuclei. Am. J. Hum. Genet. **57:** 1143–1150.
14. MORLEY, A.A., S. COX & R. HOLLIDAY. 1982. Human lymphocytes resistant to 6-thioguanine increase with age. Mech. Ageing Dev. **19:** 21–26.
15. TRAINOR, K.J., D.J. WIGMORE, A. CHRYSOSTOMOU, et al. 1984. Mutation frequency in human lymphocytes increases with age. Mech. Ageing Dev. **27:** 83–86.
16. MARTIN, G.M., C.E. OGBURN, L.M. COLGIN, et al. 1996. Somatic mutations are frequent and increase with age in human kidney epithelial cells. Hum. Mol. Genet. **5:** 215–221.
17. INAMIZU, T., N. KINOHARA, M.P. CHANG & T. MAKINODAN. 1986. Frequency of 6-thioguanine T-cells is inversely related to the declining T-cell activities in aging mice. Proc. Natl. Acad. Sci. USA **83:** 2488–2491.
18. DEMPSEY, J.L., M. PFEIFFER & A.A. MORELY. 1993. Effect of dietary restriction on in vivo somatic mutation in mice. Mut. Res. **291:** 141–145.
19. HOOK, E.B. 1981. Rates of chromosome abnormalities at different maternal ages. Obstet. Gynecol. **58:** 282–285.
20. VOGEL, F. & R. RATHENBERG. 1975. Spontaneous mutation in man. Adv. Hum. Genet. **4:** 223–318.
21. LEE, A.T., C. DESIMONE, A. CERAMI & R. BUCALA. 1994. Comparative analysis of DNA mutations in lacI transgenic mice with age. FASEB J. **8:** 545–550.

22. DOLLE, M.E.T., H. GIESE, C.L. HOPKINS, et al. 1997. Rapid accumulation of genome rearrangements in liver but not in brain of old mice. Nature Genet. **17:** 431–434.
23. WALTER, C.A., G.W., INTANO, J.R. MCCARREY, et al. 1998. Mutation frequency declines during spermatogenesis in young mice but increases in old mice. Proc. Natl. Acad. Sci. USA **95:** 10015–10019.
24. MASORO, E.J. 1988. Food restriction in rodents: an evaluation of its role in the study of aging. J. Gerontol. **43:** B59–B64.
25. CHUNG, M.H., H. KASAI, S. NISHIMURA & B.P. YU. 1992. Protection of DNA damage by dietary restriction. Free Rad. Biol. Med. **12:** 523–525.
26. SOHAL, R.S., S. AGARWAL, M. CANDAS, et al. 1994. Effect of age and caloric restriction on DNA oxidative damage in different tissue of C57BL/6 mice. Mech. Ageing Dev. **76:** 215–224.
27. STUART, G.R., O. YOSHIMITSU, J.G. DE BOER, & B.W. GLICKMAN. 2000. No change in spontaneous mutation frequency or specificity in dietary restricted mice. Carcinogenesis **21:** 317–319.
28. ADRIAN, G.S., B.H. BOWMAN, D.C. HERBERT, et al. 1990. Human transferrin: expression and iron modulation of chimeric genes in transgenic mice. J. Biol. Chem. **265:** 13344–13350.
29. BOWMAN, B.H., L. JANSEN, F. YANG, et al. 1995. Discovery of a brain promoter from the human transferrin gene and its utilization for development of transgenic mice that express human apolipoprotein E alleles. Proc. Natl. Acad. Sci. USA **92:** 12115–12119.
30. WALTER, C.A., J. LU, M. BHAKTA, S. MITRA, et al. 1993. Brain and liver targeted overexpression of O^6-methylguanine-DNA methyltransferase in transgenic mice. Carcinogenesis **14:** 1537–1543.
31. ZHOU, Z.-Q., D. MANGUINO, G.W. INTANO, et al. 2000. Spontaneous hepatocellular carcinoma is reduced in transgenic mice overexpressing human O^6-methylguanine-DNA methyltransferase. Submitted.
32. WASHINGTON, W.J., R.S. FOOTE, W.C. DUNN, et al. 1989. Age-dependent modulation of tissue-specific repair activity for 3-methyladenine and O^6-methylguanine in DNA in inbred mice. Mech. Ageing Dev. **48:** 43–52.
33. LINDAMOOD III, C., M.A. BEDELL, K.C. BILINGS, et al. 1983 O^6-alkylguanine alkyl receptor protein activity in hepatocytes of C3H and C57BL mice during dimethylnitrosamine exposure. Chem.-Biol. Interact. **45:** 381–385.

Inhibition Mechanisms of Bioflavonoids Extracted from the Bark of *Pinus maritima* on the Expression of Proinflammatory Cytokines

KYUNG-JOO CHO,[a] CHANG-HYUN YUN,[a] LESTER PACKER,[b] AND AN-SIK CHUNG[a,c]

[a]*Department of Biological Sciences, Korea Advanced Institute of Science and Technology, Kusong-dong 373-1, Yusong-gu, Taejon, 305-701, Korea*

[b]*Department of Molecular Pharmacology and Toxicology, University of Southern California, Los Angeles, California 90089-9121, USA*

ABSTRACT: The effect of bioflavonoids extracted from the bark of *Pinus maritima*, Pycnogenol (PYC), on gene expression of the proinflammatory cytokines interleukin-1β (IL-1β) and interleukin-2 (IL-2) were investigated in RAW 264.7 cells and Jurkat E6.1 cells, respectively. PYC exerted strong scavenging activities against reactive oxygen species (ROS) generated by H_2O_2 in RAW 264.7. *In situ* ELISA, immunoblot analysis, and competitive RT-PCR demonstrated that pretreatment of LPS-stimulated RAW 264.7 cells with PYC dose-dependently reduced both the production of IL-1β and its mRNA levels. Furthermore, in the same cells, PYC blocked the activation of nuclear factor κB (NF-κB) and activator protein-1 (AP-1), two major transcription factors centrally involved in IL-1β gene expression. Concordantly, pretreatment of the cells with PYC abolished the LPS-induced IκB degradation. We also investigated the effect of PYC on IL-2 gene expression in phorbol 12-myristate 13acetate plus ionomycin (PMA/Io)-stimulated human T-cell line Jurkat E6.1. PYC inhibited the PMA/Io-induced IL-2 mRNA expression. However, as demonstrated in a reporter gene assay system, the mechanism of IL-2 gene transcriptional regulation by PYC was different from the regulation of IL-1β. PYC inhibited both NF-AT and AP-1 chloramphenicol acetyltransferase (CAT) activities in transiently transfected Jurkat E6.1, but not NF-κB CAT activity. We also found that PYC can destabilize PMA/Io-induced IL-2 mRNA by posttranscriptional regulation. All these results suggest that bioflavonoids can be useful therapeutic agents in treating many inflammatory, autoimmune, and cardiovascular diseases based on its diverse action mechanisms.

KEYWORDS: Pycnogenol; Anti-inflammation; NF-κB; NF-AT; AP-1; IL-1; IL-2

There is increasing interest in the biological activities of plant extracts, especially that obtained from the bark of the French maritime pine, *Pinus maritima*. Pycnogenol (PYC) is a unique mixture of phenols and polyphenols, broadly divided into monomers such as catechin, epicatechin, and taxifolin and condensed flavonoids

---

[c]Address for correspondence: Dr. An-Sik Chung, Department of Biological Sciences, Korea Advanced Institute of Science and Technology, Kusong-dong 373-1, Yusong-gu, Taejon, 305-701, Korea. Voice: 82-42-869-2625; fax: 82-42-869-2610.
aschung@sorak.kaist.ac.kr.

such as procyanidin B1, B3, B7, and others. PYC also contains phenolic acids such as caffeic, ferulic, and *p*-hydroxybenzoic acid as minor constituents.[1] Several studies indicate that PYC participates in the cellular antioxidant network as indicated by its ability to prolong the lifetime of the ascorbyl radical[2] and to protect endogenous vitamin E[3] and glutathione[4] in human endothelial cells from oxidative stress. PYC also modulates nitric oxide metabolism in stimulated macrophages by inhibiting both iNOS mRNA expression and its activity.[5] However, little is known about the anti-inflammatory property of PYC.

During the inflammatory process, disruption of local tissue function induced by an inflammatory exudate was inevitably accompanied by margination and firm adhesion of leukocytes to the vascular endothelium, culminating in accumulation of large numbers of migrating leukocytes in the edematous extravascular tissues. The presence of these cells may add to tissue damage either by releasing degradative enzymes or by a variety of other mediators that have been assigned "proinflammatory" functions.[6]

Interleukin-1 (IL-1) is a multifunctional cytokine that is responsible for mediating a variety of processes in host defense, inflammation, and response to injury. IL-1 is produced by macrophages and many other cell types by the actions of various stimuli such as viruses, lipopolysaccharides, and phorbol esters. Biologically active IL-1β is a 17.5-kDa protein resulting from cleavage of an inactive 31-kDa proIL-1β. IL-1β has been shown to act as a growth factor for a variety of cell types including fibroblasts and keratinocytes.[7] Various studies have demonstrated that a LPS-responsive enhancer region is located between positions -3134 and -2729 in the IL-1β gene promoter, which includes the potential binding sites for NF-κB and AP-1.[8] Both NF-κB and AP-1 are implicated in the inducible expression of a variety of genes in response to oxidative stress.[9] Reactive oxygen and nitrogen species are commonly produced during the inflammatory response and are involved in the production of inflammatory cytokines.[10] Because IL-1 is a highly proinflammatory cytokine, agents that reduce the production and/or activity of IL-1 might be of a particular pharmacological and clinical interest.

Effective immune responses against pathogens require the migration of diverse sets of lymphoid cells into tissues, which occurs both under homeostatic conditions and during inflammation associated with infection. Most mature naïve T cells recirculate from the blood into secondary lymphoid organs. This recirculation provides the naïve T cell access to the organs of the body that collect antigen from epithelial surfaces, somatic tissues, and blood. Once T cells respond to antigen, become activated, proliferate, and eventually develop into memory cells, they exhibit different trafficking behaviors, preferentially homing to extralymphoid sites of inflammation. The interaction of T cells with antigens triggers a complex signaling cascade that switches on the gene program leading to T-cell activation. During this process, T cells express the autocrine growth factor interleukin-2 (IL-2).[11] IL-2 gene, which is highly regulated and exhibits virtually no basal levels of expression in resting cells, is rapidly induced upon T-cell activation. IL-2 transcription is controlled by a number of *cis*-acting elements directly upstream of the promotor and mainly controlled by a 326-bp upstream region of the transcription start site. The promotor consists of several *cis*-acting sites for transcription factors, such as NF-AT, AP-1, NF-κB, Oct, and CD28 response elements to which each transcription factor binds cooperatively and induces maximal IL-2 transcription.[12]

In addition to transcriptional regulation, the IL-2 mRNA level can be regulated posttranscriptionally. IL-2 has a short half-life, and its level rapidly increased after stimulation with mitogen such as PMA, followed by an equally rapid decline.[13] A group of AU-rich elements found in the 3′-untranslated region (3′-UTR) of IL-2 mRNA has been known to be a target for rapid and selective degradation.[14] Both a transcription inhibitor, actinomycin D (Act D), and a translation inhibitor, cycloheximide (CHX), have been reported to inhibit IL-2 mRNA degradation by interfering with the transcription and translation of the degradative machinery, respectively. As well as its inhibitory effect on IL-2 transcription, cyclosporin A, a well-known immunosuppressive drug, has been known to lead to a rapid destabilization of IL-2 mRNA, as well as its inhibitory effect on IL-2 transcription.[13] In spite of the importance of posttranscriptional regulation of cytokine genes in inflammatory diseases, however, little is known about the effect of bioflavonoids on cytokine gene stability. Therefore, in this study, the mode of action of PYC on LPS-induced IL-1β gene expression and PMA/Io-induced IL-2 gene expression has been studied.

MATERIALS AND METHODS

Reagents

LPS (from *Escherichia coli* serotype 0127:B8) and PMA were obtained from Sigma (St. Louis, MO). Fetal bovine serum (FBS), Hank's buffered salt solution (HBSS), DMEM, and RPMI 1640 were purchased from GIBCO-BRL (Grand Island, NY). 2′,7′-dichlorofluorescin-diacetate was obtained from Fluka (Germany), and PCR reagents were from Promega (Madison, WI). Rabbit anti-murine IL-1β antibody was purchased from Pepro Tech EC Ltd (London, England). Anti-murine IκBα antibody was obtained from Santa Cruz Biotechnology Inc. (Santa Cruz, CA). Pine bark extract (Pycnogenol) was a gift from Horphag Research Ltd. (Guernsey, FRA).

Cell Culture

The murine cell lines of monocyte-macrophages RAW 264.7 (ATCC TIB 71) and human T lymphocyte Jurkat E6.1 (ATCC TIB 152) were maintained at 37°C, 5% CO_2, respectively, in DMEM and RPMI 1640 containing 10% heat-inactivated FBS and 50 μg/ml gentamicin. All experiments were performed under conditions in which over 85% cell viability was maintained in all treatment groups, measured by using a WST-1 assay kit (Cat. No. 1 644 807, Boehringer Mannheim, Germany).

DCFH-DA Assay

The ROS-scavenging activity of PYC was measured using the oxidant-sensitive fluorescent probe 2′,7′-dichlorofluorescin diacetate (DCFH-DA). 2′,7′-Dichlorofluorescin (DCFH) converted from DCFH-DA by deacetylase within the cells is oxidized by a variety of intracellular ROS to 2′,7′-dichlorofluorescein (DCF), a highly fluorescent compound. RAW 264.7 cells (1×10^6 cells/ml) were preincubated with PYC (1, 5, 10, 20, or 50 μg/ml) in HBSS for 15 minutes at 37°C in a water bath. Then, 20 μM DCFH-DA was added, and an additional 15-min incubation was performed. After stimulation with 250 μM H_2O_2 for 10 minutes, the relative green DCF fluorescence within living cells was measured using a flow cytometer (FACS caliber, Becton Dickinson, USA). There was no interference between PYC and DCFH-DA.

Detection of Intracellular proIL-1β Using in Situ ELISA

After LPS stimulation, RAW 264.7 cells were washed with 200 µl of assay buffer (PBS containing 0.05% BSA and 0.02% sodium azide) and fixed with 1.5% paraformaldehyde for 15 minutes on ice. One hundred microliters of permeabilization buffer (PBS containing 0.1% saponin and 0.05% sodium azide) was added to the wells and incubated for 30 minutes. Following the addition of rabbit anti-murine IL-1β antibody (2 µg/ml) for 30 minutes, cells were washed twice with the assay buffer and then incubated with 100 µl of goat anti-rabbit IgG antibody conjugated with alkaline phosphatase (Sigma) for 30 minutes. Samples were washed twice with PBS-0.05% Tween 20, and 100 µl of substrate (*p*-nitrophenylphosphate disodium) was added. The absorbance was read at 405 nm using an ELISA microplate reader (Molecular Devices, Sunnyvale, CA).

Preparation of DNA Competitor/Competitive RT-PCR

DNA competitor containing specific PCR primer sequences for IL-1β was constructed using a competitive DNA construction kit (TaKaRa Shuzo Co., Japan). The primer sequences from 5' to 3', designed for preparation of internal standard, are forward primer 5'-TGC AGA GTT CCC CAA CTG GTA CAT CGT ACG GTC ATC TGA CAC-3' and reverse primer 5'-GTG CTG CCT AAT GTC CCC TTG AAT CAG AGT TTC TGC GGC AGT TAA-3'. The PCR reaction was performed with 30 cycles of amplification (94°C for 30 sec, 60°C for 30 sec, and 72°C for 30 sec). To purify the amplified competitor, the excess primers and dNTPs were removed using SUPREC^{TM}-02 (TaKaRa).

RNA was isolated using Trizol reagent (Molecular Research Center, Cincinnati, OH) six hours after stimulating RAW 264.7 cells with LPS as described by the company's manual. One microgram of total RNA was reverse-transcribed into cDNA using a reverse transcriptase (BM). Twenty microliters of the RT mixture was incubated at 42°C for 90 min and then heated at 90°C for 10 min. Competitive PCR was performed in a 20-µl mixture containing 3 µl of RT product, 3 µl of DNA competitor (4.05×10^{11} copies/µl), 1 × reaction buffer, 250 µM dNTP, 1 µM of each primer, and 1 unit Taq DNA polymerase (TaKaRa) with the following oligonucleotide primers: 5'-TGC AGA GTT CCC CAA CTG GTA CAT C-3' and 5'-GTG CTG CCT AAT GTC CCC TTG AAT C-3'. After an initial denaturation for 2 min at 94°C, 30 cycles of amplification (55°C for 1 min, 72°C for 1.5 min, and 94°C for 1 min) were performed followed by a 10-min extension at 72°C. A 10-µl aliquot from each PCR reaction was electrophoresed in an 8% polyacrylamide gel and visualized by ethidium bromide staining. The relative IL-1β signal was normalized against the DNA competitor, and the data were expressed as the IL-1β/DNA competitor.

Electrophoretic Mobility Shift Assay (EMSA)

Cells were lysed with hypotonic buffer (10 mM HEPES and 1.5 mM $MgCl_2$, pH 7.5), and the nuclei were pelleted by centrifugation at $3,000 \times g$ for 5 min. Nuclear lysis was performed using a hypertonic buffer (30 mM HEPES, 1.5 mM $MgCl_2$,

450 mM KCl, 0.3 mM EDTA, 10% glycerol, 1 mM DTT, 1 mM phenylmethylsulfonyl fluoride (PMSF), 1 µg/ml of aprotinin, and 1 µg/ml of leupeptin). Following lysis, the samples were centrifuged at 13,000 × g for 10 minutes, and the supernatant was retained for use in the DNA-binding assay. Two double-stranded deoxyoligonucleotides were end-labeled with [γ-^{32}P]ATP. Nuclear extracts (7.5 µg) were incubated with poly (dI-dC) and ^{32}P-labeled DNA probe in binding buffer (100 mM KCl, 30 mM HEPES, 1.5 mM MgCl$_2$, 0.3 mM EDTA, 10% glycerol, 1 mM DTT, 1 mM PMSF, 1 µg/ml of aprotinin, and 1 µg/ml of leupeptin) for 15 min. DNA binding activity was separated from the free probe using 5% polyacrylamide gel in 0.5 × TBE buffer (44.5 mM Tris, 44.5 mM boric acid, and 1 mM EDTA). Following electrophoresis, the gel was dried and subjected to autoradiography.

Immunoblot Analysis of IL-1β and IκBα

Cytosolic proteins (10 µg) were separated by 10% SDS-PAGE, then electrotransfered to a nitrocellulose membrane (Amersham, UK). The nitrocellulose membrane was preincubated for 2 hours in PBS containing 0.05% Tween-20 and 3% gelatin at room temperature. The nitrocellulose membrane was then incubated with rabbit polyclonal IgG against IκBα, actin, or IL-1β followed by an incubation with horseradish peroxidase-conjugated anti-rabbit IgG antibody. Immunoreactive bands were visualized with the enhanced chemiluminescence reagents (Amersham).

Semiquantitative RT-PCR in Jurkat E6.1 Cells

Total RNA was isolated using Trizol reagent (MRC) after stimulating Jurkat E6.1 cells with PMA/Io (100 nM/0.5 µM) as described by the company's manual. RT-PCR was performed as described in the previous section on competitive RT-PCR in the absence of DNA competitor with the following oligonucleotide primers: IL-2 (product length, 496 bp), primer 1, 5'-CAA ACT CAC CAG GAT GCT CA-3'; primer 2, 5'-AGA GCC CCT AGG GCT TAC AA-3'. GAPDH (product length, 400 bp), primer 1, 5'-ACC CAG AAG ACT GTG GAT GG-3'; primer 2, 5'-TGA GCT TGA CAA AGT GGT CG-3'. The relative IL-2 levels were determined by normalization of the intensity of IL-2 mRNA signals against those obtained for GAPDH.

Transfection and CAT Assay

pGL2-promoter vectors (Promega) containing three copies of NF-κB, AP-1, NF-AT, and Oct-1 binding sequences were kindly provided by Dr. Han, and transient transfections were performed using a general DEAE-dextran method with slight modifications.[15] Jurkat E6.1 cells (3 × 10^7 cells) were transfected, divided into six groups, plated at 5 × 10^5 cells/ml on 100-mm tissue culture plates, and incubated for 23 hours. The transfectants were treated with or without PYC, and a half hour later PMA/Io (100 nM/0.5 µM) were added. Eighteen hours later, the cells were washed with ice-cold PBS, resuspended in 0.25 mM Tris (pH 7.8), and subjected to three cycles of freezing and thawing. The lysates were centrifuged (12,000 × g for 10 min at 4°C), and the supernatant was assayed for CAT activity by the thin-layer chromatography method.[15] For quantitative analysis of radioactivity, the amount of radioactivity was determined by an image analyzer (Phospho Imager, Molecular Dynamics, Sunnyvale, CA).

Statistical Analysis

One-way analysis of variance (ANOVA) followed by the Scheffé multiple-range test was used for statistical analysis. All values are expressed as mean ± standard deviation (SD). Differences were considered significant if $p < 0.05$.

RESULTS

Intracellular Radical Scavenging Activity of PYC in RAW 264.7 Macrophages

The intracellular radical scavenging activity of a given substance can be evaluated using a DCFH-DA assay. RAW 264.7 macrophages showed relatively low levels of basal fluorescence in the absence of H_2O_2 (FIG. 1). When cells were treated with 250 μM H_2O_2 for 10 min, a marked increase in the fluorescence was evident. However, the DCF fluorescence of H_2O_2-challenged macrophages decreased significantly in a dose-dependent manner as a result of the PYC pretreatment. At the highest PYC concentration, a 65% reduction in the DCF signal was shown compared to control cells.

Inhibition of proIL-1β Production in RAW 264.7 Cells

After synthesis, proIL-1β remains primarily cytosolic until it is cleaved and transported out of the cells. The amount of proIL-1β was measured using two different approaches, namely, ELISA and immunoblotting. As shown in FIGURE 2A, stimulation of macrophages with LPS strongly increased in proIL-1β production, whereas pretreatment of the cells with PYC (20 or 50 μg/ml) significantly inhibited the LPS-induced proIL-1β production by 25% and 40%, respectively. A similar result was obtained from the immunoblotting method, which clearly demonstrated that PYC dose-dependently counteracted the proIL-1β production in RAW 264.7 cells stimulated with LPS (FIG. 2B).

Inhibition of IL-1β mRNA Expression in RAW 264.7 Cells

Since pretreatment of macrophages with PYC resulted in a substantial decrease in the production of proIL-1β, it is of particular interest whether this effect is related to change in the level of gene transcription. In nonstimulated macrophages, there was no detectable gene expression of IL-1β. After stimulation of RAW 264.7 cells with LPS for 6 hours, the expressional level of IL-1β significantly increased. As shown in the ELISA and immunoblot experiments, pretreatment of LPS-stimulated macrophages with PYC (1, 10, or 50 μg/ml) resulted in a dose-dependent decrease in IL-1β mRNA levels (FIG. 3).

Inhibitions of Both NF-κB and AP-1 Activations in RAW 264.7 Cells

The induction of proinflammatory cytokines such as IL-1β is partially controlled through the two transcription factors NF-κB and AP-1. Therefore, we investigated whether the observed inhibition of LPS-mediated IL-1β mRNA expression and its production were related to changes in NF-κB and AP-1 DNA binding activity. The stimulation of RAW 264.7 cells with LPS resulted in marked increases in both NF-κB and AP-1 binding to their cognate sites, which could be visualized as distinct

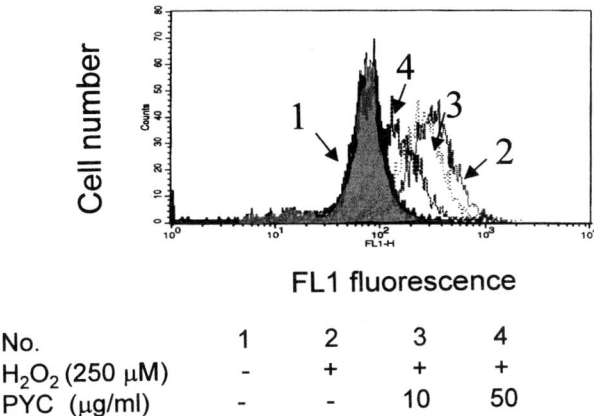
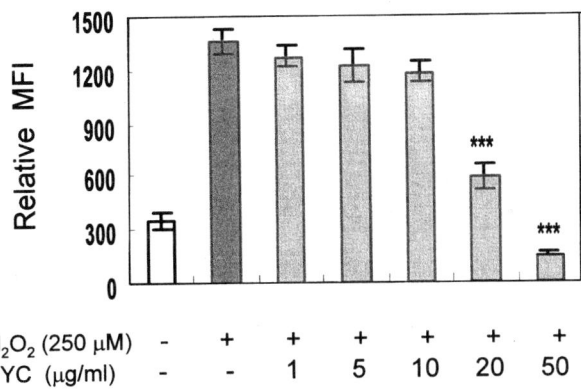

FIGURE 1. Inhibition of H_2O_2-induced ROS generation by PYC in RAW 264.7 macrophages. Cells were pretreated with PYC (0–50 μg/ml) after stimulation with 250 μM H_2O_2 for 10 min; the relative mean fluorescence intensity (MFI) was measured by using a FACS calibur (BD). Fluorescence histograms (**A**) are shown for untreated cells (1), H_2O_2-treated cells (2), and cells pretreated with PYC (10 or 50 μg/ml) before the treatment of H_2O_2 (3 or 4). (**B**) Each bar represents the mean ± SD of three independent determinations (*** $p < 0.001$).

bands in the EMSA. NF-κB and AP-1 binding were specific as demonstrated by competition assays with 100-fold molar excess amounts of ^{32}P-unlabeled NF-κB or AP-1 probes, respectively. PYC at 10 or 50 μg/ml strongly inhibited the specific binding of NF-κB and AP-1 to their consensus DNA sequences (FIG. 4A).

Since LPS-mediated activation of NF-κB is associated with the hyperphosphorylation of IκBα as well as its subsequent degradation, the cytosolic amount of IκBα was also investigated. When RAW 264.7 cells were activated with LPS, IκB largely

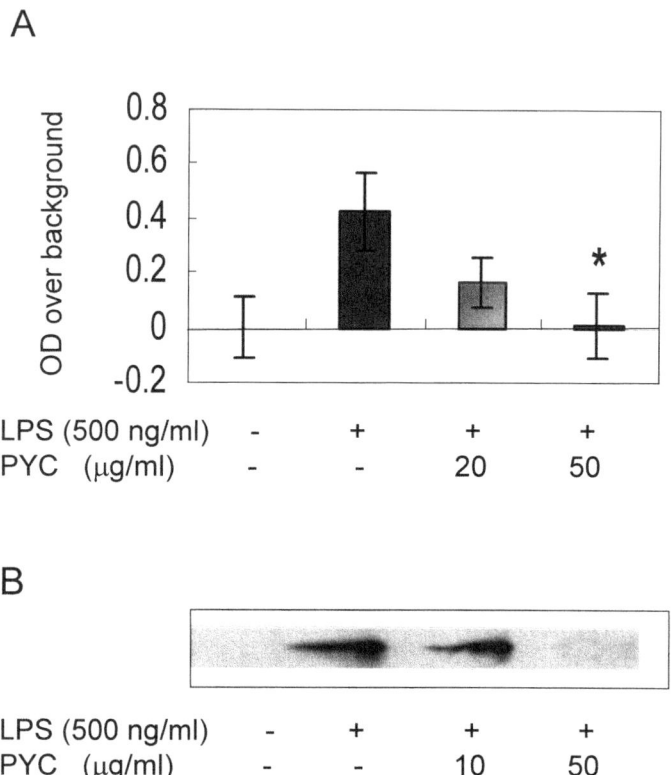

FIGURE 2. Effect of PYC on proIL-1b production in RAW 264.7 cells. Cells (5×10^5 cells/ml) were plated in a 96-well microtiter plate (**A**) or 100-mm culture plates (**B**) pretreated with PYC (20 and 50 μg/ml) for 30 min and then stimulated with LPS (500 ng/ml) for 6 hr. After LPS stimuation, the production of proIL-1β was measured using *in situ* ELISA (**A**) or immunoblotting (**B**) (* $p < 0.05$).

disappeared from cytosolic fraction. As shown in FIGURE 4B, however, pretreatment of RAW 264.7 cells with PYC abolished the LPS-induced IκB degradation.

Effects of PYC on IL-2 mRNA Expression and Its Stability

In nonstimulated Jurkat E6.1, there was no detectable gene expression of IL-2. From 3 to 24 hours of stimulation of Jurkat E6.1 with PMA/Io, the expression level of IL-2 increased time-dependently, and at 7 hours the level of IL-2 mRNA peaked (data not shown). However, pretreatment of PYC (20 or 50 μg/ml) or EGCG (50 or 100 μM) remarkably decreased the IL-2 mRNA level (FIG. 5).

To better understand the molecular mechanisms by which PYC inhibits IL-2 gene expression, we studied the posttranscriptional effect of PYC on IL-2 gene expression. After stimulation of Jurkat E6.1 with PMA/Io for 3 hours, the IL-2 mRNA level was detectable. With removal of PMA/Io after a 3-hour stimulation, however, the IL-2 mRNA level decreased time-dependently until 4 hours, after which time the level

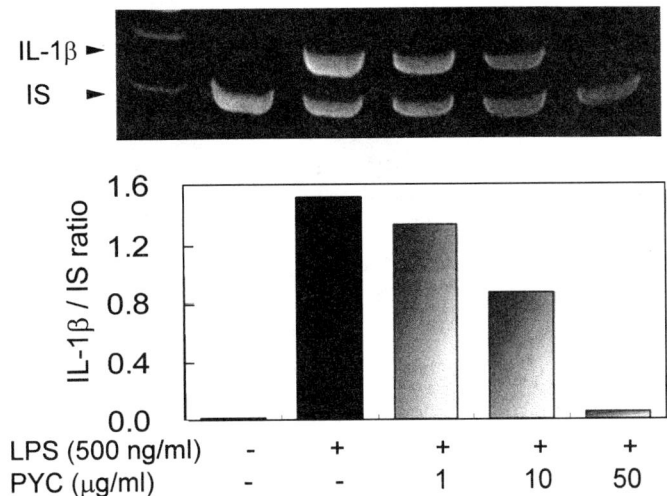

FIGURE 3. Inhibition of IL-1b mRNA expression by PYC in RAW 264.7 macrophages. Cells (5×10^6 cells) were pretreated with PYC (1, 10, or 50 μg/ml) for 30 min, then stimulated with LPS for 6 hr. Total RNA was isolated and reverse-transcribed as described in MATERIALS AND METHODS. The *upper panel* shows a gel photograph of PCR-amplified cDNA from IL-1β and DNA competitor (IS). The *lower panel* shows the densitometric analysis of the gel photograph. One representative experiment of at least three is presented.

of IL-2 mRNA declined to a low steady state (data not shown). Furthermore, in the presence of CHX or Act D, IL-2 mRNA was superinduced, and these levels were maintained up to 4 hours after removal of PMA/Io. When PYC (but not EGCG) was co-treated with Act D, the level of IL-2 mRNA decreased again (FIG. 6). This result suggests that destabilization of IL-2 mRNA may be one of the IL-2 gene regulation mechanisms of PYC.

Effects of PYC on the Activities of NF-κB, NF-AT, AP-1, and Oct-1

To evaluate the impact of PYC-mediated modulation of transcription factor DNA binding activity on gene transactivation, the effects of PYC on the following reporter gene constructs p(NF-κB)$_3$-CAT, p(NF-AT)$_3$-CAT, p(AP-1)$_3$-CAT, and p(Oct-1)$_3$-CAT were investigated. PYC inhibited NF-AT and AP-1 promoter activities in a dose-dependent manner (FIG. 7). PYC had no effect on NF-κB promoter activity nor on Oct-1 promoter activity, which coincided with the results of EMSA (data not shown). On the other hand, EGCG (20, 50, or 100 μM) can inhibit NF-κB DNA binding activity as well as that of NF-AT and AP-1 (data not shown), indicating a different regulation mechanism of PCY from that of EGCG.

DISCUSSION

Cytokines such as IL-1 and IL-2 have beneficial or detrimental effects, depending on the context and amount in which they are produced. During infection, they are

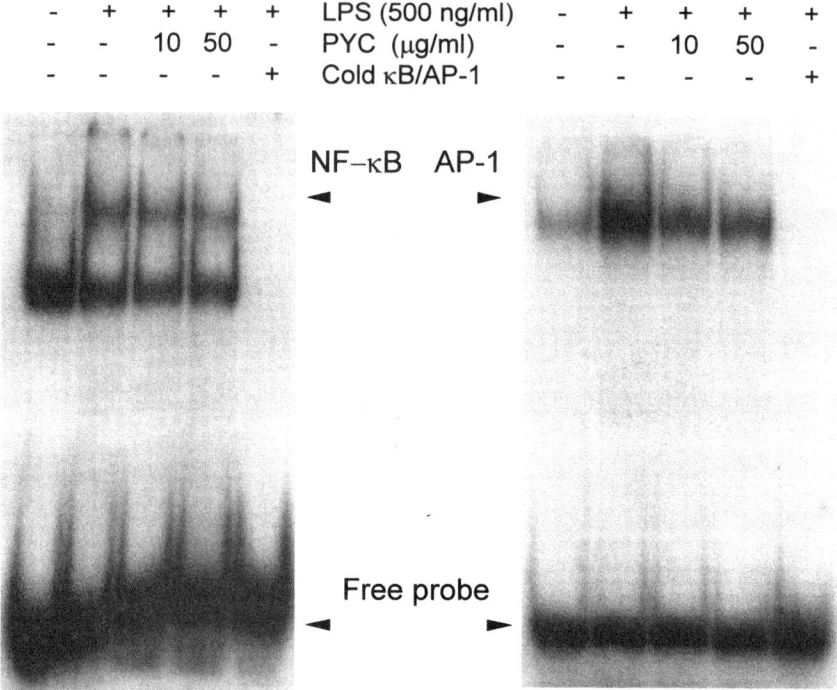

FIGURE 4A. Inhibitory effect of PYC on the DNA-binding activities of NF-kB and AP-1 in RAW 264.7 macrophages. Cells (5×10^6) were pretreated with PYC for 30 min, then stimulated with LPS (500 ng/ml) for 90 min. Nuclear extracts were isolated and incubated with the ^{32}P-labeled oligonucleotides containing either NF-κB or AP-1 consensus recognition motif. One representative experiment of at least three is presented.

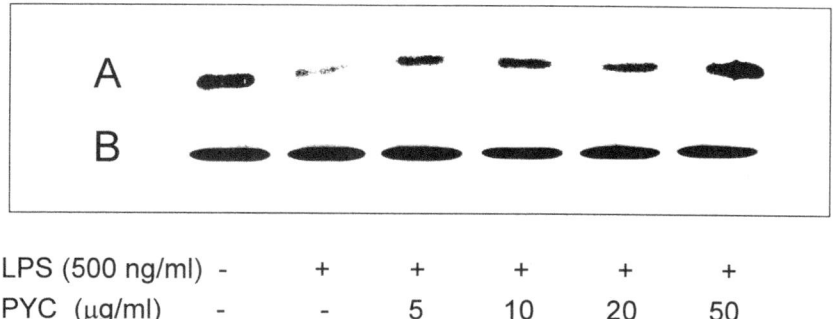

FIGURE 4B. Inhibition of the degradation of IkBa by PYC in LPS-stimulated RAW 264.7 macrophages. Cells (5×10^6) were pretreated with PYC for 30 min, then stimulated with LPS (500 ng/ml) for 90 min. Cytosolic extracts (10 µg) were prepared, then subjected to immunoblot analysis using an anti-IκBα antibody (**A**) or an anti-actin antibody (**B**). One representative experiment of at least three is presented.

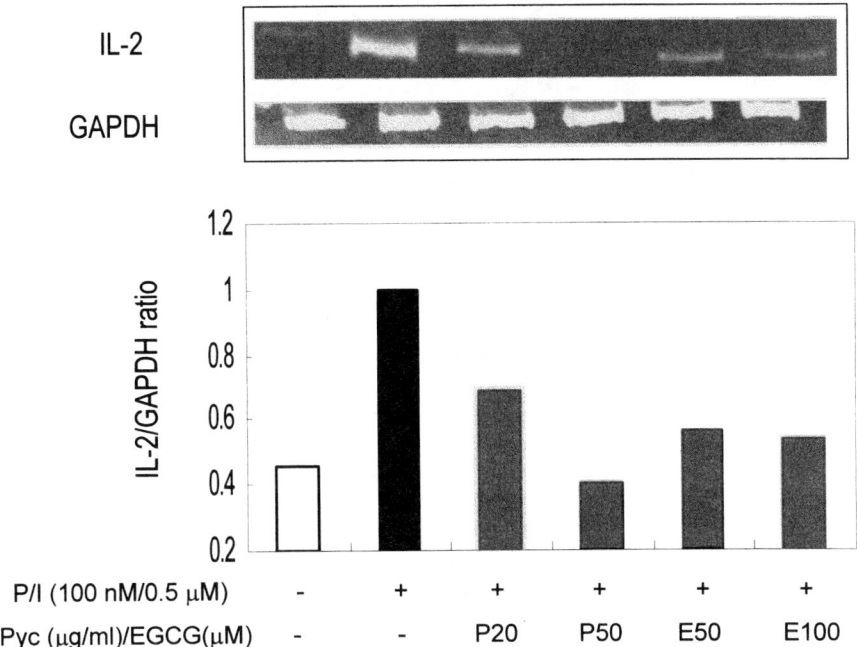

FIGURE 5. Inhibition of IL-2 mRNA expression by PYC in Jurkat E6.1 T lymphocytes. Cells (5×10^6) were pretreated with PYC (20 or 50 μg/ml) or EGCG (50 or 100 μM) for 30 min, then stimulated with PMA/Io for 7 hr. Total RNA was isolated and reverse-transcribed as described in MATERIALS AND METHODS. The *upper* and *lower panels* show gel photographs of PCR-amplified cDNAs from IL-2 or GAPDH and the densitometric analysis of the gel photograph, respectively. One representative experiment of at least three is presented.

mostly beneficial but in the case of cancer and chronic inflammatory diseases, they may be detrimental. Therefore, cellular manipulation of the production of proinflammatory cytokines such as IL-1 and IL-2 are of importance in determining the outcome of the inflammatory response.[16] In this study, it has been demonstrated for the first time that the complex mixture of bioflavonoids extracted from the bark of *Pinus maritima* significantly affected both IL-1β and IL-2 gene expressions, respectively, in RAW 364.7 cells and Jurkat E6.1, which are possibly the best characterized cell lines in terms of cytokine production.

In H_2O_2-challenged macrophages, PYC exerted a potent dose-dependent radical scavenging activity. These findings in RAW 264.7 cells are in agreement with previous *in vitro* studies utilizing ESR techniques and suggest that PYC is an efficient hydroxyl and superoxide anion scavenger.[17] Under the investigated conditions, PYC, as a mixture, displayed greater antioxidant activity than its purified catechin component did individually (data not shown), indicating that various components of PYC may interact synergistically. Especially procyanidin dimers and trimers, major constituents of PYC, have been recently shown to have strong antioxidant properties particularly in the aqueous phase.[18] These antioxidant properties of PYC might also

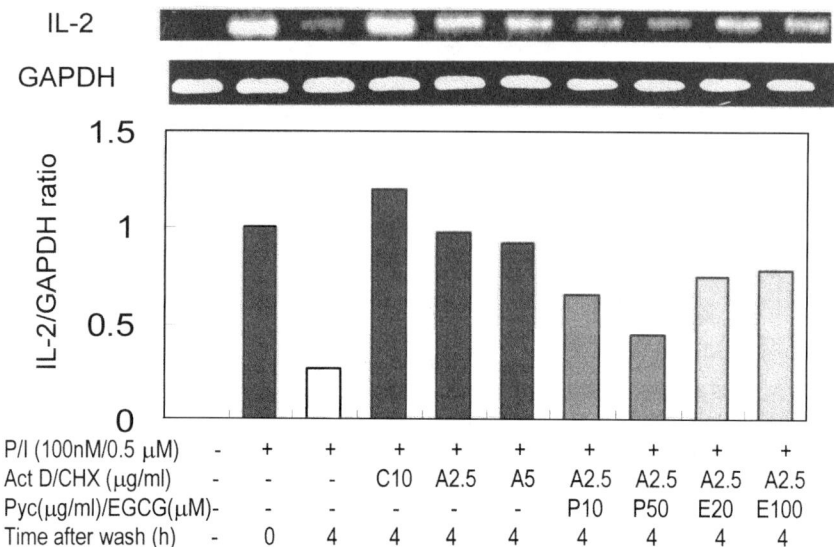

FIGURE 6. Effect of PYC on the IL-2 mRNA stability in Jurkat E6.1 cells. Cells (2.5 × 10^6 cells) were stimulated with PMA/Io for 3 hr. After washing away the supernatant, Act D (2.5 or 5 µg/ml) or CHX (10 µg/ml) was treated in the absence or presence of PYC (10 or 50 µg/ml) or EGCG (50 or 100 µM). Total RNA was isolated and reverse-transcribed as described in MATERIALS AND METHODS, and a 10-µl aliquot from each PCR reaction was electrophoresed in an 2% agarose gel and visualized by ethidium bromide staining. The *upper* and *lower panels* show gel photographs of PCR-amplified cDNA from IL-2 or GAPDH and the densitometric analysis of the gel photograph, respectively.

be an important determinant in its ability to block both NF-κB and AP-1 activation in macrophages and thereby downregulate IL-1 gene expression and production.

The activity of NF-κB is induced by a wide variety of agents, including reactive oxygen species, TNF-α, LPS, viral infection, UV irradiation, phorbol esters, and nitric oxide (NO).[19] Although no common second messenger has yet been identified, most NF-κB-activating signals can be inhibited by antioxidants.[20,21] Similar to the present data with PYC, green tea polyphenols have recently been reported to block NF-κB activation in LPS-stimulated RAW 264.7 macrophages, indicating that polyphenols might have the potential to modulate NF-κB-dependent gene expression already on the transcriptional level.[22] However, the exact underlying mechanisms by which bioflavonoids in general and PYC in particular affect LPS-mediated NF-κB activation are still not clear. Except the direct antioxidant property, it might also be possible that PYC blocks the interaction of LPS with its receptor, thereby creating a "sealing effect."[23] To test whether PYC may affect LPS-inducible phosphorylation and/or degradation of IκBα, the levels of IκBα in the cytoplasm of the macrophages pretreated with increasing concentrations of PYC and then stimulated with LPS were analyzed using a specific IκBα antibody. Stimulation of RAW 264.7 cells with LPS leads to a rapid loss of IκBα from the cytoplasm. However, PYC stabilized IκBα in a dose-dependent manner. This effect of PYC on levels of IκBα pro-

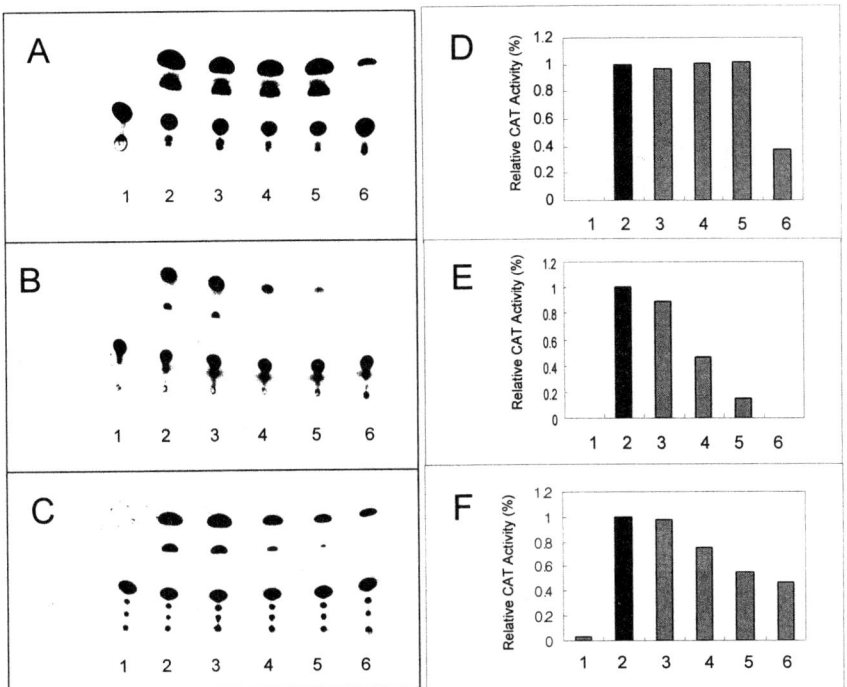

FIGURE 7. The effects of PYC on NF-kB (**A** and **D**), AP-1 (**B** and **E**) and NF-AT (**C** and **F**) CAT activities in transiently transfected Jurkat E6.1 cells. The transfected cells (5 × 10⁶ cells) were pretreated with PYC (10, 20, and 50 μg/ml), PDTC (500 μM), or fisetin (50 μM) and stimulated with PMA/Io (100 nM/0.5 μM) for 18 hr. Then, the CAT activity of each treatment group was analyzed. The relative CAT activity was normalized to the amount of CAT activity of PAM/Io-treated group (D, E, and F).

tein could be due to an inhibition of IκB phosphorylation either by inhibiting tyrosine kinase as well as IκB kinases or by blocking the degradation of IκB, which is currently being investigated in our laboratory. Because PYC inhibits NF-κB signaling in LPS-stimulated macrophages, it would affect NF-κB-dependent gene expressions of many other important mediators of inflammation in a variety of other cell types. In this regard, it has been recently demonstrated that PYC is able to normalize the increase of interleukin-6 and interleukin-10 isolated from mouse splenocytes either infected with the LP-BM5 retrovirus or fed with ethanol.[24]

Like the activation of NF-κB, the transcription factor AP-1 is redox regulated. AP-1 is a dimer composed of proteins from the Fos and Jun families with recognition sites in the promoter region of genes involved in inflammation (e.g., IL-1α, IL-1β, TNF-α), immune response, cell proliferation, and cell transformation. Under the investigated conditions, pretreatment of LPS-stimulated RAW 264.7 macrophages with PYC resulted in a significant inhibition of AP-1 binding to its consensus DNA sequences. The precise underlying mechanism regarding ROS-dependent AP-1 activation is still not clear. The perturbation of the cellular thiol redox status has been suggested to be an important signal that can be implicated in the induction of c-fos and c-jun expression caused by asbestos-induced oxidative stress in mesothelial cells.[25] In support of this, high intracellular glutathione disulfide levels have been shown to be involved in AP-1 activation.[26] Interestingly, PYC significantly protected ECV304 cells against glutathione depletion induced by different oxidative stressors.[4] Thus PYC-induced changes in GSH homeostasis might have partially counteracted LPS-induced activation of AP-1; this is currently under investigation in our laboratory. It has also been demonstrated that AP-1 activation under oxidative conditions is mediated by phosphorylation of Jun proteins.[27] Recent studies in cultured cells have shown that green tea polyphenols[28] as well as silymarin[29] suppress the activation of AP-1 through the inhibition of c-jun NH_2-terminal kinase and mitogen-activated protein kinase kinase activity. Nardini and co-workers[30] recently studied the effect of PYC on the activities of various protein kinases such as phosphorylase kinase, protein kinase A, and protein kinase C. Most remarkably, PYC displayed the ability to strongly inhibit the activity of the previous three enzymes. Thus, it appears that inhibition of specific kinases due to PYC may also play a role in preventing AP-1 DNA binding.

We also demonstrated that PYC inhibited IL-2 gene transcription in Jurkat E6.1 cells. The regulatory region of IL-2 gene contains two NF-AT sites, of which the NF-AT distal motif from IL-2 promoter site is flanked by an AP-1-like site, through which AP-1 complexes help to stabilize NF-AT binding; two additional AP-1-like sites, an NF-κB site, and two Oct-binding sites.[31] In activated T cells, cytoplasmic NF-AT is dephosphorylated by the Ca^{2+}-dependent phosphatase calcineurin to facilitate nuclear translocation and association with the AP-1 proteins Fra-1 and JunB to form the upper of the two NF-AT binding complexes.[32] When transiently transfected with $p(NF-AT)_3$-CAT and $p(AP-1)_3$-CAT, and activated by PMA/Io in Jurkat E6.1 cells, PYC significantly inhibited both NF-AT and AP-1 CAT activities. These results suggest that PYC can modulate the NF-AT pathway directly and/or via the regulation of the AP-1 pathway. In contrast to the regulation of PYC in RAW 264.7 cells, however, PYC did not affect both NF-κB DNA-binding activity and its CAT activity in Jurkat E6.1 cells. The difference in both cell lines (RAW 264.7 versus Jurkat E6.1) and mitogens (LPS versus PMA/Io) may explain the difference in the regulation of NF-κB pathway by PYC.

Regulation of mRNA stability is particularly important for short-lived cytokine mRNAs including IL-2.[33] Studies involving the induction of IL-2 gene transcription have demonstrated that the decline in IL-2 mRNA level occurs considerably faster than does the decline in transcription rate during the later stages of T-cell activation.[34] This suggests that mRNA degradation would be critical for control of mRNA levels during the later stages of T-cell activation. Up to now, transcriptional regulation of cytokine genes by various bioflavonoids has been well defined, but little is known about their posttranscriptional regulation. Here, we have found that PYC can destabilize IL-2 mRNA, which is superinduced by Act D after removal of PMA/Io. However, this result supports the possibility of posttranscriptioanl regulation of the IL-2 gene by other bioflavonoids, which are being used in many diseases.

In conclusion, present data clearly demonstrate that PYC blocks both NF-κB and AP-1 activation in LPS-stimulated RAW 264.7 cells. Thereby, PYC possibly leads to downregulation of proinflammatory cytokine IL-1β gene expression and production in macrophages. On the other hand, PYC blocks IL-2 gene expression in PMA/ Io-stimulated Jurkat E6.1 cells via posttranscriptional regulation as well as transcriptional regulation by NF-AT and AP-1. The study presented here may make a contribution to our understanding of how bioflavonoids prevent inflammatory diseases by acting as free radical scavengers and further as regulators of inflammatory cytokine gene expression.

ACKNOWLEDGMENTS

This study was supported by grants from the Ministry of Science and Technology (Molecular Medicine Program) in the Republic of Korea.

REFERENCES

1. PACKER, L., G. RIMBACH & F. VIRGILI. 1999. Antioxidant activity and biological properties of a procyanidin-rich extract from pine (*Pinus maritima*) bark, Pycnogenol. Free Radic. Biol. Med. **27:** 704–724.
2. COSSINS, E., R. LEE & L. PACKER. 1998. ESR studies of vitamin C regeneration, order of reactivity of natural source phytochemical preparations. Biochem. Mol. Biol. Intern. **45:** 583–597.
3. VIRGILI, F., D. KIM & L. PACKER. 1998. Procyanidins extracted from pine bark protect alpha.-tocopherol in ECV 304 endothelial cells challenged by activated RAW 264.7 macrophages: role of nitric oxide and peroxynitrite. FEBS Lett. **431:** 315–318.
4. RIMBACH, G., F. VIRGILI, Y.C. PARK & L. PACKER. 1999. Effect of procyanidins from *Pinus maritima* on glutathione levels in endothelial cells challenged by 3-morpholinosyndonimine or activated macrophages. Redox Rep. **4:** 171–177.
5. VIRGILI, F., H. KOBUCHI & L. PACKER. 1998. Procyanidins extracted from *Pinus maritima* (Pycnogenol): scavengers of free radical species and modulators of nitrogen monoxide metabolism in activated murine RAW 264.7 macrophages. Free Radic. Biol. Med. **24:** 1120–129.
6. KIMBALL, E.S., Ed. 1991. Cytokines as mediators of chronic inflammatory disease. *In* Cytokines and Inflammation. C.J. Dunn, Ed.: 1–3. CRC Press. Boca Raton, FL.
7. DINARELLO, C.A. 1996. Biologic basis for interleukin-1 in disease. Blood **87:** 2095–2147.
8. TSUKADA, J., M. MISAGO, Y. SERINO, *et al.* 1997. Human T-cell leukemia virus type I Tax transactivates the promoter of human prointerleukin-1beta gene through association with two transcription factors, nuclear factor-interleukin-6 and Spi-1. Blood **90:** 3142–3153.
9. PINKUS, R., L.M. WEINER & V. DANIEL. 1996. Role of oxidants and antioxidants in the induction of AP-1, NF-κB, and glutathione S-transferase gene expression. J. Biol. Chem. **271:** 13422–13429.
10. GOSSART, S., C. CAMBON, C. ORFILA, *et al.* 1996. Reactive oxygen intermediates as regulators of TNF-α production in rat lung inflammation induced by silica. J. Immunol. **156:** 1540–1548.
11. SERHAN, C.N. & P.A. WARD, Eds. 1999. Recruitment of γ/δ T-cells and other T-cell subsets to sites of inflammation. *In* Molecular and Cellular Basis of Inflammation. M.A. Jutila, Ed.: 193–214. Humana Press. Totowa, NJ.
12. JAIN, J. & C. LOH. 1995. Transcriptional regulation of the IL-2 gene. Curr. Opin. Immunol. **7:** 333–342.
13. SHAW, J., K. MEEROVITCH, R. BLEACKLEY & V. PAETKAU. 1988. Mechanisms regulating the level of IL-2 mRNA in T lymphocytes. J. Immunol. **140:** 2243–2248.
14. CHEN, C.-Y.A. & A.-B. SHYU. 1995. AU-rich elements: characterization and importance in mRNA degradation. TIBS **20:** 465–470.

15. HAN, S.H., S.S. YEA, Y.J. JEON, et al. 1998. Transforming growth factor-β1 (TGF-β1) promotes IL-2 mRNA expression through the up-regulation of NF-κB, AP-1 and NF-AT in EL4 cells. J. Pharmacol. Exp. Ther. **287:** 1105–1112.
16. GRIMBLE, R.F. 1998. Nutritional modulation of cytokine biology. Nutrition **14:** 634–640.
17. NODA, Y., K. ANZAI, A. MORI, et al. 1997. Hydroxyl and superoxide anion radical scavenging activities of natural source antioxidants using the computerized JES-FR30 ESR spectrometer system. Biochem. Mol. Biol. Intern. **42:** 35–44.
18. PLUMB, G.W., S. DE PASCUAL-TERESA, C. SANTOS-BUELGA, et al. 1998. Antioxidant properties of catechins and proanthocyanidins: effect of polymerisation, galloylation and glycosylation. Free Radic. Res. **29:** 351–358.
19. FLOHE, L., R. BRIGELIUS-FLOHE, C. SALIOU, et al. 1997. Redox regulation of NF-κB activation. Free Radic. Biol. Med. **22:** 1115–1126.
20. SALIOU, C., B. RIHN, J. CILLARD, et al. 1998. Selective inhibition of NF-κB activation by the flavonoid hepatoprotector silymarin in HepG2. Evidence for different activating pathways. FEBS Lett. **440:** 8–12.
21. SALIOU, C., M. KITAZAWA, L. MCLAUGHLIN, et al. 1999. Antioxidants modulate acute solar ultraviolet radiation-induced NF-κB activation in a human keratinocyte cell line. Free Radic. Biol. Med. **26:** 174–183.
22. YANG, F., W.J. DE VILLIERS, C.J. MCCLAIN & G.W. VARILEK. 1998. Green tea polyphenols block endotoxin-induced tumor necrosis factor-production and lethality in a murine model. J. Nutr. **128:** 2334–2340.
23. LIN, Y.L. & J.K. LIN. 1997. (−)-Epigallocatechin-3-gallate blocks the induction of nitric oxide synthase by down-regulating lipopolysaccharide-induced activity of transcription factor nuclear factor-κB. Mol. Pharmacol. **52:** 465–472.
24. CHESHIER, J.E., S. ARDESTANI-KABOUDANIAN, B. LIANG, et al. 1996. Immunomodulation by Pycnogenol in retrovirus-infected or ethanol-fed mice. Life Sci. **58:** 87–96.
25. JANSSEN, Y.M., N.H. HEINTZ & B.T. MOSSMAN. 1995. Induction of c-fos and c-jun proto-oncogene expression by asbestos is ameliorated by N-acetyl-L-cysteine in mesothelial cells. Cancer Res. **55:** 2085–2089.
26. GALTER, D., S. MIHM & W. DROGE. 1994. Distinct effects of glutathione disulphide on the nuclear transcription factor kappa B and the activator protein-1. Eur. J. Biochem. **221:** 639–648.
27. BAUSKIN, A.R., I. ALKALAY & Y. BEN-NERIAH. 1991. Redox regulation of a protein tyrosine kinase in the endoplasmic reticulum. Cell **66:** 685–696.
28. CHUNG, J.Y., C. HUANG, X. MENG, et al. 1999. Inhibition of activator protein 1 activity and cell growth by purified green tea and black tea polyphenol in H-ras-transformed cells: structure–activity relationship and mechanisms involved. Cancer Res. **59:** 4610–4617.
29. MANNA, S.K., A. MUKHOPADHYAY, N.T. VAN & B.B. AGGARWAL. 1999. Silymarin suppresses TNF-induced activation of NF-κB, c-Jun N-terminal kinase, and apoptosis. J. Immunol. **163:** 6800–6809.
30. NARDINI, M., C. SCACCINI, L. PACKER & F. VIRGILI, F. 2000. In vitro inhibition of the activity of phosphorylase kinase, protein kinase C and protein kinase A by a caffeic acid and a procyanidin rich pine bark (*Pinus maritima*) extract. Biochim. Biophys. Acta **1474:** 219–225.
31. SERFLING, E., A. AVOTS & M. NEUMANN. 1995. The architecture of the interleukin-2 promoter: a reflection of T-lymphocyte activation. Biochim. Biophys. Acta **1263:** 181–200.
32. CLIPSTONE, N.A. & G.R. CRABTREE. 1992. Identification of calcineurin as a key signalling enzyme in T-lymphocyte activation. Nature **357:** 695–697.
33. ROSS, J. 1996. mRNA stability in mammalian cells. Microbiol. Rev. **59:** 423–450.
34. UMLAUF, S.W., B. BEVERLY, O. LANTZ & R.H. SCHWARTZ. 1995. Regulation of interleukin-2 gene expression by CD28 costimulation in mouse T-cell clones: both nuclear and cytoplasmic RNAs are regulated with complex kinetics. Mol. Cell. Biol. **15:** 3197–3205.

Gene Expression and Regulation in the Extended Longevity Phenotypes of *Drosophila*

ROBERT ARKING[a]

Department of Biological Sciences, Wayne State University, Detroit, Michigan 48202, USA

ABSTRACT: We used both selection and single-gene mutagenesis studies to identify the mechanisms underlying the genetic control of longevity in *Drosophila*. The expression of the extended longevity phenotype (ELP) in our forward-selected strains depends on an early and specific upregulation of the antioxidant defense system (ADS) genes and enzymes, which results in decreased oxidative damage levels and a delayed onset of senescence. This mechanism does not alter metabolic rate and is itself reversed by a reverse selection regime. Single-gene mutational analysis of the regulatory genes controlling ADS gene expression show they are under the positive and negative control of several such genes, each of which can bring about the expression/repression of the ELP. Sister strains with identical ELPs have different patterns of ADS gene expression, showing that phenotypic equivalence does not require molecular equivalence. The organism may have multiple genetic strategies to cope with similar levels of oxidative stress.

KEYWORDS: Aging; Oxidative stress; CuZnSOD; MnSOD; Catalase; *Drosophila*; Regulatory genes

INTRODUCTION

Construction of the Strains and Adoption of an Investigative Strategy

Aging is a complex phenotype. Determining the causal factors underlying the expression of such a phenotype is a difficult problem. Genetic approaches are particularly well suited for such a task. Consequently, we decided some years ago to use artificial selection to generate long-lived strains of *Drosophila*, with the eventual goal of comparing them to their normal-lived progenitor strains in order to deduce which processes had been significantly altered and therefore might play an important role in the expression of the extended longevity phenotype.

The details of these selection experiments have been reported elsewhere.[1,2] Selection was rapidly successful, significant increases in longevity being noted by the F9 and 40–50% increases in both mean and maximum lifespan observed by the F22.[2] Recent current longevity data for the two sister lines of the normal-lived (R) and long-lived (L) strains are shown in FIGURE 1. It should be noted that the normal-lived

---

[a]Address for correspondence: Robert Arking, Visiting Professor, Department of Molecular Biology, College of Natural Sciences, Pusan National University, Pusan 609-735, Korea Voice: 82-051-510-2256; fax: 82-051-513-9258.

rarking@biology.biosci.wayne.edu

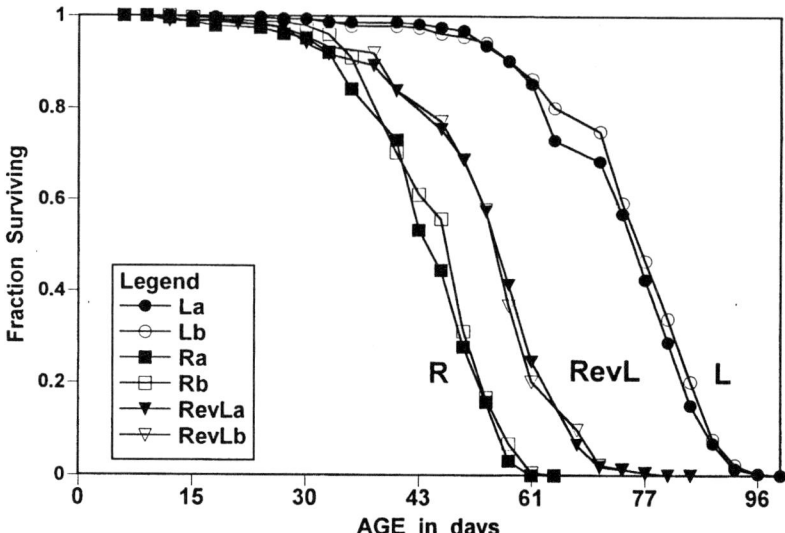

FIGURE 1. Survival curves of representative generations of the selected strains used in our studies.[12] There is a significant difference between the Ra and La curves, and between the La curves and the RevLa curves. The Ra and Rb curves are statistically identical, as are the La and Lb curves. Each survival curve is based on the age-specific values obtained from two or three replicate cohorts consisting of at least 250 mixed-sex individuals each.

progenitor R strains were maintained under conditions such that they were not subjected to selection; thus their lifespan has remained more or less constant,[3] and it is reasonable to presume that their molecular characteristics have not changed that much as well.

Having generated these long-lived strains, the question arose as to which investigative strategy—genetic or molecular—would be most effective for this complex phenotype. An examination of a two-dimensional gel of some of the proteins present in the young adult males of the Ra and La strains (FIG. 2) revealed hundreds of proteins, some of which showed apparent quantitative or qualitative differences between the strains. A few could be tentatively identified, but contemplation of these gels soon convinced us that we did not possess sufficient information to adopt an effective molecular approach. Thus we opted to ask the animals a series of genetic questions so that we might attain a better understanding of the processes underlying the extended longevity phenotype.

The results of four such experiments were particularly informative.

- First, we measured the lifetime, age-specific metabolic rates of the Ra and La strains under a variety of ambient temperatures.[4] Both strains had statistically identical mean daily metabolic rates, allowing us to conclude that the long life of the La strain was not due to a significantly lowered metabolic rate relative to the Ra strain. Thus, the rate-of-living theory as classically described did not apply to our animals.[5] This meant we could proceed with our analysis unham-

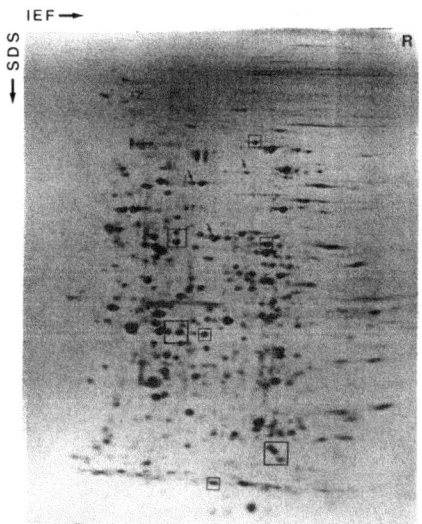 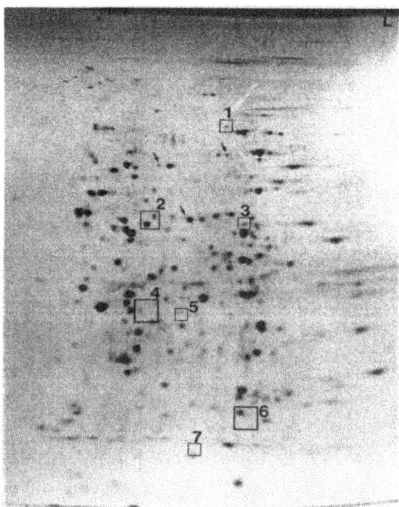

FIGURE 2. Ten-day-old males of the Ra (*left*) and La (*right*) strains were labeled with 35S methionine. Equal amounts of protein were loaded onto each gel. The pH range for the gels is ca. 3.5–8.0. Proteins 1, 3, 7, and those indicated by arrows show quantitative changes, while 2, 4, and 6 show qualitative changes. The labeling and gel were graciously done by James Fleming in 1988. See text for discussion.

pered by the complicating presence of any interactions between metabolic rate and longevity.[6]

- Second, we measured the animals' age-specific loss of performance in several unrelated, and therefore presumably independent, processes.[7] The data allowed us to conclude that (a) the La strain animals had the same pattern of senescence as did the Ra animals, and (b) the defining characteristic of the La animals' extended longevity was that they had a significantly delayed onset of senescence, which was tightly coupled to events that began at about day 5–7 of adult life.

- Third, we performed a controlled chromosome replacement study in which we substituted Ra strain chromosomes for La strain chromosomes (and vice versa) and then measured the longevity of the resulting 27 isochromosomal lines.[8] The data showed that the extended longevity phenotype was significantly dependent on genes located on the third chromosome (c3), and a mapping experiment showed that the required region was on c3L and included the copper–zinc superoxide dismutase (CuZnSOD) and catalase (Cat) loci. In addition, the data also showed that the expression of the genes on c3 was significantly modulated by (then) unknown genes located on chromosome 2 (c2).

- Fourth, the only physiological factor that robustly separated all of our various long-lived strains from all of our various normal-lived strains was that of paraquat (PQ) resistance.[9] In addition, PQ resistance was the first biomarker

TABLE 1. Summary of data from experiments testing the process underlying delayed onset of senescence[a]

Strain	Metabolic rate (Ref. 4)	Oxidative stress resistance (Ref. 9)	CuZn SOD activity (Ref.12)	CuZn SOD protein (Refs. 12,28)	ADS mRNA CuZnSOD MnSOD Cat (Ref. 12)	Non-ADS mRNAs (Ref. 11)	Oxidative damage: lipid protein (Ref. 12)	Longevity (Refs. 2,12)
La	1.04	1.64	1.49	2.06	3.45 4.61 2.63	0.95	0.56 0.82	1.67
Ra	1.00	1.00	1.00	1.00	1.00 1.00 1.00	1.00	1.00 1.00	1.00

[a] All data normalized to control values.

to be differentially affected in the two strains, and this difference first appeared at ca. 5–7 days, an age coincident with the beginning of the delayed onset of senescence. Because this bipyridyl herbicide generates free radicals in the cell and is used as an index of resistance to oxidative stress,[10] then these findings suggested that the delayed onset of senescence noted above probably involved resistance to oxidative stress.

Forward Selection and Gene Expression

If the above conclusions are correct, then one would predict that the young La adults would have a significantly increased expression of their antioxidant defense system (ADS) genes relative to the young Ra adults. This experiment was done.[11] The data unequivocally showed that the 5- to 7-day-old La animals had a significant overexpression of certain ADS mRNAs and ADS enzyme activities relative to their Ra controls. There was no difference between the two strains with regard to non-ADS genes, thus indicating that the ADS genes were being specifically upregulated[11] (also see Table 1 of Ref. 12).

As a result of these experiments, it was reasonable to conclude that the specific upregulation of the ADS genes, and its presumed effect of increasing resistance to oxidative stress, was likely to be the major process underlying the La strain's delayed onset of senescence. We have done many experiments in an effort to critically test this hypothesis. A summary of some of our data to date is presented in TABLE 1, and a summary of the ADS mRNA levels over the lifespan of the Ra and La animals is shown in FIGURE 6A. It may be seen that the specific upregulation of the ADS genes is accompanied by an increase in the animals' resistance to exogenous oxidative stress (e.e., paraquat), coupled with a decrease in its own production of endogenous reactive oxygen species (ROS) and a decrease in its own levels of oxidative damage to lipids and proteins. These changes appear to be linked to longevity. Although plausible, this is essentially correlative data and does not prove that resistance to oxidative stress plays a causal role in bringing about the expression of the extended longevity phenotype. After all, both variables may have changed as a result of alterations in a third unknown variable. A more powerful method of testing this log-

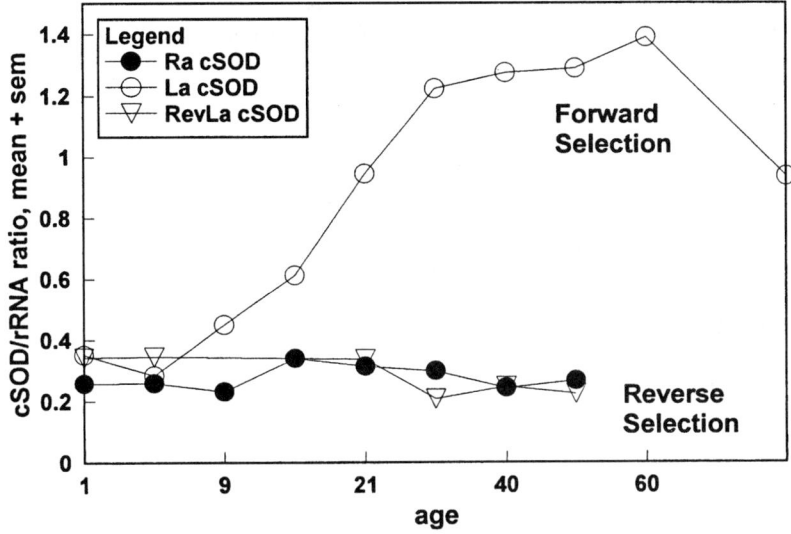

FIGURE 3. The age-related changes in the mean (± SD) CuZnSOD enzyme activity measured in males of the Ra, La, and reverse-selected RevLa strains. The La strains generally have a higher specific activity than do their Ra controls, although the early and late periods of elevated activity are obvious in both strains. The RevLa strains have a shortened lifespan (FIG. 1); reverse selection has brought about a decrease in this ADS enzyme activity such that it is now comparable to their normal-lived Ra strain animals. Each point is the mean of 3–5 replicates; points without visible error bars are those where the variance is so small that it is hidden by the data symbol. (From Arking et al.[12]; used with permission.)

ical objection was needed. Once again, two independent genetic methods provided the lever we needed.

Reverse Selection and Gene Expression

If there is a causal connection between extended longevity and ADS gene expression, then reverse selecting the La strain for a short life span should eventually yield shorter lived animals with a decreased ADS level relative to their parental La strain. In this experiment, then, we manipulated longevity and assayed for ADS levels. We did this experiment,[12] and the data for the reverse-selected RevLa strain is also shown in FIGURE 1. The survival curve of the RevLa strain is significantly different from its progenitor La strain as well as from the normal-lived Ra strain; however, the important point is that reverse selection was successful and the RevLa strain is much more like the Ra strain than the La strain. The effect of this reverse selection on the animals' ADS gene expression patterns is shown in FIGURE 3. The age-specific levels of the *CuZnSOD* and *Cat* mRNA levels in the RevLa strain are significantly different from that characteristic of the La strain and have reverted to the low and constant levels generally characteristic of the Ra normal-lived strains.[12] The changes observed in the ADS system are an order of magnitude greater than those observed with 17 other non-ADS enzymes,[12] thus indicating that these changes are very spe-

TABLE 2. Relationships between longevity, resistance to oxidative stress, ADS activity, and oxidative damage in representative mutants affecting *trans*-acting genes regulating the *ADS* genes

Specific Mutant	Longevity (relative to control)	Paraquat resistance status (relative to control)	ADS activity (relative to control)	Oxidative damage (oxidized lipid, relative to control)	Role of wild-type allele of gene in control animal	Total No. of similar mutants isolated (see text)
Mutant # 1367	0.60 ± 0.46	0.53	0.70 ± 0.18	2.42 ± 0.41	Positive regulator	5
Mutant # 0907	1.20 ± 0.36	1.20	1.63 ± 0.01	0.61 ± 0.01	Negative regulator	2
Long-lived strain (control)	1.00 ± 0.175	1.00 ± 0.17	1.00 ± 0.15	1.00 ± 0.28	—	—

SOURCE: From Ref. 15; used with permission.

cific and are not merely the by-product of a general metabolic alteration. The tight linkage between the levels of ADS gene expression and longevity strongly suggests that the former plays an important role in bringing about the latter.

Mutational Analysis of ADS Gene Regulation

Prior data suggested that the ADS genes were modulated via a *trans*-acting gene network centered on c2.[8,13,14] We searched for such genes by performing insertional mutagenesis with the *P[lacW]* transposon on the c2 of our selected high ADS-expressing La strain and screened for homozygous, robustly viable mutants with altered sensitivity to the free radical–generating compound paraquat.[15] These mutants were then tested for their effects on the ADS genes and on longevity. In this experiment, then, we manipulated ADS levels and assayed for longevity. We detected six mutants identifying at least five different genes on c2 which act in *trans* to increase or to reduce the transcription of the CuZnSOD and Cat ADS genes on c3. These same mutants alter longevity in a corresponding manner. Thus, some La mutants have only control (i.e., normal) levels of ADS gene expression, oxidative damage, and life span; others have super-elevated levels of ADS gene expression, super-low levels of oxidative damage and a super-long life (TABLE 2). Reversion of the mutation restores the normal paraquat resistance and ADS enzyme activity levels, proving that the mutant effects are linked to the inactivation of the affected gene.[15] Two of these mutants are particularly interesting, one (A0907) coordinately upregulating, and the other (A1367) coordinately downregulating, both copper–zinc superoxide dismutase (CuZnSOD) and catalase (Cat) and altering the phenotype accordingly, as shown in TABLE 2. A similar mutant has been identified by Lin *et al.*[16] on chromosome 1.

In addition, there is a significant positive correlation between ADS levels and life span in these several mutants (FIG. 4), and there is a significant negative correlation between oxidative damage and life span in these same mutants (FIG. 5). These are

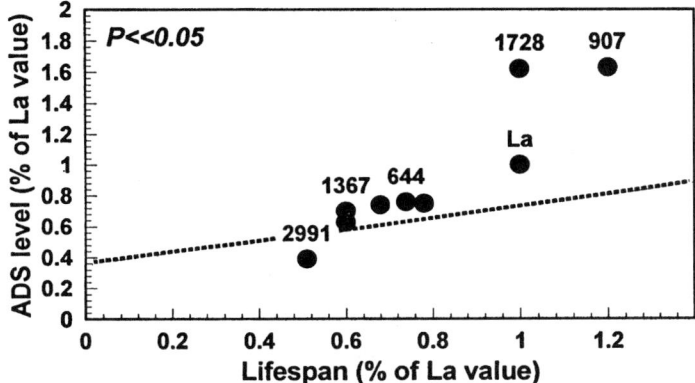

FIGURE 4. There exists a positive correlation between the mean life span of our several P-element mutants (numbers) and the La control strain, and the mean CuZnSOD enzyme activity as measured in young (ca. 7-day-old) adult males of each strain. (From Feldman et al.[15]; used with permission.)

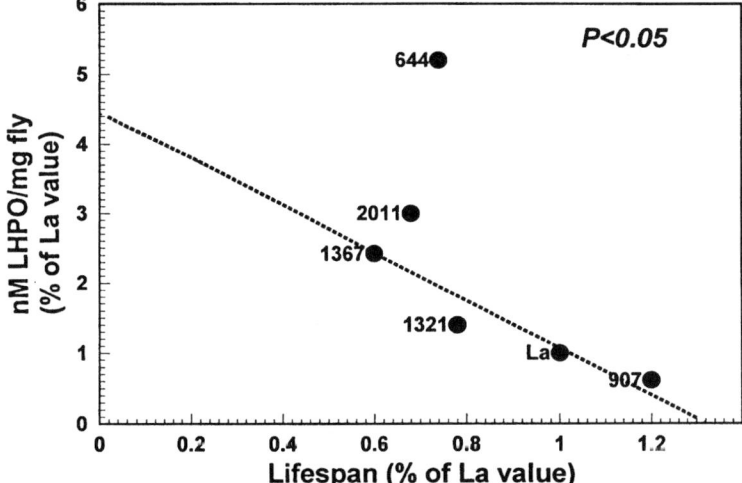

FIGURE 5. There exists a negative correlation between the mean life span of our several P-element mutants (numbers) and the La control strain, and the mean value of the lipid hydroperoxide content as measured in young (ca. 7-day-old) adult males of each strain. (From Feldman et al.[15]; used with permission.)

exactly the relationships one would expect if a specific upregulation of the ADS genes first led to an enhanced resistance to oxidative stress, then to a decreased age-specific level of oxidative damage, and this then led to a delayed onset of senescence. Thus, independently designed and executed mutation experiments, forward and reverse selection experiments, physiological experiments, and biomarker experiments have each led us to conclude that the causal connection between ADS levels and longevity lies in the relationship between the former and the age-specific levels of oxidative damage within the organism.

Several authors have suggested that a generalized stress resistance is a prerequisite for the expression of the extended longevity phenotype.[17,18] However, the empirical data suggest that it is specifically the resistance to oxidative stress that constitutes the operative factor.[12,19–22] We have other data that bears on this point. As noted above, the La animals were derived from the Ra strain and are resistant to paraquat, have enhanced ADS enzyme activities, and live long. When we employed a direct selection regime on the Ra animals, we created a new strain (PQR) of flies that is extraordinarily resistant to paraquat but that have elevated P450 enzyme levels and depressed ADS enzyme activity levels.[23,24] This PQR strain shows a normal longevity and is statistically indistinguishable from the Ra strain. In addition, we have evidence showing that the La strain animals do not possess a generalized resistance to diverse environmental stresses.[25,26] We believe that these data taken together allow us to conclude that it is probably the specific protective effects of the enhanced ADS enzymes that actually produce the extended longevity in this model system.

Phenotype Equivalence Does Not Mean Molecular Equivalence

We initially developed several sister lines of the R strain (known as Ra, Rb, etc.), and these gave rise via forward selection to several sister lines of the L strain (known as La, Lb, etc.). All of the work described above was done with the Ra, La, and Rev-La strains. The La and Lb strains have statistically identical life spans, as do the Ra and Rb strains (FIG. 1; Ref. 27). They also have statistically identical PQ resistance phenotypes.[9] The phenotypic equivalence of the La and Lb strains led to the assumption that the two strains were also equivalent at the molecular genetic level as well. We decided to critically test this assumption by determining the expression levels for three important ADS genes in the Lb strain and compare it to that of the La strain.[27] The results of this investigation are shown in FIGURE 6. The two sister strains are characterized by significantly different mechanisms and patterns of antioxidant gene expression as well as significantly different patterns of antioxidant enzyme activity and oxidative damage (not shown, see Ref. 27). We find that the La strain appears to depend on the transcriptional activation primarily of the *CuZnSOD* and *MnSOD* genes, whereas the Lb strain appears to depend on the transcriptional activation primarily of the *Cat* gene. Note that the La strain does not appear to rely on the *Cat* gene nor does the Lb strain appear to rely on the *CuZnSOD* or *MnSOD* genes. Thus the Lb strain relies on different ADS genes than does the La strain, and vice-versa.. Other differences are noted in Arking *et al.*[27] The phenotypic equivalence observed at the organism level need not hold at the molecular genetic level. This finding suggests that there is more than one molecular mechanism by which ADS genes can bring about an increased resistance to oxidative stress.

There may well be more than the two such mechanisms we have described (i.e., a putative *SOD*-dependent and a putative *Cat*-dependent process), and the cataloging of these different molecular strategies may well be an important step in our achieving a full understanding of the processes. It is also likely that the identification of forbidden or rare molecular strategies may be equally fruitful.

Finally, transcriptional changes affecting the expression of the ADS genes are often assumed to be the primary means of effectively extending longevity. However,

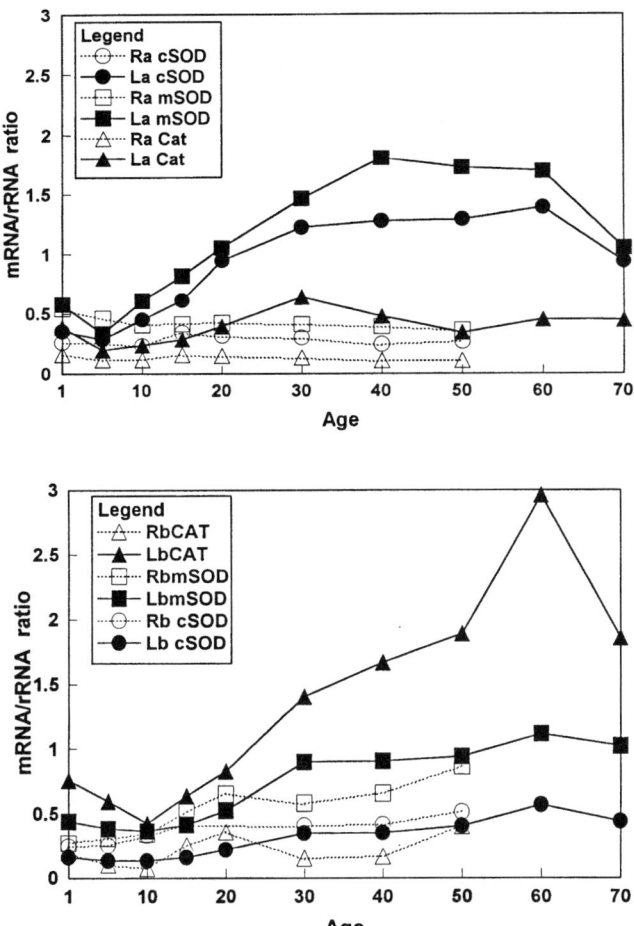

FIGURE 6. The age-specific mRNA prevalence for the *CuZnSOD*, *MnSOD*, and *Cat* genes is shown over the life span of the Ra/La strains (**A**) and the Rb/Lb strains (**B**). Error bars have been omitted for clarity but are presented in Arking *et al.*[12,27] Both graphs are to the same scale. Note that the La strain mostly upregulates the *CuZnSOD* and *Cat* genes, whereas the Lb strain mostly upregulates the *Cat* gene. There are also smaller but significant differences in the ADS gene expression patterns of the Ra and Rb strains (see Ref. 27 for discussion of this point).

we have evidence showing that the CuZnSOD enzyme activity is subject to post-translational regulation.[12,27] Understanding how this mechanism works may provide us with an additional level of intervention.

Regulatory Genes and Different Patterns of ADS Gene Expression

Antioxidant defenses protect cells from oxidative damage. The cellular response to oxidative stress is complicated. Much work has been done by a number of groups testing whether some particular ADS gene plays a role in the extended longevity phenotype. Our work with the La and Lb strains summarized above shows that presumably small genetic differences present in two supposedly identical "sister" strains subjected to the same selection regime can result in dramatically different molecular outcomes. Presumably these small starting differences, when subjected to the pressures of forward selection, bring about rather large differences in the types and expression levels of ADS genes found in the final products (FIG. 6). It is likely that these different outcomes are the result of a differential activation of the *trans*-acting regulatory gene network controlling the ADS genes, some of which we have discussed above, by these small starting differences. Thus the organism may have multiple genetic strategies to cope with slightly different patterns of oxidative stress as interpreted by the organism in the light of its own particular genetic and physiological patterns. Understanding the processes by which these strain- (and tissue?) specific ADS gene patterns are modulated should provide us with much useful information as well as potential mechanisms for intervention into the aging process.

ACKNOWLEDGMENTS

None of this work would have been possible without the dedicated efforts of many colleagues and students, especially Steven Buck, Steven Dudas, Elliott Feldman, Allen Force, Ibrahim Kadura, and John Vettraino. Supported in part by WSU research funds and in part by NIH.

REFERENCES

1. LUCKINBILL, L.S., R. ARKING, M.J. CLARE, *et al.* 1984. Selection for delayed senescence in *Drosophila melanogaster*. Evolution **38**: 996–1004.
2. ARKING, R. 1987. Successful selection for increased longevity in *Drosophila*: analysis of the survival data and presentation of a hypothesis on the genetic regulation of longevity. Exp. Gerontol. **22**: 199–220.
3. BUCK, S. & R. ARKING. 1995. Selection for increased longevity in *Drosophila melanogaster*: a reply to Lints. Gerontology **41**: 69–76.
4. ARKING, R., S. BUCK, R.A. WELLS & R. PRETZLAFF. 1988. Metabolic rates in genetically based long-lived strains of *Drosophila*. Exp. Gerontol. **23**: 59–76.
5. LINTS, F.A. 1989. The rate of living theory revisited. Gerontology **35**: 36–57.
6. VAN VOORHIES, W.A. & S. WARD. 1999. Genetic and environmental conditions that increase longevity in *Caenorhabditis elegans* decrease metabolic rate. Proc. Natl. Acad. Sci. USA **96**: 11399–11403.
7. ARKING, R. & R.A. WELLS. 1990. Genetic alteration of normal aging processes is responsible for extended longevity in *Drosophila*. Dev. Genet. **11**: 141–148.
8. BUCK, S., R.A. WELLS, S.P. DUDAS, *et al.* 1993. Chromosomal localization and regulation of the longvity determinant genes in a selected strain of *Drosophila melanogaster*. Heredity **71**: 11–22.
9. FORCE, A.G., T. STAPLES, S. SOLIMAN & R. ARKING. 1995. Comparative biochemical and stress analysis of genetically selected *Drosophila* strains with different longevities. Dev. Genet. **17**: 340–351.
10. ARKING, R., S. BUCK, A. BERRIOS, *et al.* 1991. Elevated antioxidant activity can be used as a bioassay for longevity in a genetically based long-lived strain of *Drosophila*. Dev. Genet. **12**: 362–370.
11. DUDAS, S.P. & R. ARKING. 1995. A coordinate upregulation of antioxidant gene activities is associated with the delayed onset of senescence in a long-lived strain of *Drosophila*. J. Gerontol. Biol. Sci. **50A**: B117–B127.

12. ARKING, R., V. BURDE, K. GRAVES, et al. 2000. Forward and reverse selection for longevity in *Drosophila* is characterized by alteration of antioxidant gene expression and oxidative damage patterns. Exp. Gerontol. **35**: 167–185.
13. GRAF, J.-D. & F.J. AYALA. 1986. Genetic variation for superoxide dismutase level in *Drosophila melanogaster*. Biochem. Genet. **24**: 153–168.
14. BEWLEY, G. & C.C. LAURIE-AHLBERG. 1984. Genetic variation affecting the xpression of catalase in *Drosophila melanogaster*: correlations with rates of enzyme synthesis and degradation. Genetics **106**: 435–448.
15. FELDMAN, E., I. KADURA & R. ARKING. 2000. Coordinate regulation of antioxidant gene expression in *Drosophila* by *trans*-acting mutants. In preparation.
16. LIN, Y-L, L. SEROUDE & S. BENZER. 1998. Extended life span and stress resistance in the *Drosophila* mutant methuselah. Science **282**: 943–946.
17. JOHNSON, T.E., G.J. LITHGOW & S. MURAKAMI. 1996. Hypothesis: interventions that increase the response to stress offer the potential for effective life prolongation and increased health. J. Gerontol. Biol. Sci. **51A**: B392–B395.
18. DJAWDAN, M., A.K. CHIPPENDALE, M.R. ROSE & T.J. BRADLEY. 1998. Metabolic reserves and evolved stress resistance in *Drosophila melanogaster*. Physiol. Zool. **71**: 584–594.
19. SOHAL, R.J., S. AGARWAL, A. DUBEY & W.C. ORR. 1993. Protein oxidative damage is associated with life expectancy of houseflies. Proc. Natl. Acad. Sci. USA **90**: 7255–7259.
20. SOHAL, R.J. & R. WEINDRUCH. 1996. Oxidative stress, caloric restriction, and aging. Science **273**: 59–63.
21. MARTIN, G.M., S.N. AUSTAD & T.E. JOHNSON. 1996. Genetic analysis of ageing: role of oxidative damage and environmental stresses. Nature Genet. **13**: 25–34.
22. TAUB, J., J.F. LAU, C. MA, et al. 1999. A cytosolic catalase is needed to extend adult lifespan in *C. elegans daf-C* and *clk-1* mutants. Nature **399**: 162–166.
23. ARKING, R. 1998. Molecular basis of extended longevity in selected *Drosophila* strains. Curr. Sci. **74**: 859–864.
24. VETTRAINO, J. & R. ARKING. 2000. Selection of a paraquat resistant strain of *Drosophila* with an enhanced cytochrome P450 content and decreased antioxidant gene expression. Submitted.
25. KUETHER, K. & R. ARKING. 2000. *Drosophila* selected for extended longevity are more sensitive to heat shock. AGE i22: 175–180.
26. BUCK, S., J. VETTRAINO, A.G. FORCE & R. ARKING. 2000. Extended longevity in *Drosophila* is consistently associated with a decrease in developmental viability. J. Gerontol. Biol. Sci. **55**: B292–B301.
27. ARKING, R., V. BURDE, K. GRAVES, et al. 2000. Identical longevity phenotypes are characterized by different patterns of gene expression and oxidative damage. Exp. Gerontol. **35**: 353–373.
28. HARI, R., V. BURDE & R. ARKING. 1998. Preparation of a synthetic antibody specific for CuZn superoxide dismutase protein of *Drosophila melanogaster*. Exp. Gerontol. **33**: 227–237.

Impairment of Learning and Memory in Rats Caused by Oxidative Stress and Aging, and Changes in Antioxidative Defense Systems

KOJI FUKUI,[a] KOJI ONODERA,[a] TADASHI SHINKAI,[b] SHOZO SUZUKI,[b] AND SHIRO URANO[a]

[a]*Department of Biological Chemistry, Shibaura Institute of Technology, 3-9-14 Shibaura, Minato-ku, Tokyo 108-8548, Japan*

[b]*Tokyo Metropolitan Institute of Gerontology, 35-2 Sakae-cho, Itabashi-ku, Tokyo 173-0015, Japan*

ABSTRACT: To elucidate the influence of oxidative stress on the brain functions during aging, the cognitive performance ability of rats was assessed by using the water-maze test as an oxidative stress before and after hyperoxia. Young rats showed significantly greater learning ability than both old rats and vitamin-E-deficient rats. Although the memory functions of all rats were impaired after oxidative stress, the memory retention of young rats was greater than those of other groups. After the stress, none of the rats recovered their learning ability. During aging and through hyperoxia, the release of acetylcholine from nerve terminals was remarkably decreased. Instead, thiobarbituric acid reactive substance (TBARS) contents in rat hippocampus and cebral cortex, and their synaptic membranes, were significantly increased during aging and by oxidative stress. The antioxidative defense system in rat brain was also changed by the stress. These results suggest that oxidative stress may contribute to learning and memory deficits following oxidative brain damage during aging.

KEYWORDS: Aging; Antioxidant; Brain function; Hyperoxia; Learning; Memory; Oxidative stress; Vitamin E

INTRODUCTION

Among several theories that explain the mechanism of aging, the nongenetic free-radical theory of aging is one of the most attractive[1] because some of the aspects can be explained experimentally. Up to the present day, many investigations have been carried out, and these have mostly supported this theory of aging. It has been thought that the degeneration of human sensibility with age, followed by neurological disorders, may be caused by an oxidative injury of the nervous system. The brain and nervous system are considered to be more susceptible to peroxidative damage than other tissues due to the high content of their polyunsaturated lipid-rich neural parenchyma, high oxygen utilization accounting for one-fifth of the total systemic consumption,

---

Address for correspondence: Dr. Shiro Urano, Department of Biological Chemistry, Shibaura Institute of Technology, 3-9-14 Shibaura, Minato-ku, Tokyo 108-8548, Japan. Phone: 81-3-5476-2429; fax: 81-3-5476-3162.

urano@sic.shibaura-it.ac.jp

and low antioxidative enzymes.[2-4] Recent studies concerning brain aging show increased oxidative damage during normal brain aging, as well as Alzheimer's disease.[5-7] Alzheimer's disease is considered to be an acceleration of normal aging in affected brain regions, which are damaged progressively by free radicals. The cerebral cortex and hippocampus, which are thought to control cognitive and motor functions, seem to be sensitive to oxidative stress, and to require antioxidants.[8] Recently we reported that when rats were subjected to hyperoxia, several morphological changes, for example, the swollen mitochondria, deformed nuclei in nerve cells, pigmentation, and the abnormal accumulation of synaptic vesicles in nerve terminals, were observed by electron-microscopy.[5,9] These findings imply a deficit in the neurotransmission function. Although the degeneration of hippocampal cholinergic neurons is recognized as a key to Alzheimer's disease, it is still unclear whether the neurodegeneration caused by oxidative stress may involve learning and memory impairment. In the present study, in order to define whether oxidative stress actually contributes to learning and memory impairment, the assessment of rat performance deficits due to hyperoxia was carried out using the water-maze task.[10] Changes in lipid peroxides and antioxidant status in the cerebral cortex and hippocampus were also analyzed.

MATERIALS AND METHODS

Animals

All experiments with animals were performed with permission by the Commission of Ethics for Experimental Animals of the Shibaura Institute of Technology. Male Wistar rats aged 3, 15, and 25 months, which were fed *ad libitum* using the standard diet, were used. In order to assess the ability to withstand oxidative stress, vitamin-E-deficient rats, which were fed a vitamin-E-deficient diet for 9 weeks, were also used. After an evaluation of the learning ability in all groups, all animals were maintained under 100% oxygen at 20°C for 48 h in the oxygen chambers that we had previously developed.[11]

Behavioral Testing

All animals were tested for learning and memory using the Morris water-maze task, as in the previous report, though with some modification.[10] The bottom of the pool (140 cm in diameter and 45 cm in height) was divided into quarters by white lines, and a submerged, transparent platform was placed in the center of one quadrant, which was maintained at 20°C. Before the training started, the rats were allowed to swim freely in the pool for 60 s without the platform. Daily training consisted of one trial in which the rats started for the fixed goal from three different starting points; this training lasted for 18 consecutive days. The time to goal and the length of swimming were measured, and the rate of a decrease in swimming time and length to the value unlearned at the first start was expressed as the learning rate. After all groups had learned completely, the rats were subjected to hyperoxia for 48 hours. The platform was removed and the animals were placed in the quadrant opposite the platform site. The percentage of time spent in the quadrant where the platform had been was used as an assessment of memory retention. After the water-maze task, rats were decapitated in order to evaluate the oxidative damage, that is, the changes in lipidperoxides and antioxidant status in the cerebral cortex and hippocampus.

Isolation of Synaptosomes from Rat Brain Cerebral Cortex and Hippocampus

According to the method that uses the discontinuous Ficol density gradient's centrifugation as previously reported,[5] synaptosomes were isolated. The synaptosomes obtained were immediately used for all studies.

Analyses of Lipidperoxides and Antioxidants

According to the earlier reports, thiobarbituric acid reactive substance (TBARS) formation was used as an index of lipid peroxidation of synapse in the cerebral cortex and hippocampus. The status of the vitamin E content, activities of superoxide dismutase, catalase, and glutathione peroxidase were analyzed by the known methods.[5]

Measurement of Acetylcholine Leakage from Synaptosomes

A synaptosome suspension in 1 mL Krebs-Ringer's buffer (10 mM Hepes, KRB, pH 7.4) was diluted with 200 mM eserine in KRB as a choline esterase inhibitor and incubated at 37°C for 30 min. The mixture was centrifuged at 2000 × g for 10 min at 4°C, and the synaptosomes were resuspended in KRB. After the addition of 140 mM KCl-KRB into the suspension as a stimulator of depolarization of synaptic plasma membrane, the mixture was incubated at 37°C for 5 min and centrifuged at 3000 × g for 6 min. The supernatant was used to analyze acetylcholine by HPLC (Nanospace SI-1, Shiseido, Tokyo) with electrochemical detection. HPLC was carried out on a 150 × 4.6 mm ACH-SC column (IRICA Inc., Kyoto) using 50 mM K_2HPO_4, pH 7.3, containing 1 mM tetramethylammonium chloride, 3.2 mM sodium 1-octanesulfonate, 30 mM EDTA-diNa as the mobile phase.

Statistical Analysis

The results were presented as mean ± SE. All data were assessed using the two-way analysis of variance (ANOVA).

RESULTS AND DISCUSSION

Cognitive Performance of Rats Through Oxidative Stress and During Aging

The learning ability of rats is shown in FIGURE 1. For the first trial, their learning rates are expressed as 0% in the figure. The young control rats reached the platform within 20 s after only 6 trials. However, it took 15-month-old rats 8 trials to learn the goal, while 24-month-old rats needed 14 trials. Vitamin-E-deficient rats also learned slowly. It was found that the learning ability of rats decreases during aging. Two-way ANOVA analysis revealed that young rats had a learning ability significantly higher

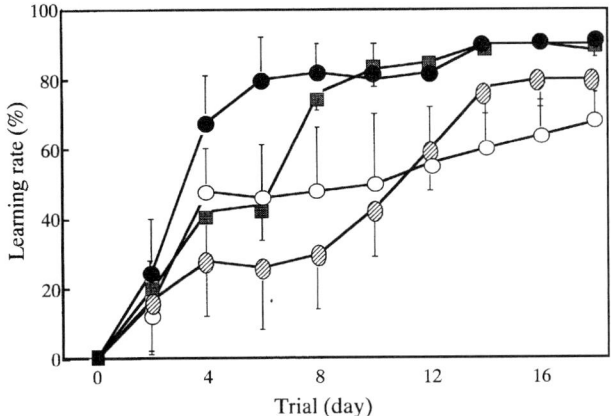

FIGURE 1. Cognitive performance of rats in learning trials. ●: 3-month-old; ■: 15-month old; ○: 24-month-old; and ○: vitamin-E-deficient rats (3 months old).

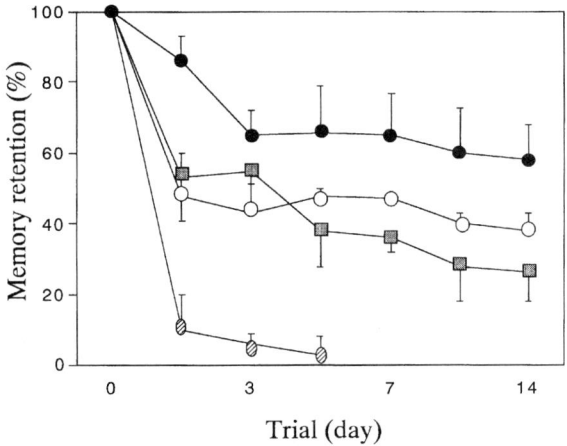

FIGURE 2. Memory retention of rats after oxidative stress in morris water maze for ●: 3-month-old; ■: 15-month-old; ○: 24-month-old; and ○: vitamin-E-deficient rats (3 months old).

than the old rats and it took vitamin-E-deficient rats 6 trials. These results imply that the learning ability of rats may be impaired during aging, and that since vitamin-E-deficient rats had poor ability, oxidative stress may involve a learning deficit.

As shown in FIGURE 2, the memory functions of all rats were remarkably impaired after hyperoxia. The young rats had higher memory retention than those in the other three groups. The ability of memory was shown to decrease during aging. Interestingly, even 10 days after hyperoxia, all the rats did not relearn again where the platform was located. These results suggest that oxidative stress contributes to the learning and memory impairment due to oxidative damage of the hippocampus and/or cerebral cortex, which are thought to control the learning and memory functions.

TABLE 1. Effect of oxidative stress on the contents of TBARS in cerebral cortex and hippocampus

	Cerebral cortex	Hippocampus
Organ		
Normal	9.27 ± 1.25^a	7.25 ± 1.58
Hyperoxia	11.47 ± 1.54	9.66 ± 3.45
Synaptic membrane		
Normal	23.83 ± 3.36^b	25.69 ± 6.57^c
Hyperoxia	73.98 ± 13.03	62.35 ± 20.88

$^a \times 10^{-10}$ mol.
$^b p < 0.002$.
$^c p < 0.05$, versus Normal.

Lipid Peroxidation of the Hippocampus and Cerebral Cortex Caused by Hyperoxia

It is implied that oxidative damage to the lipids in the brain is accompanied by an increase in thiobarbituric acid reactive substance (TBARS) values. To confirm whether the impaired cognitive function of rats is related to lipid peroxidation of the brain, changes in the lipid contents in the brain caused by hyperoxia were investigated. TABLE 1 shows the TBARS contents in the hippocampus and cerebral cortex and their synaptic membranes. Either TBARS values of both organs or their synaptic plasma membranes were increased significantly through hyperoxia. As shown in FIGURE 3, the TBARS value in the synaptic membranes from the hippocumpus increased during aging and through hyperoxia. Interestingly, the TBARS value of the synaptic membranes from young rats subjected to hyperoxia was similar to that observed in the aged rats that had not been exposed to oxygen (15 months old). These results reveal that the nerve terminals of old rats may be more susceptible to oxidative stress than are those of the young rats, and that lipid peroxidation of the synapse may be enhanced during aging, resulting in a deterioration of the nerve terminal functions. Therefore, the learning and memory functions were impaired through oxidative stress and aging.

The Release of Acetylcholine from Synaptosomes Isolated from Hippocampus

Based on the phenomenon of the abnormal accumulation of synaptic vesicles in the nerve terminals cause by hyperoxia,[9] it is thought that neurotransmitter release from the neuroterminal membranes can be impaired by the oxidative injury of synapse. To confirm this consideration, synaptosomes isolated from rat brain were incubated with potassium chloride, which stimulates the release of acetylcholine from synaptosomes. Acetylcholine release outside the membrane was then measured by HPLC. As shown in FIGURE 4, it was found that acetylcholine release from synaptosomes of oxygen-exposed rats was significantly less than that from the unexposed

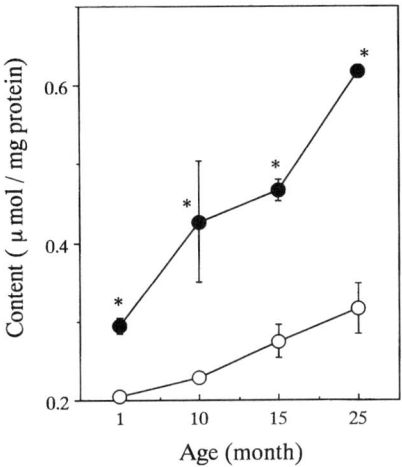

FIGURE 3. Changes in the TBARS value of synaptic membranes in the hippocampus caused by hyperoxia and during aging. Rats were maintained under air (○) or exposed to 100% oxygen (●) for 48 hours.

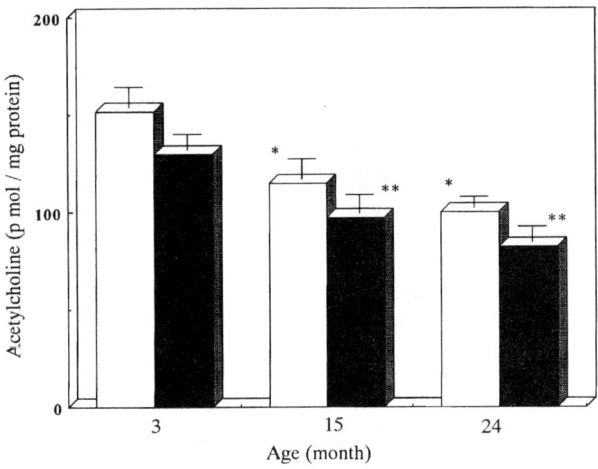

FIGURE 4. Influence of hyperoxia on acetylcholine release from synaptosomes. *Open bars*: rats maintained in air; *dotted bars*: rats subjected to hyperoxia. $*p < 0.01$ vs. 3 months in air; $** p < 0.05$ vs. 3 months hyperoxia.

rats in each age group ($P < 0.05$). The leakage decreased remarkably during aging. This supports the hypothesis that the abnormal accumulation of synaptic vesicles in nerve terminals caused by oxidative stress may be related to the deterioration of neurotransmission in the terminal.

TABLE 2. Vitamin E content and activities of antioxidative enzymes in synapse of cerebral cortex and hippocampus

	Cerebral cortex	Hippocampus
Vitamin E[a]		
Normal	2.82 ± 0.63	1.78 ± 0.56
Hyperoxia	1.91 ± 0.31[e]	1.08 ± 0.13
SOD[b]		
Normal	6.46 ± 0.512	7.87 ± 1.34
Hyperoxia	10.76 ± 0.88	9.56 ± 0.88
CAT[c]		
Normal	8.61 ± 1.05	9.32 ± 1.97
Hyperoxia	5.76 ± 0.77	6.74 ± 1.18
GSHPx[d]		
Normal	0.03 ± 0.003	0.05 ± 0.02
Hyperoxia	0.05 ± 0.01	0.11 ± 0.01*

[a] $\times 10^{-10}$ mol.
[b] U/mg protein.
[c] μ mol/mg protein.
[d] Δ 340 nm/min/mg protein.
[e] $p < 0.05$, versus Normal.

Changes in Antioxidative Defense Systems Through Hyperoxia

As shown in TABLE 2, it was found that vitamin E (α-tocopherol) contents in the synaptic membrane in the hippocampus and cerebral cortex were decreased significantly through hyperoxia. Oxidative stress lowered the contents in synaptic membranes from vitamin-E-deficient rats to a level of about 60% of the starting levels (data not shown). These results imply that vitamin E may contribute to the inhibition of the oxidative impairment of the learning and memory functions during aging.

It has been reported that the activity of SOD in synapse from the whole brain in oxygen-exposed rats was lowered significantly compared with the normal rats, and that there was no significant change in the activity of CAT.[9] In the present study, the activities of SOD and GSHPx in synapse from the hippocampus and cerebral cortex were increased under hyperoxia. On the other hand, the activity of CAT was decreased remarkably (TABLE 2). These discrepancies are presumed to be caused by the regional difference in the ability of each organ to withstand oxidative stress.

In conclusion, oxidative stress may contribute to the impairment of rat cognitive function, for example, learning and memory deficit. The deficits observed in this study are thought to be caused by the oxidative damage of the hippocampus and cerebral cortex in rats during aging and oxidative stress. Thus, in order to protect the neurodegeneration caused by the oxidative injury of the brain during aging, the antioxidant status might be changed significantly. Further studies should be carried out to define whether oxidative stress through aging actually contributes to the impairment of cognitive functions.

REFERENCES

1. HARMAN, D. 1992. Free radical theory of aging. Mutat. Res. **257:** 257–266.
2. HALLIWELL, B. 1989. Oxidant and the central nervous system: some fundamental questions. Acta Neurol. Scand. **126:** 23–33.
3. PATOLE, M.S. & T. RAMASARMA. 1988. Occurrence of lipid peroxidation in brain microsomes in the presence of NADH and Vanadate. J. Neurochem. **51:** 491–496.
4. ROUACH, H., *et al.* 1987. Lipid peroxidation and brain mitochondrial damage induced by ethanol. Bioelectronchem. Bioeng. **18:** 211–217.
5. URANO, S., *et al.* 1998. Aging and oxidative tress in neurodegeneration. BioFactors 103–112.
6. OLANOW, C. & G. ARENDASH. 1994. Metals and free radicals in neurodegeneration. Curr. Opin. Neurol. **7:** 548–558.
7. STRONG, R., M. MATTAMAL & A. ANDORN. 1993. Free radicals, the aging brain and age-related neurodegenerative disorders. *In* Free Radicals in Aging. B.P. Yu, Ed.: 223–246. CRC Press, Boca Ranton, FL.
8. STADTMAN, E. 1992. Free radicals in the genesis of Alzheimer's disease. Ann. N.Y. Acad. Sci. **695:** 73–76.
9. URANO, S., *et al.* 1997. Oxidative injury of synapse and alteration of antioxidative defense systems in rats, and its prevention by vitamin E. Eur. J. Biochem. **245:** 64–70.
10. MORRIS, R.G.M. 1984. Developments of water-maze procedure for studying spacial learning in the rats. J. Neurosci. Methods **11:** 47–60.
11. GOMI, F., M.M. DOOLEY & M. MATSUO. 1988. Antioxidant capacity of rat tissues and aging II. Biomed. Gerontol. **12:** 51–52.

Translocational Inefficiency of Intracellular Proteins in Senescence of Human Diploid Fibroblasts

IN KYOUNG LIM,[a,b] KWANG WON HONG, IN HAE KWAK, GYESOON YOON, AND SANG CHUL PARK[c]

[a]*Department of Biochemistry and Molecular Biology, Ajou University School of Medicine, Suwon, 442-721, Korea*

[c]*Department of Biochemistry, College of Medicine, and WHO Collaborating Center of Physical Culture and Aging Research for Health Promotion, Seoul National University, Seoul 110-799, Korea*

ABSTRACT: In order to investigate signal transduction pathways and related changes of actin cytoskeleton organization in cellular senescence, H-ras double mutants—V12S35, V12G37, and V12C40—were constitutively expressed in human foreskin fibroblast (HDF). Senescent HDF cells as well as the H-ras mutant expressers accumulated p-Erk1/2 in the cytoplasm with increased MEK activity and failed to translocate it to nuclei on EGF stimulation. Senescent HDF cells, V12S35 and V12G37 expressers, revealed a failure to export actin fiber from nucleus to cytoplasm and also to form stress fibers. Perinuclear expression of Rac1 was prominent in the HDF cells and V12C40 expresser; however, in the V12S35 expresser, translocation of Rac1 from perinucleus to nucleus and strong expression of RhoA were obvious. In summary, the H-ras double mutant expressers induced premature senescence through the MEK pathway, accompanied by nuclear accumulation of actin and Rac1 proteins, cytoplasmic retention of p-Erk1/2, and marked induction of RhoA expression, suggesting the translocational inefficiency of the intracellular proteins in the senescent HDF cells.

KEYWORDS: Signal transduction pathways; Senescent cells

Decreased growth rate and limited cell division, flat and large cell shapes, and tight binding of the cells to culture dish[1] are well-known characteristics of replicative senescent cells. Moreover premature senescence is known to be accelerated in response to constitutive MEK/MAPK mitogenic signaling,[2] accompanied with various changes in actin cytoskeleton organization, focal adhesions, and related signal transductions. Therefore, it might be interesting to elucidate the interactions of the signal transduction system with the cytoskeletal changes during premature senes-

---

[b]Address for correspondence: In Kyoung Lim, Department of Biochemistry and Molecular Biology, Ajou University School of Medicine, Suwon, 442-721, Korea. Voice: +82-31-219-5051; fax: +82-31-219-5059.
  iklim@madang.ajou.ac.kr

cence. Rho family proteins are regulators of signaling pathways for the organization of the actin cytoskeleton and are members of the Ras superfamily of small GTPases,[3] including RhoA, RhoB, RhoC, RhoG, and Rac1/CDC42, affecting both gene induction and actin-based cytoskeletal changes.[4] H-Ras double mutants such as V12S35, V12C40, and V12G37 are suggested to interact preferentially with specific Ras effector proteins.[5] The V12S35 binds preferentially to Raf-1 and activates MAPK without any effect on membrane ruffling;[5] the V12C40 associates with PI(3)K (Akt kinase) and promotes membrane ruffling and cell survival independent of Raf-1;[6] and the V12G37 binds Ral-GDS but fails to bind Raf-1 or PI(3)K.[5] PI3K phosphorylates Rac1 at serine 71 with a consensus sequence of xxRxRxxSYp and then inhibits GTP binding to Rac1 without a decrease of GTPase activity.[7]

In order to describe changes in the actin cytoskeleton that occurred during the accelerated cellular senescence in response to constitutive expression of H-ras mutant proteins, we have established human diploid fibroblasts, HDF, control cells, and various H-ras mutants, such as V12S35, V12G37, and V12C40, expressing stable cell lines by retrovirus infection to HDF cells. During the prolonged passages of these cell lines, changes in the actin cytoskeleton, MAPK isoforms (Erk1/2), and small G-protein RacI and RhoA expressions were examined by immunocytochemistry, Western blot analyses, and morphological studies.

We reported here that, in senescent HDF cells, cytoplasmic accumulation of p-Erk1/2 and concomitant loss of nuclear translocation occurred in response to EGF stimulation, and actin failed to translocate from nucleus to cytoplasm. Moreover, constitutive expression of V12S35 in HDF cells by retrovirus infection developed premature senescence primarily via activation of the MEK pathway and translocation of Rac1 from perinucleus to nucleus as well as overexpression of RhoA protein in both cytoplasm and nucleus.

INDUCTION OF PREMATURE SENESCENCE

Because induction of senescence is known to require wt p53 and p16ink4a expressions, it was of prime importance to examine whether p53 was wild type or not. Irradiation of the HDF cells significantly induced p53 as well as p21waf1 expressions, indicating p53 wild type in the cells. By retrovirus infection, we also prepared HDF cells that expressed H-ras double mutants. However, prior to use of the cells, constitutive expression of H-ras proteins was examined by Western blot analysis, and it was found that the three cell lines transduced with V12S35, V12G37, or V12C40 constitutively expressed H-ras proteins. Mutations at T35S, E37G, and Y40C were confirmed by genomic DNA sequencing with the automatic DNA sequencer (ABI 377). As compared with small and young control HDF cells at the PD48, virus-infected cells of the V12C40, V12G37, and V12S35 expressers revealed large and flat morphologies at the PD47 and PD42, respectively. The V12S35 expresser produced long filopodia, whereas lamellipodia were produced in the V12C40 expresser. The growth rate of the mutant ras overexpressers was much slower than the control HDF cells; however, the V12S35 expresser clearly showed the most growth retardation among the other mutant expressers as well as the control HDF cells. As one of the additional senescence markers, the expression of SA-β-galactosidase was examined in the control HDF and H-ras mutant expressers, and the rate of the expression was calculated as a percent of total cells grown. As shown in

TABLE 1. Premature senescence of HDF cells that constitutively express mutant RAS protein[a]

	Expression of SA-β-Galactosidase (Percent of total cells)			
No. of PDs	Control	V12C40	V12G37	V12S35
40	0	0	0	6.7 ± 2.9
42	0	0	0	12.3 ± 4.2
44	0	0	0	19.3 ± 3.3
45	0	0	5.4 ± 3.8	
47	0	0	20.0 ± 5.7	
50	0	8.5 ± 5.4		
59	3.3 ± 1.5			
63	21.1 ± 3.3			

[a]Data indicate mean ± SD from three independent experiments. Constant numbers of mutant cells were plated in a 60 mm flask and maintained until the cells were confluent on the bottom of the flask.

TABLE 1, the numbers of PD with SA-β-galactosidase positive cells were 59 in the control, 50 in the V12C40, 45 in the V12G37, and less than 40 in the V12S35 mutant.

HYSTERESIS OF THE SIGNAL TRANSDUCTION PATHWAY

Since it has been known that V12S35 binds preferentially to Raf-1 and activates MAPK with no effect on membrane ruffling,[5] we examined the level of p-Erk1/2 expression in young and old HDF cells. The p-Erk1/2 expression was significantly induced in PD50 HDF cells but not in PD30, whereas the V12S35 expresser strongly produced p-Erk1/2 at the earlier PD36. These findings were also confirmed by immunocytochemical staining of the early and late passage of the control HDF cells, showing a high level of p-Erk1/2 protein in the senescent cells. Treatment of PD39 HDF cells with EGF induced p-Erk expression both in cytoplasm and nucleus; however, PD59 HDF cells failed to translocate the p-Erk1/2 protein into the nucleus in response to EGF treatment. Not only the senescent HDF control cells but also the V12S35 and V12G37 expressers showed the high level of p-Erk1/2 expression as compared with HDF control and V12C40 cells.

In order to investigate the biochemical mechanism of Erk activation in senescent cells, PD66 HDF cells were pretreated with the MEK inhibitor PD98059. Inhibition of MEK activity significantly reduced phosphorylation of Erk after EGF stimulation, indicating that the highly induced expression of p-Erk1/2 in senescent cells was strongly related to activation of MEK (Erk1/2 kinase). Kinetic studies showed that the age-related impairments reduced both the level and duration of MAPK activation.[8] In brain, the constitutive activation of MAP kinases declined with age, although Erk1/2 and JNK/SAPK protein levels were not significantly altered during development or aging.[9] In our experiment, induction of activated Erk1/2 expression by EGF treatment was significantly decreased in old HDF cells as compared with that in the young. However, the old HDF cells have much higher levels of consecutively expressed p-Erk1/2 proteins than their young counterpart cells with constitutive MEK activity, suggesting the hysteresis of signal transduction modulation in the senescent cells: a higher basal-activated form versus lower inducibility.

FAILURE OF INTRACELLULAR PROTEIN TRANSLOCATION

To investigate changes of cytoskeleton organization during cellular senescence, actin expression was immunocytochemically studied. Actin was absent in the nucleus of control HDF and the V12C40 expresser at PD35, whereas V12G37 and V12S35 expressers revealed strong expression of actin in both cytoplasm and nucleus. On the other hand, HDF control cells of PD47 also strongly expressed actin in nucleus as well as cytoplasm. Therefore, all three RAS mutants and control HDF cells of the PD42-48 revealed failure of nuclear export of actin and stress fiber formation.

Actin is present in almost all eukaryotic cells and is essential for cytokinesis, cell locomotion, cell motility, cell morphology, cell growth, and other crucial events.[10] Isoforms of actin—alpha, beta, and gamma—contain leucine-rich nuclear export sequences (NES), such as -xLxxxIxxLxLx- and -xIxxxLxxVxLx-, responsible for the export of monomeric actin from nucleus to cytoplasm. Moreover, NES-disrupted actin mutants, but not of wild-type actin, induced a decrease in the proliferative potential of the cells.[11] These earlier reports support our present observation that senescent HDF cells as well as premature senescent cells, induced by H-ras double mutants, revealed an accumulation of actin in the nucleus.

Nuclear translocation of MAPK isoforms by EGF stimulation has been reported to require an intact actin cytoskeleton. Therefore, actin depolymerization significantly inhibits p-Erk1/2 transport from cytoplasm to nucleus.[12] Phosphorylated Erk1/2 in the resting cells are retained in the cytoplasm, presumably via a cytoplasmic anchoring complex composed of MEK and bound Erk1/2,[13] whereas MEK that contains a Erk1/2 docking site at the extreme N-terminus is permanently excluded from the nucleus by a nuclear export signal.[14] In our study, senescent HDF cells as well as prematurely senescent H-ras double mutant expressers failed to translocate p-Erk1/2 proteins on EGF stimulation with concomitantly increased MEK activity. These observations strongly suggest that phosphatase activity in the senescent cells might have been significantly reduced; therefore, actin-mobilizing proteins such as cofilin could not be activated, accompanied by nuclear accumulation of G actin. The defect of the actin cytoskeleton induced failure of p-Erk1/2 translocation from cytoplasm to nucleus and also decreased cellular response to mitogenic signals through MEK/MAPK pathways.

It has been known that activated RAS stimulated Rac1, and the Rac1 stimulated RhoA expressions.[3] In our experiment, Rac1 was located in perinucleus of the control and V12C40 cells, whereas it was translocated into nucleus of the V12S35 expresser at PD33 cells. RhoA was mainly expressed in nucleus of the control, V12C40 and V12G37 cells, as opposed to highly induced in both nucleus and cytoplasm of the V12S35 expresser.

It has also been reported that treatment of NIH3T3 cells with lipopolysaccharide revealed colocalization of ERM (ezrin, radixin, and moesin) proteins and F-actin in membrane protrusions. Radixin with F-actin localized in apical membrane protrusions in the presence of activated RhoA (RhoAV14), but not activated Rac (RacV12)

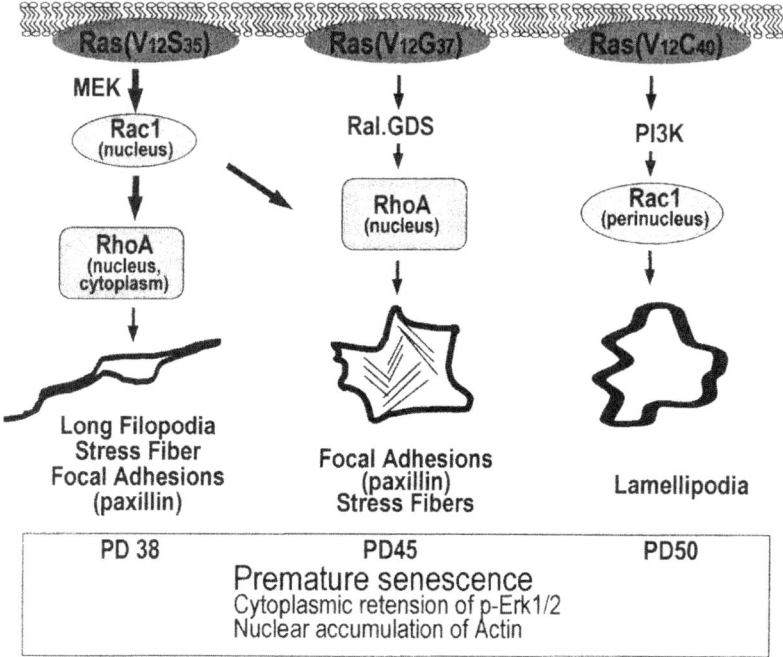

FIGURE 1. Proposed signal transduction pathways regulating premature senescence in the V12S35, V12G37, and V12C40 expressing HDF cells at PD38, PD45, and PD50, respectively, as compared with PD59 in the control HDF cells. Premature senescence induced cytoplasmic retention of p-Erk1/2 and nuclear accumulation of actin proteins, mainly through the H-rasV12S35/MEK/Rac1/RhoA. There was cross talk between the V12S35 and V12G37 pathways.

or activated CDC42. However, pretreatment with C3 transferase blocked subsequent lipopolysaccharide-induced relocalization of radixin in NIH3T3 cells, and the mitogen induced phosphorylation of serine/threonine residues of radixin. A novel function of RhoA in induction of apical membrane/actin protrusions presents a possibility that, through RhoA-dependent phosphorylation, ERM proteins may be critical regulators and components of these structures.[15]

In conclusion, premature senescence might result from failure of G-actin transport from nucleus to cytoplasm and accompanying failure of nuclear translocation of p-Erk1/2 proteins from cytoplasm in response to MEK activity. Through MEK activation, senescence pathway induced Rac1 translocation from perinucleus to nucleus, and the activated Rac1 stimulated RhoA expression in both nucleus and cytoplasm. Translocation of Rac1 from perinucleus to nucleus was most prominent in the V12S35 expresser, and partially in the V12G37 expresser. Overexpression of V12S35 produced senescent HDF cells with very long filopodia and paxillin induction with stress fiber formations. Signals induced by V12S35 have a cross talk with those that are from the V12G37 expression for regulation of actin cytoskeleton organizations (FIG. 1).

ACKNOWLEDGMENT

This study was supported by a grant (HMP-98-MS-0001) from the Good Health R & D Project, Ministry of Health and Welfare, Republic of Korea, to In K. Lim.

REFERENCES

1. MACIEIRA-COELHO, A., E. LORIA & L. BERUMEN. 1975. Relationship between cell kinetic changes and metabolic events during cell senescense *in vitro*. Adv. Exp. Med. Biol. **53:** 51– 65.
2. LIN, A.W., M. BARRADAS, J.C. STONE, L. VAN AELST, M. SERRANO & S.W. LOWE. 1998. Premature senescence involving p53 and p16 is activated in response to constitutive MEK/MAPK mitogenic signaling. Genes **12:** 3008–3019.
3. ZOHN, I.M., S.L. CAMPBELL, R. KHOSRAVI-FAR, K.L. ROSSMAN & C.J. DER. 1998. Rho family proteins and Ras transformation: the RHOad less traveled gets congested. Oncogene **17:** 1415–1438.
4. WHITEHEAD, I.P., K. ABE, J.L. GORSKI & C.J. DER. 1998. CDC42 and FGD1 cause distinct signaling and transforming activities. Mol. Cell. Biol. **18:** 4689–4697.
5. WHITE, M.A., C. NICOLETTE, A. MINDEN, A. POLVERINO, L. VAN AELST, M. KARIN & M.H. WIGLER. 1995. Multiple Ras functions can contribute to mammalian cell transformation. Cell **80:** 533–541.
6. RODRIGUEZ-VICIANA, P., P.H. WARNE, A. KHWAJA, B.M. MARTE, D. PAPPIN, P. DAS, M.D. WATERFIELD, A. RIDLEY & J. DOWNWARD. 1997. Role of phosphoinositide 3-OH kinase in cell transformation and control of the actin cytoskeleton by Ras. Cell **89:** 457–467.
7. KWON, T., D.Y. KWON, J. CHUN, J.H. KIM & S.S. KANG. 2000. Akt protein kinase inhibits Rac1-GTP binding through phosphorylation at serine 71 of Rac1. J. Biol. Chem. **275:** 423–428.
8. WHISLER, R.L., Y.G. NEWHOUSE & S.E. BAGENSTOSE. 1996. Age-related reductions in the activation of mitogen-activated protein kinases p44mapk/ERK1 and p42mapk/ERK2 in human T cells stimulated via ligation of the T cell receptor complex. Cell Immunol. **168:** 201–210.
9. HU, Y., G. SCHETT, Y. ZOU, H. DIETRICH & Q. XU. 1998. Abundance of platelet-derived growth factors (PDGFs), PDGF receptors and activation of mitogen-activated protein kinases in brain decline with age. Brain Res. Mol. Brain Res. **53:** 252–259.
10. MITCHISON, T.J. & L.P. CRAMER. 1996. Actin-based cell mobility and cell locomotion. Cell **84:** 371–379.
11. WADA, A., M. FUKUDA, M. MISHIMA & E. NISHIDA. 1998. Nuclear export of actin: a novel mechanism regulating the subcellular localization of a major cytoskeleton protein. EMBO J. **17:** 1635–1641.
12. ARNAUTOV, A.M. & N.N. NIKOL'SKII. 1998. Transport into the cell nucleus of p42 and p44 isoforms of MAP kinase induced by epidermal growth factor requires the presence of intact active cytoskeleton. Tsitologiia **40:** 639–647.
13. LENORMAND, P., J-M. BRONDELLO, A. BRUNET & J. POUYSSEGUR. 1998. Growth factor-induced p42/p44 MAPK nuclear translocation and retention requires both MAPK activation and neosynthesis of nuclear anchoring proteins. J. Cell Biol. **142:** 625–633.
14. JAARO, H., H. RUBINFELD, T. HANOCH & R. SEGER. 1997. Nuclear translocation of mitogen-activated protein kinase kinase (MEK1) in response to mitogenic stimulation. Proc. Natl. Acad. Sci. USA **94:** 3742–3747.
15. SHAW, R.J., M. HENRY, F. SOLOMON & T. JACKS. 1998. RhoA-dependent phosphorylation and relocalization of ERM proteins into apical membrane/actin protrusions in fibroblasts. Mol. Biol. Cell **9:** 403–419.

Oxidative Stress and Neurodegeneration in Prion Diseases

JAE-IL KIM,[a] SEUNG-IL CHOI,[a] NAM-HO KIM, [a] JAE-KWANG JIN,[a] EUN-KYOUNG CHOI,[a] RICHARD I. CARP,[c] AND YONG-SUN KIM[a,b,d]

[a]*Institute of Environment & Life Science and* [b]*Department of Microbiology, College of Medicine, Hallym University, Chuncheon, Kangwon-do 200-702, South Korea*

[c]*NYS Institute for Basic Research in Developmental Disabilities, Staten Island, New York 10314, USA*

ABSTRACT: Transmissible spongiform encephalopathies (TSEs), also termed prion diseases, are a group of fatal neurodegenerative diseases that affect humans and a number of other animal species. The etiology of these diseases is thought to be associated with the conversion of a normal protein, PrPC, into an infectious, pathogenic form, PrPSc. The PrPSc form shows greater protease resistance than PrPC and accumulates in affected individuals, often in the form of extracellular plaques. The pathogenesis and the molecular basis of neuronal cell death in these diseases are not well understood. Oxidative stress has been proposed to play an important role in the pathogenesis of several neurodegenerative disorders. In the present study, evidence of oxidative stress in scrapie, the archetype disease of the TSEs, is discussed. In addition, the mechanisms whereby oxidative stress could lead to neuronal degeneration are described.

KEYWORDS: Neurodegeneration, oxidative stress, prion diseases

The spongiform encephalopathies (prion disorders) are a group of transmissible diseases with common pathological changes of the central nervous system (CNS), including neuronal cell loss, vacuolation, astrocytosis, and, frequently, the presence of amyloid plaques.[1–3] Creutzfeldt-Jakob disease (CJD) in humans, scrapie in sheep, and bovine spongiform encephalopathy (BSE) in cows are the most extensively studied prion diseases.[1–3] The pathogenesis and molecular basis of neuronal cell death in these diseases remain unclear. Oxidative stress is induced by reactive oxygen species (ROS) or free radicals, and has been proposed to play an important role in the pathogenesis of several neurodegenerative disorders including Alzheimer's disease.[4] In addition to the well-known toxic nature of ROS, low concentrations of these compounds can cause small perturbations in the cellular redox state and may function as intracellular effectors of gene transcription.[5,6] In the present study, we have focused on the possible implication of oxidative stress in the mechanism of neuronal cell loss in scrapie with respect to its role in both neurotoxicity and intracellular signaling.

---

[d]Address for correspondence: Dr. Yong-Sun Kim, Institute of Environment & Life Science and Department of Microbiology, College of Medicine, Hallym University, 1 Ockcheon-dong, Chuncheon, Kangwon-do 200-702, South Korea.Voice: 82-33-240-1951; fax: 82-33-241-3422.
yskim@sun.hallym.ac.kr

First, we evaluated *in vivo* oxidative damage by examining the markers for oxidative stress in the brains of control and scrapie-infected animals. Significant increases in the level of malondialdehyde (MDA) and in the rate of generation of free radicals, including superoxide anion (O_2^-), were observed in the brains of scrapie-infected animals.[7–9] The activity of Cu/Zn-superoxide dismutase (SOD), one of the antioxidative enzymes responsible for scavenging ROS, was not affected by scrapie infection; however, Mn-SOD activity was markedly decreased in the infected group.[7,8] Based on the fact that Mn-SOD is a mitochondrial enzyme that is ordinarily involved in scavenging superoxide anion, it was presumed that there would be mitochondrial abnormalities in the brains of infected animals. This concept was supported by the observation of significant decreases in the activity of cytochrome c oxidase (complex IV) and ATPase (complex V) in the cerebral mitochondria from infected animals;[7] structural abnormalities of neuronal mitochondria from these animals were also observed by electron microscopy.[7,8]

The effect of oxidative stress in human disease has often been linked to the selective accumulation of iron in pathological regions; in this scenario, iron potentiates oxygen toxicity via a reaction termed the iron-catalyzed Harber-Weiss reaction.[10] In the presence of iron, superoxide anion and hydrogen peroxide can easily be converted to more dangerous species, such as highly reactive hydroxyl (·OH) radical.[10] In this regard, we examined the changes in the iron levels in the brains of scrapie-infected animals by spectrophotometry and histochemistry. In the scrapie-infected group, both the level of total iron and the intensity of Fe^{3+} staining were significantly increased compared to the results observed in the control group.[11] In addition, a shift in the ratio of Fe^{2+}/Fe^{3+} was observed in the brains of infected animals.[11] A change of iron redox state in favor of ferric iron (Fe^{3+}) is known to be a condition for participation of iron in hydroxyl radical formation and lipid peroxidation.[12] Therefore, these results suggest that elevated ROS generation, the changes in iron levels and in iron redox states, and lowered scavenging activity in mitochondria might lead to free radical damage to neuronal cells. Such deleterious changes are likely to be involved in the neurodegeneration observed in the brains of scrapie-infected animals.

As described earlier, it has been suggested that ROS may serve as intracellular effectors in gene regulation and may be involved in signal transduction pathways.[5,6] Among the most important pathways affected by oxidants are the nuclear factor kappa B (NF-κB) signaling pathways.[5,6] The NF-κB/Rel family of transcription factors is important in the regulation of numerous genes involved in mediating inflammation caused by viral and bacterial infections, and other stress stimuli.[13] ROS activate NF-κB, and in many types of cells a variety of structurally unrelated antioxidative compounds diminish or completely eliminate NF-κB activation.[5,6,14] As in most immunoreactive cells, the target genes for NF-κB in brain encode proteins with immune and inflammatory activities.[15] In this connection, glial cytokines and acute phase proteins have been reported in the brains of animals and humans with prion disease; it has been suggested that these are important pathogenic factors in the progression of neuropathological changes and neurodegeneration in these diseases.[16–18] From the preceding observations, we propose that the increased oxidative stress induced by scrapie infection may also be involved in NF-κB signaling functions and in the activation of cerebral inflammatory processes.

In electrophoretic mobility shift assays (EMSA) and immunohistochemical studies, NF-κB activity was significantly increased in the brains of infected animals.[9] As

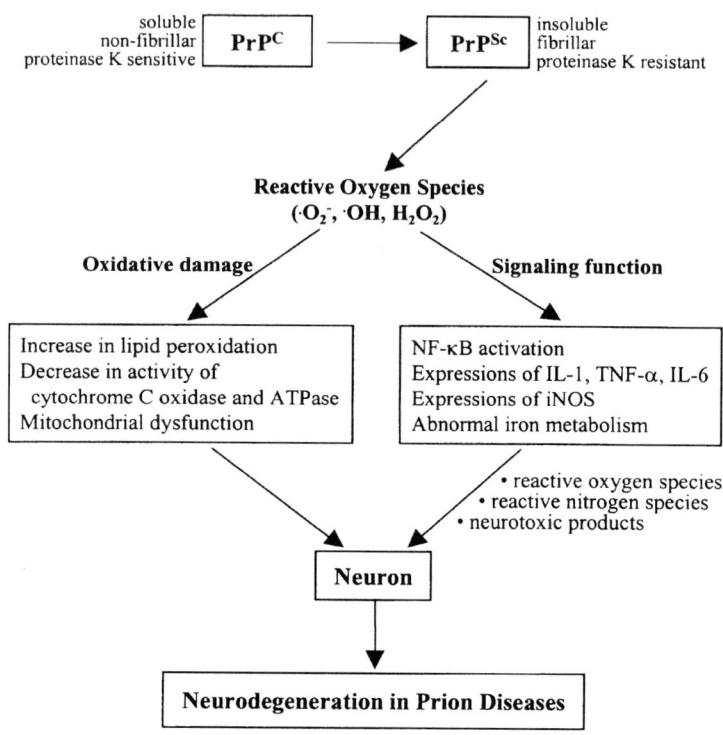

FIGURE 1. Possible implication of oxidative stress in neurodegeneration in prion diseases.

noted earlier, NF-κB is known to be a major transcriptional activator for inflammatory mediators in a variety of cells, including those in the brain; we therefore analyzed the induction of proinflammatory cytokine genes and found that interleukin-1α/β and TNF-α mRNAs were expressed only in the brains of the scrapie-infected group.[9] In double-immunohistochemical studies, immunoreactivity of NF-κB was colocalized in GFAP-positive astrocytes.[9] Prion protein is known to accumulate in astrocytes prior to the cardinal neuropathological changes in scrapie.[19] Therefore, the increase in NF-κB activity might be the result of the accumulation of prion protein in astrocytes via the increase of ROS formation. This concept is supported further by our findings that there was induction of two representative target genes of NF-κB activation, interleukin-6 and iNOS, in brain astrocytes of scrapie-infected anmials.[9,20]

To conclude, it is proposed that prion infection in brain induces oxidative stress and changes in iron metabolism. This increase in oxidative stress would directly damage neuronal cells and indirectly affect the signaling function in glial cells, resulting in indirect neuronal cell loss through the production of cytotoxic mediators (FIG. 1).

ACKNOWLEDGMENT

This work was supported by Grant 1999-1-205-005-3 from the interdisciplinary research program of the KOSEF.

REFERENCES

1. CARP, R.I., X. YE, R.J. KASCSAK & R. RUBENSTEIN. 1995. The nature of the scrapie agent. Biological characteristics of scrapie in different scrapie strain-host combinations. Ann. N.Y. Acad. Sci. **724:** 221–234.
2. CARP, R.I., R.J. KASCSAK, R. RUBENSTEIN & P.A. MERZ. 1994. The puzzle of PrP^{Sc} and infectivity: do the pieces fit? Trends Neurosci. **17:** 148–149.
3. PRUSINER, S.B. 1998. Prions. Proc. Natl. Acad. Sci. USA **95:** 13363–13383.
4. BEAL, M.F. 1995. Aging, energy, and oxidative stress in neurodegenerative diseases. Ann. Neurol. **38:** 357–366.
5. KALTSCHMIDT, B., P.A. BAEUERLE & C. KALTSCHMIDT. 1993. Potential involvement of the transcription factor NF-κB in neurological disorders. Molec. Aspects Med. **14:** 171–190.
6. ALLEN, R.G. & M. TRESINI. 2000. Oxidative stress and gene regulation. Free Radic. Biol. Med. **28:** 463–499.
7. CHOI, S.I., W.K. JU, E.K. CHOI, J. KIM, H.Z. LEA, R.I. CARP, H.M. WISNIEWSKI & Y.S. KIM. 1998. Mitochondrial dysfunction induced by oxidative stress in the brains of hamsters infected with the 263K scrapie agent. Acta Neuropathol. **96:** 279–286.
8. LEE, D.W., H.O. SOHN, H.B. LIM, Y.G. LEE, Y.S. KIM, R.I. CARP & H.M. WISNIEWSKI. 1999. Alteration of free radical metabolism in the brain of mice infected with scrapie agent. Free Radical Res. **30:** 499–507.
9. KIM, J.I., W.K. JU, J.H. CHOI, J. KIM, E.K. CHOI, R.I. CARP, H.M. WISNIEWSKI & Y.S. KIM. 1999. Expression of cytokine genes and increased nuclear factor-kappa B activity in the brains of scrapie-infected mice. Mol. Brain Res. **73:** 17–27.
10. HALLIWELL, B., J.M.C. GUTTERIDGE & C.E. CROSS. 1992. Free radicals, antioxidants, and human disease: where are we now? J. Lab Clin. Med. **119:** 598–620.
11. KIM, N.H., J.K. JIN, M.S. KWON, E.K. CHOI, R.I. CARP, H.M. WISNIEWSKI & Y.S. KIM. 2000. Increased ferric iron content and iron-induced oxidative stress in the brains of scrapie-infected mice. Brain Res. **884:** 98–103.
12. BEN-SHACHAR, D., P. RIEDERER & M.B.H. YOUDIM. 1991. Iron-melanin interaction and lipid peroxidation: implications for Parkinson's disease. J. Neurochem. **57:** 1609–1614.
13. BAEUERLE, P.A. & T. HENKEL. 1994. Function and activation of NF-κB in the immune system. Annu. Rev. Immunol. **12:** 141–179.
14. SCHRECK, R., P. RIEBER & P.A. BAEUERLE. 1991. Reactive oxygen intermediates as apparently widely used messengers in the activation of the NF-κB transcription factor and HIV-1. EMBO J. **10:** 2247–2258.
15. LIPTON, S.A. 1997. Janus faces of NF-κB: neurodestruction versus neuroprotection. Nat. Med. **3:** 19–22.
16. WILLIAMS, A., A.-M. VAN DAM, D. RITCHIE, P. EIKELENBOOM & H. FRASER. 1997. Immunocytochemical appearance of cytokines, prostaglandin E2 and lipocortin-1 in the CNS during the incubation period of murine scrapie correlates with progressive PrP accumulations. Brain Res. **754:** 171–180.
17. KORDEK, R., V.R. NERURKAR, P.P. LIBERSKI, S. ISAACSON, R. YANAGIHARA & D.C. GAJDUSEK. 1996. Heightened expression of tumor necrosis factor alpha, interleukin 1 alpha, and glial fibrillary acidic protein in experimental Creutzfeldt-Jakob disease in mice. Proc. Natl. Acad. Sci. USA **93:** 9754–9758.
18. MCGEER, P.L. & E.G. MCGEER. 1995. The inflammatory response system of brain: implications for therapy of Alzheimer and other neurodegenerative disease. Brain Res. Rev. **21:** 195–218.

19. DIEDRICH, J.F., P.E. BENDHEIM, Y.S. KIM, R.I. CARP & A.T. HAASE. 1991. Scrapie-associated prion protein accumulates in astrocytes during scrapie infection. Proc. Natl. Acad. Sci. USA **88:** 375–379.
20. JU, W.K., K.J. PARK, E.K. CHOI, J. KIM, R.I. CARP, H.M. WISNIEWSKI & Y.S. KIM. 1998. Expression of inducible nitric oxide synthase in the brains of scrapie-infected mice. J. Neurovirol. **4:** 445–450.

On the True Role of Oxygen Free Radicals in the Living State, Aging, and Degenerative Disorders

IMRE ZS.-NAGY

Department of Gerontology (VILEG Hungarian Section), University of Debrecen, Medical and Health Science Center, Debrecen, H-4012, Hungary

ABSTRACT: Oxyradicals are generally considered harmful byproducts of oxidative metabolism, causing molecular damage in living systems. They are implicated in various processes such as mutagenesis, aging, and series of pathological events. Although all this may be justified, evidence is accumulating that it is an oversimplified view of the real situation. We can assume nowadays that the living state of cells and organisms implicitly requires the production of oxyradicals. This idea is supported by experimental facts and arguments as follows. (1) Complete inhibition of the oxyradical production by KCN (or by any block of respiration) kills the living organisms much before the energy reserves would be exhausted. (2) Construction of the supramolecular organization of the cells (especially of their membranous compounds) requires the cross-linking effect of oxyradicals, particularly that of $OH\cdot$ radicals. (3) Blast type cells produce much fewer oxyradicals than do differentiated ones, and interventions increasing the production of $OH\cdot$ radicals induce differentiation of various lines of leukemic (HL-60 and K562) and normal (fibroblasts, chondroblasts, etc.) cells, while SOD expression increases greatly. (4) It is reasonable to assume that the continuous flux of $OH\cdot$ radicals is prerequisite to maintenance of constant electron delocalization on the proteins, which is a semiconductive phenomenon suggested in 1941 by Szent-Györgyi, but it has never been proven experimentally. It is theoretically possible to describe the function of the synapses as that of a single p-n-p transistor, assuming that the free radical flux maintains electron movements on the subsynaptic structures, while the actual membrane potential is governing the electron flux. This theoretical approach may open completely new possibilities for our understanding of the normal functions of living organisms, such as basic memory mechanisms in brain cells, their aging processes, and therapeutic approaches to many degenerative disorders, such as various types of dementia.

KEYWORDS: Oxygen free radicals; Aging; Degenerative diseases

INTRODUCTION

The history of discovery of oxygen free radicals in the biomedical sciences goes back to the mid-1950s, when these radicals had been proposed to play a causal role

---

Address for correspondence: Imre Zs.-Nagy, Department of Gerontology (VILEG Hungarian Section), University of Debrecen, Medical and Health Science Center, POB 50, Debrecen, H-4012, Hungary. Voice/fax: +(36-52)-418-470.
izsnagy@jaguar.dote.hu

in biological aging.[1] This idea has still not been completely accepted by many biochemists despite accumulating evidence demonstrating that these radicals do occur in biological systems and represent a real danger to macromolecular integrity.

The free radical theory of aging, elaborated and first investigated mainly by Harman[1-8] and later by many others, suggests that oxygen free radicals are harmful byproducts of aerobic life and as such represent the basic cause of aging and numerous diseases.

This concept has been implicated in numerous biological phenomena such as cellular aging, mutagenesis, inflammation, and other pathologies.[9-16] Unfortunately, however, despite the rather wide acceptance of this concept, a deeper level of analysis reveals many contradictions, unexplained problems, and paradoxical situations.

I began to point out the contradictions of the free radical theory of aging about 15 years ago[11,17-21] and during the fourth IABG Congress of Ancona suggested explicitly that the biological role of oxygen free radicals in cell differentiation and aging be reconsidered.[22] Moreover, I revisited the original ideas of Szent-Györgyi[23,24] proposing the semiconduction of proteins as an attribute of the living state in light of recent knowledge about the semiconductive properties of carbon compounds and oxygen free radicals.[25]

Although many contemporary scientists in frequent personal discussions have judged these ideas as important and exciting new avenues, to the best of my knowledge, no one has ever taken an experimental approach. Therefore, the central dogma of free-radical biology has remained unchanged; namely, most investigators suppose even today that oxygen free radicals are only harmful byproducts, and we have to fight for their elimination in order to assure a longer and healthier human life. Therefore, I would like to summarize once again the main contradictions of free-radical biology and to propose the application of the semiconductive principles of Szent-Györgyi[23,24] for the function of synapses. The main purpose is to stimulate the design and realization of new experiments in this field, which may be helpful in expanding our understanding of the living state.

THE MAIN CONTRADICTIONS IN FREE RADICAL BIOLOGY

The Paradox of the Free Radical Theory of Aging

It is well known that young individuals consume more oxygen per unit of mass and time than do old ones. Therefore, there must be a more intense radical formation in younger systems than in older ones. Despite this situation, young cells and organisms can grow and differentiate, whereas older cells progressively deteriorate in structure and functional performance. This has been termed the paradox of the free radical theory of aging.[17] The general belief that aging is caused by oxygen free radicals remains shaky unless the aforementioned discrepancy finds an acceptable explanation in the biological structure itself.

The paradox of the free radical theory of aging was explained by the membrane hypothesis of aging[26] on the basis of the age-dependent increase in the physical density of living systems. This process causes a lifelong increase in the damaging efficiency of the cross-linking effect of oxygen free radicals. In other words, even the lower level of oxygen free radicals in older systems may represent a more serious danger, because at higher physical density even fewer radicals may produce more intermolecular cross-linking. Unfortunately, most of the scientists working in this field are simply unaware of this physicochemical interrelationship.

Complete Inhibition of Oxygen Free Radical Production Is Lethal

Complete inhibition of oxygen free radical production can be achieved by various methods. For example, the first effect of KCN is to block the oxygen supply from the hemoglobin to the tissues in virtually zero time. It therefore immediately stops the formation of oxygen free radicals. This possibility deserves serious attention, because this substance is widely recognized as one of the most toxic, causing the immediate death of the organism. It is generally believed that the immediate lethal effect of KCN is due to blockage of ATP synthesis, that is, the cause of death is energy shortage. However, this explanation is probably untrue, because ATP reserves at the time of death would still be sufficient for a considerably longer time (5–10 minutes) even in the brain. Because there are virtually no oxyradical reserves, the consequences of their lack are much more immediate than the exhaustion of ATP reserves. To the best of my knowledge, no one has ever explained the role of KCN as the quickest and most perfect oxygen radical scavenger, although such an interpretation may be justified.

It is extremely intriguing that death by suffocation may be interpreted in the same way, that is, due to blockage of oxygen radical formation, with the only difference from KCN intoxication being that it is less immediate, because the oxygen reserves in the lung and blood can still be utilized for maintenance of radical flux for 2–3 minutes. In any case, even death from suffocation occurs long before exhaustion of ATP reserves in the brain.

The foregoing facts need explanation. It seems that a continuous oxygen supply for living beings is necessary not only to produce ATP, but also to maintain a "supply voltage" for living cells through continuous electron delocalization on the proteins, as will be explained. This is a completely new suggestion. This idea implicitly contradicts the simpleminded central dogma of free radical biology, according to which oxygen free radicals are considered only as harmful byproducts. It must be emphasized, however, that this concept does not deny the possibility of damaging side effects of these radicals, but it offers a much wider basis for interpretation of radical functions. The situation in living beings can be considered similar to that of electronic devices: in the latter, the supply current is an absolute prerequisite for their function, whereas the same current may cause breakdowns in some components of the system through nondesired effects such as heating and crystal melting. In other words, the free radical theory of aging may remain valid; however, we should not fight against any free radical, but only against those site-specific radical events that prove to be destructive, keeping in mind that without oxyradical formation, the living state is not possible.

Role of Oxygen Free Radicals in the Supramolecular Organization of Living Systems

Contemporary biological research is concerned mainly with molecular genetics. Therefore, few people are interested in the supramolecular organization of living material. The main question to be asked is, what kind of forces bring about, maintain, and stabilize the supramolecular and cellular organization of macromolecules? This question is justified, because the genetic code contains information only for the amino acid sequence of the protein chain; although this sequence may largely determine the coiling of the chain and even the final conformation of the macromolecule, it is scarcely known how the intermolecular bonds stabilizing the supramolecular organization of well-defined structural entities such as membranes, sarcomeres, and synapses come into being. The situation is similar to that in which we have all the components for constructing a house, but do not know how to put together and strengthen the parts to make a stable house. One can speak of hydrogen bonds, hydrophobic interactions, and other "weak" interactions, for example, that are certainly involved in the construction of the cell structure; nevertheless, they are most probably not sufficient for this purpose. Therefore, we have to assume that more stable intermolecular bonds, such as covalent cross-links, should also play a role in the relatively high level of physiologically necessary stabilization of living structures.

If the foregoing assumption is accepted, oxygen free radicals of cross-linking effect, especially the OH· free radicals, may be thought to be involved in this process. That is, we have to reconsider their role on this basis, which has so far been classified only as a damaging one. Some experimental data have shown that oxygen free radicals are involved in cell differentiation and maturation of various cultured cell lines of the blast type.[27–32] All these data suggest that the oxyradicals are much more important for living beings than was originally thought. Such an approach may shed new light into the functional interpretation of the elements of the so-called radical-defense mechanism, such as SOD and catalase. The known facts and the theoretical possibilities relevant to this idea were summarized by this author[22,26] and therefore will not be repeated in detail here.

Why Do We Have to Assume a Useful Role of Oxygen Free Radicals in the Functional Processes of Living Systems?

A further consideration is the possibility that OH· free radicals may not only produce covalent cross-links between adjacent protein and other molecules, but also contribute to the formation of protein radicals of various life spans. The involvement of such radicals in biological catalysis has already been suggested.[33] However, we have to assume the existence of a series of other important roles for OH· radicals. For example, their formation and reactions are sufficiently fast to assume their involvement in brain memory formation. If we consider that the brain is practically devoid of catalase, it seems logical to assume that most of the hydrogen peroxide formed in the brain is directed toward OH· radical production; if this is true, these radicals may have roles other than the assumed damaging roles. Although currently this is only speculation, it may be worthy of further exploration if we consider the almost complete lack of secure knowledge about brain memory mechanisms.

Semiconductive Properties of Proteins in Relation to the Flux of OH· Free Radicals

All of the preceding led me to the conviction that the role of oxyradicals should be analyzed on a much wider basis than the simpleminded damaging factor hypothesis. It seemed to me worthwhile to reconsider some older suggestions[23,34] regarding the semiconductive properties of proteins in the living state.[25] Because this idea may be completely new for most scientists working in biomedical research, the main points will also be explained.

FACTS AND PROBLEMS RELATED TO PROTEIN SEMICONDUCTION

Using methods of preparative and analytical biochemistry, the molecular components of living systems can be isolated in pure form and put in test tubes. However, life itself is lost during such purification, because the living state is bound to a supramolecular organization and interaction of the compounds within the cellular structure. The supramolecular organization is created through certain intermolecular reactions that are based on the interactions of the external electron orbits of the macromolecules. From these and many other theoretical considerations, Szent-Györgyi[23,24,34,35] concluded that the living state is bound to particularly organized functions of certain electron orbits. Consequently, it is plausible that the processes of biological maturation and aging are also related to alterations of those electron orbits of the macromolecules. Because free radical reactions usually take place on external electron orbits, these ideas and free radical biology obviously have a number of common aspects.

About 60 years ago, Szent-Györgyi[23,24] explicitly suggested that the living state involves most probably a semiconductor function of the proteins in cells. Although this was a very attractive hypothesis, it did not get accepted at that time for two main reasons. (1) Most of the contemporary biochemists could not understand the essence of this proposal, because the field of "semiconduction" was almost completely unknown for them. (2) Because at that time semiconductive phenomena were largely unexplored, even in solid state physics, the hypothesis of Szent-Györgyi[23,24] was unanimously rejected by contemporary physicists on an apparently solid, "theoretically established" basis. The main argument against this idea was that semiconduction of carbon compounds is simply not possible, because so-called valency and conduction bands in carbon compounds are energetically too far from each other. As a matter of fact, 5.5 eV energy would be required to push an electron from the valency band to the conduction band in carbon compounds (in Si, this energy gap is only 1.1 eV).[36,37] Because the only way for electron "excitation" in semiconductors at that time was assumed to be exclusively heat agitation, the hypothesis of Szent-Györgyi was unanimously rejected.[35]

This objection of physicists, although seemingly solid and convincing, did not prove to be true for carbon compounds in general. As a matter of fact, diamond transistors were soon developed in which thin layers of artificial diamond crystals doped with the trivalent boron atoms resulted in excellent semiconductor properties.[36,37] We can conclude from these achievements that (1) despite "theoretically" established barriers, semiconduction of carbon compounds is possible if the structure and the circumstances are properly designed; and (2) these kinds of "theoretical" predictions are obviously always of limited value until a question is not explored sufficiently in its physical reality.

Szent-Györgyi[34,35] took very seriously the objection of physicists to his hypothesis. Nevertheless, he believed that despite the mentioned energetic barrier, a proper mechanism may exist in living cells that can assure the formation of electron holes on proteins. In the event we can identify such mechanisms, proteins can well function as semiconductors. He assumed in general terms that if suitable electron acceptors take over electrons from protein molecules, causing "electron desaturation" of proteins, semiconduction may be realized. In this assumed process, he attributed the main role to a "one by one" electron transport where the terminal acceptor would be, for example, some carbonyl groups. He supposed the existence of a charge-transfer process maintained by compounds such as methylglyoxal. Although he and his coworkers presented extensive experimental evidence to support this concept,[34,38–42] it could not prove unanimously the basic hypothesis, mainly because of quantitative problems. As a matter of fact, semiconduction can be imagined only, if electron desaturation takes place continuously at a proper speed. Therefore, the idea of protein semiconduction in the living state was practically forgotten after the death of Szent-Györgyi.

ON THE LINK BETWEEN SEMICONDUCTION OF PROTEINS AND OXYRADICAL BIOLOGY

Szent-Györgyi[34,35] felt that a link between the semiconduction hypothesis and the existence of free radicals should exist. He described that a living mouse put into a properly designed ESR spectrometer sends a very complex ESR signal, and this signal immediately disappears when the animal is killed by KCN. This fact was considered by Szent-Györgyi as an argument for the existence of life-bound electron transitions.

There is another possibility, however, that has not been recognized by Szent-Györgyi,[34,35] namely, that the electron desaturation of proteins may well be caused and maintained by the continuous flux of OH· free radicals. This means that the practically continuous suction of electrons by OH· radicals may represent the ubiquitous mechanisms that help to overcome the energetic barrier between the valency and the conductive bands of the protein molecules. If this assumption is accepted, the continuous radical flux becomes as important for maintenance of the living state as the supply voltage is for the computers. Considering equation 1

$$OH\cdot + RH \xrightarrow{k} R\cdot + OH\cdot \quad (1)$$

where RH may represent any organic compound,[43] the estimates for k are in the range of 10^7–10^{10} M^{-1}s^{-1}. This implies that the OH· free radicals, formed continuously via O_2^--SOD-H_2O_2-Fenton reaction, pick up an electron from any of the surrounding molecules extremely quickly, in the upper range of k within about 2 molecular collisions. Although it is true that practically all organic molecules react with the OH· radicals, the rate of such reactions may be different by about 3 orders of magnitude for various components of the living material. Experimental evidence for the biological reality of the Fenton reaction is strong: (1) sufficient amounts of Fe^{2+} are available even *in vivo*;[44] and (2) OH· radicals formed by this reaction can attack practically all the amino acids and proteins even under mild chemical conditions.[45–47]

The very quick electron delocalization caused by OH· radicals may provoke some molecular alterations of RH· in the living system, as detailed before.[26] For example, formation of covalent cross-links or the formation of protein radicals of various life spans (involved in catalysis[33] or functioning as second messengers[48]). Nevertheless, from the point of view of the semiconduction hypothesis, the most important possibility is that the electron hole of R· can be refilled from the next adjacent available electron shell, resulting in a new hole, which is refilled from another shell, etc. This kind of repetition may create a situation in which the hole is moving from one place to another. This is nothing other than a semiconductive phenomenon on the protein structure, suggested by Szent-Györgyi.[23,24]

A TENTATIVE SEMICONDUCTIVE MODEL OF SYNAPSES

Obviously we have to try to outline some models of the living structure and its function in which semiconduction "makes sense" in physiologic terms. It is evident that the OH· radicals rape electrons aspecifically; therefore, the protein structure itself must play the decisive role in regulating electron movements. An attempt will be described to interpret the synaptic function in terms of the assumed "p" type semiconduction.

A plausible approach might be to describe the synaptic contacts as single transistors. To understand such a model at an elementary level, we have to summarize the basic structure and function of a transistor. The semiconductive layers (or crystals) used in electronic devices are designated as "p" or "n" types, indicating that the overall charge in them is positive or negative, respectively. A so-called p-n-p transistor used in technology is shown in FIGURE 1. Such a transistor consists of three properly constructed crystal layers put together so that between two "p" type layers we find an "n" layer, and all three layers have a self-standing electric contact with the outside world. These contacts are named emitter (E) (going to the p_1 layer), collector (C) (going to the p_2 layer), and base (B) (going to the n layer). We have to apply two different "batteries," called B-E and B-C circuits, as shown in FIGURE 1.

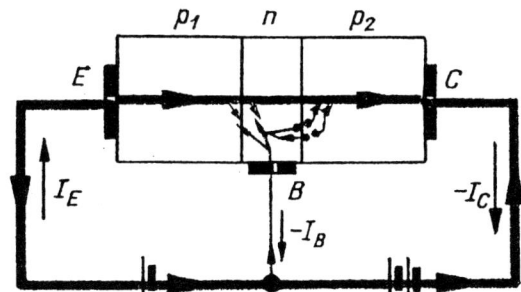

FIGURE 1. A schematic drawing of a p-n-p transistor, as explained in the text. The thick line indicates the movement of charges (holes are moving inside the p-n-p layers, while electrons are moving in the outside wires; therefore, the directions are opposite). I_E, $-I_B$, and $-I_C$ indicate the corresponding current directions, defined in technical terms. For further explanations, see text.

The simplest functions of the transistor can be defined as having two states, namely, an open one (E and C are connected to each other) or a closed one (E and C are disconnected from each other). The presence of either of these two states depends on the voltage applied on B. If the B voltage is in the range of –40–100 mV, the transistor is open, whereas in the case of nearly zero or somewhat positive B voltage, the transistor is closed. Obviously, the transition from the open to the closed state or vice versa can take place as a single event or it can be repeated with very high frequency, and in this case the transistor may transmit very high frequencies. The great advantage of the use of such semiconductive devices is that minor voltage changes on B may result in large voltage changes on the E-C contacts, that is, we can amplify electric signals to any extent. The transistors may also be of the n-p-n type, when the semiconductive layers are built up as a mirror image of the p-n-p transistor, and consequently, B voltage must be positive for opening and zero or slightly negative for closing the transistor.

Before trying to apply the semiconductive model to the synapses, we need to summarize our actual knowledge about the membrane potential of the cells. FIGURE 2 shows two essentially identical original models of the membrane potential. The model of Hodgkin and Huxley[49] demonstrates that the membrane potential (V) is about –64 mV in the resting state, and this increases to zero (or up to a low positive voltage) during the action potential due mainly to increased inward Na^+-influx (g_{Na}) under the effects of neurotransmitters (e.g., acetylcholine). This Na^+-influx is then reversed by the active pumping out of Na^+ by the Na^+-K^+-dependent ATPase. The whole process takes place within a 1–3–msec time interval. The second model is from Eccles[50] who gave the same description and detailed also the contributions of

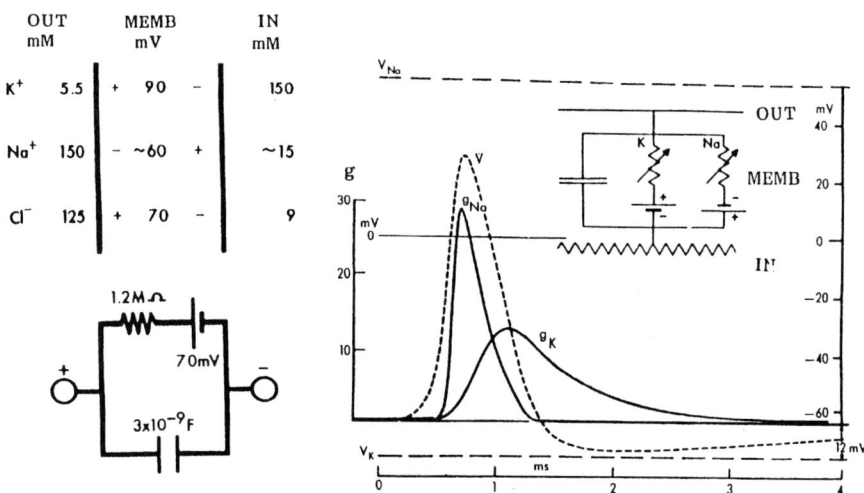

FIGURE 2. Two essentially identical electric models of membrane potential. On the left side, the (slightly modified) model from Eccles[50] with the contribution of the extra- and intracellular monovalent ion concentrations. On the *right side*, another aspect of the same membrane potential according to Hodgkin and Huxley,[49] indicating also the time scale, voltage, and ion-current changes during an action potential. Other explanations in the text.

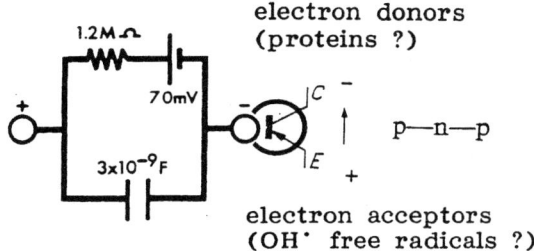

FIGURE 3. Proposed interpretation of the synapse as an elementary p-n-p transistor. In the upper part of the figure, we demonstrate an Si transistor as usual in the electronics, while the lower part depicts a synapse where the B electrode is replaced by the membrane potential in the sense as shown in FIGURE 2. C and E of the transistor are imagined as components of the subsynaptic structure and the OH· radicals, respectively. The *arrow* indicates the flow of the "hole" current between E and C in the open state of the transistor. For further explanations, see text.

various extra- and intracellular concentrations of the ions as well as their contribution to the actual membrane potential.

If we assume "p" type semiconduction for biological materials, a synapse can be imagined as shown in FIGURE 3. The role of the regulating electrode (B) can be attributed to the presynaptic membrane potential, as just described. It is very intriguing that the resting membrane potential falls exactly in the range of the opening voltage of a technical p-n-p transistor, whereas during an excitation pulse this voltage drops to a level that may result in the closure of such a transistor. If we assume that electrodes C and E are located in postsynaptic structures, C could be some of the subsynaptic proteins bearing a proper amount of delocalizable electrons, and E can be represented by the OH· free radicals.

The function of this model can be imagined as follows. In the resting state the synapses (= transistors) are open, and therefore a certain dislocation of electrons is taking place on the protein structure. This flux of electrons derives from the substrates of food (such as those that maintain energy production) and ends on OH· free radicals, that is, it disappears in water. This would mean a perfect "battery" for the living system, because there is practically no ballast to be eliminated by any special mechanisms.

Let's see what may happen during an action potential. The negative voltage on the base goes near to or above zero, that is, short closure of the transistor comes into being, during which electron flux between the collector and the emitter may be stopped and/or deviated to some other places, as compared to the resting state. Such a deviation of the electrons may create more or less persistent changes of the protein molecular conformation, and such changes may represent the elementary material basis of a kind of immediate (short-term) memory imprint.

The foregoing assumption requires further elaboration, namely, we have to find the mechanism of long-term memory. If short-term memory content is written into proteins by a kind of semiconductive mechanism due to the much shorter lifetime of proteins compared to the individual itself, there must be another way of assuring the maintenance of memory content independently from the rather quick protein decomposition. Theoretically speaking, we have to suppose the existence of a kind of reverse translation and transcription that is writing backwards the altered protein structure in some way into the genome. This part of the information should then be transcribed again to RNA and translated into new proteins, the incorporation of which to the proper place in given nerve cells may assure the long-term persistence of the memory contents. The imperfections of human memory, that is, a considerable loss of content with time, may well be explained by a statistically predictable incompleteness of such a replacement of the damaged proteins. An even more attractive fact is that we need to switch off our brain from time to time, that is, we have to go to sleep. This may be necessary to assure the time to elaborate the information having filled in our "primary memory table" during the day and transfer its contents into the long-term memory compartments.

This concept assumes a kind of reverse flow of genetic information from the proteins to DNA, which in reality is not completely unfounded even at the present level of knowledge. Molecular genetics has already discovered a process called "retroposition,"[51,52] which is nothing else than a reverse flow of genetic information from RNA to DNA. The result of this process is the formation of retroposons, which are classified into viral and nonviral superfamilies.[53] An extraordinary variety of nonviral retroposons has been described, all of them corresponding to a partial or complete DNA copy of a cellular RNA species.[53] It seems worth mentioning that although some believe that the retroposons represent a sort of molecular parasitism,[54–56] they can also confer a selective advantage on their host,[57] that is, they cannot be regarded only as a ballast. Therefore, we have to accept that retroposition can shape and reshape the eukaryotic genome in various ways, which may exactly represent a part of the just outlined, imaginary process of reverse flow of genetic information in relation to the long-term memory content. The missing link is how the primary information can really be stored by proteins.

Two important facts must be emphasized: (1) The brain accounts for 2.0–2.5% of the total human body weight, but it consumes about 20% of the total oxygen intake of the body. (2) The brain is very rich in SOD, but it is almost completely devoid of catalase, and its GPO activity is also relatively low. This fact may be explained by the necessity of brain cells to produce more OH· free radicals via SOD–H_2O_2–Fenton reaction than, for example, liver cells, in agreement with the assumption that OH· free radicals are of particular importance in quantitative terms for synaptic function and for maintenance of memory function.

POSSIBILITIES OF EXPERIMENTAL TESTING

As pointed out earlier,[25] the semiconductive properties of proteins as a basic phenomenon could be tested using the atomic force microscope (AFM).[58–60] AFM offers atomic resolution of the molecular structures in dimensions that have never been explored by any kind of optical or electron microscopy. It reveals visual information regarding the electron clouds surrounding atoms and molecules. Unfortunately, however, so far we have not been able to obtain the necessary financial support for such experiments.

REFERENCES

1. HARMAN, D. 1956. Aging: a theory based on free radical and radiation chemistry. J. Gerontol. **11:** 298–300.
2. HARMAN, D. 1957. Prolongation of the normal life span by radiation protection chemicals. J. Gerontol. **12:** 257–263.
3. HARMAN, D. 1961. Mutation, cancer and aging. Lancet **1:** 200–201.
4. HARMAN, D. 1961. Prolongation of the normal life span and inhibition of spontaneous cancer by antioxidants. J. Gerontol. **16:** 147–154.
5. HARMAN, D. 1981. The aging process. Proc. Natl. Acad. Sci. USA **78:** 7124–7128.
6. HARMAN, D. 1988. Free radical theory of aging, current status. In Lipofuscin – 1987, State of the Art. I. Zs.-Nagy, Ed. :3–21. Akadémiai Kiadò, Budapest; Elsevier Science Publishers, Amsterdam.
7. HARMAN, D. 1992. Role of free radicals in aging and disease. Ann. N.Y. Acad. Sci. **673:** 126–141.
8. HARMAN, D. 1994. Free radical theory of aging. Increasing the functional life span. Ann. N.Y. Acad. Sci. **717:** 1–15.
9. NAQUI, A., B. CHANCE & E. CADENAS. 1986. Reactive oxygen intermediates in biochemistry. Annu. Rev. Biochem. **55:** 137–166.
10. JAMIESON, D., B. CHANCE, E. CADENAS & A. BOVERIS. 1986. The relation of free radical production to hyperoxia. Annu. Rev. Physiol. **48:** 703–719.
11. ZS.-NAGY, I. 1989. Functional consequences of free radical damage to cell membranes. In CRC Handbook of Free Radicals and Antioxidants in Biomedicine. J. Miquel, A.T. Quintanilha & H. Weber, Eds. Vol. I.: 199–207. CRC Press, Inc. Boca Raton, FL.
12. CADENAS, E. 1989. Biochemistry of oxygen toxicity. Annu. Rev. Biochem. **58:** 79–110.
13. JAMIESON, D. 1989. Oxygen toxicity and reactive oxygen metabolites in mammals. Free Radic. Biol. Med. **7:** 87–108.
14. SIESJÖ, B.K., C.-D. AGARDH & F. BENGTSSON. 1989. Free radicals and brain damage. Cerebrovasc. Brain Metab. Rev. **1:** 165–211.
15. VOLICER, L. & P.B. CRINO. 1990. Involvement of free radicals in dementia of the Alzheimer type: a hypothesis. Neurobiol. Aging **11:** 567–571.
16. BEYER, W., J. IMLAY & I. FRIDOVICH. 1991. Superoxide dismutases. Progr. Nucleic Acid Res. Mol. Biol. **40:** 221–253.
17. ZS.-NAGY, I. 1986. Common mechanisms of cellular aging in brain and liver in the light of the membrane hypothesis of aging. In Liver and Aging – 1986, Liver and Brain. K. Kitani, Ed.: 373–387. Elsevier Science Publishers. Amsterdam.
18. ZS.-NAGY, I. 1987. An attempt to answer the questions of theoretical gerontology on the basis of the membrane hypothesis of aging. Adv. Biosci. **64:** 393–413.
19. ZS.-NAGY, I. 1991. Dietary antioxidants and brain aging: hopes and facts. In The Potential for Nutritional Modulation of Aging Processes. D.K. Ingram, G. Baker & N. Schock, Eds.: 379–399. Food and Nutrition Press, Inc. Trumbull, CT, USA.
20. ZS.-NAGY, I. 1989. Centrophenoxine as OH· free radical scavenger. In CRC Handbook of Free Radicals and Antioxidants in Biomedicine. J. Miquel, A.T. Quintanilha & H. Weber, Eds. Vol. II.: 87–94. CRC Press, Inc. Boca Raton, FL.

21. ZS.-NAGY, I. 1991. A review on the recent advances in the membrane hypothesis of aging. *In* Liver and Aging – 1990. K. Kitani, Ed.: 321–334. Elsevier Science Publishers. Amsterdam.
22. ZS.-NAGY, I. 1992. A proposal for reconsideration of the role of oxygen free radicals in cell differentiation and aging. Ann. N.Y. Acad. Sci. **673:** 142–159.
23. SZENT-GYÖRGYI, A. 1941. Study of energy levels in biochemistry. Nature **148:** 157–159.
24. SZENT-GYÖRGYI, A. 1941. Towards a new biochemistry? Science **93:** 609–611.
25. ZS.-NAGY, I. 1995. Semiconduction of proteins as an attribute of the living state: the ideas of Albert Szent-Györgyi revisited in the light of the recent knowledge regarding oxygen free radicals. Exp. Gerontol. **30:** 327–335.
26. ZS.-NAGY, I. 1994. The Membrane Hypothesis of Aging. CRC Press. Boca Raton, FL.
27. ZSUPÁN, I., CS. HADHÁZY, V. ZS.-NAGY, F. JENEY & I. ZS.-NAGY. 1987. The effect of OH· radicals generated by Fenton reaction on the growth and cartilage differentiation in limb bud cell culture. J. Submicrosc. Cytol. **19:** 445–455.
28. NAGY, K., G. PÁSTI, L. BENE & I. ZS.-NAGY. 1993. Induction of granulocytic maturation of HL-60 human leukemia cells by free radicals. A hypothesis of cell differentiation involving hydroxyl radicals. Free Rad. Res. Commun. **19:** 1–15.
29. NAGY, K., G. PÁSTI, L. BENE & I. ZS.-NAGY. 1995. Involvement of Fenton reaction products in differentiation induction of K562 human leukemia cells. Leuk. Res. **19:** 203–212.
30. JENEY, F. J. SZABÓ, K. NAGY, K. ORAVECZ & I. ZS.-NAGY. 1997. The effect of OH· free radicals deriving from Fenton reaction on the growth characteristics of human retrobulbar fibroblast cultures. Presented at the 13th AESF Meeting, Dec. 4–6, München, FRG.
31. JENEY, F., J. SZABÓ, K. ORAVECZ, E. BAZSÓ-DOMBI & I. ZS.-NAGY. 1998. Studies on the spontaneous and free radical-induced differentiation of the orbital fibroblasts in Graves' ophthalmopathy. Presented at the 14th AESF Meeting, Dec. 10–12, Ratzeburg, FRG.
32. CHÉNAIS, B., M. ANDRIOLLO, P. GUIRAUD, R. BELHOUSSINE & P. JEANNESSON. 2000. Oxidative stress involvement in chemically induced differentiation of K562 cells. Free Radical Biol. & Med. **28:** 18–27.
33. STUBBE, J.A. 1989. Protein radical involvement in biological catalysis? Annu. Rev. Biochem. **58:** 257–285.
34. SZENT-GYÖRGYI, A. 1977. The living state and cancer. Proc. Natl. Acad. Sci. USA **74:** 2844–2847.
35. SZENT-GYÖRGYI, A. 1978. The Living State and Cancer. Marcel Dekker, Inc. New York and Basel.
36. ANGUS, J.C. & C.C. HAYMAN. 1988. Low-pressure, metastable growth of diamond and "diamondlike" phases. Science **241:** 913–921.
37. GEIS, M.W. & J.C. ANGUS. 1992. Diamond film semiconductors. Thin sheets of diamond grown from low pressure gas and doped with impurities may serve as the basis for a new generation of electronic devices. Sci. Am. **267:** 64–69.
38. EGYÜD, L. & A. SZENT-GYÖRGYI. 1966. Cell division, SH, ketoaldehydes, and cancer. Proc. Natl. Acad. Sci. USA **55:** 388–393.
39. PETHIG, R. & A. SZENT-GYÖRGYI. 1977. Electronic properties of the casein-methylglyoxal complex. Proc. Natl. Acad. Sci. USA **74:** 226–228.
40. POHL, H.A., P.R.C. GASCOGNE & A. SZENT-GYÖRGYI. 1977. Electron spin resonance absorption of tissue constituents. Proc. Natl. Acad. Sci. USA **74:** 1558–1560.
41. BONE, S., T.J. LEWIS, R. PETHIG & A. SZENT-GYÖRGYI. 1978. Electric properties of some protein-methylglyoxal complexes. Proc. Natl. Acad. Sci. USA **75:** 315–318.
42. FODOR, G., R. MUJUMDAR & A. SZENT-GYÖRGYI. 1978. Isolation of methylglyoxal from liver. Proc. Natl. Acad. Sci. USA **75:** 4317–4319.
43. WALLING, C. 1975. Fenton's reagent revisited. Acc. Chem. Res. **8:** 125–131.
44. FLOYD, R.A. AND C.A. LEWIS. 1983. Hydroxyl free radical formation from hydrogen peroxide by ferrous iron- nucleotide complexes. Biochemistry **22:** 2645–2649.
45. ZS.-NAGY, I. AND K. NAGY. 1980. On the role of cross-linking of cellular proteins in aging. Mech. Ageing Dev. **14:** 245–251.

46. Zs.-Nagy, I. and R.A. Floyd. 1984. Hydroxyl free radical reactions with amino acids and proteins studied by electron spin resonance spectroscopy and spin trapping. Biochim. Biophys. Acta **790**: 238–250.
47. Floyd, R.A. and I. Zs.-Nagy. 1984. Formation of long-lived hydroxyl free radical adducts of proline and hydroxyproline in a Fenton reaction. Biochim. Biophys. Acta **790**: 94–97.
48. Schreck, R. and P.A. Bauerle. 1991. A role for oxygen radicals as second messengers. Trends in Cell Biol. **1**: 39–42.
49. Hodgkin, A.L., A.F. Huxley. 1952. A quantitative description of membrane current and its application to conduction and excitation in nerve. J. Physiol. (London) **117**: 500–544.
50. Eccles, J.C. 1957. The Physiology of Nerve Cells. Baltimore. Johns-Hopkins University Press.
51. Rogers, J. 1983. CACA sequences – the ends and the means. Nature **305**: 101–102.
52. Rogers, J. 1985. The origin and evolution of retroposons. Int. Rev. Cytol. **93**: 187–279.
53. Weiner, A.M., P.L. Deininger & A. Efstratiadis. 1986. Nonviral retroposons, genes, pseudogenes, and transposable elements generated by the reverse flow of genetic information. Annu. Rev. Biochem. **55**: 631–661.
54. Doolittle, W.F. and C. Sapienza. 1980. Selfish genes, the phenotype paradigm and genome evolution. Nature **284**: 601–603.
55. Orgel, L.E. & F.H.C. Crick. 1980. Selfish DNA, the ultimate parasite. Nature **284**: 604–607.
56. Wichman, H.A., S.S. Potter & D.S. Pine. 1985. Mys, a family of mammalian transposable elements isolated by phylogenetic screening. Nature **317**: 77–81.
57. Hartl, D.L., D.E. Dykhuizen, R.D. Miller, L. Green & J. De Framond. 1983. Transposable element IS50 improves growth rate of E. coli cells without transposition. Cell **35**: 503–510.
58. Binning, G., C.F. Quate & Ch. Gerber. 1986. Atomic force microscope. Phys. Rev. Lett. **56**: 930–933.
59. Rugar, D. & P. Hansma. 1990. Atomic force microscopy. Physics Today, October 1990: 23–30.
60. Ohnesorge, F. & G. Binning, G. 1993. True atomic resolution by atomic force microscopy through repulsive and attractive forces. Science **260**: 1451–1456.

Cellular and Molecular Pathogenic Mechanisms of Insulin-Dependent Diabetes Mellitus

JI-WON YOON[a–c] AND HEE-SOOK JUN[b]

[a]*Department of Microbiology and Infectious Disease,* [b]*Laboratory of Viral and Immunopathogenesis of Diabetes, Julia McFarlane Diabetes Research Centre, Faculty of Medicine, The University of Calgary, 3330 Hospital Drive N.W., Calgary, Alberta T2N 4N1, Canada*

[c]*Department of Endocrinology, College of Medicine and Laboratory of Endocrinology, Institute for Medical Science, Ajou University, 5 Wonchon-Dong, Paldal-Gu, Suwon, Korea*

ABSTRACT: Insulin-dependent diabetes mellitus (IDDM), also known as type 1 diabetes, is an organ-specific autoimmune disease resulting from the destruction of insulin-producing pancreatic β cells. The hypothesis that IDDM is an autoimmune disease has been considerably strengthened by the study of animal models such as the BioBreeding (BB) rat and the nonobese diabetic (NOD) mouse, both of which spontaneously develop a diabetic syndrome similar to human IDDM. β cell autoantigens, macrophages, dendritic cells, B lymphocytes, and T cells have been shown to be involved in the pathogenesis of autoimmune diabetes. Among the β cell autoantigens identified, glutamic acid decarboxylase (GAD) has been extensively studied and is the best characterized. β cell-specific suppression of GAD expression in NOD mice results in the prevention of IDDM. Macrophages and/or dendritic cells are the first cell types to infiltrate the pancreatic islets. Macrophages play an essential role in the development and activation of β cell-cytotoxic T cells. B lymphocytes play a role as antigen-presenting cells, and T cells have been shown to play a critical role as final effectors that kill β cells. Cytokines secreted by immunocytes, including macrophages and T cells, may regulate the direction of the immune response toward Th1 or Th2 as well as cytotoxic effector cell or suppressor cell dominance. β cells are destroyed by apoptosis through Fas-Fas ligand and TNF-TNF receptor interactions and by granzymes and perforin released from cytotoxic effector T cells. Therefore, the activated macrophages and T cells, and cytokines secreted from these immunocytes, act synergistically to destroy β cells, resulting in the development of autoimmune IDDM.

KEYWORDS: Autoimmune diseases; Diabetes mellitus, insulin-dependent; IDDM; Insulin-dependent diabetes mellitus;

Address for correspondence: J.W. Yoon, Department of Microbiology and Infectious Disease, Laboratory of Viral and Immunopathogenesis of Diabetes, Julia McFarlane Diabetes Research Centre, Faculty of Medicine, University of Calgary, 3330 Hospital Dr. N.W., Calgary, Alberta, Canada T2N 4N1. Voice: 403-220-4569; fax: 403-270-7526.

yoon@ucalgary.ca

INTRODUCTION

The development of insulin-dependent diabetes mellitus (IDDM) results from the destruction of pancreatic β cells by a complicated and chronic pathogenic process of islet-specific autoimmune reactions. Studies on β-cell–specific autoimmunity using two animal models of human IDDM, the nonobese diabetic (NOD) mouse and the BioBreeding (BB) rat, have greatly enhanced our understanding of the pathogenesis of autoimmune diabetes.[1] Cumulative evidence indicates that β–cell autoantigens, macrophages/dendritic cells, B lymphocytes, and T lymphocytes are clearly involved in the complicated pathogenic process of this disease. In this review, we discuss the role of β-cell autoantigens and these immune cells in the pathogenesis of autoimmune IDDM, particularly the results obtained from studies on NOD mice.

ROLE OF β-CELL AUTOANTIGENS

β-cell autoantigens, which are the targets of autoimmune attack in IDDM, have proven difficult to identify. The specificity of circulating autoantibodies present in the sera of IDDM patients and diabetic animals has been investigated extensively. Over 20 years ago, Bottazzo et al.[2] and MacCuish et al.[3] first detected antibodies directed against the pancreatic islets. Since that time, many studies have revealed that islet cell antibodies are prevalent in patients with IDDM. It is known that peripheral CD4+ T cells from prediabetic and early diabetic patients proliferate in response to islet autoantigens, which react with IDDM-associated autoantibodies. Autoantigens identified in humans, NOD mice, and BB rats include islet cell autoantigens, thought to possess the properties of sialic acid containing glycolipid; insulin; the insulin receptor; a 52-kD protein; a 69-kD protein, glutamic acid decarboxylase (GAD); IA-2, 37/40kD tryptic fragments of a 64-kD antigen (different from GAD); heat shock protein 65 (HSP65); carboxypeptidase H (CPH); the glucose transporter; and a 38-kD autoantigen.[4] The precise role that these autoantigens play in IDDM is not fully understood. Many different approaches have been attempted in order to study the role of β-cell autoantigens, particularly GAD and insulin, which are considered to be the most important autoantigens in IDDM.

GAD. It is believed that GAD is a major islet cell autoantigen; thus, GAD has been extensively studied. In 1990 Baekkeskov et al.[5] identified this 64-kD antigen in the pancreatic β cells of IDDM patients as glutamic acid decarboxylase, the biosynthetic enzyme of the inhibitory neurotransmitter gamma-amino-butyric acid (GABA). GAD is mainly localized to synaptic-like microvesicles in β cells. In addition to its presence in β cells, GAD is expressed in the testes, ovaries, thymus, stomach, and brain of mammals as well as in human pancreatic α, δ, and polypeptide producing (pp) cells. However, the role played by GAD in human IDDM remains unknown. To date, two distinct forms of GAD, GAD67 and GAD65, have been identified. These two forms of GAD are encoded by two different genes. The amino acid sequences of GAD67 and GAD65 are approximately 70% homologous. There is a strong variation in the expression of the two isoforms of GAD in the pancreatic islets depending on the species of animal examined.[6,7] Both human and rat islets predominantly express GAD65, whereas GAD67 is predominantly expressed in mouse islets.[7]

Immunization of NOD mice with purified GAD results in the tolerization of GAD-reactive T cells and blocks the development of T-cell responses to other β cell antigens, thus preventing insulitis and diabetes.[8,9] In their 1993 study, Kaufman et al.[8] stated that the initial immune response directed against pancreatic islets in NOD mice was a Th1 response to a confined region of GAD (amino acids 509-528 and 524-543), and later responses were directed against another region of GAD (amino acids 246-266) and other autoantigens, such as HSP65 and insulin. Although no GAD-reactive CD8+ T cells have been isolated from NOD mice, GAD-reactive CD4+ Th1 cells isolated from diabetic NOD mice induced diabetes in NOD.severe combined immunodeficiency disease (*scid*) mice.[10] These results suggest that GAD plays an important role in the pathogenesis of autoimmune diabetes. However, controversy surrounds the role played by GAD in the pathogenesis of IDDM. Chen et al.[11] have studied the reactivity of T cells to a GAD65-derived peptide, GAD65 residue 524-543, in NOD mice and two congenic NOD strains, B10.H-2^{g7} and NOD.B6$^{I12-Tshb}$. They demonstrated that the response to GAD65 524-543 was MHC class II-restricted and that T-cell responses to GAD-derived peptides can be elicited in mice resistant to the development of spontaneous IDDM. Thus, Chen et al. suggested that peripheral tolerance to GAD is not associated with the prevention of diabetes. To further investigate the role of GAD in the pathogenesis of IDDM, transgenic strategies have been used. The overall expression of GAD, after the cloning of GAD65 under the MHC class I promoter in NOD mice, accelerated the onset and increased the incidence of the disease.[12] In addition, transgenic NOD mice that express GAD65 in the β cells were established. One line, which showed high expression of GAD65, showed a preventive effect on diabetes, but another line showed no difference from control NOD mice.[13] Therefore, the role of GAD remains uncertain. To determine the role of GAD, we selectively suppressed GAD expression in the β cells of diabetes-prone NOD mice and observed whether this resulted in the prevention of autoimmune IDDM. Our recent study showed that β cell-specific suppression of GAD expression in two lines of antisense GAD transgenic mice resulted in the prevention of autoimmune diabetes, whereas any level of GAD expression in the β cells in other lines of antisense GAD transgenic NOD mice resulted in the development of autoimmune diabetes, similar to that seen in transgene-negative NOD mice.[14] These results indicate that GAD may be a triggering autoantigen in the development of autoimmune IDDM in NOD mice.

Insulin. Insulin is a logical candidate for an autoantigen of IDDM, because insulin is the only known β-cell–specific antigen related to IDDM. It has been reported that the oral intake of insulin retards disease progression in the NOD mouse as a result of the induction of immunoregulatory T cells.[15] In addition, the intrathymic injection or the subcutaneous or intranasal administration of the insulin B chain in NOD mice prevents diabetes.[16] Metabolically inactive insulin obtained by changing one amino acid in the B chain also has a preventive effect.[16] Insulin B chain-specific CD4+ T cell clones identified in NOD mice accelerate diabetes in young NOD mice and adoptively transfer the disease in NOD.*scid* mice.[17] Regulatory T cells reactive to insulin have been isolated and shown to have a preventive effect in NOD mice. More recently, a diabetogenic CD8+ T cell clone, which causes diabetes in neonatal NOD mice, was found to recognize insulin B chain amino acids 15-23.[18] These results indicate that insulin plays an important role as an autoantigen in IDDM in NOD mice. Anti-insulin antibodies (IAAs) have been detected in more than 59% of patients diagnosed with late preclinical/recent onset IDDM. However, the pathogenic role of IAAs and insulin-reactive T cells needs further investigation. There is an interesting report that examines cross-reactivity between insulin and the islet-expressed retroviral antigen p73.[19] However, the role of this cross-reactivity in the pathogenesis of autoimmune IDDM is not known.

38-kD Antigen. Anti-38-kD autoantibodies were originally identified in human diabetic sera. Roep *et al.*[20] identified a 38-kD antigen, which was recognized by a T-cell clone established from newly diagnosed IDDM patients, from the insulin secretory granule. Recently, these researchers cloned and sequenced a novel murine cDNA encoding this antigen, named imogen 38.[20] We found that the 38-kD antigen in BB rats is the only delayed-expressed islet cell autoantigen whose antibody is consistently found in acutely diabetic DP-BB rats.[21] As a result of its delayed expression, this 38-kD autoantigen may be considered 'nonself,' which may trigger β cell-specific autoimmunity. Whether there are any molecular similarities between imogen 38 and our delayed-expressed 38-kD islet cell autoantigen remains to be determined. Interestingly, we found that CMV induces antibodies directed against the 38-kD antigen in humans[22] but in this instance the role of the 38-kD autoantigen remains to be determined.

IA-2 Autoantigen (37/40kD Tryptic Fragment). IA-2 is a newly discovered member of the protein tyrosine phosphatase (PTP) family and is considered to be one of the major autoantigens of IDDM. The IA-2 protein is the precursor to the 37 and/or 40-kD islet tryptic fragment.[23] Autoantibodies directed against IA-2 have been detected in 70% of IDDM patients. But these autoantibodies are not detected in NOD mice or BB rats. The IA-2 autoantigen from a rat β-cell line (RIN5AH) reacts with sera from IDDM patients.[23] Antibodies to the IA-2 autoantigen, but not anti-GAD antibodies, react with ICAs in patients that rapidly developed IDDM.[24] However, the precise role of the IA-2 antigen in the pathogenesis of IDDM is unknown.

ROLE OF MACROPHAGES

The major populations of cells infiltrating the islets during the early stage of insulitis in BB rats and NOD mice have been shown to be macrophages and dendritic cells.[25] This infiltration precedes invasion of the islets by T lymphocytes, natural killer (NK) cells, and B lymphocytes. In addition, electron microscopy has revealed that most of the single cells present at an early stage of insulitis in BB rats are macrophages.[26] The inactivation of macrophages in NOD mice and BB rats with silica, a substance that is toxic to macrophages, results in the near complete prevention of insulitis and diabetes. This result suggests that macrophages play an important role in the development of insulitis and diabetes in these animal models. However, the precise role of macrophages in T-cell–mediated autoimmune diabetes remains unknown.

We first examined whether macrophages are required for the development of the effector T cells that destroy β cells. Splenocytes from macrophage-depleted NOD mice by liposomal dichloromethylene diphosphonate (lip-Cl$_2$MDP) did not transfer diabetes to NOD.*scid* mice, whereas those from control NOD mice in which macrophages were present did, indicating that macrophages are required for the development of β-cell–cytotoxic effector T cells in NOD mice. Our further study showed that T cells in the macrophage-depleted NOD recipients did not destroy the transplanted NOD islets, indicating that T cells in a macrophage-depleted environment lose their ability to differentiate into cytotoxic T cells that can destroy pancreatic β cells.[27] However, these T cells regained their β-cell cytotoxic potential when returned to a macrophage-containing environment.

To learn why T cells in a macrophage-depleted environment lose their ability to kill β cells, we examined the islet antigen-specific immune response and T-cell activation in macrophage-depleted NOD mice. There was a shift in the immune balance, a decrease in the Th1 immune response, and an increase in the Th2 immune response due to the reduced expression of the macrophage-derived cytokine interleukin (IL)-12. Moreover, there was a deficit in T-cell activation evidenced by significant decreases in the expression of Fas ligand and perforin. The administration of IL-12 substantially reversed the prevention of diabetes in NOD mice conferred by macrophage depletion.[27] We conclude that macrophages play an essential role in the development and activation of β-cell–cytotoxic T cells that cause β-cell destruction, resulting in autoimmune diabetes in NOD mice.

In addition, we investigated the role of macrophages in the development and activation of β-cell cytotoxic CD8$^+$ T cells in T cell-receptor (TCR)-transgenic NOD mice by the adoptive transfer of splenic T cells from macrophage-depleted TCR-β transgenic NOD mice into NOD.*scid* mice.[28] We found that none of the NOD.*scid* recipients developed diabetes up to 10 weeks after transfer, whereas most of the NOD.*scid* recipients of splenic T cells from age-matched control TCR-β transgenic NOD mice became diabetic. When intact NOD islets were transplanted under the renal capsule of macrophage-depleted 8.3-TCR-β transgenic NOD mice, most of the grafted islets remained intact, whereas most of the islets grafted into age-matched, control 8.3-TCR-β transgenic NOD mice were destroyed within 3 weeks after transplantation. The depletion of macrophages in these mice resulted in a decrease in the Th1 immune response along with an increase in the Th2 immune response and a decrease in β-cell–specific T-cell activation, as shown by significant decreases in the expression of FasL, CD40 ligand (CD40L), and perforin, as compared with control mice. As shown in NOD mice, macrophages are absolutely required for the development and activation of β-cell–cytotoxic CD8$^+$ T cells that cause β–cell destruction, which leads to diabetes in 8.3-TCR-β transgenic NOD mice.[28]

Although further studies to elucidate the precise mechanism of the involvement of macrophages in T-cell activation remain to be performed, our studies have shown that IL-12 secreted by macrophages may activate Th1-type CD4$^+$ T cells, and subsequently, the IL-2 and interferon (IFN)-γ produced by these activated CD4$^+$ T cells may assist in maximizing the activation of CD8$^+$ T cells. The downregulation of islet cell-specific T-cell activation may be another major factor contributing to the impairment of the capability of T cells to kill β cells in macrophage-depleted NOD mice.

In addition to the role of macrophages in the T-cell–mediated destruction of β cells, we also examined other factors that may be involved in the destruction of these cells. These include macrophage-derived soluble mediators such as oxygen-free radicals and other cytokines including IL-1β, tumor necrosis factor (TNF)-α, and IFN-γ. We found that expression of cytokines IL-1β, TNF-α, and IFN-γ was significantly decreased in macrophage-depleted NOD mice as compared with PBS-treated control NOD mice. These cytokines, which are released from activated macrophages, are believed to be toxic to β cells.[29,30] The toxic effect produced by activated macrophages on β cells is thought to be mediated by the superoxide anion and hydrogen peroxide. The β cell is very sensitive to the production of free radicals because islet cells exhibit very low free radical scavenging activity. Cytokines produced by islet-infiltrating macrophages may contribute to β–cell damage by inducing the production of oxygen-free radicals in the islets.[31]

ROLE OF B CELLS

Converging data suggest that B cells play a critical role as antigen-presenting cells (APCs) of β-cell autoantigens in the pathogenesis of autoimmune diabetes in NOD mice. Previously, the function of B cells was analyzed as the production of autoantibodies against β-cell autoantigens, which is considered to be a secondary phenomenon of β-cell destruction. T lymphocytes from diabetic NOD mice transfer diabetes to neonatal recipients in the absence of B cells, indicating that B cells are not required for the destruction of β cells after diabetogenic effector T cells are generated. However, later studies demonstrated that B cells are critical APCs for the initiation of T-cell–mediated autoimmune diabetes in NOD mice. B-cell–deficient NOD mice did not develop diabetes,[32] and the depletion of B cells by anti-u antibody treatment completely abrogated the development of insulitis.[33] More recently, it was reported that B-cell–specific I-A^{g7}-deficient NOD mice showed peri-insulitis, but converted to destructive insulitis after cyclophosphamide (CY) treatment. This result suggests that I-A^{g7}-mediated β–cell autoantigen presentation by B cells is critical in overcoming a checkpoint in T-cell tolerance to pancreatic β cells after their initial targeting has occurred.[34]

ROLE OF T CELLS

Substantial evidence from studies using BB rats and NOD mice supports a critical role of T cells in the pathogenesis of autoimmune type I diabetes. It has been shown that the development of diabetes was prevented by neonatal thymectomy in BB rats,[35] and BB rats treated with monoclonal antibodies (OX-19) directed against the antigens expressed on the surface of all T cells do not develop diabetes, indicating that T cells play an important role in the destruction of β cells.[36] In addition, lymphocytes from diabetic BB rats transfer the disease to young diabetes-prone BB rats.

In the NOD mouse model, it is clear that T cells play a critical role in the development of autoimmune diabetes. Athymic NOD mice and NOD.*scid* mice do not develop insulitis or diabetes.[37,38] Treatment of NOD mice with anti-CD3 antibodies inhibits the development of diabetes.[38] In addition, most transfer studies of NOD splenic T cells into NOD mice show that the transfer of diabetes requires both CD4$^+$ and CD8$^+$ T cells.[40,41] Islet cell-specific T-cell clones have been isolated from insulitic lesions and the splenocytes of both prediabetic and diabetic NOD mice. Some CD4$^+$ islet-specific T-cell clones[42] accelerate the development of diabetes in young

NOD mice and destroy islet grafts in CD8+ T-cell–depleted diabetes-resistant mice. The BDC2.5/NOD transgenic mouse, which expresses the rearranged T-cell receptor (TCR) α and β chain genes of this CD4+ T cell clone (BDC2.5),[42] exhibits an increased incidence of diabetes.[43]

In addition to CD4+ T cell involvement in β–cell destruction, experimental evidence reveals that CD8+ T cells play a role as effector cells in the destruction of β cells in the NOD mouse. CD8+ cytotoxic T cell clones (CTLs), isolated from the islets of diabetic NOD mice, destroy β cells *in vitro* and transfer diabetes *in vivo* with the help of CD4+ T cells.[44] Some CD8+ T cell clones have been shown to destroy β cells without the help of CD4+ T cells.[45] We have cloned a dozen islet-reactive CD4+ and CD8+ T cells from the lymphocytes infiltrating the pancreatic islets of NOD mice.[44] All CD4+ T cells are restricted to MHC class II of NOD, I-A^{g7}. One of our CD4+ T cell clones (NY4.1) responded only to islet cells from NOD mice, indicating that the NY4.1 clones recognize the islet antigen with a unique I-A^{nod} molecule on the islet cell or the intrinsic APCs. The remaining CD4+ T cell clones showed a proliferative response to both islet cells and spleen cells from NOD mice, but not from other strains of mice including SJL, C3H, C57BL/6, and DBA/2 mice, indicating that these clones are I-A^{g7} reactive T cells (autoreactive T cells). None of these CD4+ T cell clones, either islet-specific or autoreactive, had any cytotoxic effect on NOD islet cells *in vitro*.[44] In contrast, the CD8+ T cell clones did exhibit cytotoxic activity to NOD islets *in vitro*. Furthermore, the proliferative response and cytotoxic activity of some CD8+ T-cell clones was blocked almost completely by anti-MHC class I D^b monoclonal antibodies and that of other CD8+ T cell clones was blocked by anti-MHC class I K^d monoclonal antibodies. These results indicate that CD8+ T cell clones respond to islet cells with the restriction of MHC class I. Electron microscopic studies revealed that islet-specific CD4+ T cells attached closely to islet cells but did not destroy them *in vitro*. In contrast, all of the CD8+ T-cell clones showed a cytotoxic effect on the islet cells and the CD8+ T cells showed pseudopod-like protrusions into the β cells, but not into α or δ cells, leading to the selective destruction of β cells *in vitro*.[44] These results suggest that CD4+ and CD8+ T cells interact differently with β cells during T-cell–mediated β–cell destruction. CD4+ T cells secrete cytokines including IL-2 and IFN-γ, which in turn help maximally activate CD8+ T cells. CD8+ T cells may act as final effector cells directly involved in β–cell destruction. As a matter of fact, CD8+ T cells produce cytokines that may upregulate Fas within the islet, and the destruction of β cells could take place both specifically in relation to the production of perforin as well as nonspecifically through the Fas/FasL interaction. However, both CD4+ and CD8+ T cells, by producing inflammatory cytokines including TNF and IFN-γ, can upregulate Fas on the islets. Once Fas is upregulated on the islets, FasL-expressing CD4+ Th1 cells and CD8+ T cells may induce apoptosis to kill β cells (FIG. 1).

Among our CD4+ and CD8+ T-cell clones, an H-2^{g7}-restricted CD4+ T cell clone, NY4.1, and an H-2K^d-restricted CD8+ T-cell clone, NY8.3, were chosen for further study. TCR transgenic NOD mice expressing the rearranged TCR-α and/or -β genes derived from the diabetogenic CD8+ T-cell clone[44] were established. The TCR-β transgenic NOD mice showed a 10-fold increase in the peripheral precursor frequency of β-cell–specific CD8+ T cells and a selective acceleration of the recruitment of CD8+ T cells to the pancreatic islets of prediabetic NOD mice.[46] The TCR-αβ trans-

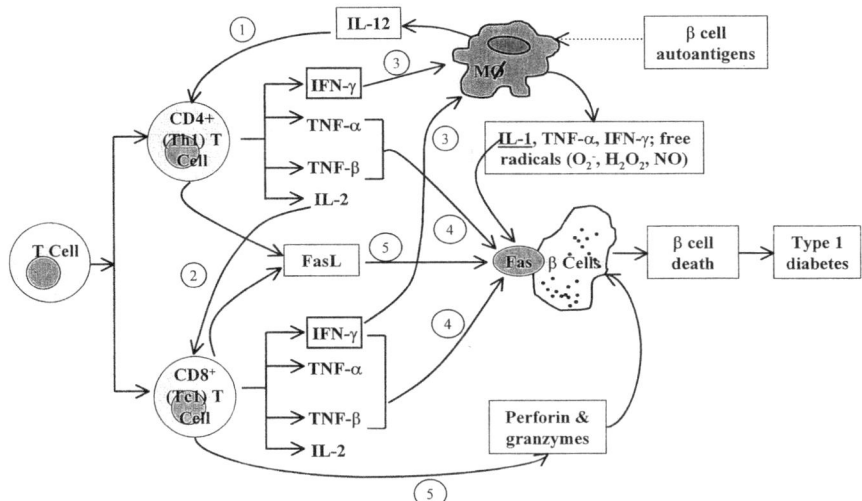

FIGURE 1. Schematic representation of the collaboration between macrophages and T cells in the destruction of pancreatic β cells. β–cell autoantigens may be released from the β cells during spontaneous turnover of β cells. The antigens are then processed by macrophages and presented to helper T cells in conjunction with MHC class II molecules. The activated macrophages may secrete IL-12, which activates Th1 type CD4+ T cells (**1**). The CD4+ T cells secrete cytokines such as IFN-γ, TNF-α, TNF-β and IL-2. While this process is taking place, β–cell-specific precytotoxic T cells may be recruited to the islets. These precytotoxic T cells may be activated by IL-2 and other cytokines released by CD4+ helper T cells to differentiate into CD8+ effector T cells (**2**). IFN-γ released by helper T cells and cytotoxic T cells may cause macrophages to become cytotoxic (**3**). These cytotoxic macrophages release substantial amounts of β cell-toxic cytokines (including IL-1β, TNF-α, and IFN-γ) and free radicals (H_2O_2, NO). Cytokines released from macrophages and T cells may induce the expression of Fas on pancreatic β cells (**4**). β cells are destroyed by Fas-mediated apoptosis (**4**) and/or granzyme and cytolysin (perforin), which are toxic to β cells (**5**).

genic NOD (8.3-NOD) mice showed a 400-fold increase in the peripheral precursor frequency of β-cell–specific CD8+ T cells and a selective acceleration of the recruitment of CD8+ T cells to the pancreatic islets of prediabetic NOD mice.[47] These mice showed an earlier onset and more rapid progression of β–cell destruction, resulting in acceleration of the onset of diabetes as compared with that in nontransgenic NOD mice. In addition, TCR transgenic NOD mice expressing the T-cell receptor (TCR)α and TCRβ chains of the CD4+ T cell clone, NY4.1, showed an accelerated onset of diabetes.[47]

Cytokines produced by T cells also play an important role in the pathogenesis of autoimmune type 1 diabetes.[48] In general, Th1 cytokines (IL-2, IFN-γ) have been shown to be involved in the development of the disease, while Th2 or Th3 cytokines (IL-4, IL-10, TGF-β) have been involved in the prevention of the disease. However, the role of cytokines in the pathogenesis of autoimmune type 1 diabetes is complex. For example, the treatment of NOD mice with anti-IFN-γ prevents the development of diabetes and the transgene expression of IFN-γ in the β cells of normal mice results in the development of type 1 diabetes. However, the genetic absence of IFN-γ in NOD mice results in a delay in the development of diabetes, but does not prevent it. The systemic administration of IL-4 or IL-10 prevents type 1 diabetes in NOD mice and the transgenic expression of IL-4 on β cells prevents the development of diabetes. However, the local expression of IL-10 in the islets accelerates the development of diabetes in NOD mice, and IL-4 knockout NOD mice did not show accelerated disease onset. Therefore, the interactions of the many different cytokines in the immune system are complicated and the development of diabetes may depend upon which way the finely tuned balance of immunoregulatory cytokines is tipped.

Recently, possible mechanisms for T-cell–mediated β–cell destruction have been elucidated. $CD8^+$ cytotoxic T cells destroy β cells through the perforin and granzyme pathway as well as through the Fas/Fas-L interaction. NOD mice lacking perforin expression were found to develop insulitis, but not diabetes.[49] Fas-deficient NOD mice were found to be free of diabetes and insulitis, and Fas-mediated apoptosis of the β cells was suggested to be the major mechanism for β–cell damage.[50,51] On the other hand, TNFα/TNFα-receptor-mediated apoptosis may also play a greater role in the destruction of β cells by $CD4^+$ T cells.[52]

CONCLUSION

Insulin-dependent diabetes mellitus (IDDM) is an autoimmune disease with a multifactorial etiology. Thus, a clear understanding of the pathogenic mechanisms involved in the etiology of this disease is not easy. Animal models such as nonobese diabetic (NOD) mice and BioBreeding (BB) rats, which spontaneously develop autoimmune diabetes similar to human autoimmune IDDM, have been used to study the pathogenic mechanisms of autoimmune IDDM. β–cell autoantigens, macrophages/dendritic cells, B cells, and T cells play important roles in the development of the disease in NOD mice. Among the β–cell autoantigens identified, glutamic acid decarboxylase (GAD) and insulin are considered to be the most important autoantigens in the development of IDDM. However, the role of these autoantigens remains to be determined. B cells clearly play a role as antigen-presenting cells, particularly of β–cell autoantigens. Macrophages, which infiltrate the islets at the early stage of insulitis, are considered to be primary contributors to the immune environment conducive for the development and activation of β-cell–cytotoxic T cells. Both $CD4^+$ and $CD8^+$ T cells play a role as final effectors in the destruction of pancreatic β cells. Although the animal models studied do not show a diabetic syndrome identical to human autoimmune IDDM, the information obtained through studies using these animal models will be invaluable for understanding the pathogenic mechanisms of human IDDM and for the development of strategies for the prevention of the disease.

ACKNOWLEDGMENTS

This work was supported by grants from the Medical Research Council of Canada, the Juvenile Diabetes Foundation International, the Alberta Heritage Foundation for Medical Research, and Grant HMP-97-B-1-002 from the Good Health Research and Development Project, Ministry of Health and Welfare, R.O.K. to J.W.Y. J.W.Y. is a Heritage Medical Scientist Awardee of the Alberta Heritage Foundation for

Medical Research. The authors gratefully acknowledge the editorial assistance of K. Clarke and A. Kyle.

REFERENCES

1. YOON, J.W. & H.S. JUN. 1998. Insulin-dependent diabetes mellitus. *In* Encyclopedia of Immunology, 2nd Ed. I.M. Riott & P.J. Delves, eds. :1390–1398. Academic Press. London, UK.
2. BOTTAZZO, G.F., A. FLORIN-CHRISTENSEN & D. DONIACH. 1974. Islet cell antibodies in diabetes mellitus with autoimmune polyendocrine deficiency. Lancet **2**: 1279–1283.
3. MACCUISH, A.C., W.J. IRVINE, E.W. BARNES & L.J. DUNCAN. 1974. Antibodies to pancreatic islet cells in insulin-dependent diabetes with coexistent autoimmune disease. Lancet **2**: 1529–1531.
4. BACH, J.F. 1995. Insulin-dependent diabetes mellitus as a β cells targeted disease of immunoregulation. J. Autoimmunol. **8**: 439–463.
5. BAEKKESKOV, S., H. JAN-AANSTOOT, S. CHRISTGAU, *et al.* 1990. Identification of the 64K autoantigen in insulin-dependent diabetes as the GABA-synthesizing enzyme glutamic acid decarboxylase. Nature **347**: 151–156.
6. FAULKNER-JONES, B.E., D.S. CRAM, J. KUN & L.C. HARRISON. 1993. Localization and quantitation of expression of two glutamate decarboxylase genes in pancreatic beta-cells and other peripheral tissues of mouse and rat. Endocrinol. **133**: 2962–2972.
7. KIM, J., W. RICHTER, H.J. AANSTOOT, *et al.* 1993. Differential expression of GAD$_{65}$ and GAD$_{67}$ in human, rat, and mouse pancreatic islets. Diabetes **42**: 1799–1808.
8. KAUFMAN, D., M. CLARE-SALZLER, J. TIAN, *et al.* 1993. Spontaneous loss of T-cell tolerance to glutamic acid decarboxylase in murine insulin-dependent diabetes. Nature **366**: 69–72.
9. ELLIOT, J.F., H.Y. QIN, S. BHATTI, *et al.* 1994. Immunization with the larger isoform of mouse glutamic acid decarboxylase (GAD67) prevents autoimmune diabetes in NOD mice. Diabetes **43**: 1494–1499.
10. ZEKZER, D., F.S. WONG, O. AYALON, *et al.* 1998. GAD-reactive CD4+ Th1 cells induce diabetes in NOD/SCID mice. J. Clin. Invest. **101**: 68–73.
11. CHEN, S.L., P.J. WHITELEY, D.C. FREED, *et al.* 1994. Responses of NOD congenic mice to a glutamic acid decarboxylase-derived peptide. J. Autoimmunol. **7**: 635–641.
12. GENG, L., M. SOLIMENA, R.A. FLAVELL, *et al.* 1998. Widespread expression of an autoantigen GAD65 transgene does not tolerize non-obese diabetic mice and can exacerbate disease. Proc. Natl. Acad. Sci. USA **95**: 10055–10060.
13. BRIDGETT, M., M. CETKOVIC-CVRLJE, R. O'ROURKE, *et al.* 1998. Differential protection in two transgenic lines of NOD/Lt mice hyperexpressing the autoantigen GAD65 in pancreatic beta-cells. Diabetes **47**: 1848–1856.
14. YOON, J.W., C.S. YOON, H.W. LIM, *et al.* 1999. Control of autoimmune diabetes in NOD mice by GAD expression or suppression in β cells. Science **284**: 1183–1187.
15. ZHANG, Z.J., L. DAVIDSEN, G.S. EISENBARTH, *et al.* 1991. Suppression of diabetes in non obese diabetic mice by oral administration of porcine insulin. Proc. Natl. Acad. Sci. USA **88**: 10252–10256.
16. WONG, F.S. & C.A. JANEWAY. 1999. Insulin-dependent diabetes mellitus and its animal models. Curr. Opin. Immunol. **11**: 643–647.
17. DANIEL, D., R.G. GILL, N. SCHLOOT & D. WEGMANN. 1994. Epitope specificity cytokine production profile and diabetogenic activity of insulin-specific T cell clones isolated from the NOD mouse. Eur. J. Immunol. **25**: 1056–1062.
18. WONG, F.S., J. KARTTUNEN, C. DUMONT, *et al.* 1999. Identification of an MHC class I-restricted autoantigen in type 1 diabetes by screening an organ-specific cDNA library. Nat. Med. **5**: 1026–1031.
19. SERREZE, D.V., E. LEITER, E.L. KUFF, *et al.* 1988. Molecular mimicry between insulin and retroviral antigen p73. Development of cross-reactive autoantibodies in sera of NOD and C57BL/KsJ db/db mice. Diabetes **37**: 351–358.

20. ARDEN, S.D., B.O. ROEP, P.I. NEOPHYTOU, et al. 1996. Imogen 38: a novel 38-kD islet mitochondrial autoantigen recognized by T cells from a newly diagnosed type I diabetic patient. J. Clin. Invest. **97**: 551–561.
21. KO, I.Y., S.H. IHM & J.W. YOON. 1991. Studies on autoimmunity for initiation of beta-cell destruction. VIII. Pancreatic beta cell dependent autoantibody to a 38 kilodalton protein precedes the clinical onset of diabetes in BB rats. Diabetologia **34**: 548–554.
22. PAK, C.Y., C.Y. CHA, R.V. RAJOTTE, et al. 1990. Human pancreatic islet cell-specific 38kD autoantigen identified by cytomegalovirus-induced monoclonal islet cell autoantibody. Diabetologia **33**: 569–572.
23. BONIFACIO, E., V. LAMPASONA, S. GENOVESE, et al. Identification of protein tyrosine phosphatase-like IA-2 (islet cell antigen 512) as the insulin dependent diabetes-related 37/40K autoantigen and a target of islet-cell antibodies. J. Immunol. **155**: 5419–5426.
24. CHRISTIE, M.R., S. GENOVESE, D. CASSIDY, et al. 1994. Antibodies to islet 37k antigen, but not to glutamate decarboxylase, discriminate rapid progression to IDDM in endocrine autoimmunity. Diabetes **43**: 1254–1259.
25. YOON, J.W., H.S. JUN & P.S. SANTAMARIA. 1998. Cellular and molecular mechanisms for the initiation and progression of β-cell destruction resulting from the collaboration between macrophages and T cells. Autoimmunity **27**: 109–122.
26. KOLB, H., G. KANTWERK, U. TREICHEL, et al. 1986. Prospective analysis of islet lesions in BB rats. Diabetologia **29** (Suppl. 1): A559.
27. JUN, H.S., C.S. YOON, L. ZBYTNUIK, et al. 1999. Role of macrophages in T cell-mediated autoimmune diabetes in NOD mice. J. Exp. Med. **189**: 347–358.
28. JUN, H.S., P.S. SANTAMARIA, H.W. LIM, et al. 1999. Absolute requirement of macrophages for the development and activation of β-cell cytotoxic CD8$^+$ T cells in T-cell receptor transgenic NOD mice. Diabetes **48**: 34–42.
29. MANDRUP-POULSEN T., K. BENDTZEN, C. DINARELLO & J. NERUP. 1987. Human tumor-necrosis factor potentiates human interleukin 1-mediated rat pancreatic beta cell-cytotoxicity. J. Immunol. **139**: 4077-4082.
30. APPELS, B., V. BURKART, M. KANTWERK-FUNKE, et al. 1989. Spontaneous cytotoxicity of macrophages against pancreatic islet cells. J. Immunol. **142**: 3803–3808.
31. CORBETT, J.A. & M.L. MCDANIEL. 1992. Does nitric oxide mediate autoimmune destruction of β cells? Possible therapeutic interventions in IDDM. Diabetes **41**: 897–903.
32. SERREZE, D.V., H.D. CHAPMAN, D.S. VARNUM, et al. 1996. B lymphocytes are essential for the initiation of T cell-mediated autoimmune diabetes: analysis of a new "speed congenic" stock of NOD.IgF^{null} mice. J. Exp. Med. **184**: 2049–2053.
33. NOORCHASHM, H., N. NOORCHASHM, J. KERN, et al. 1997. B-cells are required for the initiation of insulitis and sialitis in nonobese diabetic mice. Diabetes **46**: 941-946.
34. NOORCHASHM, H., Y.K. LIEU, N. NOORCHASHM, et al. 1999. I-Ag7-mediated antigen presentation by B lymphocytes is critical in overcoming a checkpoint in T cell tolerance to islet β cells of nonobese diabetic mice. J. Immunol. **163**: 743–750.
35. LIKE, A.A., E. KISLAUSKIS, R.M. WILLIAMS & A.A. ROSSINI. 1982. Neonatal thymectomy prevents spontaneous diabetes mellitus in the BB/W rat. Science **216**: 644–646.
36. LIKE, A.A., C.A. BIRON, E.J. WERINGER, et al. 1986. Prevention of diabetes in Biobreeding/Worcester rats with monoclonal antibodies that recognize T-lymphocytes or natural killer cells. J. Exp. Med. **164**: 1145–1159.
37. OGAWA, M., T. MARUYAMA, T. HASEGAWA, et al. 1985. The inhibitory effect of neonatal thymectomy on the incidence of insulitis in non-obese diabetes (NOD) mice. Biomed. Res. **6**: 103–106.
38. MAKINO, S., M. HARADA, Y. KISHIMOTO & Y. HAYASHI. 1986. Absence of insulitis and overt diabetes in athymic nude mice with NOD genetic background. Exp. Anim. **35**: 495–499.
39. HAYWARD, A.R. & M. SHREIBER. 1989. Neonatal injection of CD3 antibody into nonobese diabetic mice reduces the incidence of insulitis and diabetes. J. Immunol. **143**: 1555–1559.
40. CHRISTIANSON, S.W., L.D. SHULTZ & E.H. LEITER. 1993. Adoptive transfer of diabetes into immunodeficient NOD-scid/scid mice. Relative contributions of CD4+ and

CD8+ T cells from diabetic versus prediabetic NOD.NON-Thy-1a donors. Diabetes **42:** 44–55.
41. BENDELAC, A., C. CARNAUD, C. BOITARD & J.F. BACH. 1987. Syngeneic transfer of autoimmune diabetes from diabetic NOD mice to healthy neonates: requirement for both L3T4+ and Lyt2+ T cells. J. Exp. Med. **166:** 823–832.
42. HASKINS, K. & M. MCDUFFIE. 1990. Acceleration of diabetes in young NOD mice with a CD4+ islet-specific T cell clone. Science **249:** 1433–1436.
43. KATZ, J.D., B. WANG, K. HASKINS, *et al.* 1993. Following a diabetogenic T cell from genesis through pathogenesis. Cell **74:** 1089–1100.
44. NAGATA, M. & J.W. YOON. 1992. Studies on autoimmunity for T-cell-mediated β cell destruction. Distinct difference in β cell destruction between CD4+ and CD8+ T cell clones derived from lymphocytes infiltrating the islets of NOD mice. Diabetes **41:** 998–1008.
45. WONG, S., I. VISINTIN, L. WEN, *et al.* 1996. CD8 T cell clones from young nonobese diabetic (NOD) islets can transfer rapid onset of diabetes in NOD mice in the absence of CD4 cells. J. Exp. Med. **183:** 67–76.
46. VERDAGUER J., J.W. YOON, N. AVERILL, *et al.* 1996. Acceleration of diabetes in TCR-β-transgenic nonobese diabetic mice by beta cell-cytotoxic T cells expressing endogenous TCR-α chains. J. Immunol. **157:** 4726–4735.
47. VERDAGUER, J., D. SCHMIDT, A. AMRANI, *et al.* 1997. Spontaneous autoimmune diabetes in monoclonal T cell nonobese diabetic mice. J. Exp. Med. **186:** 1663–1676.
48. RABINOVITCH, A. 1998. An update on cytokines in the pathogenesis of insulin-dependent diabetes mellitus. Diabetes Metab. Rev. **14:** 129–151.
49. KAGI, D., B. ODERMATT, P. SEILER, *et al.* 1997. Reduced incidence and delayed onset of diabetes in perforin-deficient nonobese diabetic mice. J. Exp. Med. **186:** 989–997.
50. ITOH, N., A. IMAGAWA, T. HANAFUSA, *et al.* 1997. Requirement of Fas for the development of autoimmune diabetes in nonobese diabetic mice. J. Exp. Med. **186:** 613–618.
51. SU, X. O. HU, J. M. KRISTAN, *et al.* 2000. Significant role for fas in the pathogenesis of autoimmune diabetes. J. Immunol. **164:** 2523–2532.
52. KURRER, M.O., S.V. PAKALA, H.L. HANSON & J.D. KATZ. 1997. Beta cell apoptosis in T cell-mediated autoimmune diabetes. Proc. Natl. Acad. Sci. USA **94:** 213–218.

Capacity for Recovery and Possible Mechanisms in Immobilization Atrophy of Young and Old Animals

N. ZARZHEVSKY,[a] O. MENASHE,[a] E. CARMELI,[b] H. STEIN,[c] AND A.Z. REZNICK[a]

[a]*Musculo-Skeletal Laboratory, Department of Anatomy and Cell Biology, The Bruce Rappaport Faculty of Medicine, Technion, Haifa, Israel*

[b]*Physical Therapy Program, Sackler Faculty of Medicine, Tel Aviv University, Tel Aviv, Israel, 61390*

[c]*Department of Orthopaedics at Rambam Medical Center, Haifa, Israel, 31096*

ABSTRACT: The effect of limb immobilization on muscle wasting and recovery of young and old rats was studied. Limb immobilization caused rapid and pronounced muscle weight loss, which was overcome efficiently in the muscles of young animals. However, muscles of old animals did not recover as well, indicating that muscle turnover (degradation and synthesis of proteins) is slower in old muscles than in young ones. The mechanisms of muscle wasting due to immobilization may involve two stages, the fast phase employing calcium-dependent proteolysis and the slower phase recruiting the lysosomal and ubiquitin-proteosome systems. The slow phase most probably involves the penetration of white cells between the muscle fibers and involves the secretion of cytokines that mediate a cascade of intracellular events, which culminates in muscle protein degradation. Thus, it was shown in our study and in other similar reports that through the influence of TNF-α and an increase in oxidative stress, there is marked activation of transcription factor NF-κB, which in turn induces many proteins to carry the signals that eventually result in protein breakdown. Because protein turnover was shown to slow down with age, it will be of great interest to study these events in aging muscles and to try to ascertain the specific events that make protein breakdown in aged muscles different from that in young ones.

KEYWORDS: Aging; Immobilization atrophy; Limb immobilization; Muscle wasting; Protein turnover

INTRODUCTION

Skeletal muscles of elderly persons and animals lose about 20–25% of their muscle mass from young to old age. This phenomenon has been termed sarcopenia of old age,[1] and the reasons for these age-related changes in skeletal muscles are multifactorial and include changes in the muscle apparatus itself, changes in the neural

---

Address for correspondence: Dr. Abraham Z. Reznick, Department of Anatomy and Cell Biology, The Bruce Rappaport Faculty of Medicine, Technion, Haifa, Israel 31096. Voice: 972-4-8295388; fax: 972-4-8295392.
reznick@technunix.technion.ac.il

system and stimuli, and the influence of external environmental factors.[2] Among the changes observed were alterations in enzymatic activity[3] and some morphologic changes.[4] Immobilization of muscles of old animals can be used to study the muscle response to trauma and stress.[5]

Reports have claimed that administration of growth hormone (GH) to aging animals and humans can improve the performance and status of skeletal muscles.[6] Indeed, using immobilized model muscles of aging rats it was possible to show that rat GH could slow down the muscle damage and muscle weight loss due to limb immobilization of old rats.[7,8] Recently, the question of how well skeletal muscle can recover from immobilization atrophy was addressed.[9] After 4 weeks of immobilization and 4 weeks of recovery, hindleg skeletal muscles of young rats did not return to their preimmobilization weights; however, biochemically and morphologically they recovered their preimmobilization levels.[9] The questions of how well muscles of old animals can recover from immobilization atrophy compared to young ones and some possible molecular events leading to muscle protein degradation are addressed in the current report.

Immobilization and other pathologic conditions, which lead to skeletal muscle protein degradation, probably start with a fast process of increased influx of Ca^{2+} ions into the sarcoplasm. This event, leading to muscle breakdown, is already taking place within 6–12 hours after muscle immobilization and involves the activation of Ca^{2+}-dependent proteases (calpains). In a recent paper, Williams *et al.*[10] showed that activation of calpains in sepsis start with z-band disintegration, which may be the initial and perhaps the rate-limiting element in the release of myofilaments, leading to muscle protein degradation. In addition, the increased activity of calpains in immobilization has been associated with increased oxidative stress and oxidative damage to muscles,[11] which could partially be prevented by the administration of vitamin E.[12] This initial phase of muscle protein degradation due to immobilization is illustrated in FIGURE 1.

About 12–24 hours after muscles are injured, immobilized, or denervated, the infiltration of white blood cells such as macrophages and monocytes into the area of damage can be observed. The newly arriving cells are added to the resident macrophages of types ED2 and ED3, which are already present in normal healthy muscles and which do not usually participate in muscle degeneration.[13,14] These resident macrophages do not phagocytose degenerating rat skeletal muscle fibers.[13] Similarly, in various inflammations such as inflammatory myopathies, dermatomyositis, and polymyositis, white blood cell infiltration is evidenced by the presence of interleukin(IL)-1 production.[15] Specifically, it has been shown that cytotoxic T cells surround and focally invade non-necrotic muscle fibers, and this lesion can be considered the hallmark of cell-mediated myocytotoxicity.

Myotubes are highly susceptible to lysis by allogeneic CD8+ cytotoxic T cells sensitized against HLA class I alloantigens.[16] Cultured myotubes are also susceptible to lysis by antigen-nonspecific natural killer cells. The work of Dalakas indicates that in inflammatory muscle disease there is expression of messenger RNA of cytokines from activated endomysial inflammatory cells.[17]

Several years ago, in a cachexia model of muscle wasting in mice, it was shown that tumor necrosis factor alpha (TNF-α) can trigger oxidative stress and expression of inducible NO synthase (iNOS), which results in an increase of NO.[18] According to these investigators, the induction of iNOS resulted in protein degradation and

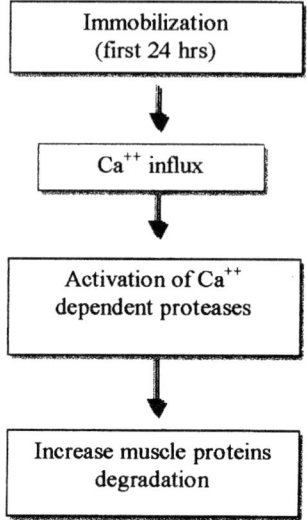

FIGURE 1. The fast phase of muscle breakdown due to immobilization.

muscle wasting. Several recent studies have shown that TNF-α, by an increase in oxidative stress, triggers the activation of transcription factor NF-κB,[19,20] which eventually results in activation of a ubiquitin-dependent proteolytic system in muscles.[21] From the foregoing discussion we would like to propose the scheme, shown in FIGURE 2, as a working molecular and cellular model for muscle wasting in limb immobilization and other muscle pathologies. It is the aim of the present report to provide experimental evidence in support of the various stages illustrated in FIGURE 2.

MATERIALS AND METHODS

Animals. The animals used in this project were young (6 months) and old (24 months) female Wistar rats. The right hindlegs of the animals were externally fixed as previously described,[5] and animals were immobilized for 4 weeks. Another group of animals were immobilized by external fixation, and subsequently the fixation was removed and the animals were allowed to recover for 4 weeks.

Body weights of the rats were determined prior to sacrifice and before hindlimb muscles (gastrocnemius, quadriceps, soleus, and plantaris) were dissected. Muscle tissues were checked using anatomic, morphologic, and biochemical parameters. The contralateral (nonimmobilized) legs were used as controls. In addition, the muscles of a third group of young and old rats served as untreated controls.

Immobilization by External Fixation.[5] Rigid immobilization was achieved by the insertion of two Kirschner wires (0.8 mm in diameter) driven through the lateral plane of the femur and tibia. Then two threaded brass rods, fitted with nuts, connected them in order to construct a rigid frame. The brass rods were 4.8 mm in diameter and 33 mm long. Each rod was cut longitudinally from both ends to an equal length

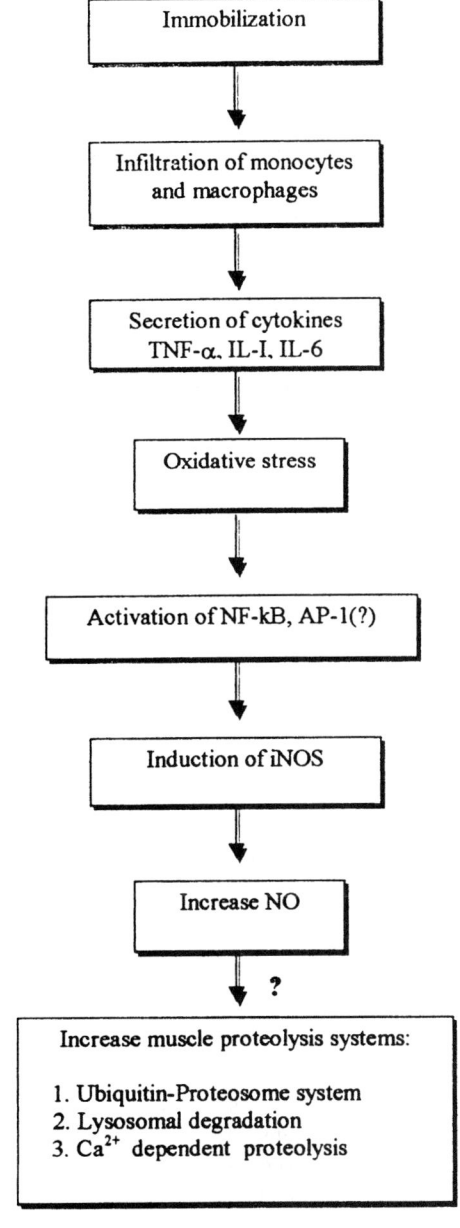

FIGURE 2. The slow phase of immobilization-associated muscle wasting.

of 13 mm. These cuts were 1–1.2 mm in width in order to contain the Kirschner wires. The overall weight of this device was 12 g.

Biochemical Studies. Animals were sacrificed by ether anesthesia at 4 weeks in Group 1 and 8 weeks in Group 2. Group 3 (untreated controls) were sacrificed at 6 or 24 months of age before experimental hindlimb immobilization. Muscle specimens for biochemical studies (200 mg each) were taken from the belly of the gastrocnemius of the right (immobilized) and left (contralateral) hindlimbs. Similarly, specimens of other muscles were taken in the same way. The muscles were immersed in 1.4 ml of 50 mM tris (hydroxymethyl) aminomethane buffer, pH 7.4, in the presence of antiproteases 1 μM phenylmethyl sulfonyl oxide (PMSF) 10 and 1 μM leupeptin. This mixture was homogenized in a polytron homogenizer (Kinematica GmbH, Lucerne, Switzerland) three times for 15 seconds. The homogenate was centrifuged for 30 minutes at 14,000 g. The supernatants were separated and utilized for enzymatic assays. Acid phosphatase activity was determined as previously described.[5] Creatine phophokinase assay was performed according to the method of Tanzar and Gilvard[22] using 0.05M glycine buffer, pH 7.4. Lipid peroxidation measurements were performed using thiobarbituric acid (TBA) according to the procedure of Ohkawa et al.[23] Protein concentration in muscle extracts was determined according to the method of Lowry et al.[24] Polyacrylamide gel electrophoresis for protein carbonyls was determined with the Oxiblot Kit using anti-DNPH antibodies (Intergen Co. Purchase, New York, USA).

Cell Cultures. The L-8 muscle myoblast cell line (produced by Prof. D. Yaffe, Weizmann Institute, Rehovot, Israel) was grown on Dulbecco's modified eagle medium (DMEM), high glucose (GibcoBRL) with the addition of fetal calf serum 15% (GibcoBRL), L-glutamine, and antibiotics. The cells were grown in a sterile incubator, with 5% CO_2 at 37°C. The medium was changed every other day. The cells were incubated with increasing H_2O_2 concentrations (500 μM, 1 mM, and 2 mM) for a 6-hour period. The incubated cells were lysed by lysis buffer: 20 mM Tris (pH = 7.5), 150 mM NaCl, 0.5 mM sodium orthovandate, 1 mM DTT, 1% triton, and 10% glycerol with the addition of protease inhibitors: 1 μM leupeptin and 1 μM PMSF. (All reagents were purchased from Sigma.)

The cell lysate proteins were run on 10% SDS polyacrylamide gel electrophoresis (PAGE) and then immunoblotted with anti-ubiquitin rat polyclonal antibody (BABCO, Richmond, California, USA).

RESULTS AND DISCUSSION

Comparison of Capacity for Recovery of Young and Old Animals

TABLE 1 shows residual muscle weights compared with contralateral controls after immobilization and recovery of various hindlimb muscles from young and old rats. The net % gain (% residual weights after recovery minus % residual weights at the end of the immobilization period) of muscle mass was far greater in young rats than in old ones. This point is illustrated clearly also in FIGURE 3.

From TABLE 1 and FIGURE 3 it can be seen that muscles of neither young nor old animals have returned to their preimmobilization weights after 4 weeks of immobilization and 4 weeks of recovery.

TABLE 1. Rat muscle weight changes during immobilaztion and recovery

Muscle	External fixation, % residual weight[a]		External fixation + recovery, % residual weight[a]		Net % gain during the recovery period[b]		Relative muscle weight gain
	Young	Old	Young	Old	Young	Old	Young/Old
Gastrocnemius	42	58.7	71.1	71.1	29.9	12.4	2.4
Quadriceps	38	56.2	57.3	66.6	19.3	10.3	1.9
Plantaris	53.5	53.4	64.3	57.7	10.9	4.3	2.5
Soleus	53.4	60.5	59	62.7	5.6	2.2	2.5

[a]% residual weight left after the period relative to control (Nonimmobilized) leg.
[b]Net % gain was determined from the difference of % residual weight at end of recovery period and the % residual weight at end of immobilization period. (The % residual weights represent the average of five different animals.)

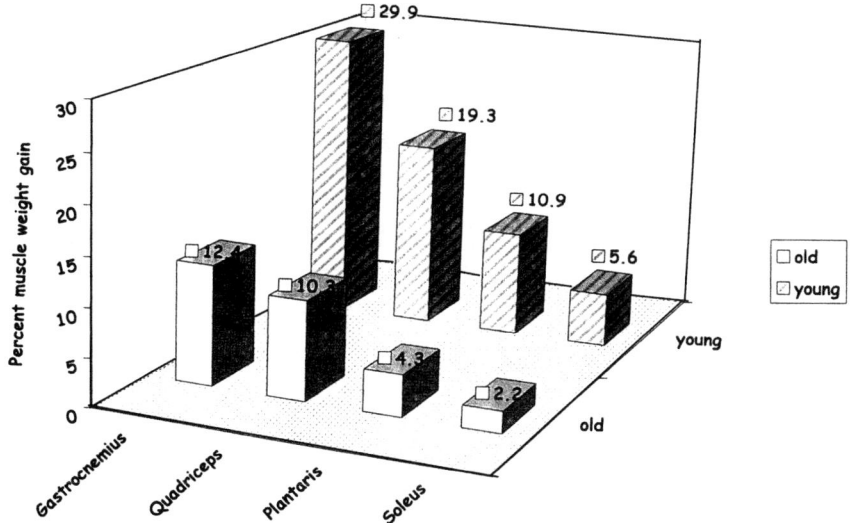

FIGURE 3. Net % change in muscle weights during immobilization and recovery. (Data were taken from Ref. 31, with permission.)

TABLE 2 compares changes in biochemical parameters in muscles of young and old animals. Whereas muscles of young rats have not returned to preimmobilization weights, the biochemical parameters have done so. In old rats, this was not the case, and all parameters measured have not returned to preimmobilization levels after 4 weeks of recovery. In addition, net % changes in biochemical parameters were greater by far in young animals than in old, as illustrated in FIGURE 4.

From these findings it can be concluded that young animals biochemically can return after 4 weeks of immobilization and 4 weeks of recovery to a preimmobilization

TABLE 2. Biochemical parameter measurements after external fixation (EF) and after EF + recovery

Biochemical parameter	External fixation, % of contralateral control		External fixation + recovery, % of contralateral control		Net % change during recovery period[a]		Relative biochemical parameter gain
	Young	Old	Young	Old	Young	Old	Young/Old
ACP activity	182.4	133.2	92.7	89.3	89.7	45.9	1.95
CPK activity	63.5	82.8	102.9	87.4	39.4	4.6	8.56
Lipid peroxidation	232.5	160	132.4	130	100.1	30.0	3.33

[a]Net % change was determined from the difference of % change afer the recovery period and the % change at end of immobilization period. (Values are averages obtained from five different animals.)

state, whereas old animals cannot. Moreover, the capacity for recovery or net % muscle gain in old animals is much lower than that in young ones, and similarly net % changes observed in the biochemical parameters were also smaller in old animals than in young ones. Altogether, these findings indicate that the ability of muscles of very old animals to repair themselves from immobization-associated damage is very poor, and therefore conditions of disuse and immobilization are detrimental to old animals and probably also to old people.

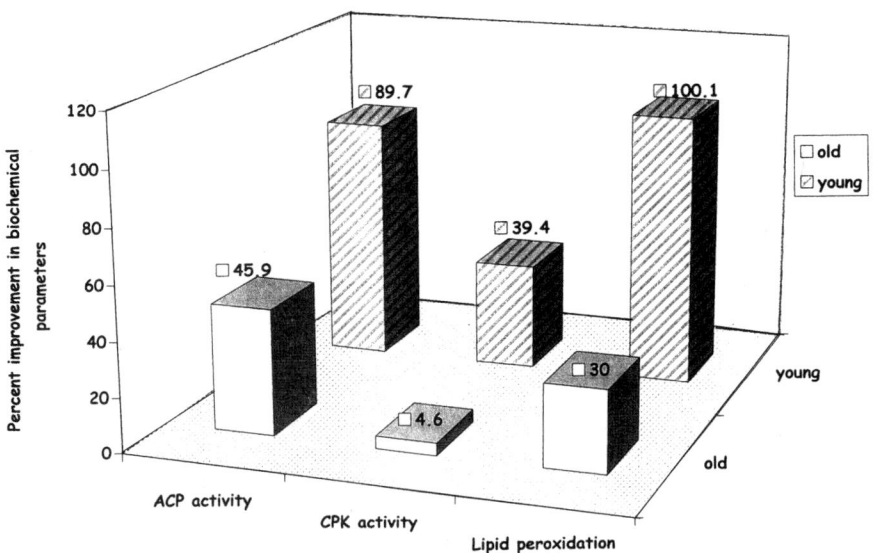

FIGURE 4. Net % change in biochemical parameters measurements after external fixation (EF) and after EF + recovery. (Data were taken from Ref. 31, with permission.)

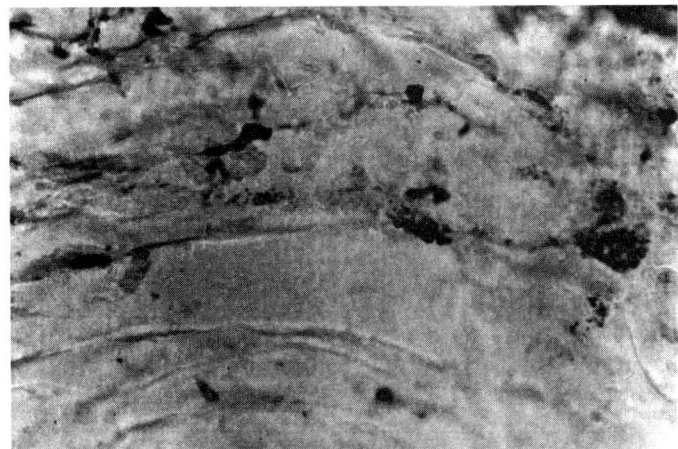

FIGURE 5. Immunohistochemistry with anti-TNF α antibody of fixated soleus muscle.

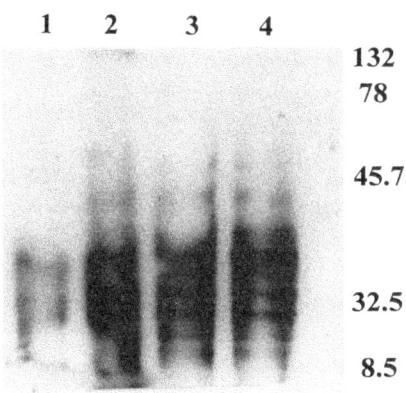

FIGURE 6. Effect of increased amounts of H_2O_2 on skeletal muscle myoblasts protein oxidation as determined by immunoblot. *Lane 1*: Level of protein oxidation in control L-8 culture (cells concentration 10^6/ml). *Lane 2*: L-8 cells incubated with presence of 0.5mM of H_2O_2. *Lane 3*: L-8 cells incubated with presence of 1mM of H_2O_2. *Lane 4*: L-8 cells incubated with presence of 2mM of H_2O_2.

Molecular and Cellular Events Leading to Muscle Wasting due to Immobilization

The cascade of events that leads to muscle wasting due to immobilization in the slow phase starts most probably with infiltration of macrophages and monocytes to the immobilized muscle tissue. This presumably is the source for cytokines such as TNF-α and other active substances. Evidence for cytokine secretion is demonstrated by immunohistochemical staining of immobilized muscle tissue with anti–TNF-α antibody (FIG. 5). The immobilized skeletal muscle demonstrates significant positive staining for TNF-α between muscle fibers. In control nonimmobilized limb muscles there was almost no staining (data not shown).

The fact that almost all staining is located outside the fibers, in the perimeter of fibers, indicates that these cytokines originate in invading macrophages which can be seen in highly degenerative muscles.[15–17]

As discussed in the introduction, TNF-α and other cytokines can elevate the intracellular oxidative status. Using Western blot analysis for protein carbonyls as a

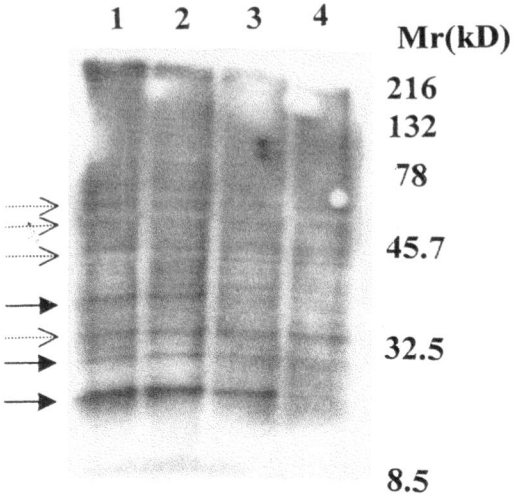

FIGURE 7. Effect of different concentrations of H_2O_2 on the level of ubiquitination of L-8 proteins. Lane 1, control L-8 cells; lanes 2–4, L-8 cells incubated with 0.5, 1.0, and 2.0 mM H_2O_2, respectively.

measure of protein oxidation, we could observe increases in protein carbonyls with increases in H_2O_2 levels (0.5–2 mM) (FIG. 6). FIGURE 6 shows that raising the level of H_2O_2 results in more oxidation of intracellular proteins of L-8 muscle cells, especially those with low molecular weights.

Raising the intracellular oxidative stress according to our model should increase the ubiquitin-dependent proteolysis. Indeed, after incubation of L-8 muscle myoblasts with various amounts of H_2O_2, we could observe that H_2O_2 had an effect on the levels of ubiquitination of L-8 proteins. Interestingly, three relatively small molecular weight proteins (*solid arrows*) could be shown to have reduced ubiquitination with increased H_2O_2 levels (FIG. 7), whereas for other proteins with relatively higher molecular weight (*dotted arrows*), the level of ubiquitination was not altered (FIG. 7).

Oxidative stress is produced in muscle tissue with activation of different factors in muscle cells, including nuclear factor-κB, which activates the induction of many enzymes, including inducible NO synthase (iNOS). Thus, we can see that there was elevation of immunohistochemical staining with anti-iNOS antibody in immobilized soleus muscle (FIG. 8A) relative to nonimmobilized soleus muscle (FIG. 8B). This pronounced staining was observed mostly between muscle fibers but occasionally also within the fibers themselves. However, direct evidence of the effect of increasing amounts of NO (using NO generator SIN-1) did not show changes in ubiquitination of L-8 proteins (data not shown). Nevertheless, a recent report by Grune et al.[25] did show that using SIN-1 and other NO donors, oxidized aconitase was degraded by the proteosome system in human cell culture of leukemia cells. Additional evidence of iNOS activation during muscle immobilization was found using the RT-PCR method for measuring mRNA of the enzyme (FIG. 9).

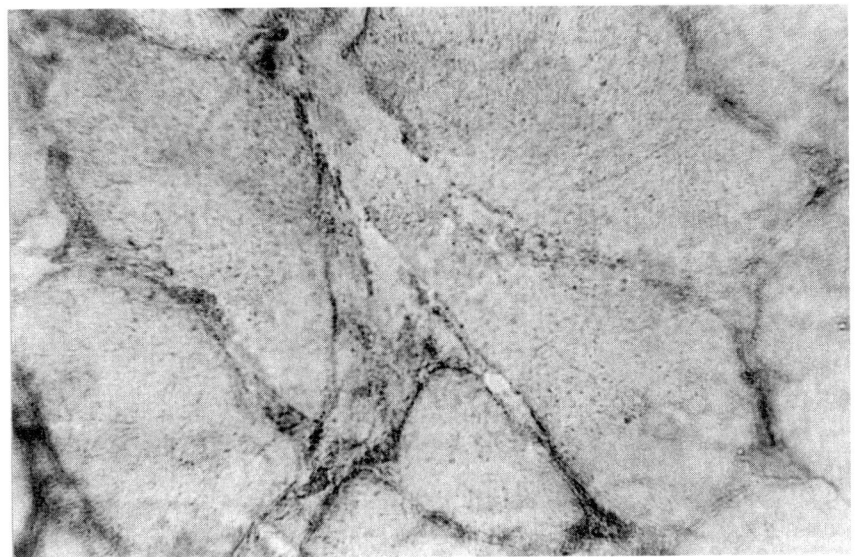

FIGURE 8A. Immunohistochmical staining for the presence of iNOS in immobilized soleus muscle (obj *100).

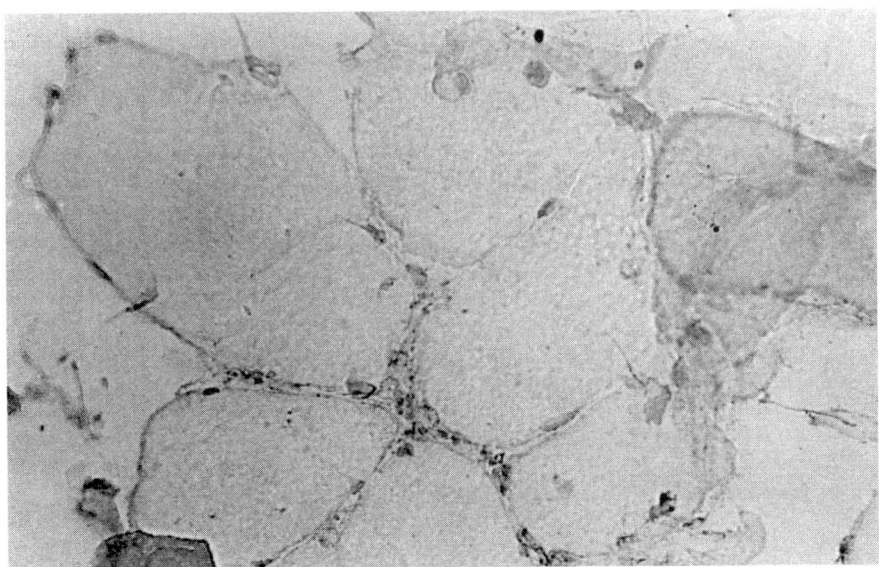

FIGURE 8B. Immunohistochmical staining for the presence of iNOS in control (non-immobilized) soleus muscle (obj *100).

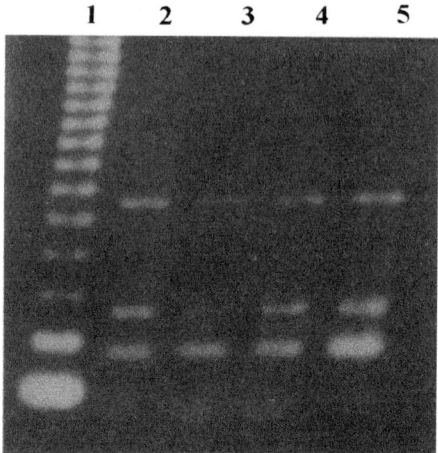

FIGURE 9. RT-PCR of mRNA of iNOS. *Line 1*: standart DNA oligonucleotides. *Line 2*: control (non-immobilized) gastrocnemius muscle. *Line 3*: immobilized gastrocnemius muscle. *Line 4*: control (nonimmobilized) quadriceps muscle. *Line 5*: immobilized quadriceps muscle.

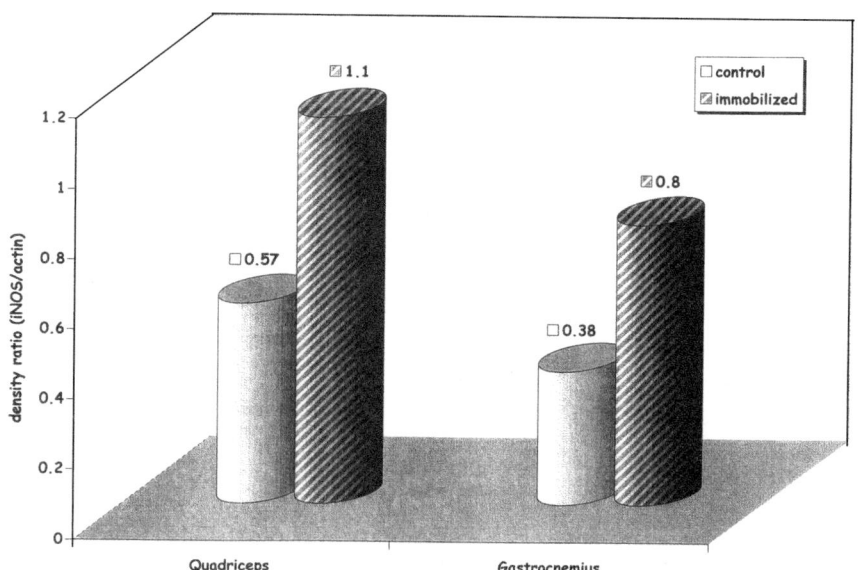

FIGURE 10. Relative band density ratio of mRNAs (iNOS/actin) in control and in immobilized quadriceps and gasrocnemius muscles.

TABLE 3. Common findings in various muscle pathologies[a]

	Cachexia[18]	Immobilization	Crush syndrome[27]	Eosinophilia myalgia syndrome[28,29]	Denervation[30]
Increased TNF-α	+	+[26]	?	+	?
Oxidative stress:					
Protein oxidation	?	+[9]	+	+	?
lipid peroxidation	+		+	+	?
Effect of Vitamin E	+	+[12]	?	?	?
					?
Increased NO synthase	+	+	+	?	?
Increased acid phosphatase	?	+[9]	+	+	+
Decreased Creatine phosphokinase	+	+[9]	+	+	+
Loss of muscle mass (protein degradation)	+	+[9]	+	+	+

[a]The numbers are from the reference list.

As seen in FIGURE 9, there was a substantial increase of c-DNA corresponding to mRNA of iNOS in the immobilized gastrocnemius and quadriceps muscles.

Using semiquantitative densitometry relative to a constitutable protein mRNA such as actin, the amount of mRNA of iNOS in immobilized muscles was about twice that found in control nonimmobilized muscles (FIG. 10).

In TABLE 3, we compare common findings that have been observed in a number of muscle pathologies. In most, there is an increase in TNF-α expression accompanied by oxidative stress and oxidative modification of lipids and proteins. Also, an increase in iNOS induction was observed in most pathologies. In addition, acid phosphatase levels were elevated in most of these muscle ailments, indicating an increase in lysosomal associated proteolysis. Finally, all of these pathologies resulted in muscle weight loss and muscle protein degradation. These observations strongly suggest that the cascade of events depicted in FIGURE 2 may serve as a common pathway by which macrophages and monocytes regulate the activation of muscle protein degradation, leading to muscle wasting and phagocytosis by invading phagocytes.

ACKNOWLEDGMENTS

This work was supported by The Krol Foundation, Lakewood, New Jersey, USA, the Israel Ministry of Health–State Bequests to the State of Israel, and a grant from the Vice Provost for Research at the Technion.

REFERENCES

1. DUTTA, C. & E.C. HADLEY. 1995. The significance of sarcopenia in old age. J. Gerontol. Series A. **50A:** 1–4.
2. CARMELI, E. & A.Z. REZNICK. 1994. The physiology and biochemistry of skeletal muscle atrophy as a function of age. Proc. Soc. Exp. Biol. Med. **206:** 103–113.
3. SAFADI, A., E. LIVNE & A.Z. REZNICK. 1997. Characterization of alkaline and acid phosphatases from skeletal muscles of young and old rats. Arch. Gerontol. Geriatr. **24:** 183–196.
4. SILBERMANN, M., S. FINKELBRAND, A. WEISS, et al. 1983. Morphometric analysis of aging skeletal muscle following endurance training. Muscle and Nerve **6:** 136–142.
5. REZNICK A.Z., G. VOLPIN, H. BEN-ARI, et al. 1995. Biochemical and morphological studies on rat skeletal muscles following prolonged immobilization of the knee joint by external fixation and plaster cast: a comparative study. Eur. J. Exp. Musculoskel. Res. **4:** 69–76.
6. REZNICK A.Z., E. CARMELI & I. ROISMAN. 1996. Effects of growth hormone on skeletal muscles of aging systems. Age **19:** 39–45.
7. CARMELI E., Z. HOCHBERG, E. LIVNE, et al. 1993. Effect of growth hormone on gastrocnemius muscle of aged rats after immobilization: biochemistry and morphology. J. Appl. Physiol. **75:** 1529–1535.
8. FUAD A.F., N. GRUENER, E. CARMELI & A.Z. REZNICK. 1996. Growth hormone (GH) retardation of muscle damage due to immobilization in old rats. Ann. N.Y. Acad. Sci. **786:** 430–443.
9. ZARZHEVSKY N., R. COLEMAN, G. VOLPIN, et al. 1999. Muscle recovery after immobilization by external fixation. J. Bone Joint Surg. [Br.] **81-B:** 896–901.
10. WILLIAMS, A.B., G.M. DECOURTEN-MYERS & J.E. FISCHER. 1999. Sepsis stimulates release of myofilaments in skeletal muscle by a calcium-dependent mechanism. FASEB J. **13:** 1435–1443.
11. KONDO, H., I. NAKAGAKI, S. SASAKI, et al. 1993. Mechanism of oxidative stress in skeletal muscle atrophied by immobilization. Am. J. Physiol. **265:** E839–E844.
12. KONDO, H., M. MIURA & Y. ITOKAWA. 1991. Oxidative stress in skeletal muscle atrophied by immobilization. Acta Physiol. Scand. **142:** 527–528.
13. MCLENNAN, I.S. 1993. Resident macrophages (ED2- and ED3-positive) do not phagocytose degenerating rat skeletal muscle fibers. Cell Tissue Res. **272:** 193–196.
14. MCLENNAN, I.S. 1996. Degenerating and regenerating skeletal muscles contain several macrophages with distinct spatial and temporal distributions. J. Anat. **188:** 17–28.
15. AUTHIER, F.J., C. MHIRI, B. CHAZAUD, et al. 1997. Interleukin-1 expression in inflammatory myopathies: evidence of marked immunoreactivity in sarcoid granulomas and muscle fibres showing ischaemic and regenerative changes. Neuropathol. Appl. Neurobiol. **23:** 132–140.
16. HOHLFELD, R., N. GOEBELS & A.G. ENGEEL. 1993. Cellular mechanisms in inflammatory myopathies. Baillières Clin. Neurol. **2:** 617–635.
17. DALAKAS, M.S. 1998. Molecular immunology and genetics of inflammatory muscle diseases. Arch. Neurol. **55:** 1509–1512.
18. BUCK, M. & M. CHOJKIER. 1996. Muscle wasting and dedifferentiation induced by oxidative stress in a murine model of cachexia is prevented by inhibitors of nitric oxide synthesis and antioxidants. EMBO J. **15:** 1753–1765.
19. SEN, C.K., S. KHANNA, A.Z. REZNICK, et al. 1997. Glutathione regulation of tumor necrosis factor α induced NF-κB activation in skeletal muscle derived L6 cells. Biochem. Biophys. Res. Commun. **237:** 645–649.
20. LI, Y.P., R.J. SCHWARTZ, I.D. WADDELL, et al. 1998. Skeletal muscle myocytes undergo protein loss and reactive oxygen-mediated NF-κB activation in response to tumor necrosis factor α. FASEB J. **12:** 871–880.
21. LLOVERA, M., C. GARCIA-MARTINEZ, N. AGELL, et al. 1997. TNF can directly induce the expression of ubiquitin-dependent proteolytic system in rat soleus muscles. Biochem. Biophys. Res. Commun. **230:** 238–244.
22. TANZAR, M.L. & C. GILVARD. 1959. Creatine kinase measurement. J. Biol. Chem. 3201–3204.

23. OHKAWA, H., N. OHISHI & K. YAGI. 1979. Assay for lipid peroxides in animal tissues by thiobarbituric acid reaction. Anal. Biochem. **95:** 351–358.
24. LOWRY, O.H., N.J. ROSEBROUGH, A.L. FARR & R.J. RANDALL. 1951. Protein measurement with the Folin phenol reagent. J. Biol. Chem. **193:** 265–275.
25. GRUENE. T., I.E. BLASIG, N. SITTE, et al. 1998. Peroxynitrite increases the degradation of aconitase and other cellular proteins by proteosome. J. Biol. Chem. **273:** 10857–10862.
26. ROISMAN, I., N. ZARZHEVSKY & A.Z. REZNICK. 1998. Effect of growth hormone on oxidative stress in immobilized muscles of old animals. *In* Oxidative Stress in Skeletal Muscle. A.Z. Reznick, I. Packer, C.K. Sen, J.O. Holloszy & M.J. Jackson, eds. :215–222. Birkhauser Verlag. Basel, Switzerland.
27. RUBINSTEIN, I., Z. ABASSI, R. COLEMAN, et al. 1998. Involvement of nitric oxide system in experimental muscle crush injury. J. Clin. Invest. **101:** 1325–1333.
28. GROSS, B., N. RONEN, S. HONIGMAN & E. LIVNE. 1999. Tryptophan toxicity-time and dose response in rats. Avd. Exp. Med. Biol. **467:** 507–516.
29. RONEN, N., E. LIVNE & B. GROSS. 1999. Oxidative damage in rat tissue following excessive L-tryptophan and atherogenic diets. Adv. Exp. Med. Biol. **467:** 497–505.
30. KALMAN, A. 1993. The effect of immobilization stress on muscles and bones of aging animals. Ph.D. dissertation. Technion-Israel Institute of Technology.
31. ZARZHEVSKY, N., E. CARMELI, D. FUCHS, et al. 2001. Recovery of muscles of old rats after hindlimb immobilization by external fixation is impaired compared with those of young rats. Exp. Gerontol. **36:** 125–140.

Nutrition Interventions in Aging and Age-Associated Disease

MOHSEN MEYDANI

Vascular Biology Program, Jean Mayer USDA-Human Nutrition Research Center on Aging at Tufts University, Tufts University, Medford, Massachusetts 02155, USA

ABSTRACT: The nutritional status and needs of elderly people are associated with age-related biological and often socioeconomic changes. Decreased food intake, a sedentary lifestyle, and reduced energy expenditure in older adults altogether become critical risk factors for malnutrition, especially protein and micronutrients. Surveys indicate that the elderly are particularly at risk for marginal deficiency of vitamins and trace elements. Changes in bodily functions, together with the malnutrition associated with advancing age, increase the risk of developing a number of age-related diseases. Chronic conditions pose difficulties for the elderly in carrying out the activities of daily living and may increase the requirements for certain nutrients due to changes in absorptive and metabolic capacity. Free radicals and oxidative stress have been recognized as important factors in the biology of aging and of many age-associated degenerative diseases. In this regard, modulation of oxidative stress by calorie restriction, as demonstrated in animal models, is suggested as one mechanism to slow the aging process and the decline of body functions. Therefore, dietary components with antioxidant activity have received particular attention because of their potential role in modulating oxidative stress associated with aging and chronic conditions. Several studies have indicated potential roles for dietary antioxidants in the reduction of degenerative disease such as vascular dementia, cardiovascular disease, and cancer. In support of epidemiological studies, our recent studies indicate that the antioxidant properties of vitamin E and polyphenols present in green tea may contribute to reducing the risk of cardiovascular disease, in part by reducing the susceptibility of low density lipoproteins to oxidation, decreasing the vascular endothelial cell expression of pro-inflammatory cytokines, and decreasing the expression of adhesion molecules and monocyte adhesion. Recently, we also demonstrated that these dietary antioxidants may have a preventive role in cancer, potentially through the suppression of angiogenesis by inhibiting interleukin-8 production and the cell junction molecule VE-cadherin. These findings concur with epidemiologic, clinical, and animal studies suggesting that the consumption of green tea and vitamin E is associated with a reduced risk of cardiovascular disease and cancer, the leading causes of morbidity and mortality among the elderly.

KEYWORDS: Aging; Antioxidants; Degenerative diseases;; Green tea; Nutrition; Oxidative stress; Vitamin E

Address for correspondence: Dr. Mohsen Meydani, Vascular Biology Program, Jean Mayer USDA-Human Nutrition Research Center on Aging at Tufts University, Boston, MA 02111. Voice: 617-556-3126; fax: 617-556-3224.
 MMeydani@HNRC.TUFTS.edu

INTRODUCTION

Aging is a complex biological phenomenon often accompanied by various socioeconomic changes that have a great impact on the nutritional status and needs of the elderly individual. The population of elderly over 65 years of age is rising in the United States and other countries. The number of older Americans has increased by 3.2 million in the last decade. This increase will be even greater in the coming years, when the "baby boom" generation arrives at old age. By 2030, there will be about 70 million elderly over the age of 65 years in the US, more than twice the number in 1998.[1] This large number of elderly is projected to constitute one fifth of the whole US population. A variety of factors, such as improved health care and diet, vaccination, and new drugs, have contributed significantly to the growth of the elderly population in the US and abroad.

With aging, however, the incidence of disability increases due to the commonly seen development of chronic conditions requiring medical attention and assistance from family or social organizations. Over one third of elderly persons are limited by chronic conditions and are unable to carry on major activities. According to recent data,[2] more than 50% of elderly over 65 years of age have one form of disability, and 33% of the elderly have at least one type of severe disability. Arthritis, hypertension, heart disease, hearing impairments, orthopedic impairments, cataracts, sinusitis, and diabetes are the most frequent health problems that pose difficulties for the elderly in carrying out activities of daily living (ADL). Therefore, it is expected that the prevalence of elderly with disabilities will increase concomitantly with the rise in the elderly population to more than 30 million in the US by the first decade of new millenium, a great responsibility to the society and younger generation. Therefore, strategies to prevent an age-related decline in mobility and reduce the prevalence of chronic disease have been recognized as important in allowing the elderly to maintain their independence and ability to carry out ADL. From an economic standpoint, preventive strategies are considered the most cost-effective solution to the problem of disability in the elderly.

NUTRITION AND AGING

Free radicals and oxidative stress have been recognized as important factors in the biology of aging and in many age-associated degenerative diseases. A time-dependent shift in the antioxidant/prooxidant balance, which leads to higher free radical generation and an increase in oxidative stress and dysregulation of cellular function, is the basis for the free radical theory of aging. This theory is commonly manifested with phenotypic changes and functional deterioration in later life. Genetic, environmental, and lifestyle factors play important roles in the rate of changes in this balance (FIG. 1) and therefore in the rates of aging and the development of age-associated diseases. Decreased food intake, a sedentary lifestyle, and reduced energy expenditure in older adults together are the risk factors for malnutrition, especially for protein and micronutrients, and may further contribute to the decline of bodily functions and the development of chronic age-associated degenerative diseases. Other factors that reduce food intake in the elderly are listed in TABLE 1. A recent survey of 40,000 subjects in 88 communities in the third National Health and Nutrition Ex-

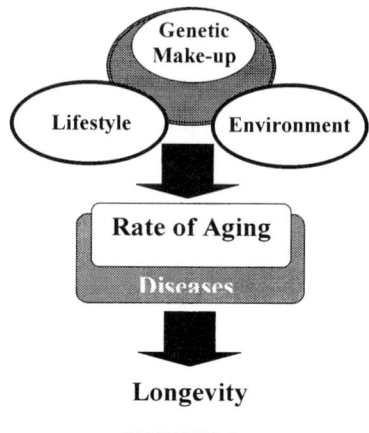

FIGURE 1.

TABLE 1. Factors increasing the risk of inadequate consumption of food by the elderly

- Diseases
- Physical disability
- Inability to chew food adequately
- Polypharmacy
- Living alone
- Limited income

amination Survey (NHANES III) in the US also included a survey of about 5,000 elderly in the US population grouped from 60–69 years, 70–79 years, and 80+ years.[3,4] This survey for the first time provided a cross-sectional health and nutrition status in the aging US population.[5] The report indicated that the median intake of total energy in elderly subjects in general is lower than the recommended 2,300 Kcal for men and 1,900 Kcal for women.[6] Caloric intake from fat by the elderly is higher than 30% of recommended allowance (RDA). Low intake of fat is widely recognized to be important for reducing the risks of obesity, coronary heart disease, and certain forms of cancer. The survey also found that elderly Americans consumed less cholesterol than 300 mg per day and more folate and B12 vitamins. They consumed enough vitamins C and A, micronutrients important for maintenance of healthy life, to meet RDA levels. However, elderly Americans appear not to be consuming sufficient calcium to meet the recommended 800 mg/day level, which is important for bone health and reducing the risk of osteoporosis and bone fracture. The survey also reported that intake of vitamin E is lower than the current recommended level (for the natural form of vitamin E), which is 15 mg/day. Vitamin E is an important antioxidant to prevent lipid peroxidation and maintain cellular membrane integrity. The NHANES III study demonstrated clearly that food insufficiency exists in the US and that its prevalence is significantly associated with the income status of the elderly

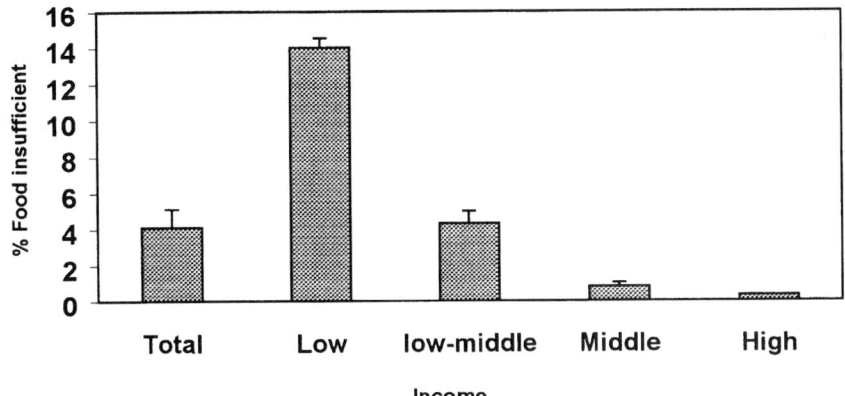

FIGURE 2. Prevalence of food insufficiency in the United States by Income Category NHANES III (1994-98).

(FIG. 2).[2] In addition to inadequate food intake and malnutrition due to income limitations, other factors listed in TABLE 1 may contribute to the risk of inadequate consumption of food in the elderly.

NUTRITION INTERVENTIONS

It is important to note that in many age-associated diseases food and nutrition play important roles (TABLE 2). Chronic conditions may also increase requirements for certain nutrients due to changes in absorption and metabolism. Mounting evidence suggests that generation of free radicals and oxidative stress is a major player in the aging process and age-associated diseases. Thus, eliminating the formation of free radicals and reducing oxidative stress, thereby increasing antioxidant defenses, are considered one means by which both the rate of aging and the risk of chronic disease can be reduced. Historically, nutrition has been recognized as an important factor in the modulation of disease and longevity. However, the only intervention shown to be effective in slowing down the aging process in animal models is caloric restric-

TABLE 2. Several age-related diseases associated with nutrition

- Cancer
- Cardiovascular disease
- Diabetes
- Osteoporosis
- Sarcopenia
- Cataract
- Macular degeneration
- Infection

tion. Caloric restriction has been proven to be an effective dietary intervention to reduce oxidative stress, improve the antioxidant defense system, and extend both median and maximum life spans in several animal models.[7] Caloric restriction has also been shown to slow the age-associated decline of bodily functions, such as those of the immune and neuronal systems,[8,9] and to delay the onset of age-related diseases such as cancer, diabetes, and cataracts.[10–12] Caloric restriction in rodent models has been shown to increase longevity when caloric restriction is introduced at any time after the animal has matured.[13] Evidence suggests that the mechanism of action of dietary restriction is mainly reduction of oxidative stress and an increase in endogenous levels of antioxidant enzymes. Restriction of caloric intake by 30–40% in humans, however, appears to be difficult, as it would require drastic behavioral modifications. This type of restriction is virtually impractical at present, except in clinical settings, and is therefore not a plausible option for increasing longevity or reducing disease risk in a population.

Because reduction of oxidative stress appears to be a main mechanism of action in dietary restriction models and is in accordance with the free radical theory of aging, it was proposed that increasing antioxidant status by feeding animals natural or synthetic antioxidants would reduce oxidative stress and thus contribute to longevity. These attempts, however, were not as successful[14–17] as the results obtained from food restriction paradigms. However, a relatively recent study demonstrated that a mixture of several dietary antioxidants, if begun early in life, might extend significantly the longevity of animals.[18] Although the results are promising, this observation needs to be reproduced by other investigators. Extension of this observation to humans, that is, long-term supplementation of a large number of human subjects with antioxidants to examine longevity, would be of great value. It would be very interesting to prove that high antioxidant capacity and low oxidative stress are a major contributing factor in the human population, in whom life expectancy according to demographic data is longer than that in others. Modification of diet without drastic reductions of caloric intake in combination with lifestyle modifications, such as exercising, abstaining from smoking, and moderating alcohol intake, together with maintenance of an individual's ideal body weight, are the factors suggested by several health organizations for upkeep of health and reduced risk of chronic diseases.

NUTRITION AND AGE-ASSOCIATED CHRONIC DISEASES

Several observational studies have shown that supplemental intake of antioxidant vitamins such as vitamins E and C is associated with reduced risk of age-associated chronic diseases such as cardiovascular disease, certain forms of cancer, cataracts, and cognitive impairment, which in turn might have contributed to the longevity and growth of the elderly population. Thus, it would be of great value to examine the potential role of supplemental intake of antioxidants vitamins in relation to the increased life expectancy observed in recent decades in the population in the US and other parts of the world.

Dietary components of foods containing antioxidant activity such as vitamin E or specific forms of fatty acids such as (n-3) polyunsaturated fatty acids (PUFA) have received particular attention because of their potential role in modulating the oxidative stress associated with aging and age-related chronic diseases. Several studies have shown a potential role of these components of the diet in the modulation of immune and inflammatory systems, which play important roles in preventing infectious and inflammatory diseases in the elderly and in reducing the risk of chronic disease such as cancer and cardiovascular disease, the two leading causes of morbidity and mortality in US and other Western societies.

Earlier, Meydani et al.[19] reported that supplementation of aged mice (24 months old) with dietary vitamin E (500 ppm) improved several indices of the immune system to levels comparable to those seen in young animals. Supplementation of aged mice with this vitamin also increased clearance of influenza virus from the lung compared with that in animals supplemented with other antioxidants such as melathonine, glutathione, or strawberry extract which contains a high level of flavonoids with antioxidant activity.[20] In a double-blind, placebo-controlled study, Meydani et al.[21,22] also reported that supplementation of elderly subjects with vitamin E for a short (1 month) or long (4.5 months) period of time also improved several in vitro and in vivo indices of immune response. The optimal immune response was observed with 200 IU of vitamin E per day in the long-term study. It is worth noting that this level of vitamin E has also been reported to be the optimal level for reducing plasma F_2-isoprostane, a reliable index of lipid peroxidation.[23] Improving the immune response in the elderly may result in a lower incidence of infections, which are prevalent among the elderly, and thus may contribute to a longer and healthier life.

Scores of observational and clinical trials have also indicated that a high intake or high plasma level of this vitamin is associated with a low risk of cardiovascular disease.[24,25] Several lines of evidence indicated that supplemental levels of vitamin E may prevent cardiovascular disease by reducing susceptibility of LDLs to oxidation,[26] reducing expression of chemokines and adhesion molecule expression and monocyte adhesion,[27] decreasing smooth muscle proliferation,[28] improving vessel relaxation,[29-31] and decreasing platelet aggregation.[32]

Marine-derived (n-3) PUFA has also been reported to contribute to cardiovascular health through its antiinflammatory properties.[33,34] Consumption of marine-derived (n-3) PUFA, which does not reduce LDL cholesterol levels, does reduce plasma levels of very low density lipoprotein (VLDL) cholesterol, and has been consistently shown to reduce plasma triglyceride levels.[35] Furthermore, marine-derived (n-3) PUFA have been shown to decrease platelet aggregation[36,37] and high blood pressure,[38] which, in part, supports the epidemiologic findings on the association of reduced risk of cardiovascular disease with fish or fish oil consumption.[33,34] In addition, the antiinflammatory characteristics of these fatty acids contribute significantly to their antiatherogenic properties. This latter effect of marine-derived (n-3) PUFA is mainly attributed to their modulation of prostanoid, leukotriene, and cytokine production, all of which participate in atherogenesis.

Supplementation with (n-3) PUFA from fish oil, however, has been reported to suppress the immune response,[39,40] which hampers enthusiasm for the use of marine-derived PUFA for its benefits in cardiovascular disease. However, the latter concern could be addressed by including the supplemental intake of vitamin E along with fish oil supplements. In a recent study, we found that supplementing elderly persons with (n-3) fatty acid of fish oil in combination with vitamin E, while maintaining the antiinflammatory properties of (n-3) PUFA, did not reduce immune indices in the elderly.[41]

Several observational studies have indicated that consumption of fruits and vegetables is associated with a lower risk of cancer.[42] Antioxidants present in fruits and vegetables in the form of antioxidant vitamins or non-nutritive polyphenols may contribute to their effect on reducing the cancer risk. Suppression of oxidative stress and prevention of DNA damages and mutation have been suggested as one of the mechanisms by which these compounds may affect cancer reduction. Another may be through inhibition of tumor growth by suppressing angiogenesis, the formation of new blood vessels from existing ones. We recently made *in vitro* observations that angiogenesis can be induced by oxidative stress induced by hydrogen peroxide, and supplementing the microvascular endothelial cells with vitamin E or green tea catechins (polyphenols with antioxidant activity) inhibits angiogenesis. Vitamin E and regular consumption of green tea have both been reported to be associated with reduced risk of cancer.[43–48] Green tea catechins have been shown to be effective in reducing angiogenesis in *in vivo* animal models.[49] Our *in vitro* studies have indicated that reductions of interleukin-8 production and disturbance in the assembly of VE-cadherin with intracellular β-catenin are some of the mechanisms by which these antioxidants modulate angiogenesis.

Decline of cognitive function with age is another factor that hinders independence and activity in the elderly. Current evidence indicates that both increased oxidative stress and antioxidant status imbalance contribute to the decline of cognitive function with age. Several studies have found associations between the decline of memory performance with age and lower status of dietary antioxidants.[50,51] The effect of dietary antioxidants on the prevention of vascular dementia, stroke, and atherosclerosis are other mechanisms by which dietary antioxidants may reduce the risk of dementia associated with vascular dysfunction and probably Alzheimer's disease. In the recent Third National Health and Nutrition Examination Survey (NHANES III), elderly over the age of 60 years were tested for their cognitive function in relation to plasma antioxidant status. The study reported that vitamins C, E, A, carotenoids, and selenium levels were correlated with memory function.[51] The survey reported that the odds ratios for poor memory performance consistently were high with low levels of plasma vitamin E. Furthermore, supplementation with vitamin E was reported to delay progression of Alzheimer's disease.[52] Experimental animal studies indicate that antioxidants present in fruits and vegetables can improve cognitive function.[53,54] Therefore, it appears that dietary antioxidants may also provide protection against oxidative damage in neuronal tissue and may prevent deterioration of the neuronal system with aging.

CONCLUSION

It is accepted that free radicals are involved in both aging and the pathology of many age-associated diseases. This concept is overwhelmingly supported by a great deal of evidence resulting from dietary restriction interventions in animal models, modulation of enzymatic and dietary antioxidant status in animal models, and observational and clinical interventions on the association of antioxidants and oxidative stress indices with chronic diseases in humans. The contribution of dietary or supplemental antioxidants during the last decades to the increase in life expectancy and growth of the elderly population is not known. However, evidence indicates that adopting a healthy lifestyle, which includes eating a balanced diet, being physically active, and abstaining from smoking, as well as the availability of better health care most likely contributes significantly to increased life expectancy. Emerging data from epidemiologic and clinical studies also emphasize the importance of micronutrients in increasing vigor of several bodily functions such as immune, cognitive, cardiovascular, and musculoskeletal functions in the elderly. In addition, supplemental intake of antioxidants and other micronutrients appears to be important in preventing or delaying the onset of several age-associated chronic diseases such as cardiovascular disease, cancer, dementia, and infections, the major cause of morbidity and mortality among the elderly. In comparison with medical care and drug treatment, nutritional interventions can more feasibly be implemented cost-effectively in every population along the age spectrum.

REFERENCES

1. FOWLES, D.G. 1999. A profile of older Americans. Program Resource Dept., Administration on Aging, US Department of Health and Human Services. Washington, DC.
2. ALAIMO, K., R.R. BRIEFEL, E.A. FRONGILLO & C.M. OLSON. 1998. Food insufficiency exists in the United States: results from the third National Health and Nutrition Examination Survey (NHANES III). Am. J. Pub. Health **88:** 419–426.
3. US DEPARTMENT OF HEALTH AND HUMAN SERVICES. 1994. Third National Health and Nutrition Examination Survey: National Center for Health Statistics.
4. NATIONAL CENTER FOR HEALTH STATISTICS. 1994. Plan and operation of the Third National Health and Nutrition Examination Survey, 1988–1994. Vital Health Statistics. Washington, DC.
5. BURT, V.L. & T. HARRIS. 1994. The third National Health and Nutrition Examination Survey: contributing data on aging and health. Gerontologist **34:** 86–90.
6. MARWICK, C. 1997. NHANES III health data relevant for aging nation. JAMA **277:** 100–102.
7. WEINDRUCH, R. 1996. The retardation of aging by caloric restriction: studies in rodents and primates. Toxicol. Pathol. **24:** 742–745.
8. FERNANDES, G., J.T. VENKATRAMAN, A. TURTURRO, et al. 1997. Effect of food restriction on life span and immune functions in long-lived Fischer-344 x Brown Norway F1 rats. J. Clin. Imuunol. **17:** 85–95.
9. BRUCE-KELLER, A.J., G. UMBERGER, R. MCFALL & M.P. MATTSON. 1999. Food restriction reduces brain damage and improves behavioral outcome following excitotoxic and metabolic insults. Ann. Neurol. **45:** 8–15.
10. WEINDRUCH, R. 1992. Effect of caloric restriction on age-associated cancers. Exp. Gerontol. **27:** 575–581.
11. NOVELLI, M., P. MASIELLO, M. BOMBARA & E. BERGAMINI. 1998. Protein glycation in the aging male Sprague-Dawley rat: effects of antiaging diet restrictions. J. Gerontol. **53:** B94–101.
12. TAYLOR, A., J. JAHNGEN-HODGE, D.E. SMITH, et al. 1995. Dietary restriction delays catract and reduces ascorbate levels in Emory mice. Exp. Eye Res. **61:** 55–62.
13. YU, BP. 1995. Modulation of oxidative stress as a means of life prolonging action of dietary restriction. *In* Oxidative Stress and Aging. R.G. Cuttler, L. Packer, J. Bertram & A. Mori, eds.: 331–342. Birkhauser Verlag. Basel.
14. HARMAN, D. 1968. Free radical theory of aging: effect of free radical inhibitors on the mortality rate of male LFA mice. J. Gerontol. **23:** 476–482.
15. COMFORT, A. 1971. Effect of ethoxyquin on the longevity of C3H mice. Nature **229:** 254–255.
16. KOHN, RR. 1971. Effect of antioxidants on life-span of C57/BL mice. J. Gerontol. **26:** 376–380.

17. HARMAN, D. 1980. Free radical theory of aging: beneficial effect of antioxidants on the lifespan of male NZB mice; role of free radical reactions in the deterioration of the immune system with age and in the pathogenesis of systemic lupus erythematosus. Age **3:** 64–73.
18. BEXLEPKIN, V.G., N.P. SIROAT & A.I. GAZIEV. 1996. The prolongation of survival in mice by dietary antioxidants depends on their age by the start of feeding this diet. Mech. Ageing Dev. **92:** 227–234.
19. MEYDANI, S.N., M. MEYDANI, C.P. VERDON, et al. 1986. Vitamin E supplementation suppresses prostaglandin E2 synthesis and enhances the immune response of aged mice. Mech. Ageing Dev. **34:** 191–201.
20. HAN, S.N., M. MEYDANI, D. WU, et al. 2000. Effect of long-term dietary antioxidant supplementation on influenza virous infection. J. Gerontol. In press.
21. MEYDANI, S.N., P.M. BARKLUND, S. LIU, et al. 1990. Vitamin E supplementation enhances cell-mediated immunity in healthy elderly subjects. Am. J. Clin. Nutr. **52:** 557–563.
22. MEYDANI, S.N., M. MEYDANI, J.B. BLUMBERG, et al. 1997. Vitamin E supplementation and in vivo immune response in healthy elderly: a randomized controlled trial. JAMA **277:** 1380–1386.
23. DILLON, G., J.A. VITA, C. LEEUWENBURGH, et al. 1998. α-Tocopherol supplementation reduces systemic markers of oxidative damage in healthy adults. Circulation **17S:** 671I.
24. MEYDANI, M. 1995. Vitamin E. Lancet **345:** 170–175.
25. MEYDANI, M. 1998. Nutrition, immune cells, and atherosclerosis. Nutr. Rev. **56** (part II): S177–182.
26. JIALAL, I., C.J. FULLER & B.A. HUET. 1995. The effect of alpha-tocopherol supplementation on LDL oxidation. Arterioscler. Thromb. Vasc. Biol. **15:** 190–198.
27. WU, D., T. KOGA, K.R. MARTIN & M. MEYDANI. 1999. Effect of vitamin E on human aortic endothelial cell production of chemokines and adhesion to monocytes. Atherosclerosis **147:** 297–307.
28. AZZI, A., D. BOSCOBOINIK, D. MARILLEY, et al. 1995. Vitamin E: A sensor and an information transducer of the cell oxidation state. Am. J. Clin. Nutr. **62** (6 Suppl): 1337S–1346S.
29. NEUNTEUFL, T., K. KOSTNER, R. KATZENSCHLAGER, et al. 1998. Additional benefit of vitamin E supplementation to simvastatin therapy on vasoreactivity of the brachial artery of hypercholesterolemic men. J. Am. Coll. Cardiol. **32:** 711–716.
30. GREEN, D., G. O'DRISCOLL, J.M. RANKIN, et al. 1998. Beneficial effect of vitamin E administration on nitric oxide function in subjects with hypercholesterolaemia. Clin. Sci. **95:** 361–367.
31. KEANEY, J.F.J., M.J. GAZIANO, A. XU, et al. 1993. Dietary antioxidants preserve endothelium-dependent vessel relaxation in cholesterol-fed rabbits. Proc. Natl. Acad. Sci. USA **90:** 11880–11884.
32. STEINER, M. 1999. Vitamin E, a modifier of platelet function: rationale and use in cardiovascular and cerebrovascular disease. Nutr. Rev. **57:** 306–309.
33. GLOMSET, J.A. 1985. Fish, fatty acids, and human health. N. Engl. J. Med. **312:** 1253–1225.
34. KINSELLA, J.E., B. LOKESH & R.A. STONE. 1990. Dietary (n-3) polyunsaturated fatty acids and amelioration of cardiovascular disease: possible mechanisms. Am. J. Clin. Nutr. **52:** 1–28.
35. HARRIS, W.S. 1997. n-3 fatty acids and serum lipoproteins: human studies. Am. J. Clin. Nutr. **65** (suppl.): 1645S–1654S.
36. HANSEN, J.B., J.O. OLSEN, L. WILSGARD, et al. 1993. Comparative effects of prolonged intake of highly purified fish oils as ethyl ester or triglyceride on lipids, haemostasis and platelet function in normolipaemic men. Eur. J. Clin. Nutr. **47:** 497–507.
37. WINTHER, K., B. MYRUP, G. HOLMAN, et al. 1993. Decreased platelet activity without change in fibrinolytic activity after low dosages of fish oil. Angiology **44:** 39–44.
38. MORRIS, M.C., F. SACKS & B. ROSNER. 1993. Does fish oil lower blood pressure? A meta-analysis of controlled trials. Circulation **88:** 523–533.

39. MEYDANI, S.N., S. ENDRES, M.N. WOODS, et al. 1991. Oral (n-3) fatty acid supplementation supresses cytokine production and lymphocyte proliferation: comparison between young and older women. J. Nutr. **121:** 547–555.
40. MEYDANI, S.N., A.H. LICHENSTEIN, S. CORNWALL, et al. 1993. Immunological effects of national cholesterol education panel (NCEP) step-2 diets with and without fish-derived (n-3) fatty acid enrichment. J. Clin. Invest. **92:** 105–113.
41. WU, D., M. MEYDANI, S.N. HAN, et al. 2000. Effect of dietary supplementation with fish oil in combination with different levels of vitamin E on immune response in healthy elderly human subjects. FASEB. J. **14:** A238.
42. AMES, B.N., M.K. SHIGENAGA & .T.M. HAGEN. 1993. Oxidants, antioxidants, and the degenerative diseases of aging. Proc Natl. Acad. Sci. USA **90:** 7915–7922.
43. NAKACHI, K., K. SUEMASU, K. SUGA et al. 1998. Influence of drinking green tea on breast cancer malignancy among Japanese patients. Jpn J. Cancer Res. **89:** 254–261.
44. MUKHTAR, H., S.K. KATIYAR & R. AGARWAL. 1994. Green tea and skin-anticarcinogenic effects. J. Invest. Dermatol. **102:** 3–7.
45. DAS, S. 1994. Vitamin E in the genesis and prevention of cancer. Acta Oncol. **33:** 615–619.
46. ATTAR, E.L. 1992. Effect of vitamin C and vitamin E on prostaglandin synthesis by fibroblasts and squamous carcinoma cells. Prostaglandins Leukotrienes Essent. Fatty Acids **47:** 253–257.
47. FLESHNER, N., W.R. FAIR, R. HURYK & W.D. HESTON. 1999. Vitamin E inhibits the high-fat diet promoted growth of established human prostate LNCaP tumors in nude mice. J. Urol. **161:** 1651–1654.
48. SHKLAR, G. & J.L. SCHWARTZ. 1996. Vitamin E inhibits experimental carcinogenesis and tumour angiogenesis. Eur. J. Cancer **32:** 114–119.
49. CAO, Y. & R. CAO. 1999. Angiogenesis inhibited by drinking tea. Nature **398:** 381.
50. PERRIG, W.J., P. PERRIG & H.B. STAVELIN. 1997. The relation between antioxdants and memory performance in the old and very old. J. Am. Geriatr. Soc. **45:** 718–724.
51. PERKINS, A., H.C. HENDRIE, C.M. CALLAHAN, et al. 1999. Association of antioxidants with memory in a multiethnic elderly sample using the Third National Health and Nutrition examination Survey. Am. J. Epidemiol. **150:** 37–44.
52. SANO, M., M.S. ERNESTO, R.G. THOMAS, et al. 1997. A controlled trial of selegiline, alpha-tocopherol, or both as treatment for Alzheimer's disease. N. Engl. J. Med. **336:** 1216–1222.
53. JOSEPH, J.A., B. SHUKITT-HALE, N.A. DENISOVA, et al. 1999. Reversals of age-related declines in neuronal signal transduction, cognitive, and motor behavioral deficits with blueberries, spinach, or strawberry dietary supplementation. J. Neurosci. **19:** 8114–8121.
54. JOSEPH, J.A., B. SHUKITT-HALE, N.A. DENISOVA, et al. 1998. Long-term dietary strawberry, spinach, or vitamin E supplementation retards the onset of age-related neuronal signal-transduction and cognitive behavioral deficits. J. Neurosci. **18:** 8047–8055.

Exercise at Old Age: Does It Increase or Alleviate Oxidative Stress?

LI LI JI

Department of Kinesiology, Nutritional Science, and Institute on Aging, University of Wisconsin-Madison, Madison, Wisconsin 53706, USA

ABSTRACT: Aging is associated with increased free radical generation in the skeletal muscle that can cause oxidative modification of protein, lipid, and DNA. Physical activity has many well-established health benefits, but strenuous exercise increases muscle oxygen flux and elicits intracellular events that can lead to increased oxidative injury. The paradox arises as to whether exercise would be advisable to aged population. Research evidence indicates that senescent organisms are more susceptible to oxidative stress during exercise because of the age-related ultrastructural and biochemical changes that facilitate formation of reactive oxygen species (ROS). Aging also increases the incidence of muscle injury, and the inflammatory response can subject senescent muscle to further oxidative stress. Furthermore, muscle repair and regeneration capacity is reduced at old age that could potentially enhance the accrual of cellular oxidative damage. Predeposition of certain age-related pathologic conditions may exacerbate the risks. In spite of these risks, the elderly who are physically active benefit from exercise-induced adaptation in cellular antioxidant defense systems. Improved muscle mechanics, strength, and endurance make them less vulnerable to acute injury and chronic inflammation. Many critical questions remain regarding the relationship of aging and exercise as we enter a new millennium. For example, how does aging alter exercise-induced intracellular and intercellular mechanisms that generate ROS? Can acute and chronic exercise modulate the declined gene expression of metabolic and antioxidant enzymes seen at old age? Does exercise prevent age-dependent muscle loss (sarcopenia)? What kinds of antioxidant supplementation, if any, do aged people who are physically active need? Answers to these questions require highly specific research in both animals and humans.

KEYWORDS: Aging; Antioxidant; Exercise; Free radical; Gene expression; Muscle; Oxidative stress

INTRODUCTION

In human population, morbidity is concentrated in the last two decades of life, beginning on the average at age 55 and increasing in frequency until the average age of death at 75.[1] The benefit of exercise is highlighted by the increase of approximately two years in longevity in physically active people as compared to less active people.[2,3] Furthermore, disability levels in a vigorously exercising population remain below that of nonexercisers, and age-related increases in disability are delayed

---

Address for correspondence: Li Li Ji, Ph.D., 2000 Observatory Drive, Madison, WI 53706. Voice: 608-262-7250; fax: 608-262-1656.

ji@soemadison.wisc.edu

by approximately 15 years.[1] These data indicate that engaging in regular physical activity would increase the age of onset of chronic illness and shorten the time between the onset of morbidity and death. This compression of the period of morbidity as a result of physical exercise would represent a significant improvement in the quality of life of the elderly and result in major reductions in the cost of treating the medical conditions of the elderly.[1] Despite these clear benefits, little is known about the adaptive mechanisms involved and the time period where major protection offered by exercise occurs. Furthermore, it is not clear whether aged individuals are more susceptible to some of the harmful effects of rigorous exercise reported in recent literature as a result of increased exposure to reactive oxygen species (ROS).[4,5]

The free radical theory of aging has allowed the establishment of a powerful link between exercise and aging research.[6] A fundamental premise for this theory is that ROS generated in normal metabolic processes are the underlying reason for cell and tissue oxidative damage seen throughout the aging process.[7] Since exercise increases metabolic rate, which is reflected by a greater amount of oxygen uptake, ROS production is also expected to increase during physical exertion. While this may seem to be detrimental to the elderly who are physically active, exercise is also known to cause adaptive responses such as improvement in antioxidant defense capacity.[5] Therefore, an important consideration in aging and exercise studies is to be able to separate the influence of exercise from those that occur solely due to aging.[6,8] Despite decades of effort, there is no uniform theory that can accurately describe the influence of exercise on aging.

In this paper, the author will consider primarily the following two factors. First, does aging increase ROS generation and oxidative damage as a result of acute unaccustomed exercise? Second, does chronic exercise (training) improve cellular and tissue resistance to age-associate oxidative stress?

EXERCISE-INDUCED ROS AND OXIDATIVE STRESS ARE GREATER AT OLD AGE

Unaccustomed strenuous exercise increases free radical generation and tissue oxidative damage in experimental animals.[9-13] The question is whether this exercise-induced oxidative stress is greater in the aged animals as compared to the young ones. Since work capacity as represented by maximal oxygen consumption (VO_2max) decreases with age, the same workload will represent a greater percentage of oxygen consumption and impose a greater stress at older age. Therefore, it is important to compare ROS generation and oxidative stress between old and young animals when they work at the same relative workload (i.e., $\%VO_2max$). Using dichlorofluorescin (DCFH) as an intracellular ROS probe, Bejma and Ji[10] have recently reported that ROS production was 77% ($p < 0.05$) higher in the deep vastus laterilas (type IIa) muscle of 25-month-old rats than 8-month-old rats at rest, and increased 50 and 38%, respectively, after one-hour treadmill running. Running speed and grade for young and old rats were adjusted so that both age groups ran at approximately 75% VO_2max. In the heart, ROS production was also increased with age, but the acute exercise bout significantly increased ROS generation only in the old rat.[14] These data clearly reveal that as animals grow older, a relatively small work task can provoke a greater ROS-generating effect in the heart and skeletal muscle, compared to when they were young.

The reason for the aged animals to increase ROS production is not entirely clear. Age-related defects in mitochondrial electron transport chain (ETC) are considered a major mechanism.[15] Mitochondria from aged animals demonstrate much lower cytochrome C oxidase (complex IV) activity than those from young ones, whereas enzyme activities in complexes I and II show lesser changes.[16] This alteration of ETC stoichiometry favors a greater electron "leakage" and formation of superoxide anion ($O_2^{\bullet-}$) found in the senescent organism. Peroxidative modification of membrane lipids has been proposed to be another major change in mitochondria at old age.[17] Higher malondialdehyde (MDA) levels were noticed in the mitochondria from aged heart and skeletal muscle.[18,19] Membrane fluidity is decreased with old age, associated with increased levels of MDA and 4-hydroxynonenol.[20,21] Biochemical and/or structural defects of membrane lipids may cause further ROS generation via enzymatic pathways involving cyclooxygenase, NADPH oxidase, and xanthine oxidase.[22] Pamplona et al.[23] recently reported that fatty acid unsaturation level was lower in heart mitochondria from long-lived pigeon (maximal life span ~35 years) than from rat (maximal life span 4 years), although the former has a similar body size and a higher metabolic rate. This difference in lipid profile was associated with a lower ROS production rate found in birds.

Since strenuous exercise greatly increases mitochondrial oxygen flux, it is often assumed that the majority of ROS production during exercise in aged animals is from the mitochondrial ETC. Unfortunately, the above assumption has never been proven experimentally. On the contrary, we have recently shown that although mitochondrial ROS production was higher in aged muscle and heart than in their young counterparts, no significant difference was observed between exercised and rested animals.[10,14] These findings suggest that another source may be important in contributing to ROS generation in aged animals.

INFLAMMATORY RESPONSE MAY BE AN IMPORTANT PATHWAY FOR ROS GENERATION

As animals grow older, there is a continuous loss of muscle size, mass, and force production, termed sarcopenia.[24] The consequences are duel, decreased performance and increased incidence of muscle injury.[2] It is well known that inflammatory cells in the injured tissues can generate ROS and reactive nitrogen species.[25,26]

Blood-borne polymorphoneutrophils (PMN) play a critical role in defending tissues from viral and bacterial invasion.[27] Activation of PMN typically starts with muscle or soft tissue damage by stretching or other mechanical force.[6,25] During acute phase response, PMN penetrate to the injured tissues and release two primary factors during phagocytosis, lysozymes and $O_2^{\bullet-}$. Lysozymes facilitate the breakdown of damaged protein and cell debris by releasing proteases. $O_2^{\bullet-}$ is produced by NADPH oxidase during a respiratory burst.[28,29] Cytoplasmic (CuZn) SOD dismutates $O_2^{\bullet-}$ to H_2O_2 that is further converted to •OH in the presence of transition metal ions, or to hypochlorous acid (HOCl) catalyzed by myeloperoxidase (FIG. 1). While this inflammatory response is considered critical in the healing from muscle injury, reactive oxidants released from neutrophils can also cause secondary damage.[6,30] Smith et al.[31] reported that one hour of moderate exercise increased neutrophil H_2O_2 generation by three-fold as well as receptor expression under *in vitro* challenge. Best

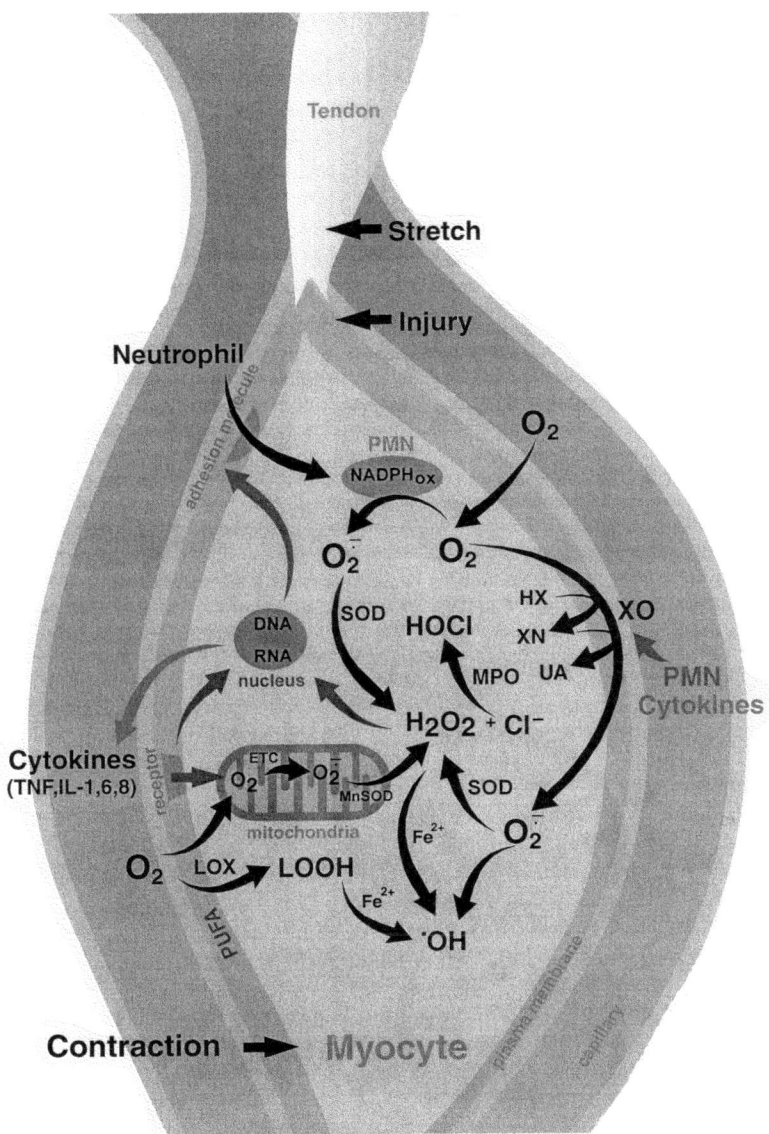

FIGURE 1. Sources of reactive oxygen species (ROS) in muscle cells during exercise and contraction-mediated injury. ETC, election transport chain; HOCl, hypochlorous acid; HX, hypoxanthine; IL, interleukine; LOX, lipooxygenase; MPO, melyeoperoxidase; PMN, polymorphoneutrophil; SOD, superoxide dismutase; TNF-α, tumor necrosis factor-α; UA, uric acid; XN, xanthine; XO, xanthine oxidase.

et al.[32] showed in an *in situ* rabbit muscle model that stretching injury caused by maximal isokinetic contraction was associated with significant ROS generation 24 h post treatment. In the injured leg there was an accumulation of PMN leukocytes, accompanied by higher GSH level and GPX and GR activities.

Strenuous exercise triggers releases of tumor necrosis factor-α (TNF-α), interleukin (IL)-1, and IL-6 from immune cells and/or damaged muscle tissue.[33] During the early phase of muscle injury, these cytokines play an important role in inflammatory responses by promoting adhesion molecule expression and nitric oxide (NO) synthase induction in the endothelial cells.[34] The resulting increase in vasodilation due to NO production facilitates PMN and circulating cytokines to migrate to the affected area. In addition, endothelial cells from injured muscle are known to secret TNF-α, IL-1, IL-6, and IL-8, although the time courses of these events are not quite clear.[35] In addition to stimulating PMN infiltration and hence ROS production, some cytokines can bind with membrane receptors and activate specific ROS-generating enzymes, such as lipooxygenase, NADPH oxidase, and xanthin oxidase.[36] Indeed, the mechanisms involving ROS generation in contraction-induced muscle injury are very complex (FIG. 1). Meydani et al.[30] showed that following an acute bout of eccentric exercise in sedentary men, circulating IL-1 levels were significantly elevated, and the urinary markers of lipid peroxidation post-exercise was attenuated by vitamin E administration. An acute bout of exhaustive exercise in human was reported to increase leukocyte, lymphocyte, and neutrophil numbers in the blood, as well as the ingestion capacity of the cells.[28] However, significant increase in $O_2^{\bullet-}$ production was noticed only at 24 h post-exercise. Bejma and Ji[10] found that ROS production from muscle mitochondrial NADPH oxidase was significantly increased after an acute bout of exercise in the young rats, but not old rats. Hellsten et al.[37] reported that plasma IL-1 concentration was significantly increased 90 min after an acute bout of strenuous one-leg eccentric exercise and remained elevated 4 days after exercise in human subjects. Muscle xanthine oxidase levels were eight-fold higher in the exercised leg, which was attributed to inflammatory response measured by leukocyte invasion.

There are currently sparse data concerning whether or not aging would increase ROS generation from inflammatory cells. However, we do know that aged individuals are more susceptible to muscle injury.[38] As compared to young animals, a much smaller workload can produce mechanical (especially eccentric) injury in the aged animals. Zerba et al.[39] showed that extensor digitalis longus (EDL) muscle from aged mice was more susceptible to lengthening contraction than that from young mice. Treatment of SOD alleviated muscle force deficit due to eccentric injury especially in the age animals. Thus, ROS generation and subsequent oxidative stress during muscle inflammation is considered a risk for aged people, especially those involving in strenuous physical exertion.

GENE EXPRESSION OF ANTIOXIDANT ENZYMES IN AGING MUSCLE

The overall cellular oxidative stress during aging is determined not only by ROS generation but also the defense capacity of antioxidant systems.[4,6,40] However, it is not an easy task to provide a general characterization of cellular antioxidant response

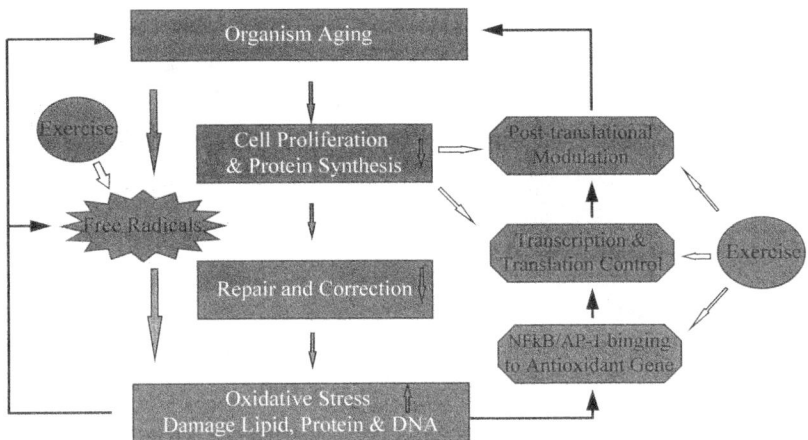

FIGURE 2. Effect of age on cellular oxidative stress and antioxidant adaptation, and the potential influence of exercise.

to aging, especially in the aging skeletal muscle. For inducible antioxidants such as antioxidant enzymes and glutathione systems, their levels are influenced by two biological forces, i.e., a general decline in cell proliferation and protein synthesis, and an age-related increase in ROS production that could potentially up-regulate antioxidant defense capacity (FIG. 2). For noninducible antioxidants such as vitamins and trace elements, diet plays a crucial role in the determination of their endogenous levels.[17] It has been well documented that skeletal muscles increase antioxidant enzyme activities as they age.[41–45] These changes occurred despite a general decline of muscle mitochondrial oxidative capacity.[46] However, aging response of antioxidant enzymes seems to be highly fiber-specific, depending on oxidative potential, recruitment pattern during exercise and intrinsic antioxidant levels of each individual muscle under investigation. Furthermore, antioxidant enzymes in different cell compartments may undergo differential changes during aging.[41] Oh-Ishi et al.[47] reported that 24-month-old rats had higher activities of CuZn SOD, Mn SOD, GPX, and CAT in soleus muscle compared with 4-month-old rats. CuZn SOD, but not MnSOD, protein content was elevated in the aged muscle. However, no significant change was noticed in the relative abundance of mRNA for both SOD isozymes. The study suggests that age-related increases in SOD activity were not caused by enhanced gene expression. To further investigate age responses of muscle antioxidant enzymes, we have recently measured gene expression products of SOD in various types (I, IIa, and IIb) of muscle fibers of old (25 month) vs. adult (8 month) rats.[48] A significant increase in MnSOD activity in gastrocnemius (mixed type II) and soleus (type I) muscles was found in old rats, whereas no significant age difference was found in MnSOD protein. Furthermore, MnSOD mRNA abundance was decreased with age in all types of muscles examined. Interestingly, binding of nuclear factor κB (NF-κB) to corresponding oligonucleotide sequences present in the MnSOD gene was decreased in gastrocnemius and soleus, whereas activator protein 1 (AP-1) binding was de-

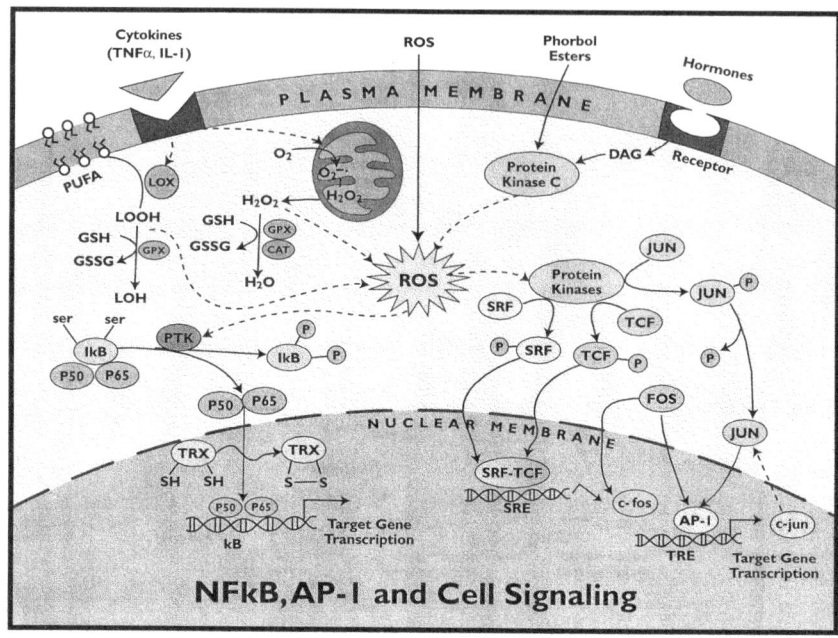

FIGURE 3. Role of NF-κB and AP-1 in the expression of MnSOD and other potential target genes. CAT, catalase; DAG, diaceylglycerol; GPX, glutathione peroxiase; IL-1, interleukin-1; LOOH, lipoperoxide; LOX, lipooxygenase; PLD, phospholipase D; PTK, protein tyrosine kinase; PUFA, polyunsaturated fatty acids; SRE, serum response element; SRF, serum response factor; SOD, superoxide dismutase; TNF-α, tumor necrosis factor-α; TRX, thioredoxin.

creased in superficial vastus lateralis (IIb) muscle.[48] In the signaling process of MnSOD gene expression, NF-κB and AP-1 play an important role (49,50). Both NF-κB and AP-1 binding sites are present in the promoter of the mammalian MnSOD gene, and oxidative stress has been shown to activate their binding[51,52] (FIG. 3). A decrease in the binding of these nuclear factors despite increased ROS generation observed in aged muscles suggest that molecular signaling of antioxidant gene expression is retarded due to aging. Thus, to the contrary of our earlier belief,[41] aging seems to decrease the ability of aged muscle to express at least MnSOD as demonstrated by lower nuclear protein binding, mRNA levels and unaltered enzyme protein. The observed increase in MnSOD activity appears to be due to a posttranslational modification (activation) of the enzyme molecules in aged muscle. In contrast to MnSOD, CuZnSOD showed increased protein content and activity with age in type II muscle in the absence of mRNA changes. Preliminary data also indicate that increased GPX activity found in aging muscle was not explained by a greater abundance of GPX mRNA.[53] Taken together, these data suggest that the widely reported increase in antioxidant enzyme activities in aging skeletal muscle are not due to enhanced gene transcription, but rather, translational and/or posttranslational mechanisms. Considering the fact that senescent skeletal muscles demonstrate augmented levels of lipid peroxidation, protein oxidation, and DNA damage, it is clear that the compensatory increases in antioxidant enzyme activity are insufficient to counterbalance increased ROS generation.

PROPER TRAINING REDUCES MUSCLE OXIDATIVE STRESS AT OLD AGE

Although aged muscles demonstrated higher levels of ROS generation when they were subjected to an acute bout of exercise at a given workload,[10] chronic exercise training with similar daily workload for 8–10 weeks resulted in lower levels of lipid peroxidation.[44] Similar training effect was found in the aged myocardium after endurance training.[19] Muscle mitochondria isolated from trained old rats showed improved respiratory control as compared to untrained old rats when challenged with external oxidants.[54] These findings demonstrate that the adaptability of muscle to training found in the young animals does not vanish at old age. However, due to the increased susceptibility of aged muscle to oxidative stress, there are some unique aspects that should be taken into consideration with regard to aged population participating in regular exercise training.

First, aging skeletal muscle is characterized with a progressive decline in oxidative enzyme levels and energy production.[55] Endurance training can effectively restore the age-associated deterioration of muscle protein content and mitochondrial oxidative capacity.[56] After training a given submaximal workload (i.e., oxygen consumption) would represent a lower relative workload (i.e., %VO_2max) as compared to before training, and therefore, impose a lower stress to the senescent muscle. The increased mitochondrial volume and protein allow oxygen consumption to be more distributed among ETC, ensuring better coupling of oxidative phosphorylation and less "spilling" of electrons.[11] Furthermore, the increased level of cytochrome C oxidase in the ETC with training decreases the likelihood of oxygen to become free radicals. Britton Chance[57] once pointed out that the best antioxidant is probably cytochrome C oxidase as it keeps $O_2^{\bullet-}$ in the bound state so that less is released into the cell media. Although not yet proven, endurance training is expected to reduce ROS generation in trained versus untrained skeletal muscle at old age at a given level of oxygen uptake.

Second, training enhances antioxidant defense capacity in aged skeletal muscle, although the results are not clear-cut. Ji et al.[58] and Hammeren et al.[59] showed that training increased muscle GPX activity along with increased mitochondrial oxidative enzymes in old rats. However, others failed to find significant adaptation of SOD, GPX, or catalase in aged muscles with training.[44,54] Based on the observation that aging decreases NF-κB and AP-1 binding, mRNA levels and energy production in muscle,[48,55] it seems that senescent muscles have more difficulty inducing antioxidant enzymes as compared to young muscles. We have recently observed that an acute bout of exercise could enhance NF-κB and AP-1 binding and activated Mn-SOD in the skeletal muscle of young rats.[60] Whether or not exercise can stimulate antioxidant enzyme gene expression at old age would be of tremendous interest in future research.

Third, rigorous training has also been found to decrease muscle GSH and vitamin E levels and to reduce mitochondrial respiratory function in skeletal muscle and heart in the young rats.[44,61,62] Starnes et al.[63] compared muscle α-tocopherol levels between trained and untrained 24-month-old rats and found a significant decrease in the trained muscle. Trained old rats also displayed a higher level of muscle thiobarbituric acid reactive substance (TBARS) when challenged by ascorbic acid and ferrous ion. These findings support a notion that heavy training may cause a deficit in muscle antioxidant reserve and protective margin.[63,64] Exercise training may potentially exacerbate this nutritional deficiency due to increased consumption or decreased dietary intake, or both. Dietary antioxidant supplementation has been shown to improve endogenous antioxidant defense, autoimmune function and increase longevity.[65]

CONCLUDING REMARKS

Exercise at old age is associated with certain risks of oxidative stress, both intrinsic and extrinsic. The intrinsic factors include an altered biochemical structure in the cell that favors ROS production during exercise, an increased fragility of muscles that frequents mechanical injury and subsequent inflammation, and a reduced cell proliferation and protein synthesis that limits antioxidant defense and repair capacity. Extrinsic factors may involve unjustified workload (over-training) and reduced dietary antioxidant intake. However, well-established benefits of regular exercise on physical and mental health undoubtedly outweigh the risks involved. Indeed, the balance of oxidants and antioxidants becomes more fragile in advance age, but as delicately outlined by B.P. Yu in this symposium,[66] moderate levels of oxidative stress are essential for the organisms to adapt and reach a new level of hormesis. As for physically active new generation of elderly population, the key is to carefully select a progressive exercise protocol and adequate antioxidant intake to minimize oxidative stress. Many critical questions remain regarding the relationship of aging and exercise as we enter a new millennium. For example, how does aging alter exercise-induced intracellular and intercellular mechanisms that generate ROS? Can acute and chronic exercise modulate the declined gene expression of metabolic and antioxidant enzymes seen at old age? Does exercise prevent age-dependent muscle loss (sarcopenia)? What kinds of antioxidant supplementation, if any, do aged people who are physically active need? Answers to these questions require highly specific research in both animals and humans.

REFERENCES

1. FRIES, J.F. 1996. Physical activity, the compression of morbidity, and the health of the elderly. J. R. Soc. Med. **89:** 64–68.
2. PAFFENBARGER, R.S., R.T. HYDE, A.L. WING, I.M. LEE, D.L. JUNG & J.B.G. KAMPERT. 1993. The association of changes in physical activity level and other lifestyle characteristics with mortality among men. N. Engl. J. Med. **328:** 538–545.
3. SANDVICK, L., J. ERIKSSEN, E. THAULOW, G. ERIKSSEN, R. MUNDAL & D. RODAHL. 1993. Physical fitness as a predictor of mortality among healthy, middle-aged Norwegian men. N. Engl. J. Med. **328:** 533–537.
4. SEN, C.K. 1995. Oxidants and antioxidants in exercise. J. Appl. Physiol. **79:** 675–686.
5. JI, L.L. 1995. Exercise and oxidative stress: role of the cellular antioxidant systems. *In* Exercise Sports Science Reviews. J.O. Holloszy, Ed.: 135–166. Williams & Wilkins. Baltimore.

6. MEYDANI, M. & W.J. EVANS. 1993. Free radicals, exercise, and aging. *In* Free Radical in Aging. B.P. Yu, Ed.: 183–204. CRC Press. Boca Raton, FL.
7. HARMAN, D. 1956. Aging: a theory based on free radical and radiation chemistry. J. Gerontol. **11:** 298–300.
8. HOLLUSZY, J.O. 1993. Exercise increases average longevity of female rats despite increased food intake and no growth retardation. J. Gerontol. **48:** B97–B100.
9. JACKSON, M.L., R.H.T. EDWARDS & M.C.R. SYMONS. 1985. Electron spin resonance studies of intact mammalian skeletal muscle. Biochim. Biophys. Acta **847:** 185–190.
10. BEJMA, J. & L.L. JI. 1999. Aging and acute exercise enhances free radical generation and oxidative damage in skeletal muscle. J. Appl. Physiol. **87:** 465–470.
11. DAVIES, K.J.A., A.T. QUANTANILLA, G.A. BROOKS & L. PACKER. 1982. Free radicals and tissue damage produced by exercise. Biochem. Biophys. Res. Commun. **107:** 1198–1205.
12. KUMAR, C.T., V.K. REDDY, M. PLASAD, K. THYAGARAJU & P. REDDANNA. 1992. Dietary supplementation of vitamin E protects heart tissue from exercise-induced oxidant stress. Mol. Cell. Biochem. **111:** 109–115.
13. O'NEILL, C.A., C.L. STEBBINS, S. BONIGUT, B. HALLIWELL & J.C. LONGHURST. 1996. Production of hydroxyl radicals in contracting skeletal muscle of cats. J. Appl. Physiol. **81:** 1197–1206.
14. BEJMA, J., P. RAMIRES & L.L. JI. 2000. Free radical generation and oxidative stress with aging and exercise: differential effects in the myocardium and liver. Acta Physiol. Scand. **169:** 343–351.
15. MIQUEL, J. & J. FLEMING. 1986. Theoretical and experimental support for an oxygen radical mitochondrial injury hypothesis of cell aging. *In* Biology of Aging. J. Johnson, R. Walford, D. Harman & J. Miquel, Eds.: 51–76. Alan R. Liss, Inc. New York.
16. NOHL, H., V. BREUNINGER & D. HEGNER. 1978. Influence of mitochondrial radical formation on energy-linked respiration. Eur. J. Biochem. **90:** 385–390.
17. YU, B.P. 1994. Cellular defenses against damage from reactive oxygen species. Physiol. Rev. **74:** 139–162.
18. JI, L.L., D. DILLON & E. WU. 1990. Alteration of antioxidant enzymes with aging in rat skeletal muscle and liver. Am. J. Physiol. **253:** R918–R923.
19. FIEBIG, R., M. GORE, R. CHANDWANEY, C. LEEUWENBURGH & L.L. JI. 1996. Alteration of myocardial antioxidant enzyme activity and glutathione content with aging and exercise training. Age **19:** 83–89.
20. CHEN, J.J. & B.P. YU. 1994. Alterations in mitochondrial membrane fluidity by lipid peroxidation products. Free Radical Biol. Med. **17:** 411–418.
21. KIM, J.D., R.J.. MCCARTER & B.P. YU. 1996. Influence of age, exercise, and dietary restriction on oxidative stress in rats. Aging Clin. Exp. Res. **8:** 123–129.
22. SAWADA, M., U. SESTER & J.C. CARLSON. 1992. Superoxide radical formation and associated biochemical alterations in the plasma membrane of brain, heart, and liver during the lifetime of the rat. J. Cell Biochem. **48:** 296–304.
23. PAMPLONA, R., M. PORTERO-OTIN, J.R. REQUENA A. HERRERO & G. BARJA. 1999. A low degree of fatty acid unsaturation leads to low lipid peroxidation lipoxidation-derived protein modification in heart mitochondria of the longeous pigeon than in the short-lived rat. Mech. Ageing Dev. **106:** 283–296.
24. ROGERS, M.A. & W.J. EVANS. 1993. Changes in skeletal muscle with aging: effects of exercise training. *In* Exercise and Sport Sciences Reviews. Vol. 21. J.O. Holloszy, Ed.: 65–102. Williams & Wilkins. Baltimore.
25. CANNON, J.G. & J.B. BLUMBERG. 1994. Acute phase immune responses in exercise. *In* Exercise and Oxygen Toxicity. C.K. Sen, L. Packer & O. Hanninen, Eds.: 447–479. Elsevier Science. New York.
26. PIZZA, F.X., I.J. HERNANDEZ & J.G. TIDBALL. 1998. Nitric oxide synthase inhibition reduces muscle inflammation and necrosis in modified muscle use. J. Leukocyte Biol. **64:** 427–433.
27. PETRONE, W.F., D.K. ENGLISH, K. WONG & J.M. MCCORD. 1980. Free radicals and inflammation: superoxide-dependent activation of a neutrophil chemotactic factor in plasma. Proc. Natl. Acad. Sci. USA **77:** 1159–1163.

28. HACK, V., G. STROBEL, J.P. RAU & H. WEICKER. 1992. The effect of maximal exercise on the activity of neutrophil granulocytes in highly trained athletes in a moderate training period. Eur. J. Appl. Physiol. Occup. Physiol. **65:** 520–524.
29. PYNE, D.B. 1994. Regulation of neutrophil function during exercise. Sports Med. **17:** 245–258.
30. MEYDANI, M., W. EVANS, G. HANDELMAN, R.A. FIELDING, S.N. MEYDANI, M.A. FIATARONE, J.B. BLUMBERG & J.G. CANNON. 1992. Antioxidant response to exercise-induced oxidative stress and protection by vitamin E. Ann. N.Y. Acad. Sci.**669:** 363–374.
31. SMITH, J.A., A.B. GRAY, D.B. PYNE, M.S. BAKER, R.D. TELFORD & M.J. WEIDEMANN. 1996. Moderate exercise triggers both priming and activation of neutrophil subpopulations. Am. J. Physiol. **39:** R838–R845.
32. BEST, T., R. FIEBIG, D.T. CORR, S. BRICKSON & L.L. JI. 1999. Free radical activity and the response of antioxidant enzymes and glutathione following acute muscle stretch injury in rabbits. J. Appl. Physiol. **87:** 74–82.
33. CANNON, J.G. & B.A. ST. PIERRE. 1998. Cytokines in exertion-induced skeletal muscle injury. Mol. Cell. Biochem. **179:** 159–167.
34. GATH, I., E.I. CLOSS, U. GODTEL-ARMBURST, S. SCHMITT, M. NAKANE, I. WESSLER & U. FORESTERMANN. 1996. Inducible NO synthase II and neuronal NO synthase I are constitutively expressed in different structures of guinea pig skeletal muscle: implications for contractile function. FASEB J. **10:** 1614–1620.
35. PEDERSEN, B.K., K. OSTROWSKI, T. ROHDE & H. RRUUNSGAARD. 1998. The cytokine response to strenuous exercise. Can. J. Physiol. Pharmacol. **76:** 505–511.
36. FLOHE, L., R. BRIGELIUS-FLOHE, C. SLIOU, M.G. TRABER & L. PACKER. 1997. Redox regulation of NF-kappa-B activation. Free Radical Biol. Med. **22:** 1115–1126.
37. HELLSTEN, Y., U. FRANDSEN, N. ORTHENBLAD, B. SJODIN & E. RICHTER. 1997. Xanthine oxidase in human skeletal muscle following eccentric exercise: a role in inflammation. J. Physiol. **498:** 239–248.
38. BROOKS, S. & J.A. FAULKNER. 1994. Skeletal muscle weakness in old age: underlying mechanisms. Med. Sci. Sports Exercise **26:** 432–439.
39. ZERBA, E., T.E. KOMOROWSKI & J.A. FAULKNER. 1990. Free radical injury to skeletal muscle of young, adult, and old mice. Am. J. Physiol. **258:** C429–C435.
40. JI, L.L. 1998. Antioxidant enzyme response to exercise and training in skeletal muscle. *In* Oxidative Stress in Skeletal Muscle. A.Z. Reznick, Ed.: 105–127. Birhauser Verlag. Basel.
41. JI, L.L., D. DILLON & E. WU. 1990. Alteration of antioxidant enzymes with aging in rat skeletal muscle and liver. Am. J. Physiol. **258:** R918–R923.
42. LAMMI-KEEFE, C.J., P.B. SWAN & P.V.J. HEGARTY. 1984. Copper-zinc and manganese superoxide dismutase activities in cardiac and skeletal muscles during aging in male rats. Gerontology **30:** 153–158.
43. LAWLER, J.M., S.K. POWERS, T. VISSER, H. VAN DIJK, M.J. KORTHUIS & L.L. JI. 1993. Acute exercise and skeletal muscle antioxidant and metabolic enzymes: effect of fiber type and age. Am. J. Physiol. **265:** R1344–R1350.
44. LEEUWENBURGH, C., R. FIEBIG, R. CHANDWANEY & L.L. JI. 1994. Aging and exercise training in skeletal muscle: response of glutathione and antioxidant enzyme systems. Am. J. Physiol. **267:** R439–R445.
45. LUHTALA, T., E.B. ROECHER, T. PUGH, R.J. FEUERS & R. WEINDRUCH. 1994. Dietary restriction attenuates age-related increases in rat skeletal muscle antioxidant enzyme activities. J. Gerontol. **49:** B321–B328.
46. JI, L. 1993. Antioxidant enzyme response to exercise and aging. Med. Sci. Sports Exercise **25:** 225–231.
47. OH-ISHI, S., T. KIZAKI, H. YAMASHITA, N. NAGATA, K. SUZUKI, N. TANIGUCHI & H. OHNO. 1996. Alteration of superoxide dismutase iso-enzyme activity, content, and mRNA expression with aging in rat skeletal muscle. Mech. Ageing Dev. **84:** 65–76.
48. HOLLANDER, J., J. BEJMA, T. OOKAWARA, H. OHNO & L.L. JI. 2000. Superoxide dismutase gene expression in skeletal muscle: fiber-specific effect of age. Mech. Ageing Dev. **116:** 35–45.

49. MEYER, M., R. SCHRECK & P.A. BAEUERLE. 1993. Hydrogen peroxide and antioxidants have opposite effects on activation of NF-κB and AP-1 in intact cells: AP-1 as secondary antioxidant-response factor. EMBO J. **12:** 2005–2015.
50. SCHRECK, R. & P.A. BAEUERLE. 1991. The role of oxygen radical as a second messenger. Trends Cell Biol. **1:** 39–42.
51. HO, Y.S., A.J. HOWARD & J.D. CRAPO. 1991. Molecular structure of a functional rat gene for manganese-containing superoxide dismutase. Am. J. Respir. Cell. Mol. Biol. **4:** 278–286.
52. WARNER, B.B., L. STUART, S. GEBB & J.R. WISPE. 1996. Redox regulation of manganese superoxide dismutase. Am. J. Physiol. **271:** L150–L158.
53. HOLLANDER, J., M. GORE, R. FIEBIG, J. BEJMA & L.L. JI. 1997. Exercise training alters superoxide dismutase gene expression in rats. FASEB J. **11:** A584.
54. CHANDWANEY, R., S. LEICHTWEIS, C. LEEUWENBURGH & L.L. JI. 1998. Oxidative stress and mitochondrial function in skeletal muscle: effects of aging and exercise training. Age **21:** 109–117.
55. HANSFORD, R.G. 1983. Bioenergetics in aging. Biochim. Biophys. Acta **726:** 41–80.
56. FITTS, R.H., J.P. TROUP & F.A. WITZMANN. 1984. The effect of aging and exercise on skeletal muscle function. Mech. Ageing Dev. **27:** 161–172.
57. NAQUI, A. & B. CHANCE. 1987. Reactive oxygen intermediates in biochemistry. Ann. Rev. Biochem. **55:** 137–166.
58. JI, L.L., E. WU & D.P. THOMAS. 1991. The effect of exercise training on metabolic and antioxidant functions in senescent rat skeletal muscle. Gerontology **37:** 317–325.
59. HAMMEREN, J., S. POWERS, J. LAWLER, D. CRISWELL, D. LOWENTHAL & M. POLLOCK. 1993. Exercise training-induced alterations in skeletal muscle oxidative and antioxidant enzyme activity in senescent rats. Int. J. Sports Med. **13:** 412–416.
60. HOLLANDER, J., R. FIEBIG, T. OOKAWARA, H. OHNO & L.L. JI. Superoxide dismutate gene expression is activated by a single bout of exercise. Pflug. Arch. In press.
61. LEICHTWEIS, S., C. LEEUWENBURGH, D. PARMELEE, R. FIEBIG & L.L. JI. 1997. Rigorous swim training deteriorates mitochondrial function in rat heart. Acta Physiol. Scand. **160:** 139–148.
62. AIKAWA, K.M., A.T. QUINTANILHA, B.O. DELUMEN, G.A. BROOKS & L. PACKER. 1984. Exercise endurance training alters vitamin E tissue levels and red blood cell hemolysis in rodents. Biosci. Rep. **4:** 253–257.
63. STARNES, J.W., G. CANTU, R.P. FARRAR & J.P. KEHRER. 1989. Skeletal muscle lipid peroxidation in exercise and food restricted rats during aging. J. Appl. Physiol. **67:** 69–75.
64. GOHIL, K., L. ROTHFUSS, J. LANG & L. PACKER. 1987. Effect of exercise training on tissue vitamin E and ubiquinone content. J. Appl. Physiol. **63:** 1638–1641.
65. MEYDANI, M. 1999. Dietary antioxidant modulation of aging and immune-endothelial cell interaction. Mech. Ageing Dev. **111:** 123–132.
66. YU, B.P. 2001. Stress resistance by caloric restriction for longevity. Ann. N.Y. Acad. Sci. This volume.

Do Antioxidant Strategies Work against Aging and Age-associated Disorders?

Propargylamines: A Possible Antioxidant Strategy

KENICHI KITANI,[a] CHIYOKO MINAMI,[a] TAKAKO YAMAMOTO,[a] WAKAKO MARUYAMA,[a] SETSUKO KANAI,[b] GWEN O. IVY,[c] AND MARIA-CRISTINA CARRILLO[d]

[a]*National Institute for Longevity Sciences, 36-3 Gengo, Moriokacho, Obu, Aichi 4748522, Japan*

[b]*Tokyo Metropolitan Institute of Gerontology, Tokyo, Japan*

[c]*Life Sciences Division, University of Toronto at Scarborough, Scarborough, Ontario, Canada, M1C 1A4*

[d]*National University of Rosario, Rosario, Argentina*

ABSTRACT: The free radical theory of aging was initially proposed by Harman[1] half a century ago primarily to explain biological aging processes. Although administration of so-called antioxidant chemicals, which have been tested in the past for several decades, turned out to be mostly ineffective in prolonging the life spans of animals,[2,3] the same theory of age-associated diseases appears to be increasingly supported in the last two decades. Despite these difficulties, the success in extending life span of 4 different animal species (mice, rats, hamsters, and dogs) with (–)deprenyl (including a study of our group) indicates that there might exist another type of antioxidant strategy in addition to a simple administration of antioxidant chemicals (for review, see Refs. 4,5). (–)Deprenyl has also been shown to increase superoxide dismutase (SOD) and catalase (CAT) activities selectively in brain dopaminergic tissues.[4,5] Interestingly, we have recently shown that another propargylamine, rasagiline not only increases antioxidant enzyme activities (CAT and SOD) in brain dopaminergic regions as (–)deprenyl does, but also increases CAT and SOD activities in extra-brain catecholaminergic systems such as the heart and kidneys as well.[6] These recent observations coupled with previous observations on the life span of animals with (–)deprenyl suggest that pharmacological modulation of endogenous antioxidant enzyme activities could be one potential antioxidant strategy against aging and age-associated disorders. If the causal relationship between the two effects of (–)deprenyl exists as we hypothesized,[4,5,7] we might be able to advance the elucidation of mechanism(s) of aging based on the free radical theory of aging.

KEYWORDS: Deprenyl; Propargylamines; Life span extension; Rats; Antioxidant enzyme upregulation

---

Address for correspondence: Kenichi Kitani, National Institute for Longevity Sciences, 36-3 Gengo, Moriokacho, Obu, Aichi 4748522, Japan. Voice: +81 562450183; fax: +81 562450184.
kitani@nils.go.jp

INTRODUCTION

The free radical theory of aging and age-associated disorders was proposed almost half a century ago and has been increasingly discussed in recent years.[1,2] Many experimental and epidemiological studies reported in the past have supported the notion that administration of antioxidant chemicals, pharmaceuticals and/or nutriceuticals can prevent the development of many age-associated disorders such as cancer,[8,9] cardiovascular disorders[10–12] (including arteriosclerosis and hypertension[10,11]), and possibly some neurodegenerative disorders such as Parkinson's disease and Alzheimer's disease.[13,14]

A recent report by Joseph and his co-workers[15] has provided further evidence that an intake of fruits and vegetables such as spinach and blueberries having potent antioxidant micro-nutrients can prevent and/or reverse age-associated declines in brain functions, including locomotive and even cognitive functions such as memory in aging rats.

In contrast, attempts to directly modify survival curves of aging rodents by means of administration of antioxidant chemicals or nutrients have not been convincingly successful. A good example is the recent study by Lipman and co-workers,[3] who have failed in prolonging the survival of C57/BL mice with the supplementation of five different antioxidants including vitamin E. The failure does not prove the invalidity of the free radical theory of aging; however, it certainly does not positively support it. A problem of this type of antioxidant strategy is that very little is known of the kinetics of these antioxidants and that we know nothing about the target organ (or tissues), or even whether such a system exists in a body for specifically regulating the life span of animals. In other words, the present state of the art of this type of antioxidant strategy against aging is a kind of "blind shooting" without knowing where the target is and further where the bullets are going. Thus, there remains to be a consensus of orthodox experimental gerontology that the only reliable means for prolonging the life span of animals is the dietary restriction (DR) paradigm.

The problem with DR is that DR changes so many different kinds of biochemical parameters in the body that there is no way to pick up the key factor(s) [mechanism(s)] which really has prolonged the life span of animals.

Another approach to prolong the life span of animals has been suggested by several groups including our group. Knoll is the first who has reported that chronic administration of a monoamine oxidase (MAO-B) inhibitor, (–)deprenyl significantly prolonged the life span of aging rats.[16] Subsequent studies[17,18] in rats including ours[18] have supported this notion, although the magnitude of its effect is quite variable depending on individual studies.[4,5,7]

Success in prolonging life span of other species such as mice,[19] hamsters,[20] and dogs[21] by (–)deprenyl has also been reported, while negative results are also found in the literature.[22–25] The mechanism(s) for prolonging life span of animals by (–)deprenyl remains unresolved. However, a severalfold increase in antioxidant enzyme activities such as superoxide dismutase (SOD) and catalase (CAT) in brain dopaminergic regions caused by the drug has been reported.[16,26–33] Our group has been extensively involved in this aspect of deprenyl's pharmacology.[26–33] Most of our study results have been reported and extensively discussed in relation to the life-prolonging effect of the drug.[4,5,7]

Deprenyl belongs to a series of propargylamines. Recently many other propargylamines[34–37] have been reported to share with deprenyl's neuroprotective and/or antiapoptotic properties. We have recently investigated the effect of rasagiline[6] on antioxidant enzyme activities and found that this property of elevating SOD and CAT activities is also shared by this propargylamine. Further, we have reported for the first time that rasagiline increases antioxidant enzyme activities not only in brain dopaminergic regions, as has been reported for (–)deprenyl (for review, see Refs. 4,5,7), but also in catecholaminergic tissues outside of the brain such as the heart and kidney.[6] We have also confirmed that this property is shared by (–)deprenyl and R-2HMP,[35,36] a prototype of series of aliphatic propargylamines (Minami et al., unpublished observations). In this paper, we summarize our past observations on this property of propargylamines and discuss the possible implication of this effect for another property of (–)deprenyl, a prolongation of life span of animals, and we propose another type of antioxidant strategy by means of modifying endogenous antioxidant enzyme activities.

MATERIALS AND METHODS

Some of the results presented here have been obtained in the Tokyo Metropolitan Institute of Gerontology (TMIG, Tokyo, Japan) using Fischer 344/Du (F-344/Du) rats originally purchased from Japan Charles River (Atsugi, Japan) and BDF1 and C57BL mice from SLC (Shizuoka, Japan).

More recent studies were performed in the National Institute for Longevity Sciences (NILS, Obu, Japan). Rats used in NILS were F-344/6JNia purchased from Harlan Sprague-Dawley (Indianapolis, IL, USA), which were raised under the contract with the National Institute on Aging (NIA, Bethesda, USA). Husbandry conditions of animals in the two institutes have been described elsewhere for TMIG[38] and NILS.[39]

Procedures for tissue preparations and enzyme activity measurements are described in detail elsewhere.[26–33] In brief, SOD activities were determined by the method described by Elster and Heupel.[40] In some recent studies, the original method of McCord and Friedowich was used.[41] Mn-SOD activities were defined as the fraction that can be inhibited by the addition of KCN at a concentration of 0.5 mM.[41] CAT activities were determined immediately after the preparation of tissue samples by the method described by Beers and Sizer.[42] Glutathione peroxidase (GSHPx) activities were determined by the method described by Paglia and Valentine.[43] Protein concentration was determined by the method of Lowry et al.[44]

RESULTS AND DISCUSSION

FIGURE 1 summarizes our initial study on SOD and CAT activities in three different groups of F-344/Du rats, which were given s.c. injections of deprenyl at a dose of 2.0 mg/kg/day for 3 consecutive weeks.[26,27] Depenyl treatment significantly increased the SOD and CAT activities in striatum of young male rats[26] but significantly decreased activities in young female rats[27] and did not modify activities in old female rats.[27]

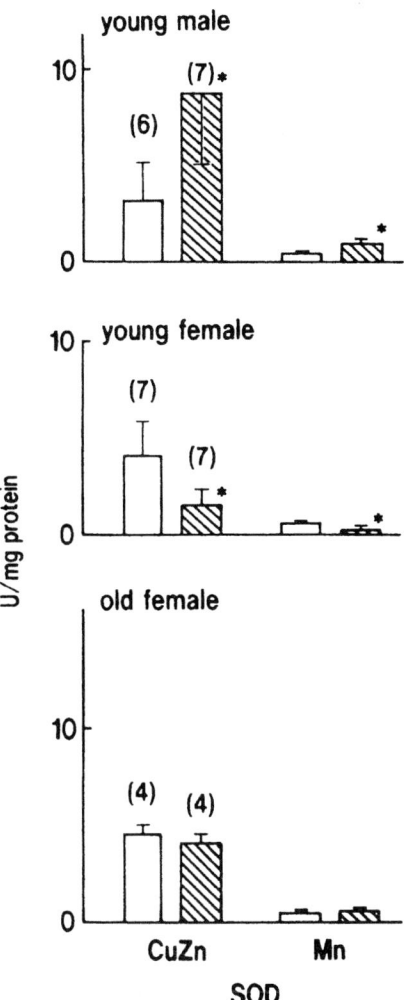

FIGURE 1. Enzyme activities of superoxide dismutase (SOD) in the striatum of control rats (*white columns*) and rats treated with s.c. injections of deprenyl for successive 21 days at a dose of 2.0 mg/kg/day (*shaded columns*). Redrawn from data previously reported by the authors for young male rats[26] and young and old female rats[27] with the permission of the publisher. Numbers in parentheses indicate the number of rats of each group. *Significantly different from corresponding control values ($p < 0.05$, t-test).

FIGURE 2 explains why we initially obtained three different and discrepant results with the same dose of the drug. This was totally due to the difference in an optimal dose among rats of different ages and sexes.[30] The mechanisms for the differences among different animal groups have been discussed in detail elsewhere.[4,5,7]

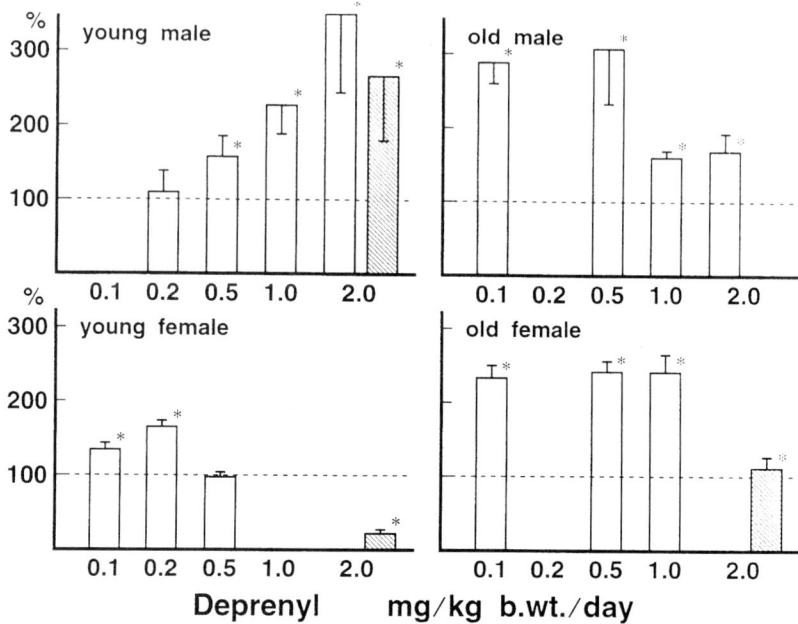

FIGURE 2. Relative enzyme activities of Mn-SOD in striata from young and old rats of both sexes treated with different doses of deprenyl. All values are expressed as percentages relative to respective control values. *White columns* indicate values in rats given 21 day s.c. continuous infusion, and *shaded columns* represent values in rats given 21 day s.c. consecutive injections. *Significantly different from respective control values ($p <0.05$). The number of rats studied in each group is 3–7 (mostly 4–5). (Reproduced from Carrillo et al.[30] with permission from *Life Sciences*.)

FIGURE 3 delineates the brain region selectivity of the drug in increasing antioxidant enzyme activities. As is clear in this figure, the drug affects activities in primarily dopaminergic tissues but not in hippocampus and cerebellum.[29] Since we also observed no effect of (–)deprenyl in antioxidant enzyme activities in the liver, we had believed that this effect of the drug is selective exclusively for dopaminergic brain regions.

FIGURE 4 shows that it was our misbelief, since rasagiline, a new analogue of (–)deprenyl, significantly increased activities not only in dopaminergic brain regions but also in catecholaminergic tissues outside of the brain such as the heart and kidneys.[6] Subsequent studies have confirmed that it is also true with (–)deprenyl and R-2HMP (Minami *et al.*, unpublished observations).

As has been discussed extensively elsewhere,[4,5,7] (–)deprenyl has at least two very unique effects to increase life span of animals as well as antioxidant enzyme activities such as SOD and CAT (but not GSHPx) selectively in regions of dopaminergic nature in the brain. A possible causal relationship between these two effects of (–)deprenyl has been discussed in detail.[4,5,7] The strongest basis for this contention by the authors is the parallelism of these two effects of the drug demonstrating an

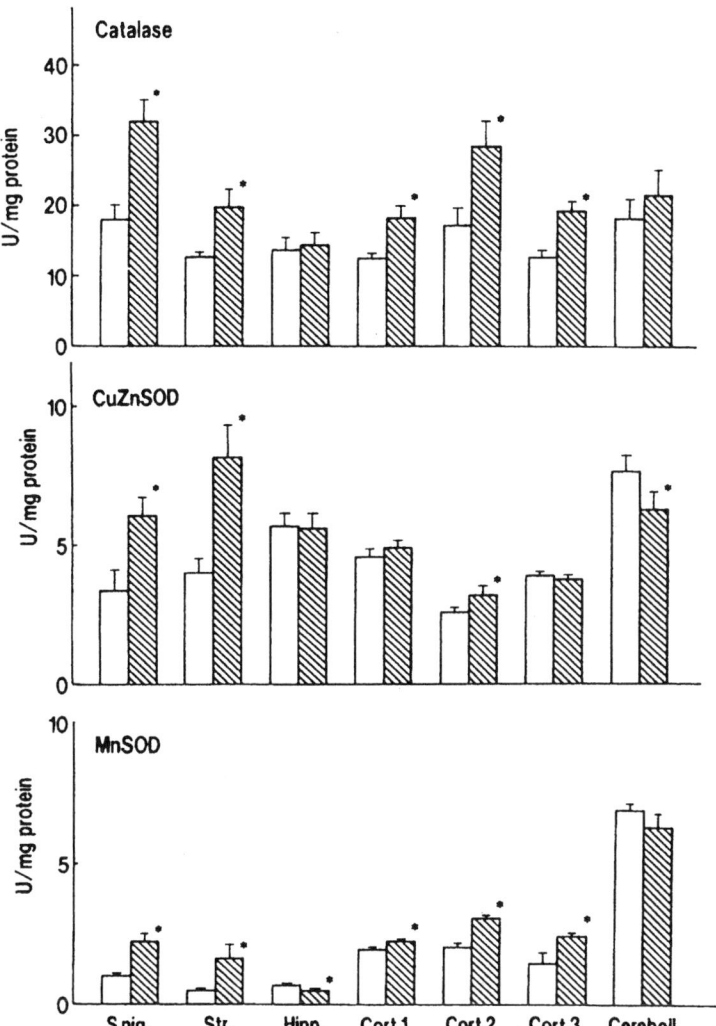

FIGURE 3. Catalase (*top panel*) and superoxide dismutase (*lower two panels*) enzyme activities in young control (*white columns*) and deprenyl-treated (*shaded columns*) male F-344 rats. The dose of deprenyl is 2.0 mg/kg/day, s.c. consecutive injections for 3 weeks. *Significantly different from respective control values ($p < 0.05$). S.nig., substantia nigra; Str., striatum; Hipp., hippocampus; Cort.1, frontal cortex; Cort.2, parietotemporal cortex; Cort.3, occipital cortex; Cerebell., cerebellum. (Reproduced from Carrillo et al.[26] with permission from *Life Sciences*.)

inverse U-shape effect. This has been clearly demonstrated for the effect on antioxidant enzyme activities (see FIG. 2 and also FIG. 6), but the evidence is not sufficient to be convincing enough for its life-prolonging effect. However, increasing evidence obtained in our life span studies on animals is strengthing this speculation.

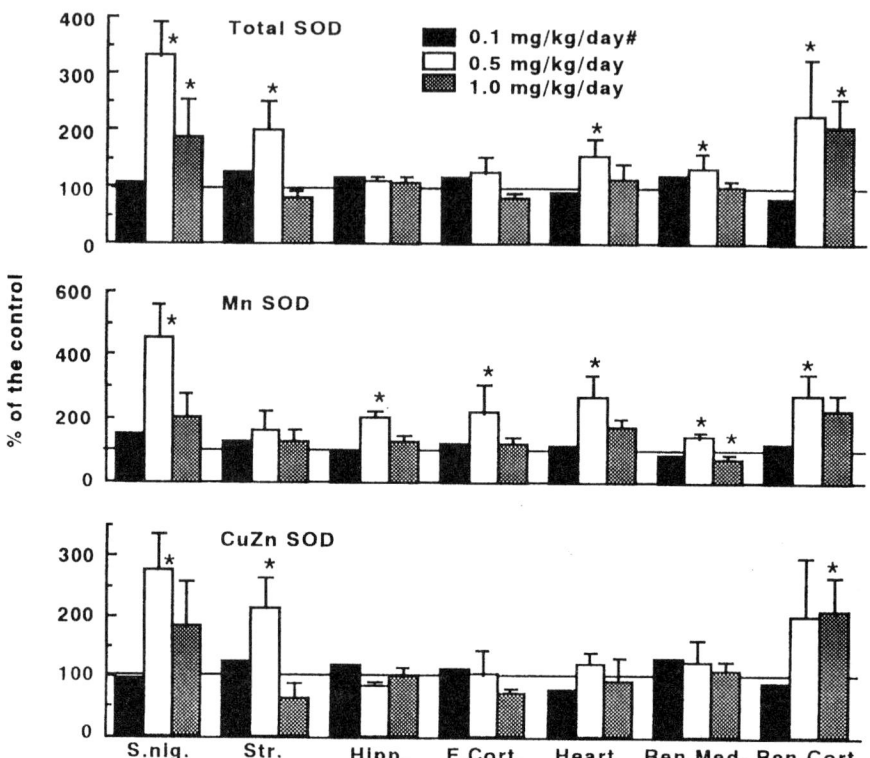

FIGURE 4. Effect of rasagiline pretreatment on superoxide dismutase activities in different tissues in male F-344 rats. All values are expressed as percentage relative to respective control values from rats given a saline solution infusion. *Significantly different from respective control values ($p < 0.05$). *Black bars* indicate values in a rat given a dose of 0.1 mg/kg/day for 3.5 weeks. *White bars* indicate values in rats given a dose of 0.5 mg/kg/day and *hatched bars* values in rats given a dose of 1.0 mg/kg/day for 3.5 weeks. S.nig., substantia nigra; Str., striatum; Hipp., hippocampus; F.Cort., frontal cortex; Ren.Med., kidney medulla; Ren.Cort., kidney cortex. (Reproduced from Carrillo *et al.*[6] with permission from *Life Sciences*.)

We have examined survivals of male F-344 rats by increasing the dose twofold from 0.5 mg/kg/injection (3 times a week) to 1.0 mg/kg/injection. To our surprise, animals who started to receive deprenyl injections at the age of 18 months started to die more quickly than saline-treated control rats, the survival at 31 months of age being only three out of twelve, while in control rats the surviving rats were seven out of twelve.[45] Although this difference in survival rate did not attain a statistical significance, such a reversed situation (i.e., a shorter life span in deprenyl-treated rats) was never observed in our previous study in which a dose of 0.5 mg/kg/injection was used.[18] Consequently, we sacrificed all surviving animals at 31 months of age after 13 months' continuous treatment. To our surprise, antioxidant enzyme activities were almost identical in any of brain regions examined for both control and

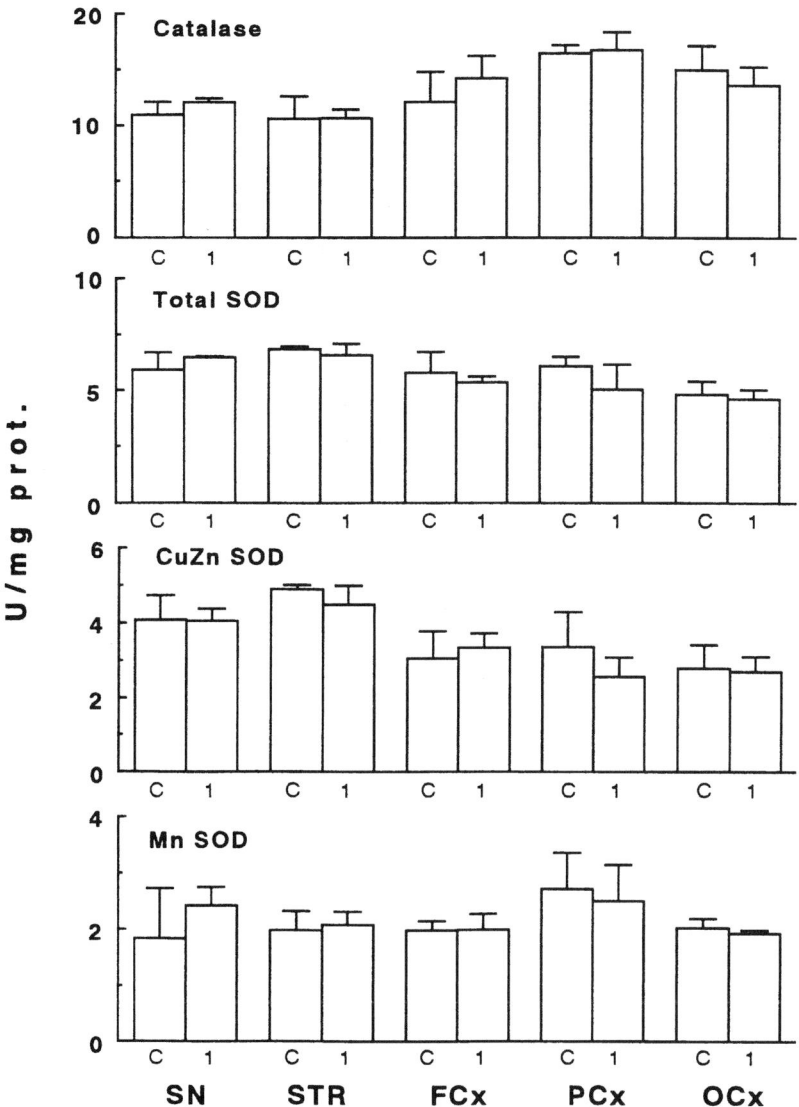

FIGURE 5. Catalase (CAT) and superoxide dismutase (SOD) activities in substantia nigra (SN), striatum (STR), frontal cortex (FCx), parietotemporal cortex (PCx), and occipital cortex (OCx) in 31-month-old male F-344 rats treated with saline (c) or deprenyl solution at a dose of 1.0 mg/kg/injection (1), three times a week for 13 months beginning at the age of 18 months. (Reproduced from Carrillo et al.[45] with permission from *Life Sciences*.)

deprenyl-treated animals (FIG. 5).[45] FIGURE 6 shows the results of our backup study in which old male rats were given s.c. injections of different doses of the drug 3 times a week only for 1 month. The dose of 1.0 mg/kg which was totally ineffective in a

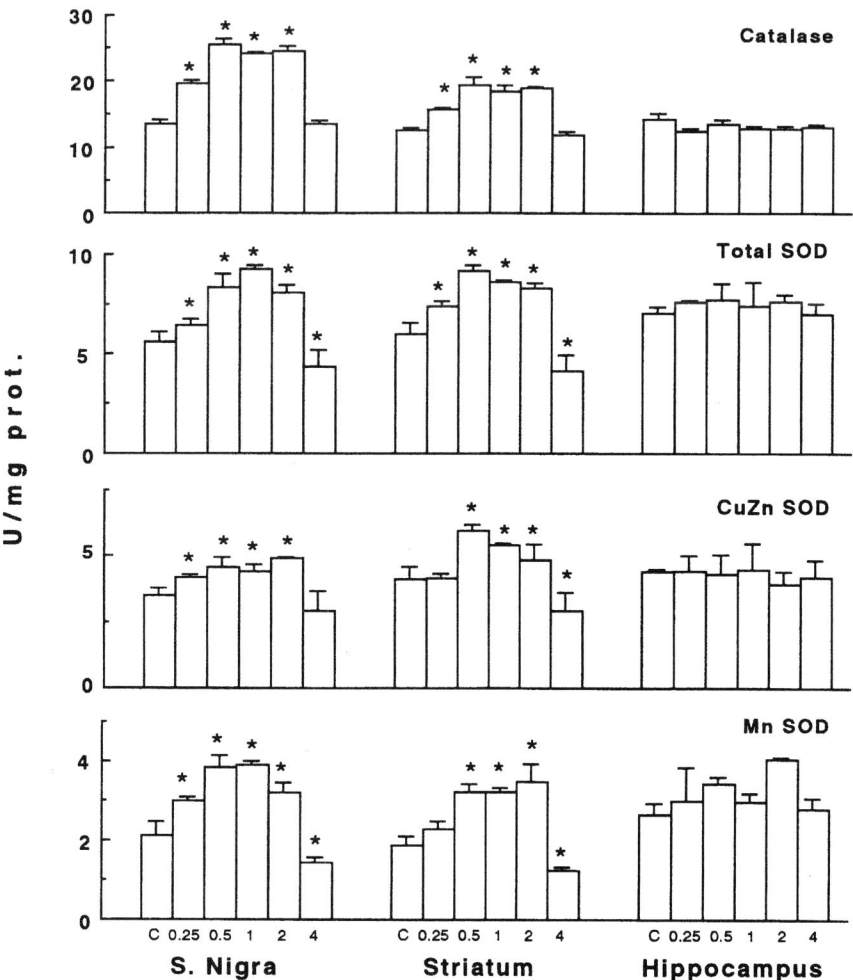

FIGURE 6. Catalase (CAT) and superoxide dismutase (SOD) activities in three different brain regions of 27-month-old male F-344 rats treated with various doses of deprenyl for one month before sacrifice. C: control rats given saline injections, 0.25-4 indicate doses of (−)deprenyl (mg/kg/injection, 3 times per week) for 1 month. *Significantly different from respective control values. ($p < 0.05$, Scheffe's F-test). (Reproduced from Carrillo et al.[45] with permission from *Life Sciences*.)

long-term study for 13 months was found to be in the middle of an optimal dose range in the 1-month study.[45]

We have suggested previously mainly based on mouse studies that a long-term treatment not only narrows the optimal dose range for increasing enzyme activities but lowers the magnitude of an increase in enzyme activities (for review, see Refs. 4,5,7). The results shown in FIGURES 5 and 6 suggest that this same pattern is evident for the effect of the drug on life span of rodents following the same rule for antioxidant enzyme activities.

The question of why the possible protection of dopaminergic tissues against oxygen-induced tissue damage due to aging can prolong the life span of animals has been extensively discussed elsewhere (for review, see Refs. 4,5,7). In brief, we have suggested that the protection of brain dopaminergic tissues by the drug may work to prolong the life span of animals possibly by means of modulating the release of humoral factors such as TNF and nerve growth factors and various cytokines including interleukins.[4,5,7]

The prolongation of survivals in female Beagle dogs achieved by (–)deprenyl administration appears to be at least partially due to the drastic decrease in the incidence of breast cancer in treated animals.[21] A similar effect may be operative in aging F-344 rats, since in this particular strain of rats, subcutaneous tumors (though benign in nature) which grow to a huge size often weighing more than 200 gr. can be an indirect cause for the death of old animals, and the development of this type of tumor appears to be prevented or at least retarded in its onset[18] by deprenyl. The antitumor effect of (–)deprenyl can be increasingly found in recent publications.[46–48]

It is also possible that some immunomodulating effect of (–)deprenyl which was clearly demonstrated by remarkably prolonging the life span of an immunodeficient mouse strain[49] is also involved in prolonging the life span of animals.

Our recent observations that a series of propargylamines including (–)deprenyl, rasagiline, and R-2HMP all increase SOD and CAT activities in organs outside of the brain such as the heart and kidneys may raise additional possibilities that the protection of these organs against age-induced tissue damage may be another factor for increasing the life span of animals. In aging rodents, nephropathy similar to human nephrotic syndorome is a common and serious lesion possibly indirectly determining life span of these species. A study by Milgram and co-workers[17] has shown that the only difference in biochemical parameters between control and long-lived deprenyl-treated rats was a significantly lower blood urea nitrogen value in the deprenyl-treated rat group. It remains to be elucidated whether (–)deprenyl and other propargylamines protect kidneys against age-induced nephropathies in rodents by means of elevating antioxidant enzyme activities in this organ. Such a nephropathy as is observed in aging rodents is not seen in aging humans. However, cardiovascular lesions including arteriosclerosis and hypertension are the primary killers of aging humans. It is well established that antioxidant strategies well designed in kinetics can efficiently prevent these cardiovascular lesions.[10–12]

It may be worthwhile to examine whether this type of indirect antioxidant strategy by means of modifying antioxidant enzymes in the cardiovascular system by propargylamines has a beneficial effect in preventing cardiovascular lesions in experimental animals as well as humans.

ACKNOWLEDGMENTS

The authors deeply acknowledge the following co-workers for their kind collaborations and useful suggestions for the works presented in this article: Drs. K. Oohashi, M. Naoi, and M.B.H. Youdim. Thanks are also due to Mrs. T. Ohara for her expert secretarial work. Part of the studies discussed in this article was supported by the grant in aid "Comprehensive Research on Aging and Health (1108)" from the Ministry of Health and Welfare.

REFERENCES

1. HARMAN, D. 1956. Aging: a theory based on free radical and radiation chemistry. J. Gerontol. **12:** 257–263.
2. HARMAN, D. 1994. Free-radical theory of aging. Increasing the functional life span. *In* Pharmacology of Aging Processes: Method of Assessment and Potential Interventions. I. Zs.-Nagy, D. Harman & K. Kitani, Eds. Ann. N.Y. Acad. Sci. **717:** 1–15.
3. LIPMAN, R.D., R.T. BRONSON, D. WU *et al.* 1998. Disease incidence and longevity are unaltered by dietary antioxidant supplementation initiated during middle age in C57BL/6 mice. Mech. Ageing Dev. **103:** 269–284.
4. KITANI, K., K. MIYASAKA, S. KANAI *et al.* 1996. Upregulation of antioxidant enzyme activities by deprenyl: implications for life span extension. Ann. N.Y. Acad. Sci. **786:** 391–409.
5. KITANI, K., S. KANAI, G.O. IVY *et al.* 1998. Assessing the effects of deprenyl on longevity and antioxidant defences in different animal models. Ann. N.Y. Acad. Sci. **854:** 291–306.
6. CARRILLO, M.C., C. MINAMI, K. KITANI *et al.* 2000. Enhancing effect of rasagiline on superoxide dismutase and catalase activities in the dopaminergic system in the rat. Life Sci. **67:** 577–585.
7. KITANI, K., S. KANAI, G.O. IVY *et al.* 1999. Pharmacological modifications of endogenous antioxidant enzymes with special reference to the effect of deprenyl: a possible antioxidant strategy. Mech. Ageing Dev. **111:** 211–221.
8. KIM, J.M., S. ARAKI, D.J. KIM *et al.* 1998. Chemopreventive effect of carotenoids and curcumins on mouse colon carcinogenesis after 1,2-dimethylhydrazine initiation. Carcinogenesis **18:** 81–85.
9. The Alpha-Tocopherol, Beta Carotene Cancer Prevention Group. 1994. The effect of vitamin E and beta carotene on the incidence of lung cancer and other cancers in male smokers. N. Engl. J. Med. **330:** 1029–1035.
10. KONDO, K., A. MATSUMOTO, H. KURATA *et al.* 1994. Inhibition of wine oxidation of low-density lipoprotein with red wine. Lancet **344:** 1152.
11. INOUE, M., N. WATANABE, K. MATSUO *et al.* 1990. Inhibition of oxygen toxicity by targeting superoxide dismutase to endothelial cell surface. FEBS Lett. **269:** 89–92.
12. YOKOZAWA, T., Z.W. LIU, & E. DONG. 1998. A study of ginsenoide-Rd in a renal ischemia-reperfusion model. Nephron **78:** 201–206.
13. The Parkinson Study Group. 1989. Effect of deprenyl on the progression of disability in early Parkinson's disease. N. Engl. J. Med. **321:** 1364–1371.
14. SANO, M., C. ERNERSTO, R.G. THOMAS *et al.* 1997. A controlled study trial of selegiline, alpha-tocopherol, or both as treatment of Alzheimer's disease. N. Engl. J. Med. **336:** 1216–1212.
15. JOSEPH, J.A., B. SHUHITT-HALE, N. DENISOVA *et al.* 1998. Long-term dietary, spinach or vitamin E, supplementation retards the onset of age-related neuronal signal-transduction and cognitive behavioral deficiting. J. Neurosci. **18:** 8047–8055.
16. KNOLL, J. 1988. The striatal dopamine dependency of life span in male rats: longevity study with (−)deprenyl. Mech. Ageing Dev. **46:** 237–262.
17. MILGRAM, N.W., R.J. RACINE, P. NELLIS *et al.* 1990. Maintenance of L-deprenyl prolongs life in aged male rats. Life Sci. **47:** 415–420.
18. KITANI, K., S. KANAI, Y. SATO *et al.* 1993. Chronic treatment of (−)deprenyl prolongs the life span of male Fischer 344 rats: further evidence. Life Sci. **52:** 281–288.
19. ARCHER, J.R. & D.E. HARRISON. 1996. L-Deprenyl treatment in aged mice slightly increases life spans, and greatly reduces fecundity by aged males. J. Gerontol. **31A:** B448–B453.

20. STOLL, S., U. HAFNER, B. KRAENZLIN et al. 1997. Chronic treatment of Syrian hamsters with low-dose selegiline increases life span in females but not males. Neurobiol. Aging **18:** 205–211.
21. RUEHL, W.W., T.L. ENTRIKEN, B.A. MUGGENBURG et al. 1997. Treatment with L-deprenyl prolongs life in elderly dogs. Life Sci. **61:** 1037–1044.
22. BICKFORD, P.C., C.E. ADAMS, S.J. BOYSON et al. 1997. Long-term treatment of male F344 rats with deprenyl: assessment of effects on longevity, behavior, and brain function. Neurobiol. Aging **18:** 309–318.
23. GALLAGHER, I.M., A. CLOW & V. GLOVER. 1998. Long term administration of (−)deprenyl increases mortality in male Wistar rats. J. Neural Transm. (Suppl.) **52:** 315–320.
24. INGRAM, D.K., H.L. WIENER, M.E. CHACHICH et al. 1993. Chronic treatment of aged mice with L-deprenyl produces marked MAO-B inhibition but no beneficial effects on survival, motor performance, or nigral lipofuscin accumulation. Neurobiol. Aging **14:** 431–440.
25. PIANTANELLI, L., A. ZAIA, G. ROSSOLINI et al. 1994. Influence of L-deprenyl treatment on mouse survival kinetics. In Pharmacology of Aging Processes: Method of Assessment and Potential Interventions. I. Zs.-Nagy, D. Harman & K. Kitani, Eds. Ann. N.Y. Acad. Sci. **717:** 72–78.
26. CARRILLO, M.C., S. KANAI & M. NOKUBO et al. 1991. Deprenyl induces activities of both superoxide dismutase and catalase but not of glutathione peroxidase in the striatum of young male rats. Life Sci. **48:** 517–521.
27. CARRILLO, M.C., S. KANAI, M. NOKUBO et al. 1992. Deprenyl increases activities of superoxide dismutase and catalase in striatum but not in hippocampus: the sex and age-related differences in the optimal dose in the rat. Exp. Neurol. **116:** 286–294.
28. CARRILLO, M.C., S. KANAI, Y. SATO et al. 1992. Sequential changes in activities of superoxide dismutase and catalase in brain regions and liver during (−)deprenyl infusion in male rats. Biochem. Pharmacol. **44:** 2185–2189.
29. CARRILLO, M.C., K. KITANI, S. KANAI et al. 1992. The ability of (−)deprenyl to increase superoxide dismutase activities in the rat is tissue and brain region selective. Life Sci. **50:** 1985–1992.
30. CARRILLO, M.C., S. KANAI, Y. SATO et al. 1993. The optimal dosage of (−)deprenyl for increasing superoxide dismutase activities in several brain regions decreases with age in male Fischer 344 rats. Life Sci. **52:** 1925–1934.
31. CARRILLO, M.C., K. KITANI, S. KANAI et al. 1994. The effect of a long term (6 months) treatment with (−)deprenyl on antioxidant enzyme activities in selective brain regions in old female F-344 rats. Biochem. Pharmacol. **47:** 1333–1338.
32. CARRILLO, M.C., K. KITANI, S. KANAI et al. 1994. (−)Deprenyl increases activities of superoxide dismutase (SOD) in striatum of dog brain. Life Sci. **54:** 1483–1489.
33. CARRILLO, M.C., K. KITANI S. KANAI et al. 1996. Long term treatment with (−)deprenyl reduces the optimal dose as well as the effective dose range for increasing antioxidant enzyme activities in old mouse brain. Life Sci. **59:** 1047–1057.
34. MARUYAMA, W. & M. NAOI. 1999. Neuroprotection by (−)deprenyl and related compounds. Mech. Ageing Dev. **111:** 189–200.
35. BOULTON, A.A., B.A. DAVIS, D.A. DURDEN et al. 1997. Aliphatic propargylamines: new antiapoptotic drugs. Drug Dev. Res. **42:** 150–156.
36. BOULTON, A.A. 1999. Symptomatic and neuroprotective properties of the aliphatic propargylamines. Mech. Ageing Dev. **111:** 187–195.
37. FINBERG, J.P.M., T. TAKASHIMA, J.M. JOHNSTON et al. 1998. Increased survival of dopaminergic neurons by rasagiline, a monoamine oxidase B inhibitor. Neuroreport **9:** 703–707.
38. NOKUBO, M. 1985. Physical-chemical and biochemical differences in liver plasma membranes in aging F-344 rats. J. Gerontol. **40:** 409–414.
39. KITANI, K., S. TANAKA, I. ZS.-NAGY. 1998. Age-dependence of the lateral diffusion coefficient of lipids and proteins in the hepatocyte plasma membrane of BN/Bi RijHsd rats as revealed by the smear FRAP technique. Arch. Gerontol. Geriatr. **26:** 257–273.
40. ELSTNER, E.F. & A. HEUPEL. 1976. Inhibition of nitrite formation from hydroxylammoniumchloride: a simple assay for superoxide dismutase. Anal. Biochem. **70:** 616–620.

41. MCCORD, E.F. & I. FRIEDOVICH. 1969. Superoxide dismutase: an enzymic function for erythrocuprein (hemocuprein). J. Biol. Chem. **244:** 6049–6055.
42. BEERS, R.F., JR. & I.W. SIZER. 1952. A spectrophotometric method for measuring the breakdown of hydrogen peroxide by catalase. J. Biol. Chem. **195:** 133–140.
43. PAGLIA, D.E. & W.N. VALENTINE. 1967. Studies on the quantitative and qualitative characterization of erythrocyte glutathione peroxidase. J. Lab. Clin. Med. **70:** 158–169.
44. LOWRY, O.H., M.J. ROSENBROUGH, A.L. FARR et al. 1951. Protein measurement with the folin phenol reagent. J. Biol. Chem. **193:** 265–275.
45. CARRILLO, M.C., S. KANAI, K. KITANI et al. 2000. A high dose of long term treatment with deprenyl loses its effect on antioxidant enzyme activities as well as on survivals of Fischer-344 rats. Life Sci. **67:** 2539–2548.
46. THYAGARAJAN, S., J. MEITES & S.K. AUADRI. 1995. Deprenyl reinitiates estrous cycles, reduces serum prolactin, and decreases the incidence of mammary and pituitary tumors in old acyclic rats. Endocrinology **136:** 1103–1110.
47. THYAGARAJAN, S., S.Y. FELTEN & D.L. FELTEN. 1998. Antitumor effect of L-deprenyl in rats with carcinogen-induced mammary tumors. Cancer Lett. **123:** 177–183.
48. THYAGARAJAN, S. & S.K. QUADRI. 1999. L-Deprenyl inhibits tumor growth, reduces serum prolactin, and suppresses brain monoamine metabolism in rats with carcinogen-induced mammary tumors. Endocrine **10:** 225–232.
49. FREISLEBEN, H.J., A. NEEB & F. LEHR. 1997. Influence of selegiline and lipoic acid in the life expectancy of immunosuppressed mice. Arzneim.-Forsch. **47:** 776–780.

Antioxidant and Immunostimulating Activities of the Fruiting Bodies of *Paecilomyces japonica*, a New Type of *Cordyceps* sp.

KUK HYUN SHIN, SOON SUNG LIM, SANG HYUN LEE, YEON SIL LEE, AND SAE YUN CHO[a]

Natural Products Research Institute, Seoul National University, Seoul, Korea

[a]*National Sericulture and Entomology Research Institute, Rural Development Administration, Korea*

ABSTRACT: *Cordyceps* is negative for its many biological activities and a tonic for restoring vital functions in traditional Chinese medicine. In an effort to evaluate the pharmacological effects, including the antiaging effect of the fruiting bodies of the cultivated *Paecilomyces japonica* fungus, a new type of *Cordyceps* sp. was investigated. This investigation was focused on ultimately revealing its biologically active principles, its effects on free-radical scavenging enzymes, lipid peroxidation, as well as its immunological functions. As a result, both water and methanol extracts were found to cause not only significant increases in rat liver cytosolic SOD, catalase, and GSEH-px activities, but also a significant decrease in MDA production in TBA reactant assay in rats. The extracts also showed immunostimulating activity as measured by carbon clearance, weight-loaded forced swimming performances, and immobilizing stress in mice. Using bioassay-guided systematic fractionation of the extracts, two pure compounds were isolated as active principles from low molecular-weight fraction, a protein-bound polysaccharide was isolated that showed a marked increase in the liver enzyme activities, as well as a significant inhibition of lipid peroxidation.

KEYWORDS: *Paecilomyces japonica*; *Cordyceps* sp.; Antioxident; Immunostimulant; Antiaging; Ergosterol; D-Mannitol; Protein-bound polysaccharide

INTRODUCTION

There is extensive evidence to implicate free radicals in the development of degenerative diseases,[1] and it is suggested that free radical damage to cells leads to the pathological changes associated with aging,[2] which can attack membrane phospholipids and ultimately cause damage to DNA and proteins. Free radicals may also be a contributory factor in a progressive decline in the function of the immune system.[3] Moreover, oxidative stress has been implicated in the development of major causes of disability such as cognitive impairment, Alzheimer's disease, impaired immune

---

Address for correspondence: Dr. Kuk Hyun Shin, Natural Products Research Institute, Seoul National University, 28, Yungun-Dong, Jongro-Ku, Seoul 110-460, Korea. Voice: 82-02-740-8919; fax: 82-02-762-8322.
khshin@plaza.snu.ac.kr

function, cataracts, and muscular degeneration in elderly people. Cooperative defense systems that protect the body from free radical damage include the antioxidant nutrients and enzymes, which are considered the first line of defense against lipid peroxidation, protecting cell membranes at an early stage of free radical attack through their free radical–scavenging activity, including enzymes, SOD, catalase, and GSH-px. Improved antioxidant status may have an immunostimulatory effect.[4-6] Identification of new antioxidants remains a highly active research area because antioxidants may reduce the risk of various chronic diseases caused by free radicals. To evaluate antiaging materials, evaluation of the scavenging activities of active oxygenes such as superoxide anions and lipid peroxides as well as inhibition of microsomal lipid peroxidation in plant resources have been studied extensively.[7]

Cordyceps sp. is recognized for its broad biological activities and as a tonic for replenishing vital function in Chinese traditional medicines, and it is expected to be developed as a preventive medicine and therapeutic agent for incurable and geriatric diseases. As an attempt to evaluate its pharmacological effects, including the antiaging effect of the fruiting bodies of cultivated fungus of *Paecilomyces japonica*, a new type of *Cordyceps* sp. that is grown on silkworm larvae, and ultimately to reveal biologically active principles, we carried out a systematic fractionation of extracts of this fungus and isolation of compounds. Their effects on free radical–scavenging enzymes, lipid peroxidation, and immune functions were investigated.

MATERIALS AND METHODS

Materials and Extraction of Samples

Dry, powdered fruiting bodies (300 g) of *P. japonica* grown on silkworm larvae were extracted 5 times with methanol and 10 times with water for primary studies on pharmacological activities. The methanol extract was concentrated to dryness under reduced pressure. In the case of water extraction, the powder was defatted 2 times with ether for 5 days by cooling and then extracted. The water extract was concentrated to dryness by lyophilization. The yield of methanol and water extract were 17.5 and 12.4%, respectively. Male Sprague-Dawley rats weighing 200–250 g and ICR mice weighing 20–30 g bred in the laboratory of the animal care facility of Natural Products Research Institute were used.

Bioassay

The antioxidant activity of the fungus was estimated by thiobarbituric acid reactant assay and by measuring free radical–scavenging enzymes and reduction of DPPH according to the method of Buege and Aust,[8] Rigo *et al.*,[9] and Blois,[10] respectively. α-Tocopherol and ascorbic acid were used as positive reference drugs. Liver injury was induced by CCl_4 in rats.

After fasting for 24 h, rats were injected sc with a mixture of CCl_4 in olive oil (1:1) at a dose of 6 mL/kg. The immunostimulating activity was evaluated by the carbon clearance test established by Wagner *et al.*[11] *in vivo* and by measuring the activity of acid phosphatase in macrophages *in vitro* by the procedure of Bergeyer *et al.*[12] The immunostimulating activity was expressed as the rate of regression coefficient of the animals treated (RCtr) to those of the control (RCc). Zymosan, dissolved in PBS solution, was used as a positive reference drug; it was injected ip at 50 µg/g body weight.

Fractionation and Isolation of Compounds

To search for active components from the fruiting bodies of *P. japonica*, bioassay-guided systematic fractionation of both methanol and water extracts and isolation and purification of compounds were performed. Methanol extract (53.0 g) suspended in water was extracted with n-hexane. Column chromatography of the *n*-hexane extract (5.62 g, 10.6%) over silica gel (*n*-hexane:EtOAc, 95:5) gave two fractions, rich in the fatty acid and the crystalline fractions. An aliquot of the fatty acid fraction was derivatized with trimethylsilane and analyzed by GC-MS. The specific major fatty acid components were identified as α-linolenic acid (18:3, 25.1% in fatty acids), which has recently been reported to be of biological interest. After recrystallization of the crystalline fraction from *n*-hexane and elucidation of the chemical structure by mass and NMR spectra, the crystalline compound was attributed to ergosterol (40 mg, 0.075%). The aqueous fractions removed from *n*-hexane were extracted subsequantly with dichloromethane (0.27 g, 0.51%), EtOAc (0.54 g, 1.02%), and *n*-butanol (3.78 g, 7.13%), and the residual fraction (42.5 g, 80.2%) was then concentrated *in vacuo*. The *n*-butanol extract was subjected to chromatography on a silica gel column (30 × 8 cm), and two needle crystalline compounds were isolated. Their major compound (7% in the methanol extract) was attributed to D-mannitol, known as cordycepic acid, and another, minor compound, identified as 1,6-dimethyl-D-mannitol.

The water extract (200 g) was systematically fractionated for isolation of polysaccharides, which were defatted with three volumes of ethanol-ether (1:1) extraction at room temperature to obtain the fatty acid fraction (PJ-FA, 48.0 g, 24%); then fatty acid–free residue was extracted with water at 100°C for 1 hour. After filtration, the filtrate was kept in cold storage, and the precipitate (PJ-PIS, 5.6 g, 2.8%) formed was separated by centrifugation. The combined supernatant was dialyzed against running water with visking cellulose tube for 2 days; the external low-molecular-weight portion (PJ-L, 15.5 g, 7.8%) and the solution in the internal tube were concentrated under reduced pressure, and three volumes of ethanol were added. The precipitate thus obtained was collected by centrifugation. The protein-bound polysaccharide (PJ-P, high molecular weight, 12.2 g, 6.1%) thus obtained was collected by separation from the yielded precipitate. Analysis of its content of hexose, hexosamine, and protein was revealed to be 75%, 17%, and 5%, respectively. The glucan moiety (PJ-1) was separated from PJ-P by ultrasonication heating at 60°C. The highest recovery of galactosamine was obtained when PJ-1–free solution was treated at pH 9.0, adjusted with 10% ammonium hydroxide. The galactosamine was confirmed to be composed of mannose, glucose, and galactose in a molar ratio of 1.00:2.88:1.83, respectively.

RESULTS AND DISCUSSION

To evaluate the antiaging effect of the fruiting bodies of cultivated fungus of *P. japonica*, the effects of their crude extracts, of various fractions, and of isolated com-

TABLE 1. Effect of fungus extracts on lipid peroxide of rat liver *in vitro*

	Concentration (μg/mL)	Lipid peroxide[a] (nmol MDA/g wet wt)	Inhibition (%)	IC_{50} (μg/mL)
Control	—	10.74	—	
Blank	—	3.43	100	
PJ-Methanol	125	6.23	61.7	85.6
	25	7.92	38.7	
	2.5	8.70	28.0	
PJ-Water	125	7.41	45.6	>125
	25	8.27	33.8	
	2.5	8.98	24.1	
	0.25	9.63	15.2	
Ascorbate	125	5.42	72.9	19.8
	25	6.23	1.7	
	2.5	10.13	8.4	
	0.25	10.62	1.6	
Glutathione	125	8.62	29.1	>125
	25	9.63	15.2	
	2.5	10.10	9.4	
	0.25	10.54	2.8	
α-Tocopherol	125	8.6	29.1	>125
	2.5	9.24	20.6	
	0.25	9.38	18.6	

NOTE: The reaction mixture of liver homogenate (1:9 volume), 8.1% sodium dodecyl sulfate (0.2 mL), TCA-thiobarbituric acid in 20% acetate buffer (2 mL, pH 3.5) was heated for 10 min in a boiling water bath. After cooling, *n*-butanol:pyridine (15:1) solution was added, centrifuged for 15 min to obtain an *n*-butanol:pyridine layer, and the absorbance was determined.

[a]The level of lipid peroxides is expressed in terms of nmol MDA/g wet wt, which was calculated from the absorbance at 532 nm using an absorption coefficient of $1.56 \times 10^5 \text{ M}^{-1}\text{cm}^{-1}\text{ L}^{-1}$.

pounds on lipid peroxidation as well as on immune functions were investigated. TABLE 1 shows the results of the effects of the fungus extracts on the production of TBA reactive substance in the rat liver homogenate *in vitro*. Although MDA production was markedly increased in the control group compared to that of the untreated group, both methanol and water extracts were shown to cause a significant decrease in MDA production in a concentration-dependent manner. The methanol extract was stronger than the water extract, as compared by their IC_{50} values, and even stronger than glutathione and α-tocopherol, typical antioxidants. Similar results were obtained in lipid peroxidation induced by Fe^{2+} and $Fe^{2+} + H_2O_2$, as shown in TABLE 2: lipid peroxide levels were progressively suppressed by the addition of increasing amounts of the fungus extracts, the inhibitory activity being a little lower than that of ascorbic acid, indicating that the fungus has a moderate antioxidant activity *in vitro*. Free radical scavenging effects of the fungus extracts on DPPH were tested; the results are indicated in TABLE 3: DPPH was reduced with the addition of both methanol and water extracts in a concentration-dependent manner. When compared by

TABLE 2. Effect of fungus extracts on lipid peroxide of rat liver induced by Fe^{2+} and $H_2O_2 + Fe^{2+}$ *in vitro*

	Conc. (μg/mL)	Fe^{2+}			$H_2O_2+Fe^{2+}$		
		Lipid peroxide [a] (nmol MDA/g wet wt.)	Inhibition (%)	IC_{50} (μg/mL)	Lipid peroxide [a] (nmol MDA/g wet wt)	Inhibition (%)	IC_{50} (μg/mL)
Control	—	12.50	—		15.90	—	
Blank	—	2.36	100		3.43	100	
Ascorbate	250	2.47	99.6	17.7	4.34	81.8	17.9
	50	2.97	94.5		4.67	79.4	
	5	11.4	6.7		13.9	15.1	
	0.5	12.0	0.1		14.6	9.8	
PJ-Methanol	250	6.53	61.2	120.5	6.40	64.3	85.5
	50	9.46	37.5		10.2	40.8	
	5	10.4	29.9		10.6	38.2	
	0.5	13.	7.8		11.3	32.8	
PJ-water	250	7.51	53.3	170.4	6.20	68.7	40.2
	50	9.10	40.4		8.72	51.1	
	5	10.0	33.1		10.5	38.6	
	0.5	10.5	29.4		11.0	34.9	

NOTE: The incubation mixture contained rat liver homogenate (0.5 mL, equivalent to 15 mg protein), 3.3 mM ferrous sulfate, or 30 mM H_2O_2 + 3.3 mM ferrous sulfate (0.3 mL) and 50 mM phosphate buffer (0.8 mL, pH 7.4) in a total volume of 1.0 mL. Incubation was carried out at 37 °C for 20 min. IC_{50} values were calculated from log-dose inhibition curves obtained with four different concentrations. The level of lipid peroxides is expressed in terms of nmol MDA/g wet wt, which was calculated from the absorbance at 532 nm, using an absorption coefficient of 1.56×10^5 $M^{-1} cm^{-1} L^{-1}$.

TABLE 3. Free radical scavenging effect of fungus extracts on DPPH

	Concentration (μg/mL)	Inhibition (%)	IC_{50} (μg/mL)
PJ-Methanol	250	67.4	130
	50	22.5	
	25	14.5	
	2.5	8.1	
PJ-Water	250	93.1	29
	50	74.1	
	25	43.7	
	2.5	9.0	
α-Tocopherol	250	91.2	27.5
	50	89.5	(64 μM)
	25	42.6	
	2.5	23.7	

NOTE: Reaction mixture (final volume, 5 mL) contained 1 mL of 1.5 mM DPPH-methanol solution, 2 mL of methanol with or without samples or α-tocopherol and 2 mL of 0.1 M sodium acetate buffer (pH 5.5). Incubation was carried out at 37°C for 30 min. Reduction of the DPPH free radical was measured at 520 nm.

TABLE 4. Effects of isolated compounds on carbon clearance in mice

Treatment	Dose (mg/kg/day, ip)	Regression coefficient (RCtr/RCc)	Index
Ergosterol	50	2.11	2
D-Mannitol	50	0.94	0
Zymosan	50	1.89	2

NOTE: Mice were administered ip with test substances for five consecutive days, and a carbon clearance test was performed 24 h after the last treatment of samples. The test methods are the same as described in the legend to FIGURE 1. Index: RCtr/RCc: $>1.5 = 2$ (very active); $<1.5 = 1$ (active); $<1.0 = 0$ (not active).

TABLE 5. Effects of isolated compounds on functions of macrophage

Treatment	Concentration(μg/mL)	Acid phosphatase (OD_{405})
Ergosterol	20	$1.108 \pm 0.067^{**}$
	4	0.965 ± 0.037
D-Mannitol	20	0.956 ± 0.021
	4	1.015 ± 0.089
LPS	—	$1.392 \pm 0.116^{***}$
Control	—	0.829 ± 0.046

NOTE: Murine macrophages (1×10^6 cells) was incubated for 24 h in the presence or absence of the samples in 0.5% DMSO at 37°C. The macrophage monolayer removed from the media was dissolved in 20 mL of Triton × 100 added with 100 mL of 15.2 mM p-nitrophenyl phosphate, 100 mL of 90 mM citrate buffer (pH 4.8) and incubated at 37°C for 1 h. The acid phosphatase activity was estimated by measuring the absorbance at 405 nm using Microwell-plate reader (Molecular Devices, USA). $**p < 0.01$; $***p < 0.001$.
Significantly different from control : $**P <0.01$; $***p <0.001$.

IC_{50}, the inhibitory potency of the water extract ($IC_{50} = 29$ μg/mL) was approximately 4.5-fold stronger than that of the methanol extract, which was equipotent to α-tocopherol ($IC_{50} = 27.5$ μg/mL). The antioxidant effects of the fungus, therefore, may be related to free radical scavenging activity and may be partly due to complex formation between Fe^{2+} ion.

The fungus extracts were also demonstrated to exhibit a significant immunostimulating activity, as measured by carbon clearance test in mice; the results are shown in FIGURES 1 and 2. Both methanol and water extracts, with three daily consecutive ip administrations at doses of 10 and 50 mg/kg, respectively, were shown to exhibit significant enhancement of phagocytosis. The potency of phagocytosis of methanol extract at 50 mg/kg, as indicated by regression coefficient (RCtr/RCc = 1.72, index = 2), was revealed to be almost the same as that of zymosan (RCtr/RCc = 1.60, index = 2), a typical phagocytosis enhancer; whereas the water extract exhibited almost twofold stronger enhancing activity at a dose of 50 mg/kg than zymosan at the same dose level.

To isolate and characterize active principles from the fungus, the water and methanol extracts were fractionated separately, and their effects on lipid peroxidation and

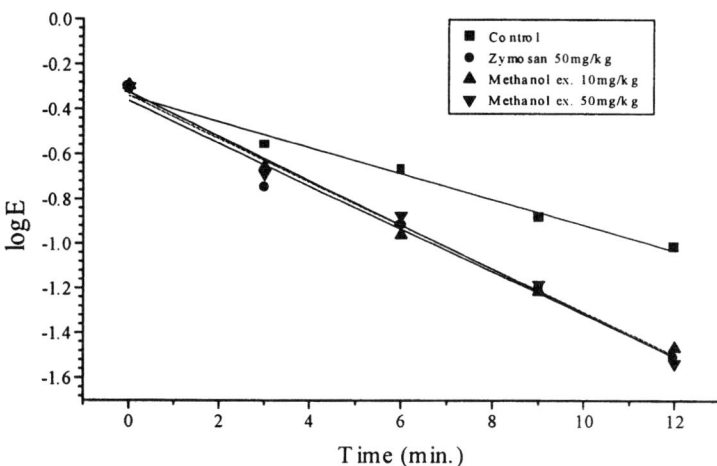

FIGURE 1. Effect of methanol extracts of the fungus on carbon clearance in mice. ICR mice weighing 20–30 g were administered ip test compounds dissolved in phosphate-buffered saline solution for three consecutive days; 24 h after the last treatment of the samples, each mouse was injected iv with carbon suspension (Rotring, diluted eight times with PBS containing 1% gelatin and warmed at 37 °C) at a dose of 10 mL/bw At 3, 6, 9, and 12 min after the injection, blood was withdrawn from the orbital vein into 0.1% sodium carbonate (2 mL), and carbon concentration in blood was estimated by determining optical density at 660 nm. From optical density, the linear regression coefficient (RC) was calculated, plotting –log E against time. The immunostimulating activity was expressed as the rate of regression coefficient of the animals treated (RCtr) to those of the control (RCc). Zymosan, known as a typical immunostimulator, was used as a positive reference compound; it was injected ip at 50 mg/kg, dissolved in PBS solution. Regression coefficient ratio (RCtr/RCc): zymosan, 1.68, very active; methanol extract, 10 mg/kg, very active; 50 mg/kg, 1.72, very active.

various free radical scavenging enzymes in the liver of CCl_4-treated rats were estimated. As shown in FIGURE 3, various fractions obtained from the methanol extract, when administered ip with a dry weight equivalent dosage of 200 mg/kg/day of total extract for seven consecutive days, were shown to cause significant inhibition of MDA production. Nonpolar fractions were stronger than polar fractions. All of the fractions from the water extract tested were shown to exhibit significant inhibition of MDA production. Associated with the inhibition of MDA production, a measure of lipid peroxides, free radical scavenging enzyme activity such as SOD, catalase, and GSH-px were significantly elevated. As shown in FIGURE 4, all fractions except the residual water fraction caused significant elevation of SOD activity. The protein-bound polysaccharides from the water extract caused only a significant elevation of the enzyme activity. Similar results were obtained in the case of catalase and GSH-px activities, as shown in FIGURES 5 and 6. FIGURE 7 shows the results of the treatment of isolated compounds on lipid peroxidation in the liver of CCl_4-treated rats. With seven daily treatments, both ergosterol and D-mannitol were observed to cause significant inhibition of MDA production; they were almost equipotent to that of α-tocopherol at the same dose level. As indicated in FIGURE 8, only ergosterol efficiently caused a significant elevation of the liver cytosolic enzyme activities.

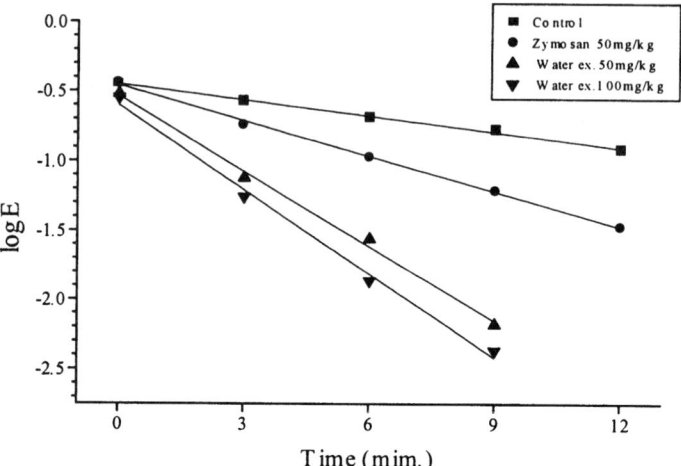

FIGURE 2. Effect of water extracts of the fungus on carbon clearance in mice. The test method is the same as that described in the legend to FIGURE 1. Regression coefficence ratio (RCtr/RCc): zymosan, 1.68, very active; water extract: 50 mg/kg, 3.23, very highly active; 100 mg/kg; 3.60, very highly active.

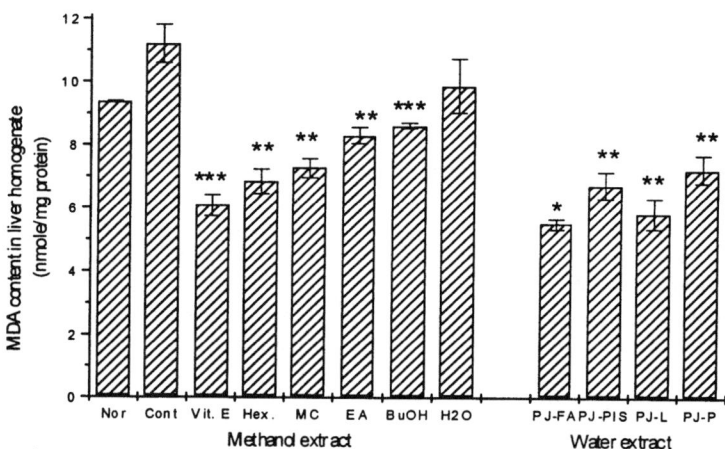

FIGURE 3. Effect of the fungus fractions on the lipid peroxidation in CCl_4-treated rats. Liver injury was induced as described in MATERIALS AND METHODS. Rats were administered ip test samples suspended in 0.5% CMC for seven consecutive days. TBA reactant assay method was the same as described in the note to TABLE 1. Significantly different from the control: * $p < 0.05$; ** $p < 0.01$.

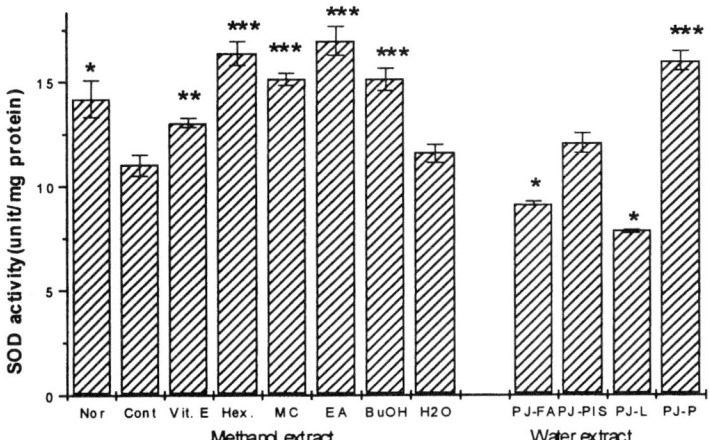

FIGURE 4. Effect of the fungus fractions on the liver cytosolic SOD activity in CCl_4-treated rats. Liver injury and treatments of test sample was performed as described in the legend to FIGURE 3. Each liver was homogenized in cold 1.15% KCl-10 mM phosphate buffer with EDTA (pH, 7.4) and centrifuged at 10,000 g for 10 min. The supernatant was further centrifuged at 40,000 g for 60 min to obtain cytosolic fractions. A mixture of 0.5 mM xanthine as a substrate (300 μL), 1% sodium deoxycholate (100 μL), 0.05 mM KCN (100 μL), xanthine oxidase (20 μL), cytosolic fraction (20 μL), 0.1mM cytochrome C (300 μL) were placed in a 1-cm cuvette, and the rate of increase in absorbance at 550 nm was recorded for 5 min. The SOD activity was expressed as unit/mg protein. Significantly different from the control : *$p < 0.05$; **$p < 0.01$; ***$p < 0.001$.

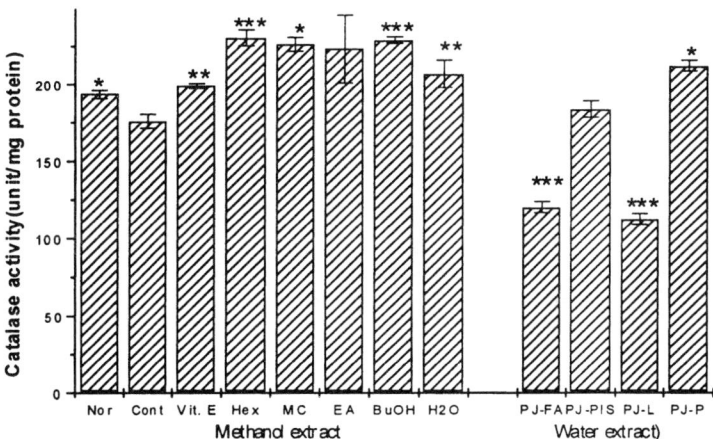

FIGURE 5. Effect of the fungus fractions of the liver cytosolic catalase activity in CCl_4-treated rats. Liver injury and treatments of test sample were performed as described in the legend to FIGURE 3. The cytosolic fraction of liver (40 μL) diluted 10 times was added with 0.13 mM phosphate buffer, pH 7.0 (500 μL), distilled water (660 μL), 15 mM H_2O_2 (1800 μL) and thoroughly mixed; the rate of changes in the absorbance at 240 nm for 5 min was recorded. The catalase activity was expressed as unit/mg protein. Significantly different from the control: * $p < 0.05$; ** $p < 0.01$; *** $p < 0.001$.

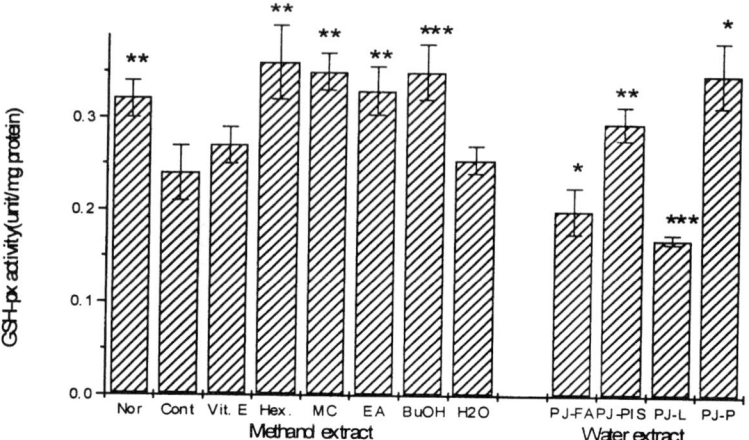

FIGURE 6. Effect of the fungus fractions on the liver cytosolic GSH-px activity in CCl_4-treated rats Liver injury and treatments of test samples were performed as described in the legend to FIGURE 3. A mixture of 0.3 mM phosphate buffer with 4.0 mM EDTA, pH 7.2 (1000 μL), 26.56 mM sodium azide (500 μL), 294.37 mM GSH (60 μL), 8.4 mM NADPH (110 μL), GSSG reductase (5 μL), cytosolic soln. (30 μL), 1 mM cumene hydroperoxide (320 μL) was placed in a 1-cm cuvette, and the rate of changes in absorbance was recorded at 340 nm at 30-s intervals for 5 min. GSH-px activity was expressed as μmol/min/g protein. Significantly different from the control: $*p < 0.05$; $** p < 0.01$.

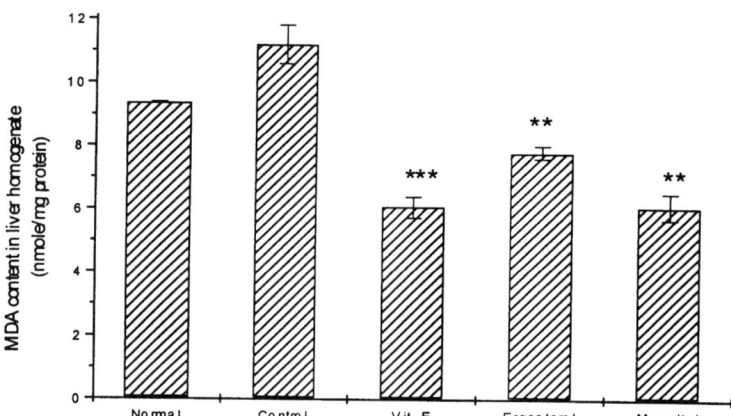

FIGURE 7. Effect of the isolated compounds on the lipid peroxidation in CCl_4-treated rats. The test methods are the same as described in the legend to FIGURE 3. Significantly different from the control: $*p < 0.05$; $** p < 0.01$.

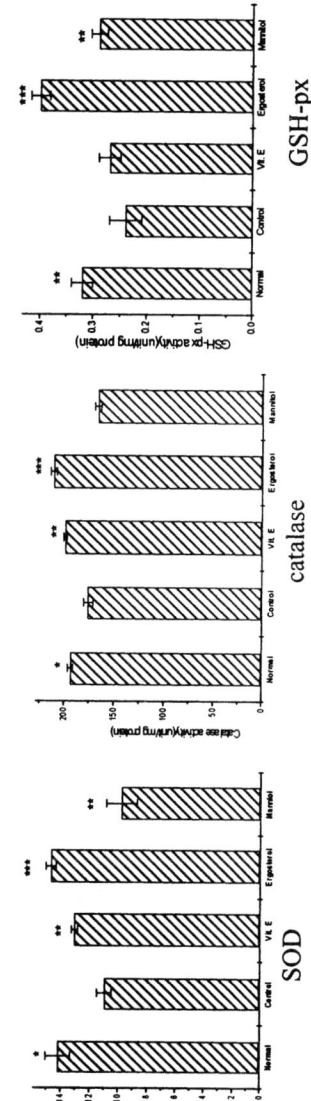

FIGURE 8. Effects of the isolated compounds on the liver cytosolic free radical scavenging enzymes in CCl_4-treated rats. The test methods are the same as described in the legend to FIGURES 4, 5, and 6. Rats were administered ip test compounds suspended in 0.5% CMC for 7 days. Significantly different from the control: $*p < 0.05$; $**p < 0.01$; $***p < 0.001$.

The effect of the compounds isolated from the fungus were tested for their effects on phagocytosis; the results are indicated in TABLE 4. Ergosterol, when administered ip at a dose of 50 mg/kg for five consecutive days, exhibited a marked enhancement of carbon clearance, its regression coefficient being 2.11; this was stronger than zymosan (RCtr/RCc = 1.89) at the same dose level. Ergosterol also showed a significant increase in acid phosphatase activity in macrophages *in vitro*, in accord with the *in vivo* results as shown in TABLE 5.

Cordyceps, particularly *Cordyceps sinensis*, is a fungus highly valued in China as a tonic and herbal medicine. Preclinical *in vitro* and *in vivo* studies show the main activities of this fungus to be in such areas as oxygen-free radical scavenging, antisenscence, hypolipidemic, antisclerotic, and sexual function–restorative activities.[13]

Because naturally occurring *Cordyceps* (the wild form of *C. sinensis*) is extremely rare, studies on the development of new fermentable strains of *C. sinensis* has been intensively pursued and have succeeded in the isolation of Cs-4, a new strain of *Cordyceps*. The purpose of the present study was to develop a new type, *Cordyceps* sp., that possesses similar biological activities from other sources of the fungal mycelia. From the fungus obtained from *P. japonica* grown on silkworm larvae we could also isolate cordycepic acid and ergosterol as main active compounds that have already been characterized as active components of *C. sinensis*.[13] It is well recognized that oxidative stress is involved in damage to biomembranes in the process known as lipid peroxidation. Vitamin E is known as a physiological antioxidant.[4,5]

Many important antioxidants, such as ascorbic acid, α-tocopherol, carotenoids, and flavonoids, that are present in many terrestrial plant sources are already well identified.[7] The present study demonstrated that the cultivated fungus from *P. japonica*, grown on silkworm larvae, new type of *Cordyceps*, possesses not only antioxidant but also immunostimulating activities. Aging is suggested to be associated with a progressive decline in the function of the immune system. Free radical generation associated with aging may be a contributory factor in the depressed immune response documented in aged animals; improved antioxidant status may have an immunostimulatory effect. The results of the present study suggest, therefore, that free radical–mediated damage can be controlled with adequate antioxidant defenses and that optimal intake of *Cordyceps* may contribute to the quality of life.

REFERENCES

1. CROSS, C.E. 1987. Oxygen radicals and human diseases. Ann. Intern. Med. **107:** 526–545.
2. BECKMAN, K.B. & B.N. AMES. 1998. The free radical theory of aging matures. Physiol. Rev. **78:** 547–581.
3. PIKE, J. & R K. CHANDRA. 1995. Effect of vitamin and trace element supplementation on immune indices in healthy elderly. Int. J. Vitam. Nutr. Res. **65:** 117–120.
4. HALLIWELL, B. 1996. Antioxidants in human health and disease. Ann. Rev. Nutr. **16:** 33–50.
5. HORWITT, M.K. 1986. Interpretations of requirements for thiamin, riboflavin, niacintryptophan and vitamin E plus comments on balance studies and vitamin B_6. Am. J. Clin. Nutr. **44:** 973–985.
6. PACKER, L. *et al.* 1995. Alpha-lipoic acid as a biological antioxidant. Free Radical Biol. Med. **19:** 227–250.

7. JOHNSON, M.K. *et al.* 1999. Potent antioxidant activity of a thiocarbamate-related compound from marine hydroid. Biochem. Pharmacol. **58:** 1313–1319 and references cited therein.
8. BUEGE, J.A. & S.D. AUST. 1978. Microsomal lipid peroxidation. Methods Enzymol. **52:** 302–306.
9. RIGO, A. & G. ROTILIO. 1977. Simultaneous determination of superoxide dismutase and catalase in biological materials by polarography. Anal. Biochem. **81:** 157–166.
10. BLOIS, M.S. 1958. Antioxidant determinations by the use of a stable free radical. Nature **26:** 1199–1200.
11. WAGNER, H. *et al.* 1985. Immunostimulierend wirkende Polysaccharide (Heteroglykane) aus hoheren Pflanzen. Arzneim-Forsch. **35:** 1069–1075.
12. BERGMEYER, H.U. *et al.* 1974. Methods of Enzymatic Analysis. Vol. **11:** 495–496. Academic Press. New York.
13. ZHU, J.S. *et al.* 1998. The scientfic rediscovery of an ancient Chinese herbal medicine: *Cordyceps sinensis*. J. Altern. Complement. Med. **4:** 289–303.

A New Function of Green Tea: Prevention of Lifestyle-related Diseases

NAOKO SUEOKA, MASAMI SUGANUMA, EISABURO SUEOKA, SACHIKO OKABE, SATORU MATSUYAMA, KAZUE IMAI, KEI NAKACHI, AND HIROTA FUJIKI

Saitama Cancer Center Research Institute, Ina, Kitaadachi-gun, Saitama 362-0806, Japan

ABSTRACT: In the normal human life span, there occur lifestyle-related diseases that may be preventable with nontoxic agents. This paper deals with the preventive activity of green tea in some lifestyle-related diseases. Green tea is one of the most practical cancer preventives, as we have shown in various *in vitro* and *in vivo* experiments, along with epidemiological studies. Among various biological effects of green tea, we have focused on its inhibitory effect on TNF-α gene expression mediated through inhibition of NF-κB and AP-1 activation. Based on our recent results with TNF-α-deficient mice, TNF-α is an endogenous tumor promoter. TNF-α is also known to be a central mediator in chronic inflammatory diseases such as rheumatoid arthritis and multiple sclerosis. We therefore hypothesized that green tea might be a preventive agent for chronic inflammatory diseases. To test this hypothesis, TNF-α transgenic mice, which overexpress TNF-α only in the lungs, were examined. The TNF-α transgenic mouse is an animal model of human idiopathic pulmonary fibrosis which also frequently develops lung cancer. Expressions of TNF-α and IL-6 were inhibited in the lungs of these mice after treatment with green tea in drinking water for 4 months. In addition, judging from the results of a prospective cohort study in Saitama Prefecture, Japan, green tea helps to prevent cardiovascular disease. In this study, a decreased relative risk of death from cardiovascular disease was found for people consuming over 10 cups of green tea a day, and green tea also had life-prolonging effects on cumulative survival. These data suggest that green tea has preventive effects on both chronic inflammatory diseases and lifestyle-related diseases (including cardiovascular disease and cancer), resulting in prolongation of life span.

KEYWORDS: Cancer prevention; TNF-α; NF–κβ; Life-prolonging effects

INTRODUCTION

In 1987, we reported the first evidence that (−)-epigallocatechin gallate (EGCG) inhibited tumor promotion in a two-stage carcinogenesis experiment on mouse skin.[1] Later, the cancer preventive effect was accepted by the scientists throughout the world.[2,3] The rodent carcinogenesis experiments showed that EGCG and green tea extract have preventive activities on carcinogenesis of various organs, such as di-

---

Address for correspondence: Hirota Fujiki, M.D., Saitama Cancer Center Research Institute, Ina, Kitaadachi-gun, Saitama 362-0806, Japan. Voice: +81 48-722-1111; fax: +81 48-722-1739.
hfujiki@cancer-c.pref.saitama.jp

gestive tract, skin, liver, pancreas, lung, prostate, and bladder, as well as pulmonary metastasis of melanoma cells.[4–6] These data have been further supported by the results of human epidemiological studies. And recently our colleagues (K.I. and K.N.) reported that their prospective cohort study found cancer preventive effects of drinking green tea on the basis of an eleven-year follow-up study among 8,552 respondents.[7]

From our intensive studies on tumor promotion with okadaic acid, we have demonstrated that TNF-α is an endogenous tumor promoter.[8] A two-stage carcinogenesis experiment on the skin of TNF-α-deficient mice clearly showed that TNF-α is an essential cytokine in tumor promotion,[9] and in a subsequent experiment, EGCG inhibited TNF-α gene expression mediated through inhibition of NF-κB and AP-1 activation.[10] TNF-α is a key cytokine not only in cancer but also in other diseases such as rheumatoid arthritis, Crohn's disease, multiple sclerosis, and idiopathic pulmonary fibrosis,[11] and TNF-α is reported to contribute to diabetes mellitus, a major lifestyle-related disease.[12] Based on accumlating evidence that TNF-α is central mediator in various diseases which frequently occur among elderly people, we hypothesized that green tea, an inhibitor of TNF-α production, might prevent the development of some of these diseases. To examine our hypothesis, we used TNF-α transgenic mice, which overexpressed TNF-α only in the lungs due to constant activation of surfactant protein-C (SP-C) promoter.[13]

In this paper, we review the cancer preventive effects of green tea and discuss its mechanisms of action from the point of view of inhibition of TNF-α as an endogenous tumor promoter. We also present the preventive effects of green tea on other TNF-α-related diseases, using results of experiments with TNF-α transgenic mice.

CANCER PREVENTIVE EFFECTS OF GREEN TEA

The key element in a cancer preventive agent is that it is nontoxic, since the target for cancer prevention is not only the high-risk group but also the general population.[14] EGCG, the main constituent of green tea, was screened from among various natural products in two-stage carcinogenesis experiments on mouse skin. Repeated topical applications of EGCG completely inhibited tumor promotion of okadaic acid, a potent tumor promoter, on mouse skin initiated with 7,12-dimethylbenz(*a*)anthracene (DMBA).[4] Since the first result published in 1987, EGCG and green tea extract have been shown to inhibit carcinogenesis of various organs of rodents, such as digestive tract including esophagus, stomach, duodenum, and colon, plus liver, lung, pancreas, and skin (TABLE 1).[4–6]

From our investigation of okadaic acid we concluded that TNF-α is an endogenous tumor promoter.[8,15] The mechanism of the action of okadaic acid is different from that of 12-*O*-tetradecanoylphorbol-13-acetate. The okadaic acid class compounds, which are potent inhibitors of protein phosphatases 1 and 2A, induced tumor promotion in three different organs—mouse skin, rat glandular stomach, and rat liver—initiated with three different initiators.[16–18] TNF-α was also induced in the target organs by the okadaic acid class compounds. And in a series of *in vitro* two-stage carcinogenesis experiments with BALB/3T3 cells initiated with 3-methylcholantrene, TNF-α induced potent tumor promoting activity.[8] To prove that TNF-α is the essential tumor promoter, we conducted a two-stage carcinogenesis experiment on skin of TNF-α-deficient mice, which were established by Lloyd J.

TABLE 1. Inhibition of carcinogenesis with EGCG and green tea extract

Organs	Species	Carcinogens	Inhibitors	Reduction of Tumor Incidence (%)
Glandular stomach	rat	MNNG	EGCG	62.0 → 31.0
Duodenum	mouse C57BL/6	ENNG	EGCG	63.0 → 20.0
Colon	rat	AOM	EGCG	77.3 → 38.1
	rat	MNU	GTE	67.0 → 33.0
Liver	mouse C3H/HeN	spontaneous	EGCG	83.8 → 52.2
Lung	mouse A/J	NNK	GTE	96.3 → 65.5
Pancreas	hamster	BOP	GTE	54.0 → 33.0
Skin	house SKG-1	UVB	GTE	67.0 → 7.0

MNNG: N-methyl-N'-nitro-N-nitrosoguanidine; ENNG:N-ethyl-N'-nitro-N-nitrosoguanidine; AOM: azoxymethane; MNU: methylnitrosourea; NNK:4-(methylnitrosoamine)-1-(3-pyridyl)-1-butanone; and BOP: N-nitrosobis-(2-oxopropyl)amine; GTE: green tea extract.

Old's research group in 1997.[19] A single application of okadaic acid to mouse skin did not induce TNF-α gene expression in skin of TNF-α-deficient mice, but it did induce TNF-α in wild mice. Repeated applications of okadaic acid did not induce any tumors in TNF-α-deficient mice initiated with DMBA by 19 weeks of tumor promotion, while 100% of the wild mice developed tumors by week 17.[9] These results clearly demonstrated that tumor promotion by okadaic acid is mediated through TNF-α, and that TNF-α is the key cytokine for tumor promotion on mouse skin. Since EGCG inhibited TNF-α gene expression in BALB/3T3 cells and KATO III cells treated with okadaic acid, EGCG's action as a cancer preventive is mediated through its inhibition of TNF-α production.[10,15]

EFFECTS OF GREEN TEA EXTRACT ON CYTOKINE PRODUCTION IN TNF-α TRANSGENIC MICE

Besides being a potent tumor promoter, TNF-α also plays an important role in the development of other diseases, including rheumatoid arthritis, multiple sclerosis, and idiopathic pulmonary fibrosis.[11,13] To examine whether green tea extract can inhibit TNF-α production in an animal model, we used TNF-α transgenic mice. These mice, which carry a chimeric gene consisting of human SP-C promoter and mouse TNF-α gene, progressively develop interstitial pneumonitis that resembles idiopathic pulmonary fibrosis in humans.[13,20] Because SP-C promoter is activated only in alveolar type II epithelial cells, TNF-α is overexpressed only in the lungs. We divided the process of interstitial pneumonitis into three stages according to histological change: early stage (1-month-old), middle stage (7-month-old), and late stage (13-month-old). In the early stage, lymphocytic dominant infiltration was observed in alveolar septa; in the middle stage this was followed by macrophage accumulation in both interstitial regions and alveolar spaces; and in the late stage, hyperplastic

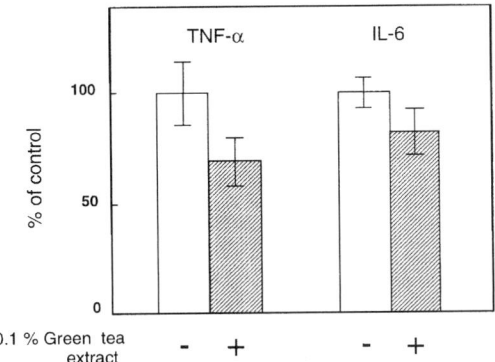

FIGURE 1. Green tea extract inhibited cytokine production. After treatment with 0.1% green tea extract in drinking water for 4 months, protein levels of TNF-α and IL-6 in the lungs were determined by enzyme-linked immunosorbent assay. The protein levels of these cytokines in the lungs of nontreated TNF-α transgenic mice were shown as 100%.

changes of bronchiolar epithelial cells were found. The TNF-α overexpression that started just after birth was continuous. IL-1α and IL-1β were overexpressed only in the early stage, while IL-6 production increased along with the progression of interstitial pneumonitis, suggesting that IL-6 contributed to the development of the disease.[20]

Based on our evidence that TNF-α is an instigator of such diseases and that green tea has inhibitory effects on TNF-α production, we hypothesized that green tea could prevent development of the diseases. To examine our hypothesis, TNF-α transgenic mice were given 0.1% green tea extract in drinking water from 10 days before birth to 4 months old. After treatment with green tea extract, protein levels of TNF-α and IL-6 were reduced by 70% and 80%, respectively (FIG. 1). The levels of mRNA expression of these cytokines were similar to those of protein levels, suggesting that green tea regulates the cytokine expression in transcriptional machinery. Since the level of SP-C mRNA did not change with treatment of green tea, the transcriptional regulation was performed in the endogenous promoter of either TNF-α or IL-6 genes (data not shown). The animal model experiment indicates that green tea has preventive effects not only on development of cancer but also on that of other TNF-α-related diseases.

PREVENTIVE EFFECTS OF GREEN TEA ON CANCER AND LIFESTYLE-RELATED DISEASES ELUCIDATED BY EPIDEMIOLOGICAL STUDIES

Along with the results of animal experiments, epidemiological studies have confirmed the preventive effects of green tea on cancer and other lifestyle-related dis-

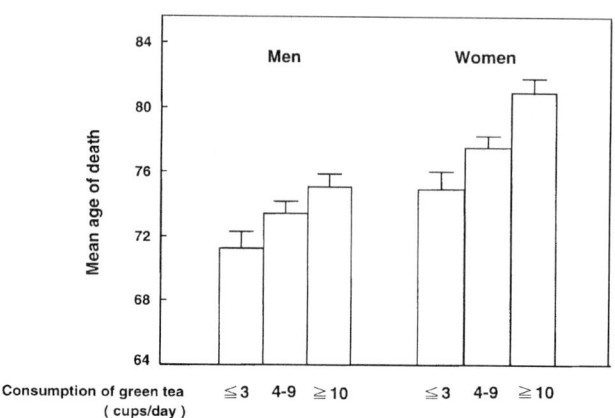

FIGURE 2. Effect of green tea on mean age of death from all causes. In the 11-year follow-up study, death from all causes was surveyed by death certificate; a total of 1,109 deaths from all causes was used in the analysis of the mean ages of death.

eases in humans. We conducted a prospective cohort study with 8,552 individuals in Yoshimi town in Saitama Prefecture beginning in 1986.[21] During an 11-year follow-up, a total of 488 cancer patients (285 males and 203 females) were determined. Respondents were divided into three groups according to daily consumption of green tea: below 3 cups, from 4 to 9 cups, and over 10 cups. Individuals who consumed over 10 cups of green tea per day showed remarkable reduction of relative risk for lung, colon, and liver cancers;[21] the relative risk of stomach cancer was also low, although not statistically significant. In addition to the cancer preventive effects, our data showed that increased green tea consumption was associated with decreased serum total cholesterol, decreased triglyceride levels, and decreased atherogenic index. Furthermore, both cardiovascular disease prevalence rate and diabetes mellitus prevalence rate were significantly lower among the population consuming over 10 cups of green tea per day.[22] Since green tea apparently helped to prevent cancer, cardiovascular disease, and diabetes mellitus, all major lifestyle-related diseases, mean age at death from all causes was compared by consumption levels of green tea. We found a higher mean age at death among men with increased consumption of green tea. Among women, the mean age at death of the population consuming over 10 cups per day was 81, which was 6 years later than that of those consuming less than 3 cups. The same tendency among both sexes (FIG. 2),[23] so these data clearly indicate that green tea reduces the risk of lifestyle-related diseases, resulting in a longer life span.

In summary, green tea, an acknowledged cancer preventive, may also prevent other lifestyle-related diseases, and other TNF-α-related diseases. We know that green tea is nontoxic, and the inference now seems clear: for a longer, healthier life, drink at least 10 cups (about 2.0 g green tea extract) every day.[24]

REFERENCES

1. YOSHIZAWA, S., T. HORIUCHI, H. FUJIKI et al. 1987. Antitumor promoting activity of (−)-epigallocatechin gallate, the main constituent of "tannin" in green tea. Phytother. Res. **1:** 44–47.
2. JANKUN, J., S.H. SELMAN, R. SWIERCZ et al. 1997. Why drinking green tea could prevent cancer. Nature **387:** 561.
3. NCI, DCPC, Chemoprevention Branch and Agent Development Committee. 1996. Clinical development plan: tea extracts green tea polyphenols epigallocatechin gallate. J. Cell. Biochem. **26S:** 236–257.
4. FUJIKI, H., A. KOMORI & M. SUGANUMA. 1997. Chemoprevention of cancer. In Comprehensive Toxicology, Vol. 12. T.G. Bowden & S.M. Fischer, Eds.: 453–471. Elsevier. Oxford.
5. WANG, Z-Y., J-Y. HONG, M-T. HUANG et al. 1992. Inhibition of N-nitrosodiethylamine- and 4(methylnitrosamino)-1-(3-pyridyl)-1-butanone-induced tumorigenesis in A/J mice by green tea and black tea. Cancer Res. **52:** 1943–1947.
6. TANIGUCHI, S., H. FUJIKI, H. KOBAYASHI et al. 1992. Effect of (−)-epigallocatechin gallate, the main constituent of green tea, on lung metastasis with mouse B16 melanoma cell lines. Cancer Lett. **65:** 51–54.
7. NAKACHI, K., K. IMAI & K. SUGA. 1997. Cancer-preventive effects of drinking green tea in a Japanese population. Proc. Am. Assoc. Cancer Res. **38:** 261.
8. KOMORI, A., J. YATSUNAMI, M. SUGANUMA et al. 1993. Tumor necrosis factor acts as a tumor promoter in BALB/3T3 cell transformation. Cancer Res. **53:** 1982–1985.
9. SUGANUMA, M., S. OKABE, M.W. MARINO et al. 1999. Essential role of tumor necrosis factor-α in tumor promotion as revealed by TNF-α-deficient mice. Cancer Res. **59:** 4516–4518.
10. OKABE, S., Y. OCHIAI, M. AIDA et al. 1999. Mechanistic aspects of green tea as cancer preventive on human stomach cancer cell lines. Jpn. J. Cancer Res. **90:** 733–739.
11. AGGARWAL, B.B. & K. NATARAJAN. 1996. Tumor necrosis factors: developments during the last decade. Eur. Cytokine Netw. **7:** 93–124.
12. HOTAMISLIGIL, G.S., N.S. SHARGILL & B.M. SPIEGELMAN. 1993. Adipose expression of tumor necrosis factor-α: direct role in obesity-linked insulin resistance. Science **259:** 87–91.
13. MIYAZAKI, Y., K. ARAKI, C. VESIN et al. 1995. Expression of a tumor necrosis factor-α transgene in murine lung causes lymphocytic and fibrosing alveolitis. J. Clin. Invest. **96:** 250–259.
14. HONG, W.K. & M.B. SPORN. 1997. Recent advances in chemoprevention of cancer. Science **278:** 1073–1077.
15. SUGANUMA, M., S. OKABE, E. SUEOKA et al. 1996. A new process of cancer prevention mediated through inhibition of tumor necrosis factor α expression. Cancer Res. **56:** 3711–3715.
16. SUGANUMA, M., H. FUJIKI, H. SUGURI et al. 1988. Okadaic acid: an additional non-phorbol-12 tetradecanoate-13-acetate-type tumor promoter. Proc. Natl. Acad. Sci. USA **85:** 1768–1771.
17. SUGANUMA, M., M. TATEMATSU, J. YATSUNAMI et al. 1992. An alternative theory of tissue specificity by tumor promotion of okadaic acid in glandular stomach of SD rats. Carcinogenesis **13:** 1841–1845.
18. OHTA, T., E. SUEOKA, N. IIDA et al. 1994. Nodularin, a potent inhibitor of protein phosphatases 1 and 2A, is a new environmental carcinogen in male F344 rat liver. Cancer Res. **54:** 6402–6406.
19. MARINO, M.W., A. DUNN, D. GRAIL et al. 1997. Characterization of tumor necrosis factor deficient mice. Proc. Natl. Acad. Sci. USA **94:** 8093–8098.
20. SUEOKA, N., E. SUEOKA, Y. MIYAZAKI et al. 1998. Molecular pathogenesis of interstitial pneunonitis with TNF-α transgenic mice. Cytokine **10:** 124–131.
21. IMAI, K., K. SUGA & K. NAKACHI. 1997. Cancer-preventive effects of drinking green tea among a Japanese population. Prev. Med. **26:** 769–775.
22. IMAI, K. & K. NAKACHI. 1995. Cross sectional study of effects of drinking green tea on cardiovascular and liver diseases. BMJ **310:** 693–696.

23. NAKACHI, K., S. MATSUYAMA, S. MIYAKE *et al.* 2000. Preventive effects of drinking green tea on cancer and cardiovascular disease: epidemiological evidence for multiple targeting prevention. Biofactors. In press.
24. FUJIKI, H. 1999. Two stages of cancer prevention with green tea. J. Cancer Res. Clin. Oncol. **125:** 589–597.

Anti-aging and Health-promoting Constituents Derived from Traditional Oriental Herbal Remedies

Information Retrieval Using the TradiMed 2000 DB

IL-MOO CHANG

Graduate Studies in Natural Products Science, Natural Products Research Institute, Seoul National University, Seoul 110-460, Korea

ABSTRACT: Asia, Korea, China, and Japan have legally adopted the traditional Oriental (Chinese) medical system along with the Western system. A number of traditional herbal drugs including the polypharmacy type of prescriptions (a combination of multiple herbs) are available and are widely dispensed. Herbal therapy used in traditional Oriental medicine appears to be quite different from its counterpart Western drug therapy. The polypharmacy type of herbal therapy generally exhibits holistic effectiveness by exerting activities to multitarget organs (organ systems) according to the principles of traditional Oriental medicine. The Traditional Oriental Medicine Database (TradiMed 2000 DB) is a unique database of traditional Oriental herbal therapy containing a variety of information such as formulae, chemical information on ingredients, botanical information on herbal materials, and a dictionary of disease classification (TOM and Western classification). A formula, namely, the Sip-Jeon-Dae-Bo-Tang consisting of 10 different herbs, was selected by retrieving information from the TradiMed 2000 DB. Then its tonic effects for elderly people were shown as an example.

KEYWORDS: Antiaging; Tonic herbs; Traditional Chinese herbal therapy; TradiMed database

A GLIMPSE AT TRADITIONAL ORIENTAL HERB THERAPY

With the use of drugs in human history, both Oriental and Occidental worlds applied a "Similia similibus" type of selection to plant and animal materials available. In other words, a single herb was used as a drug to remedy human ailments. Later, a polypharmacy type of herbal therapy was introduced (a combination of multiple herbal materials in a single formula). At the present time, approximately 100,000 polypharmacy type prescriptions have been recorded in the literature. These vast numbers of polypharmacy herbal prescriptions are a characteristic feature of traditional Oriental (Chinese) herbal therapy. In the long course of its development, Chinese herbal therapists employed a unique doctrine or grand hypothesis, the so-

---

Address for correspondence: Professor Il-Moo Chang, Graduate Studies in Natural Products Science, Natural Products Research Institute, Seoul National University, Seoul 110-460, Korea. Voice: +82 2-763-2055; fax: +82 2-745-1015.
changim@snu.ac.kr

called "Yin-Yang and Five Elements" theory to justify and explain their findings. This grand hypothesis was believed to control all natural phenomena including human life and all other organisms.[1]

The principles of prescribing polypharmacy remedies was designed to maintain a balance between Yin and Yang in the interaction of the Five Elements (five organ systems: the heart, kidney, liver, lung, and spleen systems) of human physiology. When pathogenic factors of either external (bad Qui) or internal factors (the seven emotions) alter the human body, Yin and Yang are said to be out of balance. To restore balance, a traditional Oriental doctor will select herbs with Yang or Yin properties. When illness results from too much Yang, a doctor prescribes an herb with Yin properties or vice versa.[2] Within this concept, about two thirds of the remedies so far reported consist of 5–6 herbal materials, while the remaining one third have more than 5–6. A few have more than two dozen separate herbal materials. Seeing such large numbers, many Western scientists become dismayed and wonder what specific pharmacological effects can be studied if any in a mixture of several dozen herbs.

To help understand these complexities, we can divide herbal materials into four groups according to their function: King, Vassal, Assistant, and Delivery servant herbs. The King group consists of the most pharmacologically active herbs. The Vassals play a role of additive action, similar in activity to the Kings but with different herbal materials. Assistants usually perform a detoxifying activity. When we consider that each herb contains a variety of constituents, both helpful and harmful to the patient, the Assistants act to nullify that harmful activity. Finally, Delivering servants help transport the active constituents existing in the King and Vassal herbal materials to target organs.

In addition to these principles, traditional Oriental doctors frequently combine two different polypharmacy formulas—one to treat a specific organ, e.g., liver, and the other to treat a related aspect such as bile. By doing this, a single polypharmacy formula can exhibit multiple treatments to several organs. Traditional Oriental herbal remedies are believed to show holistic effects for precisely this reason. Information on the King herbs in certain polypharmacy formulas has drawn the attention of modern pharmacologists and phytochemists, because there is a higher possibility of isolating active constituents from herbal materials identified as King herbs. For example, ephedrine, artemisin, and shizandrin were all isolated from the Oriental herbs Ephedrae Herba, Artemisiae Folium, and Shizandrae Fructus, respectively. They are all used in modern drugs.

HERBAL REMEDIES FOR THE ELDERLY

By the physiological view based on the doctrine of Yin-Yang and Five Elements, the functions of the kidney system and Qui circulation work less effectively in most elderly persons. The Oriental term for the kidney system represents a group of human organs including the kidney, reproductive-sexual organs, and bladder. This system functions in controlling hormones and other body fluids. The Oriental term of Qui is a concept that perhaps can be best translated, as the vital energy needed to maintain normal body health. Qui is believed to be derived from a combination of Heaven Qui (air needed for respiration) and Earth Qui (nutritional sources from food). Qui circulates through meridian paths throughout the body to supply vital energy.[3] However, its existence has not yet been proved by experiment. When the circulation of Qui is impeded due to aging or a shortage of Qui results from illness, various ailments and reduced body functions manifest themselves. In the case of the elderly, tonic type formulas are usually given in order to elevate the state of Qui to a sufficient rate of circulation.

Several hundred traditional Oriental herbal remedies for elderly persons are available. For the current discussion, I wish to present examples of typical tonic remedies: one is to increase the Qui activity, and the other is to replenish the functions of kidney system.

INFORMATION RETRIEVAL USING THE TRADIMED 2000 DB

The contents of the Traditional Oriental Medicine Database (TradiMed 2000 DB) can be accounted as a comprehensive treatise of traditional Oriental herbal therapy. The DB offers six groups of information as follows: (1) a total of 12,634 titles of herbal formulas, dosage, indication, meridian target organs, bibliographic citations, etc.; (2) botanical and taxonomical information on herbal materials and original plants with full-color photo images; (3) chemical information on constituents with analytical data; chemical formulas with drawings of chemical structures, melting points, optical rotations, spectral data of infrared, ultraviolet, mass spectra and nuclear magnetic resonance spectra; (4) a dictionary of disease classification in terms of Oriental medicine and equivalent modern pathological terms and total 4,080 diseases with detailed descriptions of symptoms; (5) traditional ways of processing methods of medicinal plants; and (6) clinical case studies (a total of 844 cases) by integrating traditional Oriental and modern medical therapies.[4]

Using the TradiMed 2000 DB, we searched for traditional Oriental formulas for elevating Qui activity and for replenishing kidney systems of the elderly. Then we searched for natural constituents in the King herb.

HERBS IDENTIFIED AS THE KING HERB REPLENISHING THE KIDNEY SYSTEM

Herbs identified as the King herb replenishing the kidney system are as follows (Herbs in Latin: Botanical names, Natural constituents):

(1) Astragali Radix : *Astragalus membranaceus*, Bunge, (Leguminosae) : Acetylsoyasaponin A5, Acetylastrogaloside I, Arginine, Arg (L-form, s-form), Astragalin, Astragaloside I, II, III, IV, V, VI, VII, VIII, Astragenol, Astramembrangenin, Astramembrannin I, II, Calycosin-7-O-β-D-glucopyranoside, Calycosin, Canavanine (s-form, L-form), Cycloastragenol, Formononetin, Isoastrogaloside I, II, Isoquercitrin, Isorhamnetin, Kaempferol, Lupeone, Methylnissolin-3-glucoside, Quercetin, Rhamnocitrin-3-O-β-D-glucopyranoside, Soyasaponin I, β-Sitosterol, γ-Aminobutyric acid.

(2) Atractylodis Rhizoma : *Atractylodes japonica*, Koidz., (Compositae) : (6E,12E)-Tetradecadiene-8,10-diyne-1,3-dioldiacetate, 3-Hydroxyatracty-

lon, 3-β-Acetoxyatractylon, Atractylenolide, Atractylodin, Atractylon, Selina-4(14),7(11)-diene-8-one.

(3) Brassocae Semen : *Brassica rapa*, L.,(Cruciferae) : 1-Cyano-3,4-epithiobutane, 1-Cyano-4,5-epithiopentane, 3-*O*-β-D-Glucopyranosylisorhamnetin, Astragalin, But-3-enyl-isothiocyanate, But-3-enylisothiocyanate, Cyanin, Dehydroascorbic acid, Goitrin, Isoquercitrin, Isoquercitrin; 7-*O*-β-D-glucopyranoside, Isorhamnetin-3,7-di-*O*-β-D-glucopyranoside, Isorhamnetin-7-*O*-β-D-glucopyranoside-3-*O*-α-D-sophoraside, Isorhamnetin-7-*O*-β-D-glucopyranoside, Kaempferol-3,7-di-*O*-β-D-glucopyranoside, Kaempferol-3-*O*-β-D-[glucopyranosyl(1-2)glucopyranosyl]-7-*O*-β-D-glucopyranoside, Kaempferol-3-*O*-β-D-sophoroside, Napoleferin, Quercetin-3-*O*-sophoroside, Quercimeritrin, Quercimeritrin; 3-*O*-sophoroside, Rubrobrassicon

(4) Calami Rhizoma : *Acorus calamus var. angustatus*, Bess., (Araceae) : (+)β-Pinene, (−)-Calamenene, 1,3,11-Elematriene, 1,4,9-Cadalatriene, 1,8-Cineole, Cineole, Cajeputol, Eucalyptol, Asarone, Elemicin, Eugenol, Eugenic acid, Linalool, Shyobunone, Terpinen-4-ol, 4-Terpineol, β-Gurjunene, β-Selinene, δ-Cadinene, γ-Asarone, *p*-Cymene, *trans*-Isoeugenolmethyl ether.

(5) Chrysanthemi Flos : *Chrysanthemum morifolium*, Ramat., (Compositae) : Caffetannic acid, 16-β-Hydroxy-3-*O*-palmitylpseudotaraxasterol, Apigenin, Apigetrin, 16-β-Hydroxypseudotaraxasterol, Chlorogenic acid, Diosmetin-7-*O*-β-D-glucopyranoside, Pseudotaraxasterol, Taraxasterol.

(6) Cuscutae Semen : *Cuscuta chinensis*, Lam., (Convolvulaceae) : Arbutin, Arbutoside, Ericolin, Astragalin, Caffeic acid, Chlorogenic acid, Caffetannic acid, Caucutoside A, B, Hyperoside, Quercetin.

(7) Lycii Fructus : *Lycium chinense*, Mill., (Solanaceae) : 1-Methoxycarbonyl-β-carboline, 24-Ethyllophenol, 24-Methyl-31-norlanost-9(11)-en-ol, 24-Methylene-cycloartanol, 24-Methylenelanost-8-en-3-β-ol, 24-α-Methyllophenol, 3-Hydroxy-7,8-dehydro-β-ionon, 31-Norlanosterol, 4-α,14-α,24-Trimethylcholesta-8,24-dien-ol, 4-α,24-Dimethylcholesta-7,24-dien-ol, Betaine, Aurantiamide acetate, Cholest-7-en-ol, Cycloartanol, Cycloeucalenone, Dehydro-α-cyperone, Diosgenin, Gramisterol, Isofucoserol, Kukoamine A, Lanost-8-en-3-β-ol, Lanosterol, Lophenol, Lupeol, Lycimamide, Lyciumin A, B, *N*-9-Formylharman, Nicotianamine, Obtusifolin, Obtusifoliol, Perlolyrine, Solavetivone, Stigmastane-3,6-dione(α5*H*), Stigmasterol, Sugiol, Vanillic acid, Withanolide A, B, β-Amyrin.

(8) Polygonati Rhizoma : *Polygonatum Kingianum*, Coll. et Hemsl, (Liliaceae) : 25(*R*)-Polygonatum saponin Po-8, Daucosterol, Funkioside C, Kingianoside A, B, C, D.

(9) Polygoni Multiflori Caulis : *Polugonum multiflorum*, Thunb., (Polygonaceae) : 1,8-Dihydroxy-3-methyl-9-anthrone, 2,3,4′,5-Tetrahydroxystilbene, 2-*O*-β-D-Glucopyranosyl-2,3-4′,5-tetrahydroxystilbene, Chrysophanic acid, Emodin-8-*O*-β-D-glucopyranoside, Emodin, Guiajaverin, Hyperoside, Polygoacetophenoside, Rhaponticin, Ponticin, Rhapontin, Rhein, β-Sitosterol.

(10) Rehmanniae Radix: *Rehmannia glutinosa*, (Gaertn.) Libosch (Scrophulariaceae): Ajugol, Catalpol, Gardoside, Glutinoside, Luteolin-3′-methyl

ether, Melittoside, Myoporoside, Rehmaglutin A, B, C, D, Rehmanioside A, B, C, D, Rehmapicroside, Verbascoside, Acteoside, Kusaginin.
(11) Sophorae Fructus : *Sophora japonica*, L., (Leguminosae) : 5,7-Dihydroxy-3',4'-methylenedioxyisoflavone, Anagyrine((−)-form), Azukisaponin, Biochanin A-7-O-β-D-xylosylglucoside, Biochanin A-7-O-gentiobioside, Biochanin A, Flemichapparin B, Genisein-7-O-β-cellobioside, Genistein, Irisilidone-7-O-β-D-glucopyranoside, Irisolidone, Isorhamnetin, Kaempferol, Kaikasponin, Matrine((+)-form, (+,−)Maackiain, Oxymatrine((+)-form), Pratensein, Quercetin, Sissotrin, Sophocarpine((−)-form), Sophojaponicin, Sophorabioside, Sophoricoside, Soyasaponin 1, Stizolamine, Syringin, Syringoside, Alyposide, Ligustrin.

HERBS IDENTIFIED AS THE KING HERB ELEVATING QUI ACTIVITIES

Herbs identified as the King herb elevating Qui activities are as follows:

(1) Acanthopanacis Cortex: *Acanthopanax sessiliflorus* (Rupr. et Maxim.) Seem. (Araliaceae).
(2) Asparagi Radix: *Asparagus cochinchinensis* Merr. (Liliaceae): Asparagoside IV, VI, VII, Asparagus saponin Asp-IV, V, VI, VII, Aspartic acid, Methylprotogracillin, Pseudoprotodioscin.
(3) Ginseng Radix: *Panax ginseng* C.A. Mey. (Araliaceae): (+)-γ-Cadinene, (20R)-Protopanaxatriol, (E)-α-Bisabolene, 1(5), 11-Guaiadiene, 1,8-Cineole, Cineole, Cajeputol, Eucalyptol, 1-Ethoxycarbonyl-β-carboline, 2,6-Dimethylpyrazine, 2-Ethyl-5-methylpyrazine, 2-Ethyl-6-methylpyrazine, 2-Isobutyl-3-methoxypyrazine, 2-Isopropyl-3-methoxypyrazine, 2-Methyl-4-pyrone-3-O-β-D-glucopyranoside, 2-*sec*-Butyl-3-methoxypyrazine, 20(R)-Protopanaxadiol, 20R-Ginsenoside Rg2, Rg3, Rh1, 20S-Ginsenoside Rg3, 20S-Glucosyl-ginsenoside Rf, 24-Methylene-cycloartanol, 3-Isopropyl-2-methoxy-5-methylpyrazine, 3-Methoxy-5-(1-O-β-D-glucopyranosyl)heptyl-2(5H)-furanone, 3-*sec*-Butyl-2-methoxy-5-methylpyrazine, 5-Ethyl-2,3-dimethylpyrazine, Biotin, Campesterol, Chloropanaxydiol, Cholesterol, Cycloartenol, Cycloeucalenol, Dihydropanaxacol dencichine, Diisopropyl sulfide, Eremophilene, Estradiol, Estrone, Ethylene, Eugenol, Eugenic acid, Falcarinol, Ferulic acid, Folic acid, Fumaric acid, Galanin, γ-Selinene, Ginsenoside F1, F2, F3, Ra1, Ra2, Rb1, Rb2, Rb3, Rc, Re, Rf, Rg1, Rg2, Rh1, Rh2, Ro, Ginsenoyne A, B, C, D, E, F, G, H, I, J, K, Glutamic acid, Gypenoside-XVII, Heptadeca-1,4-diene-6,8-diyne-3,10-diol, Heptadeca-1,9-dien-4,6-diyn-3-ol; (s)-(z)-form, Heptadeca-1-en-4,6-diyn-3,9-diol, Heptadeca-1-*trans*-8-diene-4,6-diyne-3,10-diol, Indole-3-acetic acid, Invertase, Isoquercitrin, Kaempferol, Leucine, Ligustrazine, Linalool, Lupeol, Lutein, (L-form), Malic acid, Malonyl Ginsenoside Rb1, Rc, Rd, Moretenol, N-9-Formylharman, Neoxanthin (all E-form), Nicotinamide, Nicotinic acid, Notoginsenoside R1, Obtusifoliol, Oleanolic acid, Panasinsanol A, B, Panax ginseng, 20(s)-Prosapogenin, Panax ginseng glycoside P1, Panax glycoprotein, Panax saponin A, B, C, Panaxacol, Panaxa-

diol, Panaxatriol, Panaxydol, Panaxydolchlorohydrine, Panaxyne epoxide, Panaxyne, Panaxytriol, Pantothenic acid, Pelargonidin-3-monoglucoside, Pelargonin, Perlolyrine, Phenylalanine, Phosphatidylcholine, Proline (S-form, L-form), Protopanaxadiol, Putrescine, Quinquenoside R1, Salicylic acid, Spathulenol, Spermidine, Spinacine (S-form), Squalene-2,3-oxide, Squalene, Stigmasterol, Trifolin, Trimethylpyrazine, Vanillic acid, Violaxanthin (all-E form), Vitamin B_{12}, α-Farnesene, α-Pinene(+,−), α-Pyrrolidone, α-Santalene, α-Selinene, α-Terpineol, β-Amyrin, β-Eudesmol, β-Farnesene, β-Guaiene, β-Gurjunene, β-Maaliene, β-Patchoulene, β-Sitosterol, δ-Cadinene, δ-Elemene, ε-Muurolene, γ-Elemene.

(4) Poria(Hoelen): *Poria cocos* Wolf (Polyporaceae): Choline, Dehydropachymic acid, Ergosterol, Pachymic acid, Polyporenic acid C, Poricoic acid A, B, Tumulosic acid.

(5) Toosendan Fructus: *Melia toosendan* Sieb. Et Zucc. (Meliaceae): Chuanliansu, Loliolide, Iso-Chuanliansu, Lipomelianol (Mixture of the 3-*O*-stearate, palmitate, myristate, laurate of melianol), Melia-inoside B, Meliaionoside A, Melianone, Toosendanoside, Toosendansterol A, B.

SUMMARY

The information retrieval system at the TradiMed 2000 DB yielded more than a dozen herbs with major anti-aging effects that are used in traditional Oriental herbal therapy and have been used for a long time. In addition, the currently known array of natural constituents was shown. This information can be utilized to verify the effectiveness of those herbal materials based on modern science and technology. The ginseng root, known as a tonic herb for years, contains more than several dozen of these constituents. However, the effective constituents have not been identified yet. There is a great opportunity for us to study traditional herbal remedies with respect to current research trends in complementary and alternative medicine.

REFERENCES

1. CHANG, I.M. & J.G. CHI. 1999. Harmonization of traditional Oriental (Chinese) medicine and modern medicine: a step forward with TradiMed Database 2000. *In* Traditional and Alternative Medicine in the 21st Century, K.-Y. Cha, Ed.: 151–160. Pochun Cha University. Seoul.
2. LIU, F. & L.Y. MAU. 1980. Chinese Medical Terminology. Commercial Press. Hong Kong.
3. XIE, Z. 1999. Selected terms in traditional Chinese medicine and their interpretations (IX). Chinese J. Integrated Trad. Western Med. **5:** 300–302.
4. CHANG, I.M. 1999. Traditional Oriental Medicine Database (TradiMed 2000 DB). Dong Bang Media. Seoul.

Caloric Restriction in Primates

M. A. LANE, A. BLACK, A. HANDY, E. M. TILMONT, D. K. INGRAM, AND G. S. ROTH

Laboratory of Neurosciences, Gerontology Research Center, National Institute on Aging, National Institutes of Health, Baltimore, Maryland 21224, USA

ABSTRACT: Caloric restriction (CR) remains the only nongenetic intervention that reproducibly extends mean and maximal life span in short-lived mammalian species. This nutritional intervention also delays the onset, or slows the progression, of many age-related disease processes. The diverse effects of CR have been demonstrated many hundreds of times in laboratory rodents and other short-lived species, such as rotifers, water fleas, fish, spiders, and hamsters. Until recently, the effects of CR in longer-lived species, more closely related to humans, remained unknown. Long-term studies of aging in nonhuman primates undergoing CR have been underway at the National Institute on Aging (NIA) and the University of Wisconsin-Madison (UW) for over a decade. A number of reports from the NIA and UW colonies have shown that monkeys on CR exhibit nearly identical physiological responses as reported in laboratory rodents. Studies of various markers related to age-related diseases suggest that CR will prevent or delay the onset of cardiovascular disease, diabetes, and perhaps cancer, and preliminary data indicate that mortality due to these and other age-associated diseases may also be reduced in monkeys on CR, compared to controls. Conclusive evidence showing that CR extends life span in primates is not presently available; however, the emerging data from the ongoing primate studies strengthens the possibility that the diverse beneficial effects of CR on aging in rodents will also apply to nonhuman primates and perhaps ultimately to humans.

KEYWORDS: Increasing life span; Insulin levels; Primates; Rodent models

INTRODUCTION

Caloric restriction (CR) or reduced feeding of an otherwise nutritionally replete diet is the most consistent and reproducible method for increasing life span and delaying the onset, or reducing the incidence, of many age-associated diseases.[1,2] Unlike many interventions that may increase average life span by reducing the negative influence of age-associated diseases or other segmental aspects of aging, CR is thought to alter fundamental biological processes that regulate aging and longevity in a variety of organisms. The effects of this nutritional intervention on life span have been reproduced many hundreds of times in laboratory rodents and other short-lived species, including rotifers, water fleas, fish, hamsters, and spiders. Until recently lit-

---

Address for correspondence: Mark A. Lane, Ph.D., Gerontology Research Center, 5600 Nathan Shock Drive, Baltimore, MD 21224. Voice: 410-558-8481; fax: 410-558-8323.
MLANE@vms.grc.nia.nih.gov

TABLE 1. Longitudinal studies of caloric restriction in nonhuman primates

Parameter	NIA[a]	UW
Age range[b]	1–2, 3–5, >15	8–14
Species		
Rhesus		
Long-term	M (60), F (60)	M (30), F (30)
Short-term/mechanistic	M (28), F (12)	M (16)
Squirrel		
Long-term	M (40)	—
Total	200	76
Diet	Semisynthetic	Synthetic
Energy conent	3.77 kcal/gram	3.91 kcal/gram
Fat content (source)	5% (soy)	10% (corn)
Vitamin supplement	Yes	Yes (since 1994)
	Premix in chow	Premix (CR only)
CR paradigm	30% of control	30% of control
Concurrent controls	Yes	Yes
Random assignment	Yes	Yes

[a] NIA, National Institute on Aging; UW, University of Wisconsin-Madison.
[b] Age at which CR was initiated.

tle was known regarding the efficacy of this intervention for alteration of aging in long-lived species more closely related to humans.

In 1987 our laboratory within the Intramural Research Program of the National Institute on Aging (NIA), USA, began the first large-scale, longitudinal study of CR in nonhuman primates.[3,4] At present, the NIA colony involves nearly two hundred rhesus (*Macaca mulatta*) and squirrel (*Saimiri sp.*) monkeys on a variety of longitudinal and short-term studies of CR and aging. A similar, but smaller, study involving about 90 rhesus monkeys was begun at the University of Wisconsin-Madison (UW) in 1989.[5] These two studies are the primary ongoing longitudinal studies of aging and CR designed to test the hypothesis that long-term CR slows aging and extends life span in nonhuman primates. Some pertinent details of these experiments are presented in TABLE 1. Several important differences between the two studies are worth noting. First, the age at onset of CR and the age ranges being studied differ. Monkeys at the NIA were begun on CR at 1–2, 3–5, or >15 years of age. The UW study focused on adult-onset (8–14 yr) CR. Together, these studies cover most of the rhesus life span. The remainder of this manuscript will summarize over a decade of research on the primate model of CR. We will focus on establishing the primate model, effects on age-related disease, and development and evaluation of candidate markers of aging.

TABLE 2. Summary of findings from primate caloric restriction studies

Finding		Agrees with Rodent Data
▼	Body weight	Yes
▼	Fat and lean mass	Yes
▼	Trunk: leg–fat ratio	NR
▼	Time to sexual maturity	Yes
▼	Time to sexual maturity	Yes
▼	Fasting glucose/insulin	Yes
▲	Insulin sensitivity	NR
▼	Metabolic rate (short term)	Yes
♦	Metabolic rate (long term)	Yes
▼	Body temperature	Yes
♦ or ▲	Locomotion	Yes
▼	Serum triglycerides	Yes
▲	Serum HDL 2B	Yes
▼	IGF-1/growth hormone	Yes
▼	IL-6	Yes
♦	Testoster-one	NR
♦	Estradiol, LH, FSH, *prog*	NR
♦	Wound closure rate	Yes
♦	Fibroblast clonal proliferation	?
♦	β-*gal* senescent cells	?
▼	Rate of decline in DHEAS	?
▼	Lymphocyte number	Yes
♦	Lymphocyte calcium response	No

SYMBOLS: ▼, decreased; ▲, increased; ♦, no effect or change; NR, not reported.

ESTABLISHING THE NONHUMAN PRIMATE MODEL OF CALORIC RESTRICTION

Prior to the initiation of these long-term studies, controlled long-term CR studies had not been conducted in species that lived longer than laboratory rodents. Thus, it became important to establish the safety and efficacy of this paradigm in this primate. To that end both the NIA and UW studies have studied many of the same parameters that had been reported in rodents. A summary of the effect of CR on these parameters and their agreement with rodent findings is presented in TABLE 2. A more detailed review of these early findings can be found elsewhere.[6]

It is readily apparent that CR has significant effects on body composition and development. Rhesus monkeys on CR in both the NIA and UW studies weigh less and have less overall body fat and lean body mass, compared to controls.[7–9] It has also been shown that monkeys on CR have less abdominal fat, compared to controls.[10] In addition, our studies at the NIA have shown that CR delays sexual maturation[11] and skeletal maturation[12] in young male monkeys.

Other findings, some of which are related to proposed mechanisms of CR, from the two primate studies, have also shown good agreement with rodent data. For example, monkeys on CR exhibit reductions in body temperature[13] and a transient lowering of 24-h metabolic rate.[13–15] Both laboratories have also invested much effort in examining the effects of CR on glucoregulation in rhesus monkeys. Despite slight differences in diet composition and overall body composition of the monkeys in the two studies, the effects of CR on glucoregulation show good agreement between the two studies and with existing rodent data as outlined in TABLE 2. Monkeys on CR have lower fasting glucose and insulin and improved insulin sensitivity, compared to controls.[7,8,16] A detailed discussion of the remaining findings presented in TABLE 2 is beyond the limited scope of this manuscript, and the reader is referred to the original references for more information. Taken together, the findings reported in TABLE 2 and in other reports[6,17] have helped to establish the nonhuman primate model of CR and strengthen the possibility that CR will extend life span in longerlived species, perhaps ultimately in humans.

EFFECTS ON AGE-RELATED DISEASES

Nonhuman primate studies of CR have also focused much attention on markers relevant to several age-related diseases, including diabetes, cardiovascular disease, and osteoporosis. As discussed above, monkeys on long-term CR exhibit significant reductions in fasting glucose and insulin levels and increased insulin sensitivity as well as changes in body composition that would be expected to reduce risk for developing cardiovascular disease and/or diabetes. Other reports from the NIA study have shown that monkeys on CR have reduced triglycerides in both male[18] and female monkeys[10,16] and that levels of a subfraction ($HDL2_B$) of "good" (HDL) cholesterol are increased in young male monkeys on CR.[18] Low levels of this particular HDL subfraction have been associated with increased risk of myocardial infarction in men.[19] In the UW study it has been reported that CR lowered serum triglycerides and that monkeys on the diet had increased amounts of lower molecular weight LDL particles, compared to controls.[20] Preliminary studies at the NIA that have examined indices of arterial stiffness, such as pulse wave velocity measured in the aorta, suggest increased vessel elasticity in CR monkeys, compared to controls.[16] Additional studies are needed to confirm this finding.

More recently, in our laboratory we have shown that these changes, particularly the effects of CR on insulin levels in monkeys occur very rapidly in response to CR.[21] FIGURE 1 shows the temporal pattern of these changes in response to CR. In these studies, older monkeys (>18 yr) in the CR group were fed progressively less (10% per month) until reaching a 30% reduction in intake and were then maintained at this level for one year. Clearly, the monkeys in the CR group showed a progressive and significant reduction in fasting insulin levels (panel A) over the course of the study. Similar changes were observed for the serum triglyceride level; however, these effects were not statistically significant (panel B). Interestingly, we observed these changes prior to the observation of any significant effects of CR on body composition, suggesting that to some extent effects of CR might be independent of such changes. These studies also showed that it might be possible to induce beneficial effects on disease risk factors even when CR is begun in older monkeys.

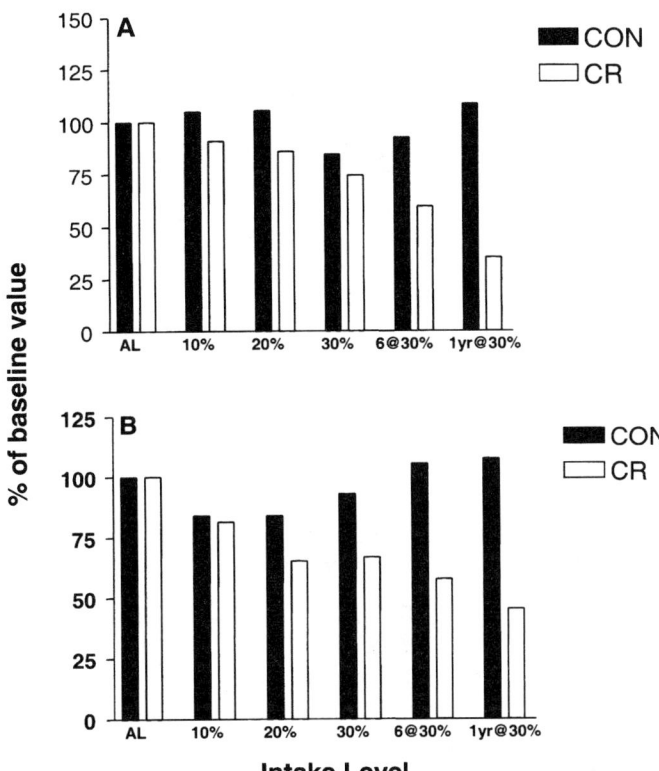

FIGURE 1. Effect of short-term caloric restriction on fasting insulin and serum triglyceride levels in old (18 yr) male rhesus monkeys. Each bar shows the average ± SEM percentage of control (baseline) levels for CON ($n = 6$) and CR ($n = 6$) monkeys at each intake level. (Adapted from Lane et al.[21])

DEVELOPING BIOMARKERS OF AGING

Rhesus monkeys (*Macaca mulatta*) are the primary species being studied in the CR experiments. The maximal life span of this species is estimated to be 40 years, with an average life span of 24 years. An effect on average and maximal life span by CR would provide conclusive evidence that CR retards aging in this model. However, given the long life span of the rhesus monkey, it is important to examine physiological markers that can be used to determine whether CR has slowed the rate of biological aging. The concept of "biomarkers of aging" remains controversial as discussed by Nakamura et al.[22,23] However, we have described a logical, statistically based strategy for evaluation and testing of candidate markers.[22,23] In brief, candidate biomarkers of aging must meet four basic criteria, including (1) a significant cross-sectional correlation with chronological age, (2) a significant longitudinal change with age that is in the same direction as the cross-sectional effect, (3) longitudinal stability of individual differences, and (4) a proportionality to species' life

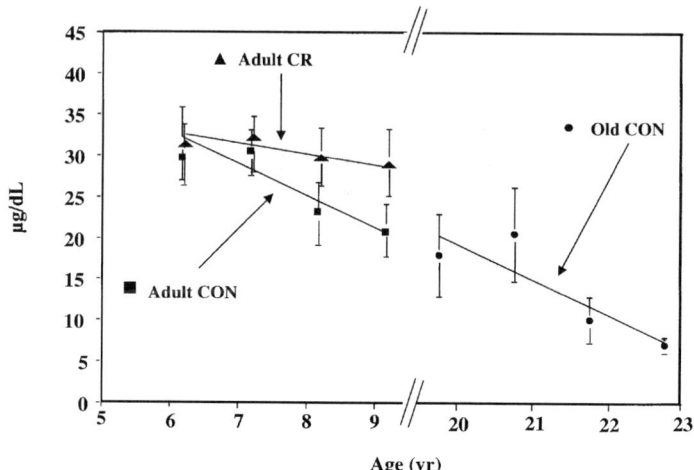

FIGURE 2. Calorie restriction slows the age-related decline in serum dehydroepiandrosterone-sulfate levels. The rate of decline as determined by the slope of the regression line was significantly less in CR monkeys compared to controls (t test; $p < 0.05$).

span. Criteria 3 and 4 require additional explanation. Criterion 3 states that when examined over time the differences between individuals for a given marker must remain stable (i.e., the rank ordering of individuals should remain mostly unchanged). This stability of interindividual variability strengthens the conclusion that changes observed are due to real physiological differences and not related to artifact. The last criterion suggests that the rate of change (criteria 1 and 2) should be proportional to the species' life span. Short-lived species must show a faster rate of change compared to longer-lived species.

We have identified several candidate markers of aging that appear to meet most of these criteria, including several blood chemistry and hematology parameters,[22,23] the accumulation of pentosidine in skin samples,[24] and serum levels of dehydroepiandrosterone-sulfate.[25] In addition to meeting all four of our primary criteria, one of these candidate markers, the decline in serum DHEAS levels, has also been shown to be responsive to CR in rhesus monkeys. FIGURE 2 shows that long-term CR slowed the rate of decline in serum DHEAS in young adult male monkeys. In this abbreviated study, serum DHEAS levels declined over 30% in control monkeys, compared to CR monkeys, the levels of which declined less than five percent. These data do not conclusively show that CR retards aging in monkeys, nor do they support that supplementation with DHEAS or other hormones prevents or retards aging. Instead, they offer proof that CR may retard postmaturational aging as measured by this index of adrenal steroid production.

Although life span data will not be available for several more years, the data presented above strongly support that CR might retard aging in long-lived species. Additional support for this conclusion comes from our preliminary studies of morbidity and mortality in our colony. TABLE 3 illustrates the effect of CR on neoplastic events in our ongoing studies. The relatively low numbers of events examined is insufficient

TABLE 3. Caloric restriction (CR) reduces neoplasia in Rhesus and squirrel monkeys

	Monkey Group	Malignant/ Premalignant	Benign	Total
Rhesus	Control	4	2	6
	CR	1	1	2
Squirrel	Control	4	0	4
	CR	0	0	0

Types of neoplasia observed

Controls
adenocarcinoma (pancreas, liver, mesentery, pelvis)
hepatocellular carcinoma
leukemia (liver, spleen, kidney, cervical lymph nodes)
seminoma (testes)
uterine leiomyoma (benign)

CR
lymphosarcoma
dermal fibroma (benign)

TABLE 4. Mortality in NIA monkeys[17]

	Rhesus		Squirrel	
Cause of death	CON[a]	CR	CON	CR
Cardio-vascular disease/diabetes	2	1	3	0
Neoplastic disease	2	1	2	0
Endome-triosis complica-tions	1	1	0	0
Kidney disease	0	1	0	0
Pneumonia	0	0	1	0
Liver failure	1	0	0	0
Total	6	4	6	0

[a] CON, control; CR, carolic restriction.

to allow statistical analyses; however, these findings clearly suggest that the number of neoplastic events is reduced in CR monkeys, compared to controls. TABLE 3 also shows that a wider variety of neoplastic events are found in controls as opposed to CR monkeys. The significance of this is not known, but this finding is consistent with a general reduction in neoplasia in CR monkeys.

TABLE 4 summarizes the effect of CR on mortality related to various disease categories in our NIA colony. It is apparent that the number of disease-related deaths is lower in CR monkeys, compared to controls. However, the relatively low numbers of deaths in our colony does not permit us to draw firm statistically based conclusions at this time.

In summary, after over a decade of research, the available data from the primate studies of CR are in good agreement with the extensive rodent literature relevant to this paradigm. We have also shown that CR reduces many risk factors of age-related disease and slows the decline in serum levels of DHEAS. The current findings do not present sufficient proof that CR slows aging in primates. However, preliminary findings related to morbidity and mortality support this notion. Conclusive proof that CR retards aging in primates, as reported extensively in rodent models, is not yet available. However, the emerging data from the ongoing studies of CR in monkeys suggest that this nutritional paradigm may be universal among species for its effects on extension of life span and retardation of aging.

ACKNOWLEDGMENTS

We would like to recognize the continuing excellence in animal care and research support from the NIA, contract, and Veterinary Resources Program staff. We also acknowledge the contributions of various collaborators who have contributed to our studies over the past decade.

REFERENCES

1. WEINDRUCH, R. & R. WALFORD. 1988. The retardation of aging and disease by dietary restriction. Charles C. Thomas. Springfield, IL.
2. YU, B.P. 1994. Modulation of aging processes by dietary restriction. CRC Press. Boca Raton, FL.
3. INGRAM, D.K. et al. 1990. Dietary restriction and aging: the initiation of a primate study. J. Gerontol. Biol. Sci. **45:** B148–63.
4. LANE, M.A. et al. 1992. Dietary Restriction in Nonhuman Primates: Progress Report on the NIA Study. Ann. N. Y. Acad. Sci. **673:** 36–45.
5. KEMNITZ, J.W. et al. 1993. Dietary restriction of adult male rhesus monkeys: Design, methodology and preliminary findings from the first year of study. J. Gerontol. Biol. Sci. **48:** B17–26.
6. LANE, M.A. et al. 1997. Beyond the rodent model: calorie restriction in rhesus monkeys. Age **20:** 39–50.
7. KEMNITZ, J.W. et al. 1994. Dietary restriction increases insulin sensitivity and lowers blood glucose in rhesus monkeys. Am. J. Physiol. (Endo. Metab.) **266:** E540–547.
8. LANE, M.A. et al. 1995. Diet restriction in rhesus monkeys lowers fasting and glucose-stimulated glucoregulatory endpoints. Am. J. Physiol. (Endo. Metab. 31) **268:** E941–E948.
9. TILMONT, E.M. et al. 1996. Calorie restriction reduces body weight, body fat, and lean mass in rhesus monkeys. Gerontologist **36** (suppl.) 19.
10. LANE, M.A. et al. 1999. Calorie restriction in nonhuman primates: effects on diabetes and cardiovascular risk. Toxicol. Sci. **52:** (Suppl.) 41–48.
11. ROTH, G.S. et al. 1993. Age-related changes in androgen levels of rhesus monkeys subjected to dietary restriction. Endocr. J. **1:** 227–234.
12. LANE, M.A. et al. 1995. Aging and food restriction alter some aspects of bone metabolism in male rhesus monkeys (*Macaca mulatta*). J. Nutr. **125** (6):1600–1610.
13. LANE, M.A. et al. 1996. Dietary restriction lowers body temperature in rhesus monkeys consistent with a postulated anti-aging mechanism in rodents. Proc. Nat. Acad. Sci. USA **93**(9): 4159–4164.
14. RAMSEY et al. Thermogenesis of adult male rhesus monkeys: results through 66 months of dietary restriction. FASEB J. **10:** A726.
15. LANE, M.A. et al. 1995. Energy balance in rhesus monkeys (*Macaca mulatta*) subjected to long-term dietary restriction. J. Gerontol. Biol. Sci. **50A:** B295–302.
16. LANE, M.A. et al. 1999. Calorie restriction in nonhuman primates: implications for age-related disease risk. J. Anti-Aging Med. **4:** 315–326.
17. ROTH, G.S. et al. 1999. Calorie restriction in primates: will it work and how will we know? J. Am. Geriatr. Soc. **47:** 896–903.

18. VERDERY, R.B. *et al.* 1997. Caloric restriction (dietary restriction without malnutrition) lowers triglyceride levels and increases HDL levels in rhesus monkeys (*Macaca mulatta*) fed low fat diets. Am. J. Physiol. **273** (Endocrinol. Metab. 36): E714–E719.
19. BURING, J.E *et al.* 1992. Decreased HDL2B and HDL3 cholesterol, apo A-I and apo A-II and increased risk of myocardial infarction. Circulation **85:** 22–29.
20. EDWARD, I.J. *et al.* 1998. Calorie restriction in rhesus monkeys reduces low density lipoprotein interaction with arterial proteoglycans. J. Gerontol. Biol. Sci. **53A** (6): B443–448.
21. LANE, M.A. *et al.* 2000. Short-term calorie restriction improves disease-related markers in older male rhesus monkeys (*Macaca mulatta*). Mech. Ageing Dev. **112**(3): 185–196.
22. NAKAMURA, E. *et al.* 1994. Evaluating measures of hematology and blood chemistry in male rhesus monkeys as biomarkers of aging. Exp. Gerontol. **29:** 151–177.
23. NAKAMURA, E. *et al.* 1998. A strategy for identifying biomarkers of aging: further evaluation of hematology and blood chemistry data from a calorie restriction study in rhesus monkeys. Exp. Gerontol. **33**(5): 421–444.
24. SELL, D.R. *et al.* 1996. 1996. Longevity and the genetic determination of glycoxidation kinetics in mammalian senescence. Proc. Natl. Acad. Sci. USA **93:** 485–490.
25. LANE, M.A. *et al.* 1997. DHEAS: A biomarker of primate aging slowed by calorie restriction. J. Clin. Endocrinol. Metab. **82**(7): 2093–2096.

Calorie Restriction Enhances the Expression of Key Metabolic Enzymes Associated with Protein Renewal during Aging

STEPHEN R. SPINDLER

Department of Biochemistry, University of California, Riverside, Riverside, California 92521, USA

ABSTRACT: Our studies show that dietary caloric restriction (CR) alters the expression of key metabolic enzymes in a manner consistent with an increased rate of extrahepatic protein turnover and renewal during aging. Of the key hepatic gluconeogenic enzyme genes affected by CR, glucose 6-phosphatase mRNA increased 1.7- and 2.3-fold in young and old CR mice. Phosphoenolpyruvate carboxykinase mRNA increased 2-fold in young mice, and its mRNA and activity increased 2.5- and 1.7-fold in old mice. These changes indicate that CR enhances the enzymatic capacity for gluconeogenesis. The carbon required for gluconeogenesis appears to be generated from peripheral protein turnover. Muscle glutamine synthetase mRNA increased 1.3- and 2.1-fold in young and old CR mice, suggesting increased disposal of nitrogen and carbon derived from protein catabolism for energy. mRNA for the key liver nitrogen disposal enzymes glutaminase, carbamyl phosphate synthase I, and tyrosine aminotransferase were increased by 2.4-, 1.8-, and 1.8-fold in CR mice. Consistent with increased hepatic nitrogen disposal, hepatic glutamine synthetase mRNA and activity were each decreased about 40% in CR mice. Together, these and our other published data suggest that CR enhances and maintains protein turnover, and thus protein renewal, into old age. These effects are likely to resist the well-documented decline in whole body protein renewal with age. Enhanced renewal may reduce the level of damaged and toxic proteins that accumulate during aging, contributing to the extension of life span by CR.

KEYWORDS: Hepatic gluconeogenesis; Nitrogen; Carbon; PEPCK; Amino acid catabolism; Oxaloacetate

INTRODUCTION

The mechanisms by which dietary caloric restriction (CR) extends life span, reduces cancer incidence, and increases the mean age of onset of age-related diseases and tumors remain the subject of both speculation and scientific inquiry.[1,2] Here we have begun to examine the hypothesis that reduction of dietary energy produces metabolic changes that play a role in the health- and life-span extending benefits of CR.

Address for correspondence: Stephen R. Spindler, Department of Biochemistry, University of California, Riverside, Riverside, California 92521. Voice: 909-787-3553; fax: 909-787-4434.
spindler@ucrac1.ucr.edu

Our studies show that CR alters the expression of key enzymes of hepatic gluconeogenesis and increases the mRNA and/or activity of key enzymes responsible for the disposal of nitrogen derived from peripheral tissue protein catabolism for energy production.[3,4] These CR-related effects oppose age-related changes in the mRNA and/or activity of many of these key metabolic enzymes.

These results are consistent with the view that CR increases the shuttling of nitrogen and carbon from the peripheral tissues to the liver, especially during the postabsorptive period following feeding. We found that CR enhances the flux of ammonia and carbon derived from extrahepatic protein turnover through the detoxification and gluconeogenic pathways of the liver. In this way, CR enhances the turnover of extrahepatic protein for energy production, extending higher levels of protein turnover into old age. These changes may result in the biochemically and physiologically younger soma associated with CR. This paper summarizes the results that support this view of CR action.

CALORIC RESTRICTION ENHANCES EXPRESSION OF KEY GLUCONEOGENIC GENES

Gluconeogenesis is the process by which the liver, and to a much more limited extent the kidney, produces glucose from substrates principally derived from protein turnover in the peripheral tissues. This process is most active between feedings, when blood insulin levels fall, blood glucagon levels rise, and glycogen stores in the liver and other tissues begin to be depleted.

Measurements of phosphoenolpyruvate carboxykinase (PEPCK) mRNA and activity are excellent indicators of the enzymatic capacity for gluconeogenesis in the liver. This enzyme catalyzes the committing step in gluconeogenesis, the conversion of oxaloacetate to PEP (FIG. 1). Committing steps in metabolic pathways are essentially irreversible. Once carbon is converted to PEP it will be converted to glucose in the liver. Because there are no known allosteric modifiers of the activity of any PEPCK isoform,[5] the activity of this enzyme is a good indicator of the enzymatic capacity available for initiating gluconeogenesis.

We found that PEPCK mRNA and activity approximately doubled in the liver of young (7 month old) and old (28 month old) mice fed a CR diet (CR mice).[4] Also, there was a small age-related decrease in PEPCK mRNA in the liver, suggesting a decline in the enzymatic capacity for *de novo* glucose production with age. A similar decrease in liver PEPCK mRNA with age has been reported in hepatocytes isolated from aging rats.[6] The mice used to generate the data described above were fasted for 23 hours before the studies were begun. This insured that the mice were well into the postabsorptive phase. Essentially all the oxaloacetate used for gluconeogenesis at that time must have been derived from peripheral tissue protein turnover. For these reasons, the results described above are consistent with the idea that aging decreases the production of glucose from amino acids derived from peripheral tissue turnover. Further, CR increased the utilization of amino acids from peripheral tissues for gluconeogenesis in the liver in young and old mice.

The results described above led us to ask, "How does feeding affect PEPCK expression in CR and control mice?" To investigate this question, CR and control mice

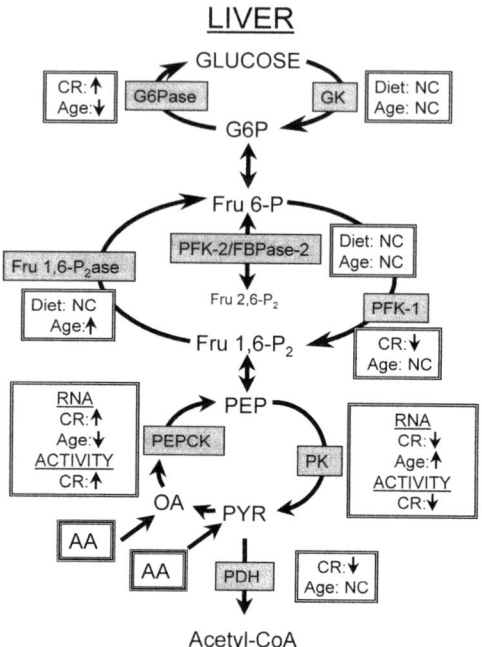

FIGURE 1. Summary of the effects of age and CR on the glycolytic and gluconeogenic pathways of the liver. Glycolytic metabolism in the liver involves three irreversible, regulated steps. Glucokinase (GK) initiates glucose metabolism by phosphorylation of C6, yielding glucose 6-phosphate (G6P). The committed step in glycolysis, and the second irreversible and regulated step, is the phosphorylation of fructose 6-phosphate (Fru 6-P) by phosphofructokinase-1 (PFK-1) to produce fructose 1,6-bisphosphate (Fru 1,6-P_2). The third irreversible step controls the outflow of the pathway. Phosphoenolpyruvate (PEP) and ADP are used by pyruvate kinase (PK) to produce pyruvate (PYR) and ATP. Pyruvate dehydrogenase (PDH) oxidatively decarboxylates pyruvate to form acetyl-CoA. Phosphoenolpyruvate carboxykinase (PEPCK) catalyzes the first committed step in gluconeogenesis. The main non-carbohydrate precursors for gluconeogenesis are amino acids from the diet, and from muscle protein breakdown. Other organs also contribute amino acids, but muscle is the major source. Most of these amino acids are converted to oxaloacetate (OA), which is metabolized to PEP by PEPCK. In the second regulated and essentially irreversible step in gluconeogenesis, fructose 1,6-bisphosphatase (Fru 1,6-P_2ase) catalyzes the formation of Fru 6-P from Fru 1,6-P_2. Finally, in the third essentially irreversible reaction of gluconeogenesis, glucose is formed by the hydrolysis of G6P in a reaction catalyzed by glucose 6-phosphatase (G6Pase). Substrates are not boxed, enzyme names are in shaded boxes, summaries of experimental results are in double-bordered boxes, and amino acids are indicated by *AA* in triple-bordered boxes. A down or up arrow indicates a general decrease or increase in the expression of the gene in CR mice. Arrows after *Age* indicate the general results for aged animals in both dietary groups. NC, no change. (Reproduced with permission from Dhahbi *et al.*[4])

were fasted for approximately 24 hours and fed their normal daily ration of food. PEPCK mRNA was reduced 1.5 hours after feeding in both control and CR mice. However, the mRNA increased rapidly by 5 hours after feeding to significantly higher levels in the CR mice.[3] It remained more elevated in these mice until 24 hours af-

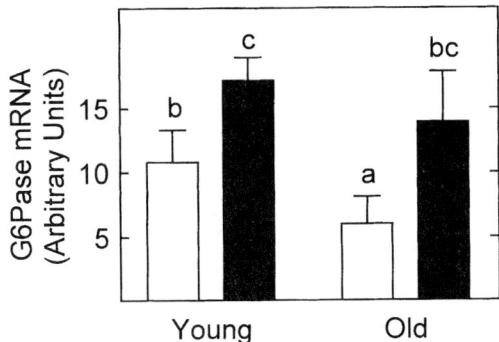

FIGURE 2. Effects of age and diet on G6Pase mRNA levels in mouse liver. G6Pase mRNA levels in the liver of young and old, control (*open bars*) and CR (*closed bars*) mice were determined ($n = 6$ mice for each dietary regimen and age group). Results are expressed as means ± SD. Message levels were assessed by 2-factor ANOVA with age and diet as factors. The significance of differences between any two groups was tested by Tukey's pairwise comparisons. Bars labeled at the top with different letters are statistically different ($p < 0.05$). (Reproduced with permission from Dhahbi et al.[4])

ter feeding. The activity of the enzyme roughly paralleled the response of PEPCK mRNA to CR and feeding.[3]

Glucose-6-phosphatase catalyzes the terminal step in hepatic glucose production, the hydrolysis of glucose 6-phosphate to glucose and inorganic phosphate (FIG. 1). This step leads to the release of glucose from the liver into the circulation when blood glucose levels would otherwise fall. We found that CR increased hepatic G6Pase mRNA abundance 1.6-fold and 2.3-fold in young and old mice, respectively (FIG. 2).[4]

G6Pase mRNA abundance was higher in CR mice during a significant part of the day.[3] The response of G6Pase mRNA to feeding was very different in CR and control mice. Feeding led to a rapid decrease in G6Pase mRNA in control mice. By contrast, feeding led to a rapid increase in G6Pase mRNA in CR mice.

We found that glycogen was deposited at the same rate and to the same final extent in control and CR mice. Therefore, the results from our G6Pase studies are consistent with the idea that the gluconeogenic capacity of CR animals remains higher throughout the day, except immediately after feeding. These data strongly suggest that more carbon from amino acid turnover in peripheral tissues is converted to glucose by the liver of CR mice. Further, CR appears to prevent an age-related decrease in this process.

CHANGES IN MUSCLE GENE EXPRESSION INDICATE THAT CALORIC RESTRICTION INCREASES AMINO ACID CATABOLISM

Our investigation of PEPCK expression in muscle provided further evidence of the influence of CR on amino acid catabolism in muscle. Initial studies were performed using mice fasted for approximately 24 hours. After this period of fasting,

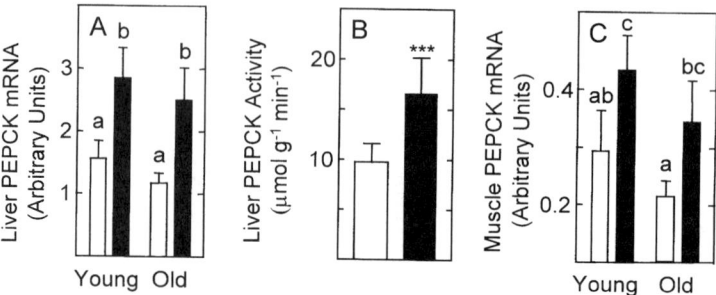

FIGURE 3. Effects of age and diet on PEPCK mRNA and activity. Liver and muscle PEPCK mRNA and liver PEPCK activity were quantified. *Panel A:* PEPCK mRNA abundance in the liver of young and old, control (*open bars*) and CR (*closed bars*) mice (6 animals from each dietary regimen for each age group). *Panel B:* liver PEPCK activity in old control and CR mice ($n = 8$ mice of each dietary group). Student's unpaired t test was used to analyze the effect of CR on hepatic PEPCK in this group of mice. Three asterisks indicate that the results are very highly significant ($p < 0.001$). *Panel C:* PEPCK mRNA levels in mixed hind leg and back muscle of individual mice from the group in *panel A*. Statistical analysis of the effects of age and diet were as in FIG. 2. The significance of differences between any two groups was tested by Tukey's pairwise comparisons. Bars labeled at the top with different letters are statistically different ($p < 0.05$). (Reproduced with permission from Dhahbi *et al.*[4])

mice are far into the postabsorptive state. At this time, the major source of extrahepatic substrates for gluconeogenesis is amino acids derived from muscle.[7] PEPCK is part of the alanine biosynthetic pathway in muscle. Carbon for alanine biosynthesis is derived primarily from the degradation of branched-chain amino acids. The alanine synthesized from this degradation is transported through the blood to the liver, where it serves as a gluconeogenic precursor.

PEPCK mRNA was significantly elevated in the muscle of young and old CR mice (FIG. 3C). This result suggests that CR is accompanied by increased catabolism of branched chain amino acids derived from turnover of peripheral tissue protein. Because turnover of muscle protein for energy production is accompanied by turnover of protein from most other organs, these data further support the idea that CR enhances whole body protein turnover.

During the postabsorptive state, muscle and other tissues use amino acids derived from protein turnover to generate energy via the TCA cycle. This amino acid catabolism is initiated in the muscle by two enzymatic steps, collectively called the transdeamination reaction (FIG. 4). Transdeamination leads to the liberation of the amino nitrogen as ammonia. Because of its extreme toxicity, this ammonia is transferred to glutamate by glutamine synthetase (GS), producing glutamine. Glutamine serves to transfer both carbon and a nitrogen to the liver. The GS reaction is the only enzymatic reaction specific to the formation of glutamine in muscle.[8]

CR decreased muscle GS mRNA in both young and old mice.[4] Because the abundance of GS mRNA declined with age in control mice, the stimulation of GS mRNA levels by CR was greatest in old mice, where it more than doubled. Thus, peripheral

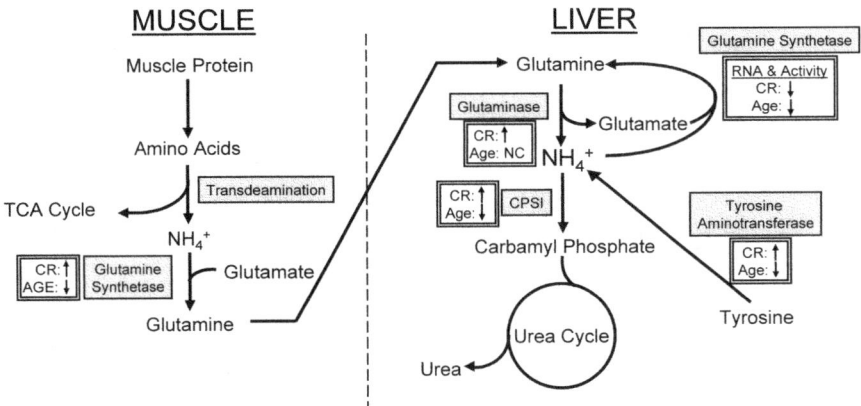

FIGURE 4. Summary of the effects of age and diet on muscle and liver nitrogen metabolism. Transdeamination of amino acids produces tricarboxylic acid cycle intermediates and ammonia in muscle. Glutamine synthetase synthesizes glutamine from glutamate and ammonia. Glutamine is transported to the liver where glutaminase releases the ammonia, regenerating glutamate. CPSI converts this ammonia to carbamyl phosphate, which is converted to urea in the uric cycle. The amino group of excess tyrosine is released by TAT as ammonia, which is also detoxified beginning with the action of CPSI. In the FIGURE, substrates are not boxed, enzyme names are in shaded boxes, and summaries of experimental results are in double-bordered boxes. A down or up arrow indicates a general decrease or increase in expression of the gene in CR mice. Arrows after "Age" indicate general results for aged animals in both dietary groups. NC is no change. (Reproduced with permission from Dhahbi et al.[4])

tissues of CR mice appear to have a greater capacity for the biosynthesis of glutamine, and the transfer of this carbon and nitrogen to the liver (FIG. 4).

LIVER GENE EXPRESSION INDICATES CALORIC RESTRICTION INCREASES PERIPHERAL TISSUE AMINO ACID CATABOLISM

In the liver, CR enhances the enzymatic capacity for catabolism of glutamine derived from extrahepatic protein turnover. The nitrogen and carbon originating from muscle protein catabolism can be returned to the glutamine pool in pericentral hepatocytes through the action of GS (FIG. 4).[9] CR significantly reduces the level of GS activity and mRNA in the liver (FIG. 5A and B). Further, feeding had little effect on the levels of GS mRNA and activity.[3] Thus, synthesis of glutamine in the liver is reduced by CR, indicating that there is a greater flux of carbon from peripheral tissues to the liver for gluconeogenesis in CR animals.

We found further evidence that CR increases the shuttling of nitrogen and carbon to the liver from the peripheral tissues. The hepatic catabolism of glutamine is initiated by glutaminase.[9] Glutaminase produces glutamate and ammonia from glutamine (FIG. 4). Because hepatic glutamine synthase activity is reduced in CR mice, the nitrogen derived from this reaction will be channeled into the disposal pathway. Glutaminase mRNA was more than twice control levels in young and old

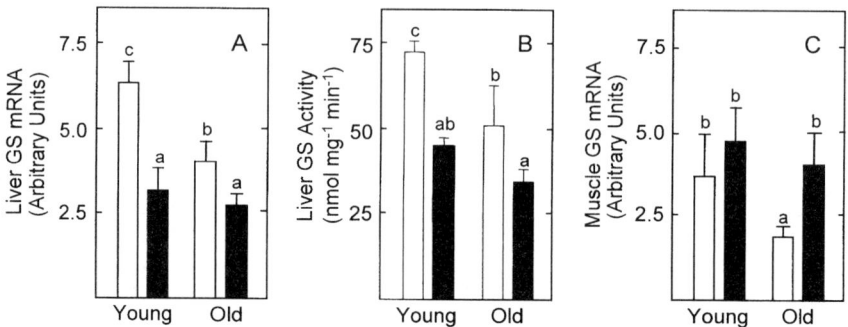

FIGURE 5. Effects of age and diet on GS mRNA and activity. Quantitation of liver GS mRNA (*panel A*), liver GS activity (*panel B*), and muscle GS mRNA (*panel C*) of young and old, control (*open bars*) and CR (*closed bars*) mice (*n* = 6 mice for each dietary regimen and age group). Statistical analysis of the effects of age and diet were as in FIG. 2. (Reproduced with permission from Dhahbi *et al*.[4])

CR mice.[4] Glutaminase mRNA levels closely reflect the levels of glutaminase activity.[10,11] Therefore, this CR-related increase in hepatic mRNA very likely leads to a congruent increase in glutaminase activity.

Ammonia production by glutaminase is coupled to urea synthesis by the enzyme carbamyl phosphate synthase I (CPSI). CPSI mRNA levels in young and old CR mice were twice that of control mice.[4] We have previously shown that the level of CPSI mRNA in CR mice reflects the level of CPSI protein and activity.[12] There was an ~20% decrease in CPSI mRNA with age, indicating that there is an age-related decrease in CPSI mRNA and activity. Together these data are further indications that CR leads to enhanced carbon flux to the liver from amino acid degradation in the peripheral tissues.

This amino acid degradation extends to tyrosine, an amino acid that requires a liver-specific enzyme, tyrosine amino transferase (TAT), for catabolism. TAT degradation of tyrosine is well-known to provide ketogenic and gluconeogenic substrates to the liver when glucose is limiting and amino acids are used as a major source of energy. TAT mRNA in fasting CR mice was approximately double the level in control mice.[3] Aging decreased TAT mRNA in the liver by an average of 37%, whereas CR returned it to youthful levels.

CONCLUSIONS AND DISCUSSION

The results described here are best understood in the context of feeding and the postabsorptive period. Feeding induces a wave of protein biosynthetic activity in cells. For several hours after feeding, the blood levels of substrates and insulin are at their highest. This combination stimulates substrate uptake and protein synthesis. In CR mice, this period is brief due to the rapid rise and fall of blood insulin and substrates.[3] As the animal enters the postabsorptive phase, insulin and substrate levels fall. Energy is produced during this time through the catabolism of glycogen, lipids, and extrahepatic protein, especially muscle protein.

Our studies of the expression of the muscle and liver enzymes indicate that CR mice have an enhanced capacity for mobilizing and transporting carbon and nitrogen products of muscle protein catabolism to the liver. CR mice also have enhanced hepatic capacity for the biosynthesis of glucose from this carbon, and for the detoxification of this nitrogen.

Because the muscles and tissues of the CR and control mice we studied are approximately at steady state (their weights are approximately constant over a period of months), it is clear that turnover of extrahepatic tissues is balanced by synthetic activity. Therefore, it seems clear that after feeding, there is a brief but intense period of biosynthesis in CR mice, followed by a higher level of protein degradation for energy generation.

Thus, probably through the effects of CR on insulin and substrate availability, CR appears to drive alternating periods of intense biosynthesis and turnover that are approximately balanced in their net effects on body weight. In this way CR may enhance protein renewal in mice of all ages, resisting the well-documented decline in peripheral tissue protein turnover with age. This effect on protein renewal may be one of the mechanisms by which CR resists the accumulation of oxidized, racemized, and damaged amino acids in proteins. This may resist the well-documented age-related accumulation of inactive and cross-linked proteins.[13,14] Enhanced protein renewal may be one of the ways CR extends life span and resists the onset of age-related diseases.

REFERENCES

1. WEINDRUCH, R. & R.L. WALFORD. 1982. Dietary restriction in mice beginning at 1 year of age: effects on life-span and spontaneous cancer incidence. Science **215:** 1415–1418.
2. WEINDRUCH, R. & R.L. WALFORD. 1988. The Retardation of Aging and Disease by Dietary Restriction. Charles C. Thomas. Springfield, IL.
3. DHAHBI, J.M., P.L. MOTE, J. WINGO, B.C. ROWLEY, S.X. CAO, R. WALFORD & S.R. SPINDLER. Calorie restriction alters the response of key metabolic enzyme genes. Mech Ageing Dev. In press.
4. DHAHBI, J.M., P.L. MOTE, J. WINGO, J.B. TILLMAN, R.L. WALFORD & S.R. SPINDLER. 1999. Calories and aging alter gene expression for gluconeogenic, glycolytic, and nitrogen-metabolizing enzymes. Am. J. Physiol. **277:** E352–E360.
5. HANSON, R.W. & L. RESHEF. 1997. Regulation of phosphoenolpyruvate carboxykinase (GTP) gene. Annu. Rev. Biochem. **66:** 581–611.
6. WIMONWATWATEE, T., A.R. HEYDARI, W.T. WU & A. RICHARDSON. 1994. Effect of age on the expression of phosphoenolpyruvate carboxykinase in rat liver. Am. J. Physiol. **267:** G201–G204.
7. FELIG, P. 1975. Amino acid metabolism in man. Annu. Rev. Biochem. **44:** 933–955.
8. KING, P.A., L. GOLDSTEIN & E.A. NEWSHOLME, 1983. Glutamine synthetase activity of muscle in acidosis. Biochem. J. **216:** 523–525.
9. MEIJER, A.J., W.H. LAMER & R.A. CHAMULEAU. 1990. Nitrogen metabolism and ornithine cycle function. Physiol. Rev. **70:** 701–748.
10. WATFORD, M., N. VINCENT, Z. ZHAN, J. FANNELLI, T. KOWALSKI & Z. KOVACEVIC. 1994. Transcriptional control of rat hepatic glutaminase expression by dietary protein level and starvation. J. Nutr. **124:** 493–499.
11. ZHAN, Z., N.C. VINCENT & M. WATFORD. 1994. Transcriptional regulation of the hepatic glutaminase gene in the streptozotocin-diabetic rat. Int. J. Biochem. **26:** 263–268.

12. TILLMAN, J.B., J.M. DHAHBI, P.L. MOTE, R.L. WALFORD & S.R. SPINDLER. 1996. Dietary calorie restriction in mice induces carbamyl phosphate synthetase I gene transcription tissue specifically. J. Biol. Chem. **271:** 3500–3506.
13. STADTMAN, E.R. 1992. Protein oxidation and aging. Science **257:** 1220–1224.
14. VAN REMMEN, H., W.F. WARD, R.V. SABIA & A. RICHARDSON. 1995. Gene expression and protein degradation. *In* Handbook of Physiology. Section **11:** Aging, E.J. MASORO, Ed.: 171–234. Oxford University Press. New York.

Caloric Restriction in Primates and Relevance to Humans

GEORGE S. ROTH, DONALD K. INGRAM, AND MARK A. LANE

Laboratory of Neurosciences, Gerontology Research Center, National Institute on Aging, National Institutes of Health, Baltimore, Maryland 21224, USA

ABSTRACT: Dietary caloric restriction (CR) is the *only* intervention conclusively and reproducibly shown to slow aging and maintain health and vitality in mammals. Although this paradigm has been known for over 60 years, its precise biological mechanisms and applicability to humans remain unknown. We began addressing the latter question in 1987 with the first controlled study of CR in primates (rhesus and squirrel monkeys, which are evolutionarily much closer to humans than the rodents most frequently employed in CR studies). To date, our results strongly suggest that the same beneficial "antiaging" and/or "antidisease" effects observed in CR rodents also occur in primates. These include lower plasma insulin levels and greater sensitivity; lower body temperatures; reduced cholesterol, triglycerides, blood pressure, and arterial stiffness; elevated HDL; and slower age-related decline in circulating levels of DHEAS. Collectively, these biomarkers suggest that CR primates will be less likely to incur diabetes, cardiovascular problems, and other age-related diseases and may in fact be aging more slowly than fully fed counterparts.

Despite these very encouraging results, it is unlikely that most humans would be willing to maintain a 30% reduced diet for the bulk of their adult life span, even if it meant more healthy years. For this reason, we have begun to explore CR mimetics, agents that might elicit the same beneficial effects as CR, *without* the necessity of dieting. Our initial studies have focused on 2-deoxyglucose (2DG), a sugar analogue with a limited metabolism that actually reduces glucose/energy flux without decreasing food intake in rats. In a six-month pilot study, 2DG lowered plasma insulin and body temperature in a manner analagous to that of CR. Thus, metabolic effects that mediate the CR mechanism can be attained pharmacologically. Doses were titrated to eliminate toxicity; a long-term longevity study is now under way. In addition, data from other laboratories suggest that at least some of the same physiological/metabolic end points that are associated with the beneficial effects of underfeeding may be obtained from other potential CR mimetic agents, some naturally occurring in food products. Much work remains to be done, but taken together, our successful results with CR in primates and 2DG administration to rats suggest that it may indeed be possible to obtain the health- and longevity-promoting effects of the former intervention without actually decreasing food intake.

KEYWORDS: Caloric Restriction; Primates; Humans

Address for correspondence: Dr. George S. Roth, Laboratory of Neurosciences, Gerontology Research Center, National Institute on Aging, National Institutes of Health, 5600 Nathan Shock Drive, Baltimore, MD 21224. Voice: 410-558-8178; fax: 410-858-8323.

geor@vax.grc.nia.nih.gov

INTRODUCTION

It has been known for over six decades that reduced caloric intake is the only conclusive and reproducible intervention shown to retard aging and extend healthy life span in mammals.[1] Dietary caloric restriction (CR) maintains physiological and behavioral functions and delays and reduces the severity of many age-related diseases in a variety of animal models.[2] These range from invertebrates to primates; data from the latter are recently beginning to suggest strong parallels between beneficial CR effects in experimental rodents and monkeys.[3]

The first large-scale controlled study of CR in primates was initiated by us at the National Institute on Aging in 1987.[4] Major objectives included determination of whether this intervention could indeed slow aging and maintain health and vitality in rhesus and squirrel monkeys in a manner analogous to its well-documented effects in rodents and, by inference, might be applicable to humans. Results from this and similar projects, subsequently begun at other institutions, bode well for the possibility that certain indices of aging and age-associated diseases may indeed be diminished by CR in humans as well.[5] These include a slower age-related decline in circulating levels of the steroid hormone dehydroepiandrosterone sulfate (DHEAS); lower plasma concentrations of glucose, insulin, cholesterol, and triglycerides; lower systolic and diastolic blood pressure as well as arterial stiffness; and increases in insulin sensitvity and levels of HDL2b.[3,5] Taken together, these findings suggest that CR primates will be less likely to contract diabetes, cardiovascular disease, cancer, and other pathologies of aging than fully fed counterparts. Thus, opportunities for an entire new area of dietary therapeutic intervention might eventually be available.

In addition, CR monkeys have lower body temperatures and initially reduced metabolic rates, symptomatic of a fundamental shift from a growth and reproductive strategy to a life-maintenance mode.[6] These physiological adaptations are also analogous to those elicited by CR in rodents, whose protective mechanisms have been enhanced, and median and maximal life spans extended.[1,2] Such alterations are undoubtedly linked with the "antidisease" effects as well and suggest possible biological mechanisms by which beneficial effects might be exerted.

Unfortunately, it is very doubtful that most humans would be willing to adopt a CR lifestyle, even with the promise of an extended, healthy life span. Difficulties with compliance and problems associated with so-called yo-yo and fad dieting are leading examples of practical arguments against CR for people. Moreover, enjoyment of food is a positive, life quality–enriching experience for most of us and renders an "appetite suppressant" strategy equally unpalatable. Thus, we have chosen to explore potential "CR mimetics" as a means of achieving the beneficial effects of restriction *without* dieting or suppressing appetite.

PHYSIOLOGICAL AND METABOLIC HALLMARKS OF CR IN RODENTS AND PRIMATES

TABLE 1 compares some of the most robust physiological and metabolic indices of the CR state in rodents and primates. Although lower plasma insulin concentrations and body temperature are probably the most reproducible of these, all are use-

TABLE 1. Summary of findings from the NIA Study of Calorie Restriction in Nonhuman Primates

Finding	Reference	Agrees with rodent data
▼ Body weight	Lane et al., J. Nutr. **125**: 1600	yes
▼ Fat and lean mass	Lane et al., Am. J. Physiol. **31**: E941	yes
▼ Trunk:leg fat radio	DeAngelis et al., Gerontologist (Oct. 98)**	NR
▼ Time to sexual maturity	Roth et al., Endocrine J. **1**: 227	yes
▼ Time to skeletal maturity	Lane et al., J. Nutr. **125**: 1600	yes
▼ Fasting glucose/insulin	Lane et al., Am. J. Physiol. **31**: E942	yes
▲ Insulin sensitivity	DeAngelis et al., Gerontologist (Oct. 98)**	NR
▼ Metabolic rate (short-term)	Lane et al., Proc. Natl. Acad. Sci. USA **93**: 4159	yes
◆ Metabolic rate (long-term)	Lane et al., J. Gerontol. Biol. Sci. **50A**: B295	yes
▼ Body temperature	Lane et al., Proc. Natl. Acad. Sci. USA **93**: 4159	yes
◆ or ▼ Locomotion	Weed et al., Physiol. Behav **62** (1): 97	yes
▼ Serum triglycerides	Verdery et al., Am. J. Physiol. **36**: E 714	yes
▲ Serum HDL 2B	Verdery et al., Am. J. Physiol. **36**: E 714	yes
▼ IGF-1/growth hormone	Cocchi et al., Neuroends. Lett **17**: 181	yes
▼ IL-6	Lane et al., J. Nutr. **125**: 1600	yes
◆ Testosterone	Unpublished	NR
◆ Estradiol, LH, FSH, prog	Handy et al., Gerontologist (Oct. 98)**	NR
◆ Wound closure rate	Roth et al., Gerontol. Biol. Sci. **52A**: B98	yes
◆ Fibroblast clonal proliferation	Pendergrass et al., J. Cell. Physiol. (in press)	?
◆ β-Gal senescent cells	Pendergrass et al., J. Cell. Physiol. (in press)	?
▼ Rate of decline in DHEAS	Lane et al., J. Clin. Endocrinol. Metb. **82** (7): 2093	?
▼ Lymphocyte number	Weindruch et al., Aging **9**(4): 304	yes
◆ Lymphocyte calcium response	Grossman et al., J. Cell Physiol. **162**: 298	no

NOTE: ▼ decreased; ▲ increased; ◆ no effect or change; NR, not reported; ** abstract.

ful and can serve as a basis for evaluating the short-term effects of potential CR mimetics. Obviously, it is too early to ascertain whether life span is extended by CR in primates, although preliminary morbidity and mortality data exhibit very promising trends in this direction.[5] Similarly, while longevity experiments with CR mimetics in rodents are quite feasible, much faster suggestive evidence as to efficacy may be obtained from shorter-term physiological assessments.

We have, therefore, sought to establish a battery of such measures in order to screen candidate CR mimetics. Our strategy is to combine and compare data from our own studies as well as the existing literature to determine what agents might be the most promising. In light of the critical relationship between glucoregulation, energy metabolism, and the beneficial effects of CR in both rodents and primates (TABLE 1), we have chosen to explore compounds that exert their initial biological effects at these levels.

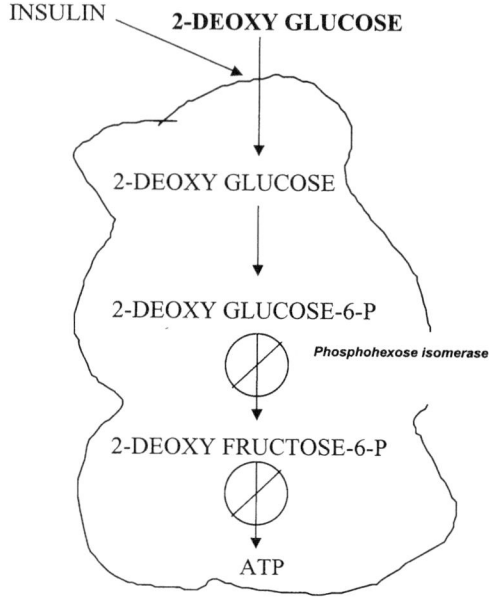

FIGURE 1. Effects of 2-deoxyglucose on cellular glucose metabolism. 2-Deoxyglucose enters the cell and is phosphorylated but is not metabolized further. 2-Deoxyglucose phosphate inhibits further metabolism of native glucose molecules.

2-DEOXYGLUCOSE—THE FIRST CANDIDATE

A substantial body of data on the physiological and metabolic effects of the glucose analogue 2-deoxyglucose (2DG) has been compiled over the last two decades. This sugar has been employed for a variety of purposes, ranging from tracing native glucose molecule transport and processing to actually blocking energy metabolism. FIGURE 1 shows a schematic of the effects of 2DG on glucose metabolism. Its primary effect is to serve as an extremely strong competitor of the enzyme phosphohexose isomerase, which converts glucose-6-phosphate to fructose-6-phosphate. As a consequence, the former phosphate builds up and is eventually excreted, while metabolism of native glucose is greatly reduced. Because of this latter effect, 2DG is quite toxic at higher concentrations.

Despite this potential toxicity, however, 2DG at lower dosages and/or in very short-term experiments has been shown to elicit some of the very same physiological and metabolic effects as CR. These include lowering body temperature[7] and reducing tumor formation[8] in rats, and elevating circulating glucocorticoid hormone concentrations in humans.[9] It was, therefore, decided to examine the longer-term effects of various concentrations of 2DG administered in chow on several metabolic hallmarks of CR in rats. TABLE 2 illustrates the design of this experiment.[10]

TABLE 2. Experimental design: 2-deoxy glucose treatment

Group	n	Treatment
Ad lib	20	Ad lib
Pair-fed	20	Pair-fed to lowest intake
0.2%	20	0.2% 2-dg in diet
0.4%	20	0.4% 2-dg in diet
0.6%	20	0.6% 2-dg in diet

EFFECTS OF SIX-MONTH 2DG ADMINISTRATION TO FISCHER RATS

The highest dose of 2DG did, indeed, prove to be toxic, as four rats in that group died in the first five weeks of the study.[10] Unfortunately, the cause of death could not be determined, although unidentifiable vacuolar inclusions were noted in some 2DG-treated animals. Since the 0.6% dose appeared to define the lower limits of the toxicity range, it was decided to administer this concentration of 2DG only every other week, leaving this experimental group untreated on alternate weeks. This strategy proved to be successful, as no further deaths occurred.

Food intake was substantively affected by 2DG only in the first month or two, as the animals adapted to the taste of the chow (mostly at the highest dose, reflecting also the toxicity discussed above).[10] Consumption by most animals was essentially identical to that of the *ad libitum* control group during the remainder of the study. Thus, the objective of maintaining nonrestricted dietary intake was indeed achieved. FIGURE 2 shows the corresponding effect of 2DG on body weight. In general, rats at the two highest concentrations exhibited slight reductions in weight over the entire six months of the experiment, in the 5–10% range.[10] Since food consumption was not significantly altered, these decreases are consistent with a CR mimetic action by the sugar analogue.

Having satisfied requirements for lack of toxicity, maintenance of food intake, and weight control, it became important to assess some metabolic indices in the experimental rats. FIGURE 3 depicts body temperature over the course of the study. Although a fair amount of variability is apparent over the relatively narrow range of physiological temperature, animals in the 0.4% and 0.6% groups did indeed exhibit reductions during most of the experiment.[10] Thus, one important metabolic index of the CR state was achieved by 2DG administration.

A consistent, but statistically nonsignificant, trend toward lower plasma glucose levels relative to controls (on the order of 5%) was also observed in the 2DG groups at 13 and 24 weeks.[10] These results are illustrated in FIGURE 4. Although reductions in blood sugar are often observed in CR rodents and primates, a much more robust metabolic hallmark is decreased insulin concentration (TABLE 1).[3,5] FIGURE 4 also shows the latter, which is reduced by about 30%, comparable to most CR studies, in the 0.4% group of rats.[10]

Taken together, the above findings demonstrated for the first time that key physiological effects of CR could indeed be achieved by long-term administration of low concentrations of 2DG to rats, *without* significantly affecting food intake. Of course, these results beg the obvious question of whether these same experimental animals

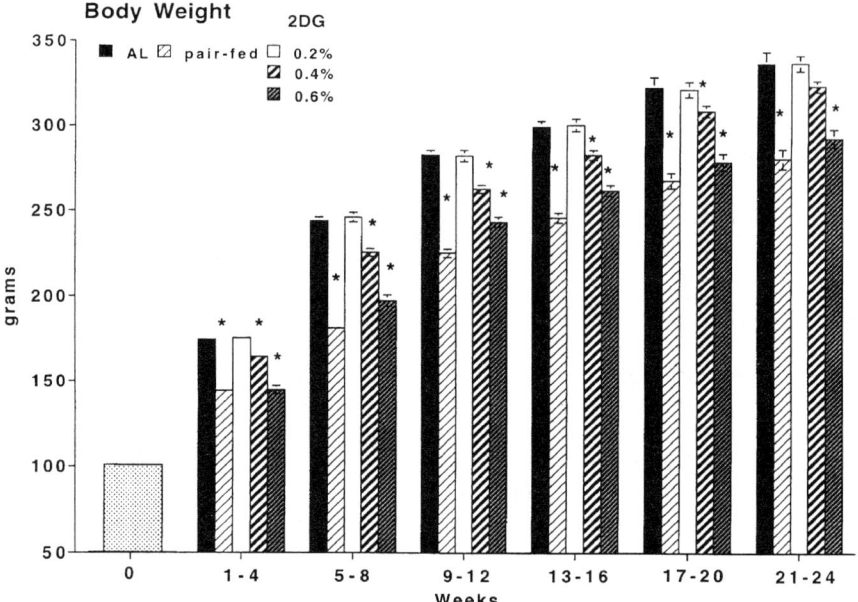

FIGURE 2. Effect of 2-deoxyglucose on body weight in Fischer-344 rats. Values are means ± standard errors. Details can be obtained from Reference 10.

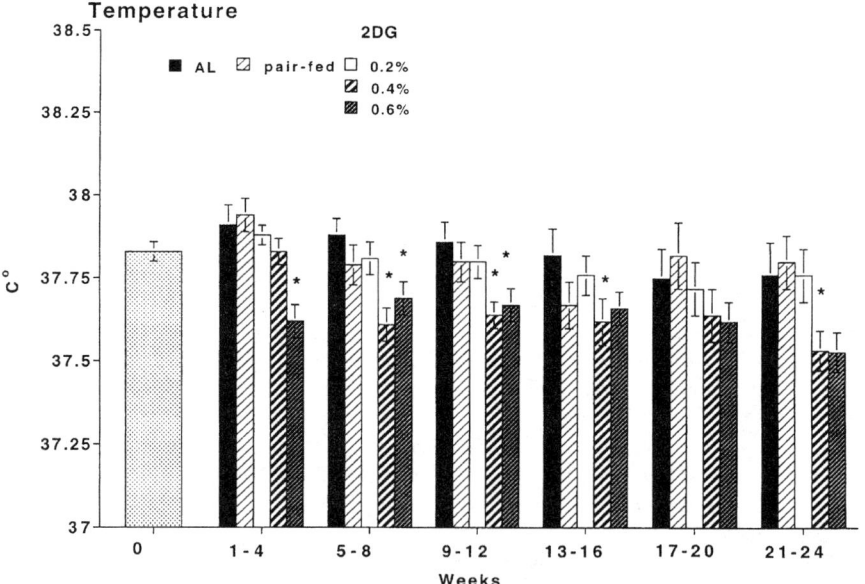

FIGURE 3. Effect of 2-deoxyglucose on temperature in Fischer-344 rats. Experimental design and data presentation are as for FIGURE 3, and details are in Reference 10.

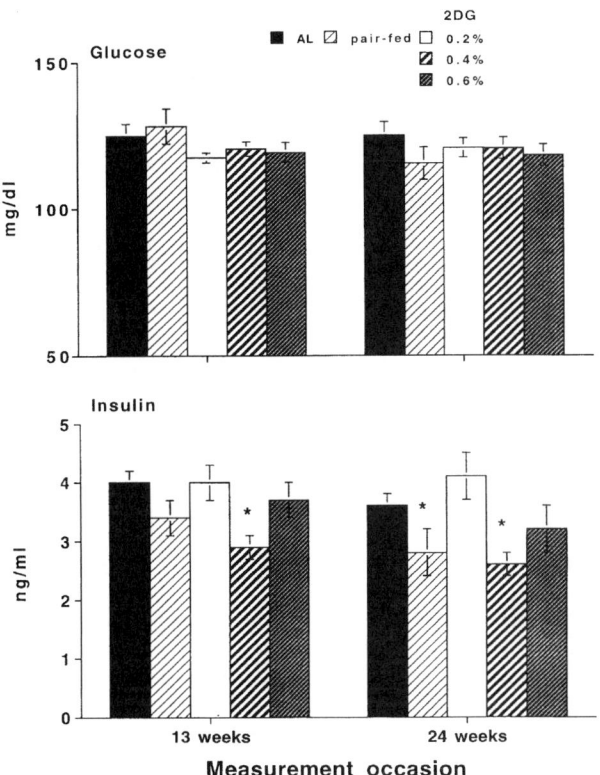

FIGURE 4. Effects of 2-deoxyglucose on plasma glucose and insulin levels in Fischer-344 rats. Details are as for FIGURES 2 and 3.

will actually age at a slower rate, incur the diseases of aging later and to a lesser extent, and live longer than *ad libitum*–fed control counterparts. The latter experiment is currently under way, having been initiated in December of 1999 with 140 additional rats and employing 2DG dosages of 0.3% and 0.4%. Various physiological/metabolic as well as extensive pathological assessments will be performed. It will take another two to three years to determine whether the sugar analogue can indeed be employed as a true CR mimetic.

OTHER POTENTIAL CR MIMETIC STRATEGIES

If the 2DG-treated rats in the ongoing longevity study do actually outlive their controls, an entire new research area will be opened, with 2DG as the "lead" compound. Of course, a wider range between the toxic and the beneficial effects of potential CR mimetic agents would be highly desirable, if not essential, if this strategy is ever to be applied to humans. Consequently, whether or not the 2DG animals ex-

TABLE 3. Inhibitory effects of gymnemoside b and gymnemic acids on the increase in serum glucose of oral glucose-loaded rats

	Increase in serum glucose (mg/dL) one half hour after oral glucose
Control	77.4 ± 7.6
Gymnemic bacid	61.2 ± 7.6
Control	62.9 ± 4.3
Gymnemic acid III	46.3 ± 6.9
Control	65.5 ± 4.7
Gymnemic acid V	41.9 ± 6.1
Control	66.9 ± 2.3
Gymnemic acid VII	51.5 ± 5.2

NOTE: Adapted from Yoshikawa et al., 1997, Clin. Pharm. Bull. **45:** 1671.

hibit increased health, vitality, and longevity, other such compounds must be identified and evaluated.

In fact, a fairly large literature (both scientific and folk/popular) exists in the area of medicinals that might elicit some of the same beneficial effects as CR. An exhaustive treatise is well beyond the scope of the present review, but a few illustrative examples can provide some perspective with regard to the possibilities.

Gymnema Sylvestre and Antidiabetics

The leaves of the Asian plant *Gymnema sylvestre*, have long been employed as a folk remedy for diabetes and its related symptoms.[11] Called "gur-mar" or "gurmara," which means "sugar destroyer" in Hindi, *Gymnema* has played an active role in Ayurvedic medicine for nearly three millenia.[12] More recently, it has been marketed as a health food/herbal medicine in Japan, where it is purported to be effective against both diabetes and obesity.[11] Although the plant and its extracts appear to exert multiple biological effects, including reducing the perception of sweetness,[13] the end point most relevant to CR mimicry is probably a reduction in blood sugar concentrations, especially following an oral glucose load.[11]

Matsuda and his colleagues have identified a number of active ingredients, falling into a broad class of triterpines called gymnemosides as well as some gymnemic acids, that elicit this particular response.[11] TABLE 3 is an adaptation of their results from the most effective of these agents, showing reductions of approximately 20 to 30% in serum glucose concentrations 30 minutes after oral administration of 100 mg per kg of body weight. The effect appears to be exerted at the level of glucose adsorption through the intestine, far removed from that of 2DG, which inhibits an enzyme early in the process of glucose metabolism. Nevertheless, lowering of serum glucose concentrations would qualify as a CR mimetic effect. Of course, a more reproducible end point would be a reduction in circulating insulin levels, but unfortunately this effect was not examined.[11]

These results do suggest, however, that certain other antidiabetic agents might mimic CR by lowering insulin concentrations and/or sensitizing target cells and tissues to its effects. A number of such agents are currently available, but again for present purposes a few examples will suffice to demonstrate possible research opportunities. Two classes of compounds with specific effects on both lipid and carbohydrate metabolism are at present prominent in this category. These are the biguanides and the thiazolidinediones. At least one study has already reported that a member of the former group, phenformin, extends both mean and maximal life span in mice.[14] Unfortunately, however, the mouse strain employed, C3H/Sn, is cancer prone, with a mean life span of only 450 days. Furthermore, food intake was not determined, so it is uncertain how much of the effect might be attributable to appetite suppression. Whether similar potential antiaging effects can be achieved with longer-lived rodent strains remains to be determined.

Another biguanide, metformin, is more commonly employed clinically. Although these agents have been available for nearly 30 years, their exact mechanism(s) of action is still uncertain. Their biological effects include lowering blood lipids, reducing gluconeogenesis (the opposite of CR), and decreasing glucose adsorption through the intestine (like the gymnemosides).[15] Their most consistent effect, however, seems to be the facilitation of glucose entry into cells,[15,16] which results in increased insulin sensitivity (like CR). The thiazolidinedione that has received the most recent attention is troglitizone. Its precise effects are even less well understood than those of the biguanides. However, it does appear to regulate certain genes involved in both lipid and carbohydrate metabolism and, like the biguanides, increases glucose entry into cells.[17] Thus, antidiabetics may indeed offer at least some of the beneficial effects of CR, probably without the same degree of restriction, but to what extent the effects are due to appetite suppression remains to be determined.

Garcinia Cambogia

One other Ayurvedic folk medicine with potential CR mimetic effects on fat metabolism is the Brindall berry, *Garcinia cambogia*.[18] This fruit has traditionally been used as a preservative for fish and condiments in Indian cooking; extracts are used as food supplements throughout the world. *Garcinia* has been alleged to exert weight control by increasing lipolysis, decreasing lipogenesis, and appetite suppression, although the latter does not appear to be an absolute requirement for the other two effects. At the biochemical level, the principal active ingredient appears to be hydroxycitrate, which inhibits isocitrate lyase.[18] This enzyme plays a key role in lipogensis, although it is not clear how its inhibition facilitates lipoylosis as well. In any case, the aggregate effects of *Garcinia* on lipid metabolism bode well for the possibility that this aspect of actual CR can indeed be mimicked by pharmacological or nutraceutical means.

SUMMARY AND CONCLUSIONS

Data from an ongoing 13-year study in monkeys strongly suggest that CR can exert the same beneficial antiaging, antidisease effects in primates as it does in rodents and lower animals. Although conclusive longevity results will not be available for a number of years, preliminary morbidity and mortality data are consistent with the possibility of both an extended life span and health span for CR primates, ultimately including humans. Unfortunately, long-term 30% restriction of food intake is beyond the capability of most people, even with the promise of such benefits.

For this reason, a more practical strategy is that of CR mimetics, to achieve the positive effects of restriction without actually reducing caloric consumption. The first candidate CR mimetic is 2-deoxyglucose, or 2DG. A six-month pilot experiment, in which it was fed to rats, demonstrated that very low dosages could be administered without significant toxicity or reduction in dietary intake yet still elicit some of the critical physiological/metabolic end points of CR. These included lower circulating insulin concentrations and lower body temperatures. A longevity study is currently under way.

Regardless of the results of the latter investigation, which is expected to take two to three years, it will be extremely useful to screen other potential CR mimetics, with wider "effective to toxic dose ranges" than 2DG. The fact that certain other pharmacological agents, as well as naturally occurring food/nutraceutical products, can achieve at least some of the same metabolic effects as CR also bodes well for the feasibility of this approach. It is expected that a number of exciting results from studies in this new area will occur in the very near future, which, it is hoped, will ultimately lead to the possibility of "eating one's cake and having it, too."

REFERENCES

1. Yu, B.P., Ed. 1994. Modulation of Aging Processes by Dietary Restriction. CRC Press. Boca Raton, FL.
2. WEINDRUCH, R. & R.W. WALFORD. 1998. The Retardation of Aging and Disease by Dietary Restriction. Thomas. Springfield, IL.
3. LANE, M.A., D.K. INGRAM & G.S. ROTH. 1997. Beyond the rodent model: caloric restriction in rhesus monkeys. Age **20:** 45–56.
4. INGRAM, D.K., R.G. CUTLER, R. WEINDRUCH et al. 1990. Dietary restriction and aging: the initiation of a primate study. J. Gerontol. **45:** B148–B163.
5. ROTH, G.S., D. INGRAM & M.A. LANE. 1999. Caloric restriction in primates: will it work and when will we know? J. Am. Geriatr. Soc. **47:** 896–903.
6. ROTH, G.S., D.K. INGRAM & M.A. LANE. 1995. Slowing aging by caloric restriction. Nature Med. **1:** 414–415.
7. STAMPER, J.L. & J. DARK. 1997. Metabolic fuel availability influences thermoregulation in deer mice (*Peromyscus maniculatus*). Physiol. Behav. **61**(4): 521–524.
8. KERN, K.A. & J.A. NORTON. 1987. Inhibition of established rat fibrosarcoma growth by glucose antagonist 2-deoxy-D-glucose. Surgery **182**(2): 380–385.
9. GOLDSTEIN, D.S., A. BRIER, O.M. WOLKOWITZ et al. 1992. Plasma levels of catecholamines and corticotrophin during acute glucopenia induced by 2-deoxy-D-glucose in normal men. Clin. Auton. Res. **2:** 359–366.
10. LANE, M.A., D.K. INGRAM & G.S. ROTH. 1998. 2-Deoxy-d-glucose feeding in rats mimics physiologic effects of calorie restriction. J. Anti-aging Med. **1:** 327–337.
11. YOSHIKAWA, M., T. MUAKAMI, M. KADOYA et al. 1997. Medicinal foodstuffs. IX. The inhibitors of glucose adsorption from the leaves of *Gymnema sylvestre* R. Br. (Asclepiadaceae): structures of gymnemosides a and b. Chem. Pharmacol. Bull. **45**(10): 1671–1676.
12. BARNETT, R.A. & J. BARONE. 1996. Ayurvedic Medicine: Ancient Roots, Modern Branches. Concorp Management. Pittsburgh, PA.
13. BRALA, P.M. & R.L. HAGAN. 1983. Effects of sweetness perception and caloric value of a preload on short term intake. Physiol. Behav. **30:** 1–9.

14. DILMAN, V.M. & V.N. ANISIMOV. 1980. Effect of treatment with phenformin, diphenylhydantoin or L-dopa on life span and tumor incidence in C3H/Sn mice. Gerontology **26**(5): 241–246.
15. M. F. MCCARTHY. 1998. Utility of metformin as an adjunct to hydroxycitrate/carnitine for reducing body fat in diabetics. Med. Hypotheses **51:** 399–403.
16. A. KLIP. 1990. Cellular mechanism of action of metformin. Diabetes Care **13:** 696–704.
17. LENHARD, J.M., S.A. KLIEWER, M.A. PAULIK *et al.* 1997. Effects of troglitizone and metformin on glucose and lipid metabolism. Biochem. Pharmacol. **54:** 801–808.
18. SULLIVAN, A.C., J.G. HAMILTON, O.N. MILLER & V. WHEATLEY. 1972. Inhibition of lipogenesis in rat liver by (-)- hydroxycitrate. Arch. Biochem. Biophys. **150:** 183–190.

Aging and Caloric Restriction in Nonhuman Primates

Behavioral and *in Vivo* Brain Imaging Studies

DONALD K. INGRAM,[a] SVETLANA CHEFER,[b] JOHN MATOCHIK,[b] TAMMY D. MOSCRIP,[c] JAMES WEED,[d] GEORGE S. ROTH,[a] EDYTHE D. LONDON[b,e] AND MARK A. LANE[a]

[a]*Laboratory of Neurosciences, Gerontology Research Center, National Institute on Aging, National Institutes of Health, 5600 Nathan Shock Drive, Baltimore, Maryland 21224, USA*

[b]*Neuroimaging Laboratory, Intramural Research Program, National Institute on Drug Abuse, National Institutes of Health, 5400 Nathan Shock Drive, Baltimore, Maryland 21224, USA*

[c]*Department of Psychology, Columbia University, 406 Schermerhorn Hall, 1190 Amsterdam Avenue, New York, New York 10027, USA*

[d]*Office of Research Services, Veterinary Resources Program, National Institutes of Health, 9000 Rockville Pike, Bethesda, Maryland 20892, USA*

ABSTRACT: In a long-term longitudinal study of aging in rhesus monkeys, a primary objective has been to determine the effects of aging and caloric restriction (CR) on behavioral and neural parameters. Through the use of automated devices, locomotor activity can be monitored in the home cages of the monkeys. Studies completed thus far indicate a clear age-related decline in activity consistent with such observations in many other species, including humans. However, no consistent effects of CR on activity have been observed. Selected groups of monkeys have also been involved in brain imaging studies, using magnetic resonance imaging (MRI) and positron emission tomography (PET). MRI studies completed thus far reveal a clear age-related decline in the volumes of the basal ganglia, the putamen, and the caudate nucleus, with no change in total brain volume. PET analysis has revealed an age-related decline in the binding potential of dopamine D_2 receptors in the same brain regions. These results are consistent with findings in humans. Although additional longitudinal analysis is needed to confirm the present results, it would appear that locomotor activity, volume of the basal ganglia, as well as dopamine D_2 receptor binding potential provide reliable, noninvasive biomarkers of aging in rhesus monkeys.

KEYWORDS: Locomotor activity; MRI; PET; Basal ganglia; Putamen; Caudate nucleus

Address for correspondence: Dr. Donald K. Ingram, Laboratory of Neurosciences, Gerontology Research Center, National Institute on Aging, National Institutes of Health, 5600 Nathan Shock Dr., Baltimore, MD 21224. Voice: 410-558-8180; fax: 410-558-8323.
doni@vax.grc.nia.nih.gov
[e]Present address: Department of Psychiatry and Biobehavioral Sciences, Neuropsychiatric Institute, University of California at Los Angeles, C8-532 NPI, UCLA-NPI Box 60, 760 Westwood Plaza, Los Angeles, CA 90024.

INTRODUCTION

In addition to beneficial effects on life span and protection against chronic diseases,[1] studies in rodents have documented a number of age-related behavioral declines that are retarded by long-term caloric restriction (CR). Among these are increased locomotor activity as well as improved performance in tasks assessing sensorimotor abilities,[2-4] motor learning,[5] avoidance learning,[2] and maze learning[3,4,6,7] observed in rodents on CR. Postmortem analyses of rat brains have demonstrated parallel neurochemical effects of CR, such as an antagonism of the decline in D_2 dopamine receptors in the neostriatum[8,9] and a suppression of age-related changes in dendritic spines.[10]

In 1987, the National Institute on Aging (NIA) initiated a study of CR in rhesus monkeys (*Macaca mulatta*) to determine whether the antiaging effects of this nutritional intervention could be observed in a long-lived species with relevance to human aging.[11] Summaries of the diverse findings from this study can be found in previous publications.[12,13] Because it is important to determine how this nutritional manipulation influences behavioral function throughout the life span, an important component of this long-term project was assessment of behavioral changes associated with CR. Potential effects on motor and cognitive performance were of particular concern. As an adjunct to behavioral analysis, direct assessments of brain structure and function were also included because *in vivo* brain imaging techniques, such as magnetic resonance imaging (MRI) and positron emission tomography (PET), allow these measurements to be made in a noninvasive manner.

In the current review, we summarize findings from the NIA study as well as other studies of primate aging regarding age-related changes in locomotor activity, volume of the basal ganglia measured by MRI, and binding potential of dopamine D_2 receptors in the basal ganglia measured by PET. These studies have been initiated only within the last few years of the NIA study because effects of CR on behavior were considered to be manifested only after long-term treatment. The objective for many of the initial studies described herein was to establish that the behavioral and imaging assays were age sensitive, and then later to extend the studies in CR groups. Thus, for many of the assays, the question of CR effects has not yet been addressed. The details on the design, husbandry, and diet in the NIA study can be found elsewhere.[11] In general, the study involved a large group of male and female rhesus monkeys that were placed at various ages on either a control diet (near ad libitum levels) or CR (30 percent less food than that provided to control monkeys of comparable age and body weight). For the data presented in this review, all monkeys had been in the study for at least five years.

LOCOMOTOR ACTIVITY

A decline in the level of general locomotor activity is one of the most sensitive and robust age-related behavioral changes.[15-17] This decline begins around reproductive maturity and progresses throughout the life span of many species, including humans.[15-17] In rodents, this age-related decline in locomotor activity can be predictive of life span.[18,19]

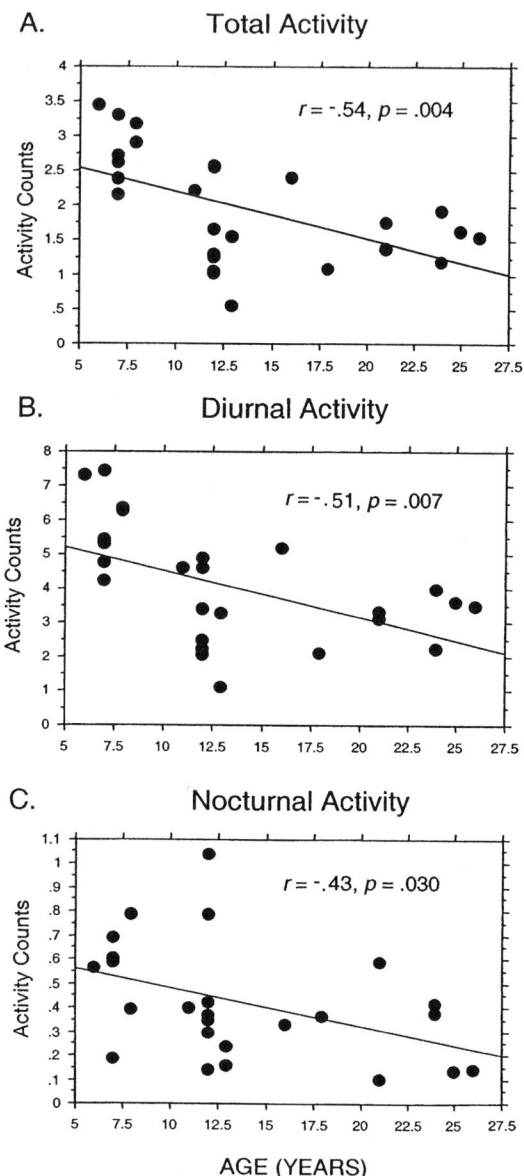

FIGURE 1. Regression of age on total activity counts for per minute for female rhesus monkeys in the control group.

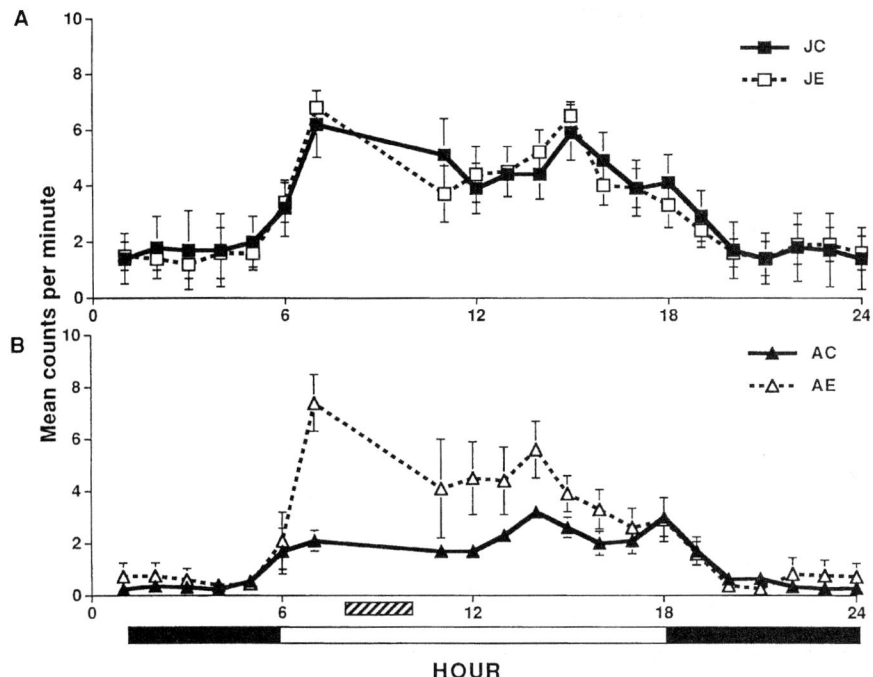

FIGURE 2. Mean (SEM) hourly activity counts over 24-h period for male rhesus monkeys in two different age groups (J = 8.2–8.4 years; A = 10–12.2 years) in control (CON) and experimental (EXP) groups. *Open bar* = lights on; *filled bar* = lights off; *striped bar* = data deleted during husbandry period.

By using automated devices, locomotor activity can be measured in a highly standardized, noninvasive manner. In the NIA study, a custom-made device can provide 24-h monitoring of locomotor activity of monkeys in their home cages. Detailed descriptions of the device and the procedure for monitoring activity are found elsewhere.[20,21] In general, activity was sampled hourly to detect gross movement in the cages and was translated into a mean activity count per minute. Analysis of repeated recordings of activity in a subsample of the monkeys has documented the high degree of reliability of the measurements as conducted.[20]

The results of these studies were straightforward with respect to age differences but not with respect to diet effects. In separate assessments of male and female rhesus monkeys, an age-related decline in locomotor activity was evident in the control groups (see females in FIG. 1). Having monitored the activity of adult male rhesus monkeys in the NIA study (FIG. 2), Weed et al.[21] reported increased activity associated with CR, but only in one group of monkeys examined (10–12.2 years) and not in a younger group (8.2–8.4 years). When comparing activity levels between control and experimental groups of female rhesus monkeys (FIG. 3), Moscrip et al.[20] noted only one significant effect of diet (FIG. 3A), which was in the youngest group of monkeys (6–8 years of age). Monkeys in the experimental group exhibited lower

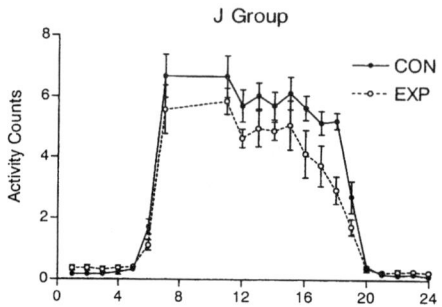

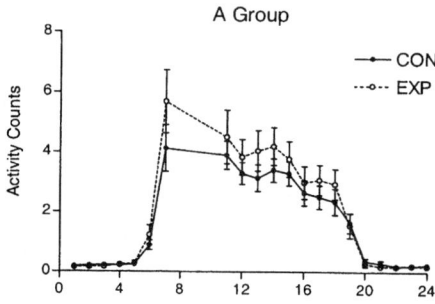

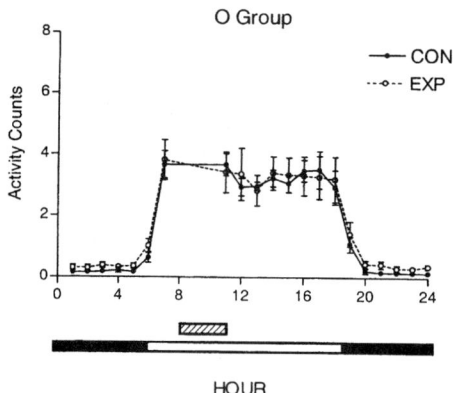

FIGURE 3. Mean (SEM) hourly activity counts over 24-h period for female rhesus monkeys in three different age groups (J = 6–8 years; A = 10–19 years; O = 18–26 years) in control (CON) and experimental (EXP) groups. *Open bar* = lights on; *filled bar* = lights off; *striped bar* = data deleted during husbandry period.

activity compared to controls. CR monkeys that were 10–19 years of age showed reduced activity, but this difference was not statistically significant (FIG. 3B). No differences in activity were apparent in the oldest group of monkeys (FIG. 3C). Thus, no clear picture of how CR affects locomotor activity has emerged from the NIA study thus far.

An age-related decline in locomotor activity was previously observed in nonhuman primates, including squirrel monkeys[22] and rhesus monkeys.[23] Tests to evaluate the effect of CR on locomotor activity have been confined largely to rodent studies. Results from studies monitoring home cage activity in mice[24,25] and rats[26,27] reveal higher levels of activity among animals on CR compared to ad libitum–fed (AL) controls. A longitudinal analysis of the home cage activity of rats confirmed the progressive activity decline in AL controls but not in CR groups.[28]

Only two other groups have employed devices and procedures similar to those used in the NIA study to examine home cage activity of male rhesus monkeys. Kemnitz et al.[29] reported that activity was reduced in adult male monkeys (9–10 years old) after one year on CR; however, after five years, the difference between control and CR groups was no longer statistically significant.[30] DeLany et al.[31] noted higher locomotor activity in a group of old (22 years old) monkeys on CR for 10 years, compared to controls.

This diversity of findings emerging from the monkey studies might be due to differences in diet composition, age, gender, length of CR, or other factors. Thus, additional longitudinal analysis will be needed to establish the possible dynamic pattern of CR effects on locomotor activity. As an example, in a longitudinal study of CR in rats, Goodrick et al.[29] noted that wheel-running activity was generally less in CR groups early in life, but ultimately greater later in life, after the control groups had exhibited a marked age-related decline in activity.

MRI ANALYSIS OF BASAL GANGLIA

Age-related decline in motor performance has been attributed in part to structural and neurochemical changes in the basal ganglia as a component of the ascending dopamine (DA) system.[33] The loss of dopamine-producing cells in the substantia nigra (SN) represents the neuropathology of Parkinson's disease.[34] In a postmortem anatomical analysis of rhesus monkey brains, Emborg et al.[23] reported an age-related decline in the number of tyrosine hydroxylase (TH)–positive neurons, which manufacture DA. Moreover, the number of DA neurons was directly correlated with the level of locomotor activity that had been recorded in these monkeys. In their investigation of squirrel monkeys, Irwin et al.[22] reported no age-related decline in the number of nigral TH-positive neurons, but did report an age-related decline in DA content of the SN (70%) and putamen (30%), but not in the caudate nucleus.

Focusing on male rhesus monkeys in the control group of the NIA study, Matochik et al.[35] used MRI to assess age differences in the volume of the basal ganglia. Significant age-related declines in the volume of the putamen (FIG. 4B) and the caudate nucleus (FIG. 4C) were observed. The age-related volumetric decline in the putamen appeared to occur earlier in life than that recorded for the caudate nucleus, which presented the appearance of a progressive change with age. These structural changes were regionally specific since total brain volume did not differ significantly with age (FIG. 4A). MRI studies in humans have confirmed the age-related decline in the volumes of the caudate and putamen.[37–39]

What remains unclear from the MRI analysis of NIA monkeys are the exact structural changes that account for the age-related volumetric declines in specific regions of the basal ganglia. Among the possible factors would be neuronal loss, neuronal

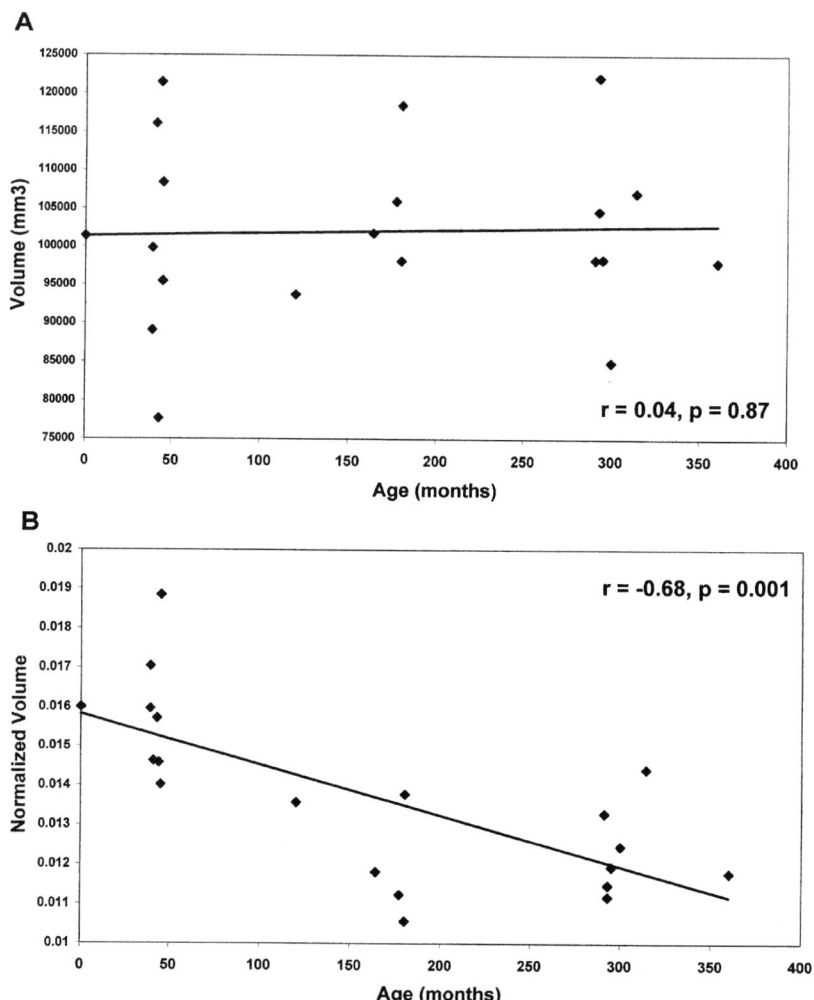

FIGURE 4. Regression of age on volumes estimated by MRI for whole brain (**A**), putamen (**B**), and caudate nucleus (**C**) in male rhesus monkeys.

atrophy, dendritic shrinkage, or reduced white matter present in these structures. In their postmortem analysis of age-related changes in the hippocampus and neocortex of rhesus monkeys, Peters et al.[40] noted that poor cognitive performance was best correlated with loss and alterations in white matter rather than counts of neurons or synapses, which showed no significant age changes based on stereological analysis. MRI analysis of aging human brain has confirmed that the age-related decline in white matter volume exceeds the volumetric loss in gray matter,[41] but this finding has not been supported in other studies.[42] Moreover, using MRI analysis of female rhesus brains, Andersen et al.[43] reported age-related decline in total brain volume

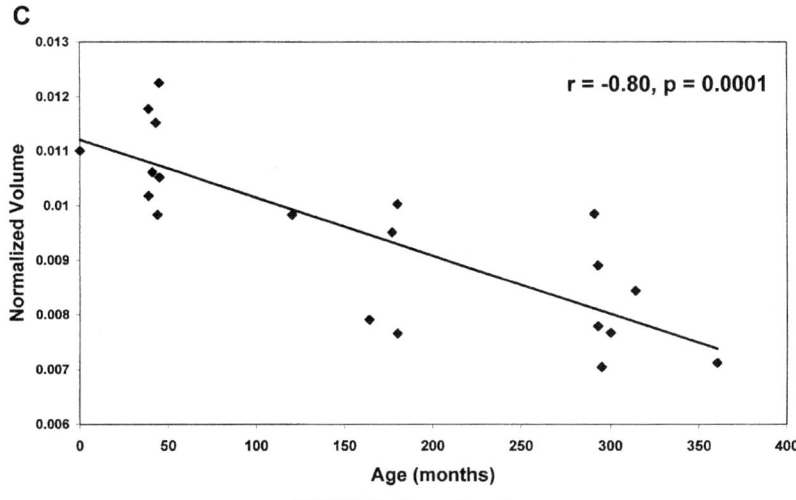

FIGURE 4 *continued.*

(in contrast to the findings on male rhesus monkeys from the NIA study), which they attributed to gray matter loss primarily.

Age changes in white matter volume are currently being investigated in the NIA study. In addition, volumetric analysis of the basal ganglia in CR monkeys is underway. Despite discrepancies among MRI studies, it would appear that age-related volumetric changes in basal ganglia are reasonable candidates as neurological biomarkers of aging and could be used to determine if the rate of brain aging is being altered in the CR monkeys.

PET ANALYSIS OF DOPAMINE D_2 RECEPTORS

Loss of striatal dopamine D_2 receptors (D_2R) is one of the most robust neurochemical changes in the aging brain.[44,45] This decline is considered to underlie the impairments observed in motor performance with increasing age.[45]

Lai et al.[46] confirmed an age-related decline in D_2R in the caudate and putamen of male rhesus monkeys by *in vitro* receptor binding assays of postmortem tissue. In humans the age-related loss of D_2R has been documented by PET, using a variety of dopamine receptor ligands.[47–50] Using PET analysis of ^{11}C raclopride binding, Morris et al.[51] evaluated the binding potential of D_2R in the NIA control male monkeys. FIGURE 5 presents the significant age-related decline observed in this parameter in the striatum, which represented both the caudate nucleus and putamen. In this study, the age effect persisted even after correction for possible confounding effects of an age-induced reduction of basal ganglia volume.

Given the age sensitivity of the PET analysis, a follow-up study is planned to determine if CR retards the age-related loss of striatal D_2R. Previous analysis of D_2R receptor binding in rats documented that CR alters the rate of aging in this neurobiological parameter.[8,9]

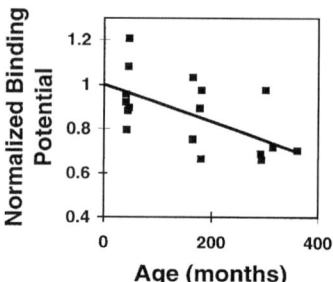

FIGURE 5. Regression of age on ^{11}C raclopride binding potential (corrected for partial volume effects) estimated by PET in male rhesus monkeys.

SUMMARY

Noninvasive procedures have been established to evaluate the effects of CR on behavioral and neurological parameters in rhesus monkeys involved in a longitudinal study. Analyses completed to date have documented age-related decline in locomotor activity accompanied by volumetric reductions in the basal ganglia and the binding potential of D_2 dopamine receptors. Additional analyses have been planned to assess whether CR alters the rate of age-related decline in these behavioral and neurobiological parameters.

REFERENCES

1. WEINDRUCH, R. & R. WALFORD. 1988. The retardation of aging and disease by dietary restriction. Charles C. Thomas. Springfield, IL.
2. DUBEY, A., M.J. FORSTER, H. LAL & R.S. SOHAL. 1996. Effect of age and caloric intake on protein oxidation in different brain regions and on behavioral functions of the mouse. Arch. Biochem. Biophys. **333:** 189–197.
3. INGRAM, D.K., R. WEINDRUCH, E.L. SPANGLER et al. 1987. Dietary restriction benefits learning and motor performance of aged mice. J. Gerontol. **42:** 78–81.
4. MEANS, L.W., J.L.HIGGINS & T.J. FERNANDEZ. 1993. Mid-life onset of dietary restriction extends life and prolongs cognitive functioning. Physiol. Behav. **54:** 503–508.
5. GOULD, T.J., K.E. BOWENKAMP, G. LARSON et al. 1995. Effects of dietary restriction on motor learning and cerebellar noradrenergic dysfunction in aged F344 rats. Brain Res. **684:** 150–158.
6. MAGNUSSON, K.R. 1998. Aging of glutamate receptors: correlations between binding and spatial memory performance in mice. Mech. Ageing Dev. **104:** 227–248.
7. PITSIKAS, N., M. CARLI, S. FIDECKA & S. ALGERI. 1990. Effect of life-long hypocaloric diet on age-related changes in motor and cognitive behavior in a rat population. Neurobiol. Aging **11:** 417–423.
8. LEVIN, P, J.K. JANDA, J.A. JOSEPH et al. 1981. Dietary restriction retards the age-associated loss of rat striatal dopaminergic receptors. Science **214:** 561–562.
9. ROTH, G.S., D.K. INGRAM & J.A. JOSEPH. 1984. Delayed loss of striatal dopamine receptors during aging of dietarily restricted rats. Brain Res. **300:** 27–32.
10. MOROI-FETTERS, S.E., R.F. MERVIS, E.D. LONDON & D.K. INGRAM. 1989. Dietary restriction suppresses age-related changes in dendritic spines. Neurobiol. Aging. **10:** 317–322.
11. INGRAM, D.K., R.G. CUTLER, R. WEINDRUCH et al. 1990. Dietary restriction and aging: the initiation of a primate study. J. Gerontol. Biol. Sci. **48:** B17–B26.

12. LANE, M.A., D. K. INGRAM, R. G. CUTLER et al. 1992. Dietary restriction in nonhuman primates: progress report on the NIA study. Ann. N.Y. Acad. Sci. **673:** 36–45.
13. LANE, M.A., D.K. INGRAM & G.S. ROTH. 1997. Beyond the rodent model: calorie restriction in rhesus monkeys. Age **20:** 45–56.
14. ROTH, G.S., D.K. INGRAM & M.A. LANE. 1999. Calorie restriction in primates: will it work and how will we know? J. Am. Geriatr. Soc. **47:** 896–903.
15. INGRAM, D.K. 2000. Age-related decline in physical activity: generalization to nonhumans. Med. Sci Sports Exerc. **32:** 1623–1629.
16. INGRAM D.K., M. JUCKER & E.L. SPANGLER. 1994. Behavioral manifestations of aging. In Pathology of Aging Animals, Vol. 1: Rat. U. Mohr, C. Capen & D. Dungworth, Eds.: 149–170. ILSI Press. Washington, DC.
17. SALLIS, J.F. Age-related decline in physical activity: a synthesis of human and animal studies. Med. Sci. Sports Exerc. **32:** 1623–1629.
18. INGRAM, D.K. & M.A. REYNOLDS. 1986. Assessing the predictive validity of psychomotor tests as measures of biological age in mice. Exp. Aging Res. **12:** 39–42.
19. WAX, T.M. & C. L. GOODRICK. 1978. Nearness to death and wheelrunning behavior in mice. Exp. Gerontol. **13:** 233–236.
20. MOSCRIP, T.D., D.K. INGRAM, M.A. LANE et al. 2000. Locomotor activity in female rhesus monkeys: assessment of age and calorie restriction effects. **54:** B407-B417.
21. WEED, J.L., M.A. LANE, G.S. ROTH et al. 1997. Activity measures in rhesus monkeys on long-term calorie restriction. Physiol. Behav. **62:** 97–103.
22. IRWIN, I., L.E. DELANNEY, T. MCNEILL et al. 1994. Aging and the nigrostriatal dopamine system: a non-human primate study. Neurodegeneration **3:** 251–265.
23. EMBORG, M.E., S.Y. MA, E.J. MUFSON et al. 1998. Age-related declines in nigral neuronal function correlate with motor impairments in rhesus monkeys. J. Comp. Neurol. **401:** 253–265.
24. DUFFY, P.H., R.J. FEUERS & R.W. HART. 1990. Effect of chronic caloric restriction on the circadian regulation of physiological and behavioral variables in old male B6C3F1. Chronobiol. Int. **7:** 291–303.
25. DUFFY, P.H., R.J. FEUERS, J.A. LEAKEY & R.W. HART. 1991. Chronic caloric restriction in old female mice: changes in circadian rhythms of physiological and behavioral variables. In Biological Effects of Dietary Restriction. L. Fishbein, Ed.: 245–263. Springer-Verlag. Berlin.
26. DUFFY, P.H., R.J. FEUERS, J.A. LEAKEY et al. 1989. Effect of caloric restriction on physiological variables related to energy metabolism in the male Fischer 344 rat. Mech. Aging Dev. **48:** 117–133.
27. DUFFY, P.H., R.J. FEUERS, K D. NAKAMURA et al. 1990. Effect of chronic caloric restriction on the synchronization of various physiological measures in old female Fischer 344 rats. Chronobiol. Int. **7:** 113–124.
28. YU, B.P., E.J. MASORO & C.A. MCMAHAN. 1985. Nutritional influences on aging of Fischer 344 rats: I. Physical, metabolic, and longevity characteristics. J. Gerontol. **40:** 657–670.
29. KEMNITZ, J.W., R. WEINDRUCH, E.B. ROECKER et al. 1993. Dietary restriction of adult rhesus monkeys: design, methodology and preliminary findings from the first year of the study. J. Gerontol. Biol. Sci. **48:** B17–B26.
30. RAMSEY, J.J., E.B. ROECKER, R. WEINDRUCH et al. 1996. Thermogenesis of adult male rhesus monkeys: results through 66 months of dietary restriction. FASEB J. **10:** A726.
31. DELANY, J.P., B.C. HANSEN, N.L. BODKIN et al. 1999. Long-term calorie restriction reduces energy expenditure in aging monkeys. J. Gerontol. Biol. Sci. **54:** B5–B11.
32. GOODRICK, C.L., D.K. INGRAM, M.A. REYNOLDS et al. 1983. Effects of intermittent feeding upon growth, activity, and lifespan in rats allowed voluntary exercise. Exp. Aging Res. **38:** 36–45.
33. HUBBLE, J.P. 1998. Aging and the basal ganglia. Neurol. Clin. **16:** 649–657.
34. TEDROFF, J.M. 1999. Functional consequences of dopaminergic degeneration in Parkinson's disease. Adv. Neurol. **80:** 67–70.
35. MATOCHIK, J., S.I. CHEFER, E.D. MORRIS et al. 1998. Age-related decline in striatal volume in monkeys as measured by magnetic resonance imaging. Neurobiol. Aging. In press.

36. GUNNING-DIXON, F.M., D. HEAD, J. MCQUAIN et al. 1998. Differential aging of the human striatum: a prospective MR imaging study. Am. J. Neuroradiol. **19:** 1501–1507.
37. KIRSHMAN, K.R., M.M. HUSAIN, W.M. MCDONALD et al. 1990. In vivo stereological assessment of caudate volume in man: effects of normal aging. Life Sci. **47:** 1325–1329.
38. MURPHY, D.G.M., C. DECARLI, M.B. SCHAPIRO et al. 1992. Age-related differences in volumes of subcortical nuclei, brain matter, and cerebrospinal fluid in healthy men as measured with magnetic resonance imaging. Arch. Neurol. **49:** 839–845.
39. RAZ, N., I.J. TORRES & J.D. ACKER. 1995. Age, gender, and hemispheric differences in human striatum: a quantitative review and new data from in vivo MRI morphometry. Neurobiol. Learn. Mem. **63:** 133–142.
40. PETERS, A., D.L. ROSENE, M.B. MOSS et al. 1996. Neurobiological bases of age-related cognitive decline in the rhesus monkey. J. Neuropathol. Exp. Neurol. **55:** 861–874.
41. GUTTMANN, C.R., F.A. JOLESZ, R. KIKINIS et al. 1998. White matter changes with normal aging. Neurology **50:** 972–978.
42. SULLIVAN, E.V., L. MARSH, D.H. MATHALON et al. 1995. Age-related decline in MRI volumes of temporal lobe gray matter but not hippocampus. Neurobiol. Aging **16:** 591–606.
43. ANDERSEN, A.H., Z. ZHANG, M. ZHANG et al. 1999. Age-associated changes in rhesus CNS composition identified by MRI. Brain Res. **829:** 90–98.
44. ROTH, G.S. 1995. Changes in tissue responsiveness to hormones and neurotransmitters during aging. Exp. Gerontol. **30:** 361–368.
45. ROTH, G.S. & J.A. JOSEPH. 1994. Cellular and molecular mechanisms of impaired dopaminergic function during aging. Ann. N.Y. Acad. Sci. **719:** 129–135.
46. LAI, H., D.M. BOWDEN & A. HORITA. 1987. Age-related decreases in dopamine receptors in the caudate nucleus and putamen of the rhesus monkey (Macaca mulatta). Neurobiol. Aging **8:** 45–49.
47. ANTONINI, A., K.L. LEENDERS, H. REIST et al. 1993. Effect of age on D_2 dopamine receptors in normal human brain measured by positron emission tomography and ^{11}C raclopride. Arch. Neurol. **50:** 474–480.
48. RINNE, J.O., J. HIETALA, U. RUOTSALAINEN et al. 1993. Decrease in human striatal dopamine D_2 receptor density with age: a PET study with ^{11}C raclopride. Cereb. Blood Flow Metab. **13:** 310–314.
49. VOLKOW, N.D., G.J. WANG, J.S. FOWLER et al. 1996. Measuring age-related changes in dopamine D_2 receptors with ^{11}C raclopride and ^{18}F-N-methylspiroperiodol. Psychiatry Res. **67:** 11–16.
50. WONG, D.F., D. YOUNG, P.D. WILSON et al. 1997. Quantification of neuroreceptors in the living human brain: III. D_2-like dopamine receptors: theory, validation, and changes during normal aging. J. Cereb. Blood Flow. Metab. **17:** 316–330.
51. MORRIS, E.D., S.I. CHEFER, M.A. LANE et al. 1999. Loss of D_2 receptor binding with age in rhesus monkeys: importance of correction for differences in striatal size. J. Cereb. Blood Flow Metab. **19:** 218–229.

The Inflammation Hypothesis of Aging

Molecular Modulation by Calorie Restriction

HAE YOUNG CHUNG, HYON JEEN KIM, JUNG WON KIM, AND BYUNG PAL YU

Department of Pharmacy, College of Pharmacy, Research Institute of Genetic Engineering, Pusan National University, Gumjung-Ku Pusan 609-735, Korea

ABSTRACT: Current evidence strongly indicates that reactive oxygen species (ROS) and reactive nitrogen species (RNS) are widely implicated in the inflammatory process. However, mechanistic information is not readily available on the extent to which ROS/RNS contributes to the proinflammatory states of the aging process. The involvement of the underlying inflammation during the aging process and the molecular delineation of anti-inflammatory action of calorie restriction (CR) is described. Age-related upregulations of NF-κB, IL-β, IL-6, TNFα, cyclooxygenase-2, and inducible NO synthase are all attenuated by CR. The suppression of the NF-κB activation was accomplished by blocking the dissociation of inhibitory IκBα and IκBβ by CR. These findings provide underlying molecular insights into the anti-inflammatory action of CR in relation to the aging process. Based on these and other available data, it is suggested that the "Inflammation Hypothesis of Aging" supports the molecular basis of the inflammatory process as a plausible cause of the aging process.

KEYWORDS: Aging; Antiaging; Anti-inflammatory; Calorie restriction; NF-κB; ROS; Inflammation; NO synthase

INTRODUCTION

Inflammation is a complex host's normal defense reaction to insult and stress, both physiological and nonphysiological, like chemicals, drugs, oxidants, or a variety of microbial entities. Inflammation responses, whether acute or chronic, are activated by well-coordinated, sequential events controlled by humoral and cellular reactions. Reactive oxygen species (ROS), such as $\cdot O_2^-$, $\cdot OH$, H_2O_2, and reactive nitrogen species (RNS), such as NO and $ONOO^-$, are heavily implicated in the inflammatory process (FIG. 1). The deleterious effects of ROS/RNS are dependent on their concentration and the microenvironment in which ROS/RNS are released. Overproduced or uncontrolled ROS/RNS are a major causative factor in tissue inflammation. As shown in FIGURE 1, the inflammatory responses usually proceed in the following sequential phases: (1) intracellular activation, (2) infiltration of proinflammatory macrophages and lymphocytes, (3) increased vascular permeability, and (4) tissue damage and cell death.[1]

Address for correspondence: Dr. Hae Young Chung, Department of Pharmacy, College of Pharmacy, Pusan National University, Gumjung-Ku Pusan 609-735, Korea. Phone: 82-51-510-2814; fax: 82-51-510-2814.
hyjung@hyowon.pusan.ac.kr

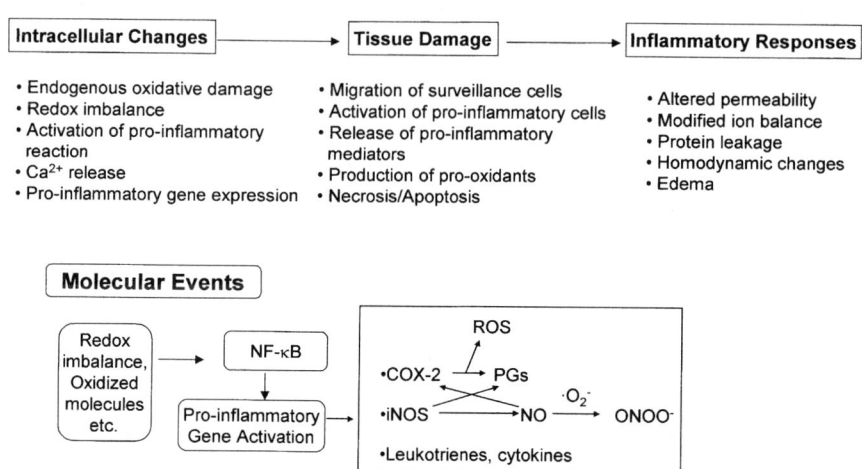

FIGURE 1. Biochemical and molecular changes leading to inflammatory responses.

The introduction of neutrophils, lymphocytes, and macrophages, which release ROS, RNS, and lytic enzymes further amplify the inflammatory reaction.[2] Furthermore, various inflammatory genes are activated by the transcription factor, NF-κB, which is extremely sensitive to oxidants and many proinflammatory substances.[3] For instance, NF-κB activates gene expression of proinflammatory cytokines, such as IL-1β,[4] IL-6,[5] and TNFα,[6] as well as the proinflammatory enzymes, cyclooxygenase-2 (COX-2)[3] and inducible nitric oxide synthase (iNOS).[7] In our recent study, we found that COX-2 and NF-κB were upregulated in rat kidney during aging,[3] and was suppressed by calorie restriction (CR). Although several pieces of evidence show that CR can modulate NF-κB activation by its antioxidative action,[8] this aspect of CR has not received much attention to date.

The involvement of the inflammatory process in several diseases has long been known, but until a recent proposal by McGeer and McGeer, its implication in the aging process has been less appreciated. Their "Inflammatory Hypothesis of Dementia" highlights the importance of inflammation in aging.[9] Other age-related inflammatory processes are the age-related alterations of vascular endothelial and smooth muscle cells, which lead to pathogenic expressions, as seen in atherosclerosis[10] and vascular dysfunctions of diabetes.[11]

The evidence accumulated to date on the beneficial, antiaging action of CR is consistent with its anti-inflammatory property. Based on reported data and new evidence obtained from our laboratory, we propose the "Inflammatory Hypothesis of Aging," to highlight the involvement of the underlying inflammation process during the aging process as discussed below. In the present report, we use the molecular mechanisms of the anti-inflammatory action of CR as the supporting basis of the proposal.

OXIDATIVE STRESS, PROSTAGLANDINS, AND INFLAMMATION

Vasoactive prostaglandins (PGs) are essential components in the regulation of vascular function under normal physiological conditions,[12] and their role in the inflammatory process has been long known. Moreover, changes in PG activities in vascular cells can have a widespread impact on vascular tone and the inflammatory response of the vasculature.

Several reports have addressed PG production during aging. Most of the data seem to indicate that the production of inflammatory PGs such as PGE_2, TXA_2, PGH_2, and PGG_2 increase with advancing age, whereas cytoprotective PGs such as PGI_2 decrease with age.[13–16] Macrophages from old mice are reported to produce more PGE_2 than young mice, indicating the dysregulation of immune cells for proinflammatory conditions with age.[17]

The PG synthesis pathway is a major ROS-generating source during the conversion of PGG_2 to PGH_2. Little information is available on how much of the PG pathway contributes to the total ROS status. At our laboratory, to estimate the extent of PG-derived ROS, ROS generation was measured in the presence of the COX inhibitor, indomethacin. ROS generation was measured by the fluorometric method using dichlorofluorescin diacetate in tissue homogenates and subcellular fraction. ROS generation in the heart,[18] kidney,[19] and brain[20] showed a gradual increase with age. COX-derived, indomethacin-inhibitable ROS increased with age. The COX-derived ROS were about 30% of total ROS.[3] COX-2 mRNA and protein levels also showed age-related increases.[3]

To obtain evidence that COX activity is related to ROS levels, we used Mn-superoxide dismutase (Mn-SOD) knockout mice to increase the oxidative stress level.[18] In heart postmitochondria and mitochondria fraction from these mice, ROS generation significantly increased compared to wild-type mice (data not shown). These increases were parallel to the marked increases in cardiac and renal COX-2 mRNA levels,[18,19] providing evidence that COX-2 expression is influenced by the ROS status. Our findings agree with the data of Feng et al.,[21] who reported that radical scavengers suppress COX-2 expression induced by IL-1, TNFα, and lipopolysaccharide (LPS). Taken together, the data suggest that COX-derived ROS are a major contributor to the inflammatory process.

iNOS IN INFLAMMATION AND AGING

The essential role of NO in normal physiological functions is firmly established. The enzyme responsible for NO has several isoforms. Among three of these isoforms, eNOS, bNOS, and iNOS, iNOS is readily induced by proinflammatory cytokines and LPS.[22]

The ability to induce iNOS, and thereby generate large amounts of NO, suggests that this isoform may play a major role, as one might expect in a chronic condition such as aging. For example, Cernadas et al. reported that the vessel walls of aging rats show an enhanced expression of eNOS and iNOS.[23] Poynter et al. also showed that the mean daily level of urinary nitrate plus nitrite excretion by young animals was lower than that secreted by aged animals, indicating increased iNOS.[24] Our laboratory recently obtained data showing that induction of iNOS gene expression in-

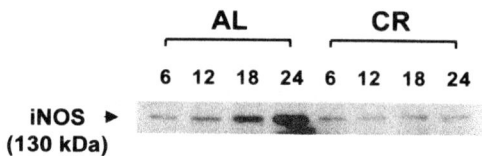

FIGURE 2. Effect of age and CR on iNOS gene expression. (ABBREVIATIONS: AL, *ad libitum*; CR, calorie restriction.)

creases during aging in the kidney of lupus-nephritis-prone mice.[25] In addition, as shown in FIGURE 2, iNOS gene expression was substantially increased in aged Fischer 344 rat kidney, showing that dysregulated NO production causes inflammatory reactions and autoimmune disease states.

PROINFLAMMATORY CYTOKINES IN THE AGING PROCESS

Cytokines are major communication channels that provide links within and between the immune system and other organs.[26] During aging, a shift occurs in the ratio of native to memory T cells, with associated changes in the cytokine profile that favor increases in inflammatory cytokines such as TNFα, IL-1, IL-6, INFγ, and TGFβ.[27–30] We should note, however, that most age-related changes in cytokine levels are investigated mainly *in vitro*, and the results are not consistent.[28,31,32]

While the production of IL-6, but not IL-1β and TNFα, by peripheral mononuclear cells were reported to increase in the elderly compared to young subjects,[31] Riancho *et al*. reported an age-related increase of IL-1 production in peripheral blood mononuclear cells in old animals.[28] On the other hand, IL-1β levels were higher and IL-6 levels were lower in the liver of old rats than young rats.[33] In a recent study in our laboratory, the levels of proinflammatory cytokines in aged and/or LPS-treated rats were measured. We found that mRNA levels of IL-1β and IL-6 showed an increase with age, which were further enhanced by LPS challenge in older rats.[33] Results showed that mRNA expressions of IL-1β and IL-6 significantly increased in LPS-treated old rats, as did the mRNA amount of TNFα in old rats. The LPS challenge that caused a significant increase in these proinflammatory proteins, especially in old rats, indicates an enhanced sensitivity to inflammation with aging.[33] It is important to note that the gene expression of these proinflammatory proteins was matched by levels of intracellular oxidative stress.[18–20]

ROLE OF NF-κB IN THE INFLAMMATORY PROCESS

NF-κB is an ubiquitous, pleiotropic transcription factor known to be extremely sensitive to various stimuli,[34,35] particularly ROS.[36] Unlike some of the other transcription factors, the NF-κB complex is held in the cytoplasm as an inactive state by the inhibitory subunit, IκB. The phosphorylation of IκB and its subsequent degradation of inhibitory IκB allows translocation of NF-κB to the nucleus.[36] This NF-κB

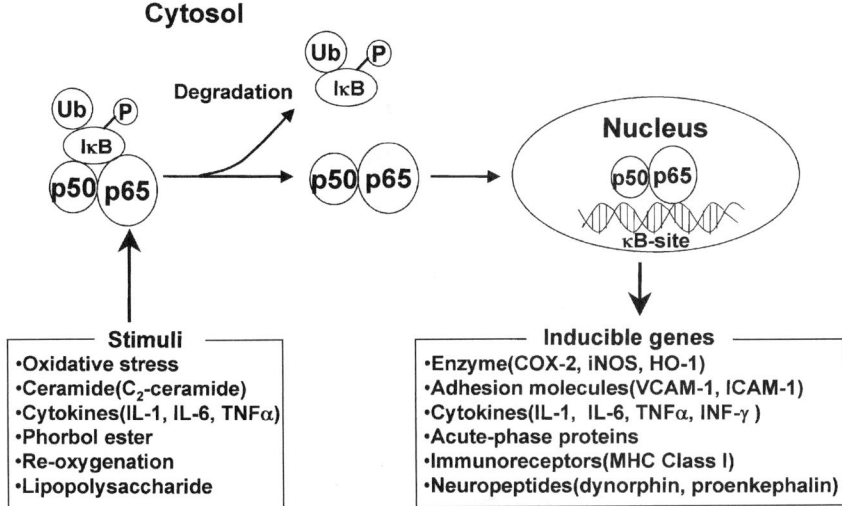

FIGURE 3. Diverse stimuli activating NF-κB and a range of genes induced through NF-κB.

transactivation can be elicited by inflammatory stimuli such as TNFα, lymphotoxin, IL-1, lipopolysaccharide, protein synthesis inhibitors, ultraviolet light, and phorbol esters [37,38] (FIG. 3).

Many researchers have looked into the age effect on the regulation of NF-κB. Existing data show that the nuclear DNA-binding activity of the NF-κB factor increases during aging in all tissues of the rats and mice tested.[39,40] Helenius et al. found that heart, liver, kidney, and brain tissues from old rodents expressed higher levels of NF-κB binding activity than tissues from young adult rodents.[39] Korhonen et al. reported a significant upregulation of NF-κB in brain samples of rat.[40] But the precise mode of age-related NF-κB activation has not been delineated. In a recent study, we found new information that activated NF-κB was due to an age-related IκBα decrease and its dissociation increase from the complex in the cytosol, allowing the nuclear translocation of NF-κB.[3] The study further indicated that anti-inflammatory CR action suppressed NF-κB (FIG. 4) through inhibiting the IκB dissociation by the upregulation of cytosolic IκBα and IκBβ.

CALORIE RESTRICTION AS A REGULATOR OF INFLAMMATION

Extensive gerontological research has confirmed that CR imposed on laboratory rodents extends their mean and maximum lifespans.[41] We investigated the effect of CR on the ROS generation specifically derived from the COX pathway of prostanoid metabolism; the results are summarized here. We found CR suppressed COX-derived ROS generation during aging. CR also blunted increases in the production of prostanoids such as seen in TXA_2, PGI_2, and PGE_2 generation. These findings are

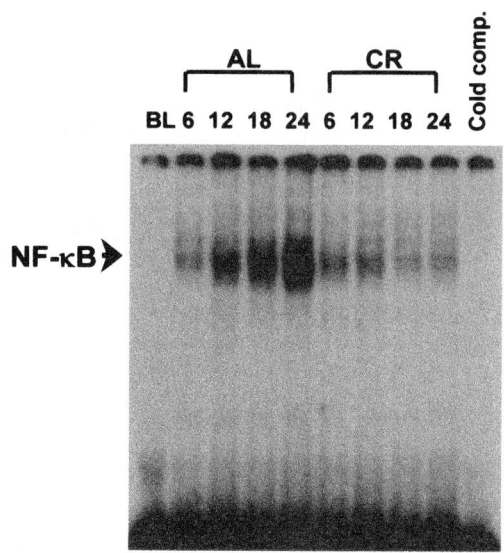

FIGURE 4. Effect of age and CR on NF-κB activity. (ABBREVIATIONS: AL, *ad libitum;* CR, calorie restriction.)

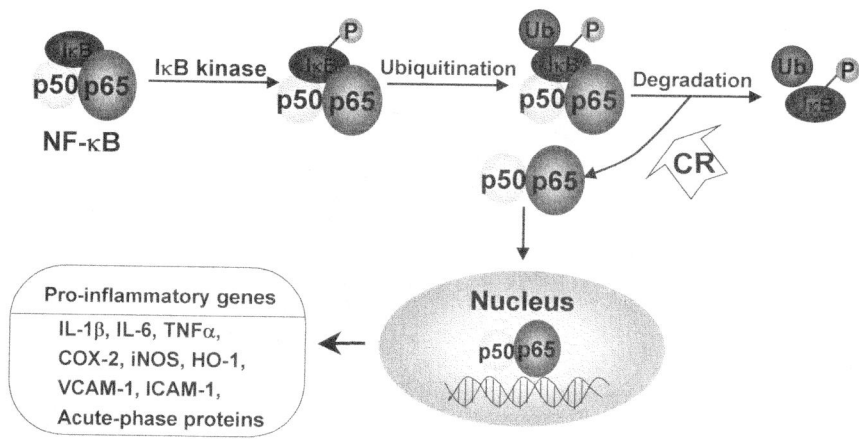

FIGURE 5. Possible active site of CR action in NF-κB activating system. (ABBREVIATION: CR, calorie restriction.)

consistent with what is known about CR's action against inflammation and oxidative stress. It is not surprising therefore to notice that in CR rats, the age-related increase in COX activity, PG synthesis, and COX-derived ROS generation were all suppressed by CR (unpublished data). The beneficial CR effects were further extended to the regulation of gene expression, as CR suppressed the increase of COX-2 mRNA and protein levels with age through the modulation of NF-κB and IκB.

In regard to CR's anti-inflammatory action, glucocorticoids should be mentioned, as they are well known for their anti-inflammatory property. Klebanov et al. showed that short-term CR animals (2 months) with elevated glucocorticoid levels were able to better manage carrageenan-induced inflammation, credited to increased glucocorticoid levels.[42] However, readers should be reminded that this experimentation was a short-term CR with an acute inflammatory response. In aged animals, glucocorticoid levels are elevated, and yet their inflammatory responses are still aggravated, indicating that the anti-inflammatory action of glucocorticoids might not be the major pathway in aged animals.

In summary, our laboratory found that CR attenuates several major proinflammatory proteins by preventing the dissociation of inhibitory IκBα and IκBβ from NF-κB complex. Other NF-κB-dependent genes—IL-1β, IL-6, TNFα, COX-2, and iNOS—are modulated in a similar fashion by CR (FIG. 5).

CONCLUSION

The implications of ROS/RNS in the tissue inflammation during the aging process are well demonstrated. Until recently, however, no quantitative information has been available on the extent of ROS/RNS generation contributing specifically to inflammatory reactions during aging.

Our laboratory obtained evidence for the first time that the activation of age-related NF-κB and the gene expression of several proinflammatory proteins are all attenuated by CR. Our data further showed that the attenuation of the NF-κB activation by CR was accomplished by blocking the dissociation of inhibitory IκBα and IκBβ. The regulation of inflammatory response by CR at molecular levels was further exhibited by the suppression of age-related increases in proinflammatory COX-2 gene expression and PG synthesis. A similar attenuation by CR was shown on other NF-κB-dependent genes, IL-1β, IL-6, TNFα, COX-2, and iNOS. Thus, a significant realization is that the inflammatory process is intricately involved in the aging process. These findings provide supportive molecular insights into the anti-inflammatory action of CR. Based on these findings and rationale, we propose the "Inflammation Hypothesis of Aging." Further molecular exploration is warranted for a better delineation of molecular interactions between normal aging and the inflammatory process.

ACKNOWLEDGMENT

This work was suppoted by Korea Research Foundation Grant (KRF-99-005-F00030).

REFERENCES

1. HUERRE, M.R. & P. GOUNON. 1996. Inflammation: patterns and new concepts. Res. Immunol. **147:** 417–434.

2. MAYERS, I. & D. JOHNSON. 1998. The nonspecific inflammatory response to injury. Can. J. Anaesth. **45:** 871–879.
3. KIM, H.J., *et al.* 2000. The effect of age on cyclooxygenase-2 gene expression: NF-κB activation and IκBα degradation. Free Radical Biol. & Med. In press.
4. GOTO, M., *et al.* 1999. Involvement of NF-κB p50/p65 heterodimer in activation of the human pro-interleukin-1beta gene at two subregions of the upstream enhancer element. Cytokine **11:** 16–28.
5. LEBERMANN, T.A. & D. BALTIMORE. 1990. Activation of the interleukin-6 gene expression through the NF-κB transcription factor. Mol. Cell. Biol. **10:** 2327–2334.
6. YAO, J., *et al.* 1997. Lipopolysaccharide induction of the tumor necrosis factor-alpha promoter in human monocytic cells. Regulation by Egr-1, c-Jun, and NF-κB transcription factors. J. Biol. Chem. **272:** 795–801.
7. TAYLOR, B.S., *et al.* 1998. Multiple NF-κB enhancer elements regulate cytokine induction of the human inducible nitric oxide synthase gene. J. Biol. Chem. **273:** 15148–15156.
8. YU, B.P. 1996. Aging and oxidative stress: modulation by dietary restriction. Free Radical Biol. & Med. **21:** 651–668.
9. MCGEER, E.G. & P.L. MCGEER. 1999. Brain inflammation in Alzheimer disease and the therapeutic implications. Curr. Pharm. Des. **5:** 821–836.
10. FIOTTI, N., *et al.* 1999. Atherosclerosis and inflammation. Patterns of cytokine regulation in patients with peripheral arterial disease. Atherosclerosis **145:** 51–60.
11. COLWELL, G.A. 1999. Inflammation and diabetic vascular complications. Diabetes Care **12:** 1927–1928.
12. MURAY, R.K., *et al.* 1993. Lipids of physiologic significance. *In* Harper's Biochemistry. Appleton and Lange, Eds.:143. Prentice Hall. London.
13. BEHARKA, A.A., *et al.* 1997. Macrophage prostaglandin production contributes to the age-associated decrease in T cell function which is reversed by the dietary antioxidant vitamin E. Mech. Ageing Dev. **93:** 59–77.
14. LEE, M. & M. FELDMAN. 1994. Age-related reductions in gastric mucosal prostaglandin levels increase susceptibility to aspirin-induced injury in rats. Gastroenterology **107:** 1746–1750.
15. HORNYCH, A., *et al.* 1991. The influence of age on renal prostaglandin synthesis in man. Prostaglandins Leukotrienes Essent. Fatty Acids **43:** 191–195.
16. NAKAJIMA, M., *et al.* 1997. Aging decreases the production of PGI2 in rat aortic endothelial cells. Exp. Gerontol. **32:** 685–693.
17. HAYEK, M.G., *et al.* 1997. Enhanced expression of inducible cyclooxygenase with age in murine macrophages. J. Immunol. **159:** 2445–2451.
18. KIM, J.W. 1998. Attenuation of free radical generation related to cardiac arachidonate cascade by dietary restriction during aging. M.S. Thesis, Pusan National Univ., Pusan, Korea.
19. KIM, H.J. 1999. Regulation of inflammatory enzymes via NF-κB in the aging process. M.S. Thesis, Pusan National Univ., Pusan, Korea.
20. BAEK, B.S., *et al.* 1999. Regional difference of ROS generation, lipid peroxidation, and antioxidant enzyme activity in rat brain and their dietary modulation. Arch. Pharm. Res. **22:** 361–366.
21. FENG, L., *et al.* 1995. Involvement of reactive oxygen intermediates in cyclooxygenase-2 expression induced by interleukin-1, tumor necrosis factor-alpha, and lipopolysaccharide. J. Clin. Invest. **95:** 1669–1675.
22. STUEHR, D.J., *et al.* 1991. Purification and characterization of the cytokine-induced macrophage nitric oxide synthase: an FAD- and FMN-containing flavoprotein. Proc. Natl. Acad. Sci. USA **88:** 7773–7777.
23. CERNADAS, M.R., *et al.* 1998. Expression of constitutive and inducible nitric oxide synthases in the vascular wall of young and aging rats. Circ. Res. **83:** 279–286.
24. POYNTER, M.E. & R.A. DAYNES. 1999. Age-associated alterations in splenic iNOS regulation: influence of constitutively expressed IFN-γ and correction following supplementation with PPARα activators or vitamin E. Cell. Immunol. **195:** 127–136.
25. KIM, Y.J. Antiaging mechanism of fish oil. M.S. Thesis, Pusan National Univ., Pusan, Korea.

26. ROITT, I.M., J. BROSTOFF & D.K. MALE. 1993. The cytokine network. *In* Immunology: 8–15. Mosby. St. Louis.
27. HOBBS, M.V., *et al.* 1993. Patterns of cytokine gene expression by CD4+ T cells from young and old mice. J. Immunol. **150:** 3602–3614.
28. RIANCHO, J.A., *et al.* 1994. Age-related differences in cytokine secretion. Gerontology **40:** 8–12.
29. MILLER, R.A. 1991. Aging and immune function. Int. Rev. Cytol. **124:** 187–215.
30. KUBO, M. & B. CINADER. 1990. Polymorphism of age-related changes in interleukin (IL) production: differential changes of T helper subpopulations, synthesizing IL-2, IL-3 and IL-4. Eur. J. Immunol. **20:** 1289–1296.
31. ROUBENOFF, R., *et al.* 1998. Monocyte cytokine production in an elderly population: effect of age and inflammation. J. Gerontol. Med. Sci. **53:** M20–M26.
32. RIKANS, L.E., *et al.* 1999. Effect of age and carbon tetrachloride on cytokine concentrations in rat liver. Mech. Ageing Dev. **108:** 173–182.
33. KWON, H.J. 2000. Gene expression of proinflammatory proteins and NF-κB activation in the aging process. M.S. Thesis, Pusan National Univ., Pusan, Korea.
34. BAEUERLE, P.A. & T. HENKEL. 1994. Function and activation of NF-κB in the immune system. Annu. Rev. Immunol. **12:** 141–179.
35. BALDWIN, A.S., JR. 1996. The NF-κB and IκB proteins: new discovers and insights. Annu. Rev. Immunol. **14:** 649–683.
36. BOWIE, A. & L.A. O'NEILL. 2000. Oxidative stress and nuclear factor-kappaB activation: a reassessment of the evidence in the light of recent discoveries. Biochem. Pharmacol. **59:** 13–23.
37. BAEUERLE, P.A. 1991. The inducible transcription activator NF-κB: regulation by distinct protein subunits. Biochim. Biophys. Acta **1072:** 63–80.
38. GRILLI, M., J.J.-S. CHIU & M.J. LEONARDO. 1993. NF-κB and Rel: participants in a multiform transcriptional regulatory system. Int. Rev. Cytol. **143:** 1–62.
39. HELENIUS, M., *et al.* 1996. Changes associated with aging and replicative senescence in the regulation of transcription factor nuclear factor-kappa B. Biochem. J. **318:** 603–608.
40. KORHONEN, P., M. HELENIUS & A. SALMINEN. 1997. Age-related changes in the regulation of transcription factor NF-κB in rat brain. Neurosci. Lett. **225:** 61–64.
41. YU, B.P. 1994. How diet influences the aging process of the rat. Proc. Soc. Exp. Biol. Med. **205:** 97–105.
42. KLEBANOV, S., *et al.* 1995. Hyper-adrenocorticism, attenuated inflammation, and the life-prolonging action of food restriction in mice. J. Gerontol. Biol. Sci. **50A:** B79–B82.

Panel Discussion

Perspectives in Aging Research in the New Millennium

SANG CHUL PARK, CHAIR

S. C. PARK (*Seoul National University College of Medicine, Seoul, South Korea*): I'd like to ask the participants to comment on the future aspects of aging research in their own fields. Afterwards, I will ask Earl Stadtman and Denham Harmon to make some general comments.

K. KITANI (*National Institute for Longevity Sciences, Aichi, Japan*): In my view aging studies so far have been a little confused because many people are mixing up the so-called public mechanism of aging and the private mechanism of aging, which was defined some years ago by George Martin in Seattle. The private mechanism applies only to certain subjects. It cannot be generalized to aging theory. On the other hand, the more important mechanism, the public mechanism, operates in a wide range of different species. When we discuss our own data or data from other studies, we have to make it clear whether we are discussing the private mechanism or are trying to make an interpretation with regard to the public mechanism of aging. The latter is what we need to start from now. Of course we have to work on the molecular, the genetic, and the cellular levels. But all of us have to keep in mind that finally what we need to do is resolve the mechanism of aging as the aging of the whole organism.

B. P. YU (*University of Texas, San Antonio, TX*): I second what Dr. Kitani was saying, but I'd like to add some remarks about the future of aging research in Korea. With limited resources, I think we should focus on certain aspects of the specific geographical areas. More than 80 percent of dementia in Korea is actually due to the vascular dementia totally different from western area. This is just the typical type of a thing that I try to use as examples. And I look at thing that with a limited resources whether we can do better or maybe help to all the knowledge about the dementia from that angles. And this of course I start from the molecular level up to the (ecological) study. So what I see this has not only the basic understanding of aging, but also imagine application to the therapeutic type of approach. So that cover that ends. Dr. Park Sang Chul and Kenichi Kitani always mention about the functional longevity. And I fully support that idea within the spirits of, this kind of application which we have to resolve what ever means we have. And doing in depth a basic and clinical research, same time we have to really look at for the extension of a function of the longevities. I think that's a key.

D. K. INGRAM (*National Institute on Aging, Baltimore, MD.*): My comments will be directed towards gerontology as a discipline and then towards the future role of genetics in our scientific pursuits. In 1975, as a graduate student at the University of Georgia, I attended my first Society for Neural Science meeting in Atlanta, Georgia. The attendance was about 800 or maybe a 1000. Last November, I attended the Society for Neural Science meeting in Miami, Florida, and the attendance was 27,000 people. Neural science 25 years ago was a hybrid science in which various disciplines were brought together to study the brain; it became a new research paradigm. Gerontology also is a hybrid science, requiring the interaction of many disciplines. I see that the attendance we've had here in Korea shows the upward curve in the dedication to this new discipline. I predict that in a couple of decades gerontology will have the power, strength, and potential that I've seen in neuroscience, as a legitimate science with incredible new interest among scientists.

Part of that interest goes back to my experience in 1978, when I finished my graduate work at the University of Georgia and took my first doctoral fellowship at the Jackson laboratory in the "Behavior Genetics" section. My major professor in psychology told me, "I don't understand how you can analyze behavior in terms of genetics." There's a far reach from psychological phenomena to gene expression. Recently I was very excited by a collaboration: we examined gene expression during a learning event in its alteration with aging. We used the emerging microarray technology, which was presented at this meeting and which some years ago I thought was not a very good approach to science. It was what we called a shotgun approach, trying to ask all the questions at once. I'm convinced now that it's not a shotgun, it's more like a cruise missile: you can knock down a number of questions you want to ask. We're very fortunate to have this powerful new technology to identify genes that are expressed during a psychological event; it opens up an incredible new frontier that will no doubt be exploited. As the genome project unfolds and we gain access to the entire human genome and the genomes of our experimental models, it will be incredibly exciting to have in our hands this new technology. This, combined with the increased interest in and demographic imperative of gerontology, indicates the field's great potential.

A. REZNICK (*Technion, Haifa, Israel*): I was asked to talk about the role of exercise and physical activity as a practical approach to aging. When we talk about genes and about molecular biology in aging, we sometimes forget that for everyday practical life we need other things, such as proper nutrition and proper exercise. Aging can be said to have extrinsic and intrinsic causes, which are interrelated. Extrinsic causes, such as environmental stresses, can be subdivided into many other categories, such as physical activity, nutrition, life habits, and psychological stresses. The intrinsic causes are programmed or random. The former have to do with the genetics of aging; the latter have to do with postsynthetic modification of proteins, random chemical modifications, and free radical changes. All of these causes of the aging process are affected by exercise.

Rats aged 6, 9, 15, and 20 months were subjected to the same running exercise for four and a half months to determine the effect on survival. Among those that started at 6 months the survival rates were 80% for the trained and 63% for the nontrained. Among those that started at 9 months the survival rates were 70% for the trained and 53% for the nontrained. Among those that started the exercise program at 15 months the survival rates for the trained and the nontrained were about the same. For those that started the exercises at 20 months the survival rate of the nontrained was much higher than that of the trained. It appears that at around 15 months a threshold is reached for a particular activity beyond which that activity is detrimental to longevity. We looked at various other parameters, such as biochemical data and enzymes, and found confirmation that there is such an age threshold for particular kinds of exercise, that the same exercise is not appropriate for all ages.

The challenge that we have is to find the right recipe for exercise for humans in old age in order to make exercise beneficial. I think exercise is beneficial and important, but it can be also very dangerous when the threshold of age is contravened. So in the next millennium we have to ask those who work in exercise and aging to find a good recipe. Also, it must be recognized that chronological age and biological age not always go together. A person can be 50 chronologically but 40 or 60 biologically. So we cannot tell a person who is 50 to do an exercise appropriate for a 50-year-old unless we know how well he is physically and whether his chronological and biological ages correspond. From that point of view, we have to be very careful when we advise people to do exercise. That's where the research has to go in the next millennium: to find the proper exercise for aging people, so that it may be beneficial to all of the elderly.

S. GOTO (*Toho University, Chiba, Japan*): I would like to make some remarks on Dr. Byung Pal Yu's talk about hormesis. I have been very interested in that approach for a number of years. For example, rather than drugs, I would like to suggest bathing in hot springs. In Korea, Japan, and perhaps in China people like to bathe in hot springs; and they live long. This is probably because bathing causes the induction of (heat shock) proteins and also perhaps the potentiation of the immune reaction under the skin, which have a protective effect on health.

I would also like to remark on the effect of alcohol. As you know, alcohol is metabolized to acetaldehyde, which may cause some modification of proteins. This may have some protective effect because the slight damage to the protein may cause some elevation of protective enzymes. Daily intake of alcohol will induce such a protective effect. I think it would be worthwhile to pursue the mechanisms of the health-promoting effect of bathing in hot springs and drinking alcohol, both of which are more pleasurable than taking a tablet or two.

Finally, the study of centenarians may be very important as we enter the next century. In Japan the number of centenarians is increasing by perhaps 2000–3000 per year, reaching nearly 11,000 as of autumn 1999. These people are a very good target for studying human longevity. We should probably study their genetic background and lifestyle. These may perhaps yield ideas on both the mechanism of aging and life extension measures.

G. S. ROTH (*National Institute on Aging, Baltimore, MD*): Some people have suggested that health span and life span may be inseparable. It's going to be very interesting to see if people who do live to great ages benefit from increased quality of life and more healthy years. Or will the very dire prediction of some be borne out that people who attain such ages will spend the last 20 or so years of life incapacitated and institutionalized. Certainly that's something none of us want. From a research point of view it hasn't really been brought up yet that we're probably going to have all of the human genome sequence in the next decade. Those of you who work on the genetic aspects of longevity know that almost every other week in *Science* and *Nature* someone with a nematode or yeast comes up with another gene for longevity. There are many there. From the standpoint of humans I think this is probably not the way we are going to extend the maximal life span. I do believe that the characterization of all these genes will probably help us alleviate many of the diseases of aging.

A former director of our institute was of the opinion that aging doesn't exist, that it really is the diseases of aging that we need to focus on. We hear very often of the concept of squaring the survival curve. We are pushing the median life span further and further out, but not necessarily the maximal life span. I think that's what the human genome project can do for us. I think that genes for diabetes, genes for cardiovascular disease, genes for cancer—all of these are going to help us square the curve. But from the standpoint of the fundamental underlying process that we call aging and that predisposes us to all of these age-related diseases, I think we can only work thermodynamically. I don't think gene therapy in a mammal is going to be practical at all. I think aging is too complex for that. I think it's a global thermodynamic disordering process. The only way we're going to effect it is by a thermodynamic intervention. Obviously we're biased, because the calorie restriction paradigm is the one intervention that has stood the test of time. It's a thermodynamic intervention. I have begun to scratch the surface with respect to ways to mimic the beneficial effects of caloric restriction without limiting food intake but also through a thermodynamic type of intervention, by slowing the energy flow.

I. Zs.-Nagy (*University of Debrecen, Debrecen, Hungary*): I'm convinced that predictions are very difficult to make. We believe that on the basis of our actual knowledge we can make predictions. We are just fooling ourselves, because the actual knowledge is always limited; and we don't know what knowledge future will bring. My dream is that in the future rationality in gerontological research will prevail. But we have to realize that gerontological research is still in the analytical phase. So we are collecting data. A lot of these data will not be significant at all in understanding the general mechanism because they are describing details that are not important from general point of view. Even if we know all the 6000 gene products that are now under exploration, we still have to return to the cell.

Cell physiology has been forgotten: one sees hardly any papers dealing with the cell as a whole. One does see molecular biological research with descriptive results, but most people don't know about the cell as a whole. So when we have come to know all of the products, we will have entered a new period, one in which we have to select what is important and what is not important from this general point of view. Then we will realize that the main common aspect of all living systems is the physical chemistry of the cell.

M. Meydani (*Tufts University, Medford, MA*): I'm here not to predict. I'm here to outline what kind of a task we have in the future; what we know, where we are, and where we are going; how to manage the aging population—how to keep them alive, healthy, and enjoying their lives by pharmacological intervention, biological intervention (maybe gene therapy, maybe not), and lifestyle intervention. I'm thinking that we can do a lot by changing lifestyle. We are soon going to know about our genetic makeup. There is a quite a bit of interaction between lifestyle and environment with these genes, and we cannot ignore that. Every day we are interacting with these genes by eating breakfast, lunch and dinner. The food we eat is getting into our cells and is interacting with our genes, stimulating or suppressing them. Nutritional intervention is practical and cheaper than pharmacological intervention or gene therapy. We can do alot with nutrition. At this point we don't know what the nutritional requirements are for people over the age of 50. The U.S. Food and Drug Administration's recommended daily allowances are set for a maximum age of 50. We need to know the nutritional requirements of older people—60, 65, even 85 or 100. We must learn what they need to remain alive and healthy. This is the big task in front of us.

J. VIJG (*University of Texas Health Science Center and Institute for Drug Development, San Antonio, TX*): It seems that there are two major conclusions that can be drawn about aging. One is that aging is really multifactorial, with many causes and many mechanisms. The second is that people's approaches to aging are not necessarily very logical: they just go off to their own pet theories. That's I think why aging research is still a young science. But it's going to be maturing. I think genome analysis is going to play a major role. The only way to get good information about what is the driving force of the aging process and the mechanisms of longevity is to do an objective screen. You can call that the genomics of aging or age genomics. Of course, even if you have the total human genome sequence, you have to search through all that raw sequence to find coding regions and identify the genes to find the pathways that drive the aging process and control longevity. First of all you can do genome typing. Once you have a consensus sequence of the human genome, you need to go after the enormous individual variation that probably determines a lot about how somebody ages. Then you would use that polymorphic variation and mobilize population genetic studies on various aspects of aging and longevity. You have to associate functional values of genes with particular function types. Finding resistance to functional decline, selecting individuals with a particularly high resistance to general or vascular decline would be interesting. I think this would give us insight into the genes or gene variants that actually control those processes. You can do that at the RNA level using microarrays or at the protein level using other technologies, such as SAGE. It's likely that these studies have already begun. Then you need to do something with this information, and this is the more exciting part. This is what you could call a functional genomics of aging and longevity. So you really have to look at function. We will see an enormous development of the technology by which we can reconstruct functional processes.

To the myriad of molecular information regarding gene variance expression patterns you can apply cluster analysis, and eventually you will be able to predict protein functions. The meaning of the slight differences among gene coding sequences must be ascertained. The second part is similar—to reconstruct functional pathways in model systems. You can use this technique to develop artificial chromosomes and cells so that you can put entire functional pathways on one particular factor and bring it into cells or other organisms. The developments here are in the realm of novel factors and delivery systems.

Finally, I think the most exciting part will be that you can eventually quit doing the experiments altogether because you can completely simulate those pathways in interaction, creating digital organisms. This is not as far away as many people think. It means that you can play with an organism, let it age, let it make all kinds of changes, and see what happens. Then you can make a practical variant of the organism by creating cells using a minimum number of genes. Eventually, you may wonder whether it's still worthwhile to get more and more information about how to alter the aging process in humans when you can simply download your brain. I guess you won't need your body any more. This may be several centuries away. But I think genomics is definitely the major key to the future in aging research.

PARK: Prevention of disease is a very important aspect of future research in gerontology. We heard a very good story about green tea. Here in Korea, as in Japan and China, we have a long history of so-called herbal, or traditional, medicine. Herbs contain a lot of very interesting, effective, useful antioxidants along with other ingredients. They appear to help prevent disease. Our familiarity with their use in medicine perhaps gives us an advantage, which I think we ought to exploit through greater research efforts. The primary goal of an experiment in gerontology is extension of the functional life span. Prevention of disease also accomplishes that goal.

YU: Scientists have a responsibility to inform the general public; scientists in the field of aging are behind in this respect. We must form a united group and put in the do a credible job, so that we have something to offer the public. To inform the public takes a lot of time and effort. Say that what they're doing is wrong and what they are doing are right. Public is completely at the loss. And I think that this is very pertinent and also essential part of the responsibility of scientists working aging.

D. HARMON (*University of Nebraska College of Medicine, Omaha, NE*): First I think we'd better keep in mind what the goal is—to make sure we can increase our healthy span and productive life. I mean by that not just the number of years, but also that we make sure that the terminal portion of life is at least satisfactory. At present there are two ways to get there. We can continue doing what we're doing, which is to try to improve our general living conditions. This includes nutrition, medical care, accident prevention, and so forth. This approach has served us very well. We have risen from an average life expectancy of 30 years in the time of ancient Rome to an average life expectancy in developed countries that is about six to nine years short of our potential maximum average life expectancy at birth. In the past we didn't necessarily know anything about aging. We just accumulated better practical knowledge: how to build better houses, and a little bit more about nutrition, for example. But from here on we're going to have to concentrate on that process that is within us, the so-called aging process. It's an innate process that kills us. There are a lot of clues as to what that process is. I need not mention to you that this research is a very uncertain enterprise. I think we should continue to do what we have been doing and cast a wide net to accept ideas from all sources.

To do that we need more money. This is a real shortcoming in the United States. We have very little money for basic research. Most of the money is going into the so-called social programs. I think we should have some appropriate funding bodies, if we can find them, who can rise above their immediate self-interest and pick out the avenues that look promising and direct more resources and effort into them. I think this is how we're going to have to go in the future. Our research is too uncertain. We have to maintain a broad approach. It will be difficult to increase our average life expectancy significantly, but there are a lot of clues out there in the research literature right now about things we can do that may have an impact on our maximum life span. I think we just have to keep our eyes open and keep working.

E. STADTMAN (*National Heart, Lung, and Blood Institute, Bethesda, MD*): The problem with aging research is that it is a multifaceted process. It depends largely on how you define aging. In general I agree with what's been said here, but when it comes to identifying the causes of aging, whether at the genetic level or another level, I think this is going to be an unsolvable problem, at least in the near future, simply because aging isn't a single thing. It's one thing in one individual, but it's a different thing in another. You can imagine, for example, that aging could result from a knockout of almost any important enzyme activity in the cell. This would have implications for signal transduction pathways, where a myriad of proteins interact with one another. My guess is that when you get to the point where you start looking for defects that lead to differences in life span in different people, you'll find many possibilities. It's already been shown that you can identify more than one gene—three or four genes have been identified—that will increase life span. But the problem is that there may be another 50 genes that can do that, too.

Trying to relate what goes on in one individual with respect to what goes on in another is where the big problem is going to come. Cells have remarkable backup systems; they have two completely different enzyme systems that can perform the same function. If a person is born with a defect in one of the two systems, then he may be more prone to degeneration as a consequence of a defect in the other, as opposed to person who is born with both genes viable. So again the question is, are we going to be able to solve the question of aging in terms of identifying specific genes? I believe it's conceivable that almost every gene can contribute to the aging process. A given gene may be more important in one individual then it is in another, depending on their genetic backgrounds.

Having said this, I'm reminded of lecture by a very prominent biochemist that I attended when I was a graduate student. He said there are two things that we will probably never understand because they're just too complicated. One is how nucleic acids are made, and the other is how proteins are made. As you all know, we now know an awful lot about the chemistry of the biosynthesis of nucleic acid and proteins. So when I say that it may be difficult or impossible to define all of the genes that are involved in aging, I may be just as far off as that guy who gave that talk when I was a graduate student.

In my talk I presented some evidence that there is an accumulation of oxidized proteins in the course of the aging process. Among the various models that have been used in this context is a rat model, in which it has been shown by a person in my laboratory that when one analyzes the carbonyl content of proteins in rats, one finds an age-related increase in the amount of oxidative damage. When we reexamined this phenomenon 10 years later, in a different context, we didn't see that same effect of aging in carbonyl content that we had observed earlier. I was concerned that maybe the original investigation was flawed. We found that we still had samples from the original study in the −80-degree deep freezer, so we reexamined them. We found the same age-related change that had been recorded earlier, so something had happened in the interim. The rats used in both studies were obtained from the same source and, we were told, had been given the same diet, the same treatment. But it was clear that after 10 years there was a difference in the animals. In fact, it was pointed out to us that those animals were now living about 30% longer than they did 10 years earlier.

This raises a very serious question: When you start looking at changes as a function of chronological age, what is the genetic background? What has been selected for over time? I think the difference between the original study and the later study comes down to the fact that over a period of 10 years there had been a selection process in the animals that had changed their responses to oxidative stress.

I agree with virtually everything said here today. We're talking about a lot of different processes and ways to look at them. I think hormesis is going to be one of the major areas of study in the future. It's quite clear already that if you expose an animal to one kind of oxidative stress at a low, nonlethal level, it can withstand an otherwise-lethal dose of that same stress. We're going to be looking at this in the future. With the new technology of the gene chip, by which you can follow the fates of genes under various conditions, we will be able to identify hundreds and thousands of the genes that are involved. Maybe there will be some surprises with respect to what happens during the aging process.

Finally, I think one of the more important things that's going to happen in the immediate future—it's happening now—is the role of alterations in the cell signal transduction pathways, leading, for example, to apoptosis and the capacity for cell regulation, will be examined. Why, for instance, do cells elect to use reactive oxygen species such as hydrogen peroxide as a signaling event for apoptosis on the one hand and for cellular replication on the other hand, when it's known that hydrogen peroxide can be very damaging? I think one scenario follows from the consideration that once a tissue has reached the adult stage, it ceases to increase in size. Very little cell division then occurs, except to the extent that there has been cellular damage that has not been gotten rid of. So, coming back to the cell signaling pathways, I wonder if it might not be that when the steady state level of hydrogen peroxide, which is normally low, starts to increase just a little bit, the cells become alarmed. They set in motion a regulatory process that would allow them to take care of the events that would happen if the level of reactive oxygen species were to continue to elevate. They set in place a mechanism for apoptosis on the one hand and a mechanism for cell replication on the other hand, in response to this slightly elevated level of hydrogen peroxide. Then, if a damaging event occurs as a consequence of the increased reactive oxygen species formation, leading to oxidation of cellular function or functional molecules such as proteins, DNA, and lipids, the apoptotic system is now active. It's ready to get rid of that damaged cell. But it's more important that, once you get rid of that dead cell, a good cell be able to replace it. You have to set in place a regulatory cell replicative capacity so that you can replace that bad cell with a good cell.

If there is any merit to this general thesis, then I think at least one aspect of aging is associated with a loss of the apoptotic capacity of cells. Indeed, when we measure oxidative damage, we may be looking at damage that has not been replaced—we are looking at cells that did not get apoptotic treatment when they should have. In any case, I think that in the area of signal transduction, the area of hormesis, coupled with the whole problem of genetic changes, is going to be the thing of the future as far as research in the aging field is concerned.

PARK: All the aspects of aging research have been discussed. I think research methods must somehow be standardized, using the same model systems or the same objects, so that data may be compared all over the world; and I think all the aspects of science should collaborate in aging research. This would do much to promote the goal of aging research, to improve the health and quality of life of the elderly.

A Thermolabile Variant of Methylenetetrahydrofolate Reductase Is a Determinant of Hyperhomocyst(e)inemia in the Elderly

JUN-HYUN YOO

Department of Family Medicine, Center for Clinical Research, Samsung Biomedical Research Institute, Samsung Medical Center, Sungkyunkwan University School of Medicine, Seoul, Korea

Hyperhomocyst(e)inemia has been recognized as an independent risk factor of occlusive vascular disease, including coronary artery disease, stroke, peripheral arterial occlusive disease. Hyperhomocyst(e)inemia, without renal dysfunction, is caused by genetic factors, nongenetic factors or a combination of both. In addition, it is understood that the presence of a genetic defect is mandatory to sustain long-term, elevated concentration of plasma homocysteine during life. Methylenetetrahydrofolate reductase (MTHFR) enzyme catalyzes the reduction of 5,10-methylenetetrahydrofolate to 5-methyltetrahydrofolate, which is the primary methyl donor for the remethylation of homocysteine to methionine. A common mutation (677 C→T) in the 5,10-methylenetetrahydrofolate reductase gene, in which a cytidine residue at nucleotide position 677 is replaced by thymidine, is associated with a reduced enzyme activity and confers a thermolabile property of the enzyme. To examine whether the MTHFR genetic polymorphism is a determinant of hyperhomocyst(e)inemia in the elderly, one hundred forty-two patients with angiographically documented coronary artery disease and 122 patients with cerebral infarction proven by magnetic resonance imaging, and 208 healthy subjects (≥65 years) were studied. Those with thyroid or renal dysfunction, cancer, or users of multivitamin or estrogen were excluded. The prevalence of hyperhomocyst(e)inemia, defined as 15.0 mol/L, was higher in subjects than in controls (25.4 versus 10.0%, $p = 0.005$). The frequency of MTHFR TT homozygotes did not differ between the diseased group and the normal group (14.5 versus 12.8%, $p < 0.05$). In the diseased group, MTHFR TT genotype had a higher total homocysteine level than those of CT or CC types (19.8 ± 7.1 versus 10.7 ± 5.6, 10.3 ± 4.6 mol/L, $p < 0.05$). In the normal group, MTHFR TT genotypes exhibited a higher tHcy level than those of CT or CC types (14.8 ± 7.3 versus 9.6 ± 4.6, 9.2 ± 4.2 mol/L, $p < 0.05$). In multiple logistic regression analysis to determine the independent effect of MTHFR genotype on homocyst(e)ine levels, TT genotype, folate, and advancing age emerged as the significant predictors of moderate hyperhomocyst(e)inemia after additional adjustment of vitamin B_{12}, smoking, and alcohol drinking. In elderly Koreans studied, this finding indicates that the MTHFR TT genotype is a major determinant of hyperhomocyst(e)inemia. The elderly bearing MTHFR TT genotype may need a higher requirement of folate to maintain the normal range of plasma homocyst(e)ine concentration.

Age-related Increase in the Expression of Heat-Shock Protein Genes in the Tissues of Unstressed Rats

RYOYA TAKAHASHI AND SATARO GOTO

Department of Biochemistry, School of Pharmaceutical Sciences, Toho University, Japan

Conformationally and functionally altered proteins accumulate in various tissues with age. We previously found that the amount of heat-labile enzymes are increased in the tissues of mice and rats with aging. Although a causal relationship between senescence and altered proteins is unclear, it is likely that their accumulation could deteriorate various cellular functions, especially the ability to cope with a variety of stresses. It is well known that heat-shock proteins (hsps) are induced by hyperthermia and other stresses. Most of these inducers share the common property of causing the accumulation of denatured proteins within cells. The results of most studies, including our own work, have indicated that the expression of hsp genes (mostly hsp70) by various inducers is reduced in *in vitro* aged cells and cells from aging animals, but little information is yet available on age-related changes in the expression of hsp genes in the tissues of unstressed animals. In this study, we investigated the effect of aging on the expression of stress-inducible hsp (hsp25 and hsp70) genes in the brain, liver, and heart of unstressed rats (F344). The steady-state levels of mRNAs and the extracts of heat-shocked rat hepatocytes (43°C, 30 min) as a positive control. Although no detectable levels of hsp70 mRNA were observed in all tissues examined from unstressed young and old rats, the amount of hsp70 in the heart of old rats was about 40% higher than that in young ones. Higher amounts of the mRNA and protein of hsp27 were observed in the heart of both young and old rats. The mRNA and protein levels of hsp27 in the heart appeared to increase with age but no statistically significant difference was observed between young and old animals. Hsp27 mRNA was not detectable in the liver and brain but, interestingly, the amount of hsp27 in both tissues increased by about twofold with age. We also measured the activity of heat shock factor (HSF), which plays a critical role in regulating the transcription of hsp genes. The activity of HSF in the liver extract from unstressed rats significantly increased with age. Increase in the level of hsps in unstressed aged animals might be a reflection of age-related accumulation of altered proteins.

Amyloid-β-Peptide 25-35 Fragment Modulates the Expression of the Mitochondrial Cytochrome Oxidase Gene

BOK-GHEE HAN, EUN HYE HAN, JEUNG YEUB AHN, AND JUNGSOON PARK

Laboratory of Degenerative Diseases, Department of Biomedical Sciences, Korean National Institute of Health, Seoul 122-701 Korea

It has been suggested that mitochondrial dysfunction is one of the causes of neurological diseases including Alzheimer's disease (AD). AD-associated mitochondrial dysfunction is well known, but the underlying mechanisms are unknown. In addition, amyloid-β-peptide (Aβ), which is an important component of neuritic plaques in an AD patient's brain, is known to be a key factor in the neuropathogenesis of AD. The purpose of this study was to assess whether Aβ-induced cytotoxicity involves mitochondrial dysfunction. When the activities of cytochrome c oxygenase (COX) as a marker of mitochondrial function were measured, a significant decrease in COX was observed in Aβ-treated SK-N-SH cells. Expression of mitochondrial DNA-encoded COX subunit genes was analyzed by quantitative RT-PCR and northern blotting. It was found that COX subunit mRNA levels decreased in Aβ-treated cells as compared with control cells. Aβ induced a significant decrease in all mitochondrial COX subunits (I, II, and III) in a dose- and time-dependent manner. A mitochondrial transcription factor, mtTF-1, mRNA level was also decreased after Aβ treatment. These results suggest that Aβ modulates the mitochondrial gene expression through the decrease of mtTF-1.

Analysis of the Cell Distribution of Endogenous Murine Leukemia Virus in the Brains of SAMR1 and SAMP8 Mice

BYUNG-HOON JEONG,[a] JAE-KWANG JIN,[a] EUN-KYOUNG CHOI,[a] H.C. MEEKER,[c] CHRISTINE A. KOZAK,[d] RICHARD I CARP,[c] AND YONG-SUN KIM[a,b]

[a]*Institute of Environment and Life Science, Hallym Academy of Sciences and*
[b]*Department of Microbiology, College of Medicine, Hallym University, Chunchon, Kangwon-Do 200-702, Korea*

[c]*Department of Virology, NYS Institute for Basic Research in Developmental Disabilities, Staten Island, NY 10314, USA*

[d]*Laboratory of Molecular Microbiology, National Institute of Allergy and Infectious Diseases, National Institutes of Health, Bethesda, Maryland 20892, USA*

Much higher levels of ecotropic murine leukemia virus (E-MuLV) are seen in the brains of accelerated senescence-prone (SAMP8) mice than in those of an accelerated senescence-resistant (SAMR1) strain. In order to investigate the cellular localization of E-MuLV in SAMP8, we determined the types of cells that express E-MuLV antigen in striatum, brainstem, hippocampus, and cerebellum of SAMR1 and SAMP8 by immunohistochemistry. E-MuLV antigen was seen in the neurons and astrocytes of brain regions of SAMP8, but not in those of SAMR1. In SAMP8, immunoreactivity of glial fibrillary acidic protein (GFAP) was significantly enhanced. Vacuolation was detected only in brains of SAMP8, but not those of SAMR1. Furthermore, we analyzed the gene expression of mRNA of E-MuLV in the brains of SAMR1 and SAMP8 by RT-PCR and found that E-MuLV mRNA was expressed at a high level in SAMP8 mice compared to SAMR1 mice. Automatic DNA sequencing of a 605-base sequence in the envelope coding region of the SAMP8-derived virus mRNA (RT transcribed) was identical to the same region of the AKV MuLV proviral gene. A restriction map of SAMP8 isolate showed no differences from that of AKV MuLV. These results suggest that E-MuLV generated from endogenous AKV provirus replicates in neurons and astrocytes in the brains of SAMP8 and could cause the neuronal cell loss, astrocytosis, and vacuolation seen in this mouse strain.

Analysis of Traditional Korean Food Patterns According to the Healthy Longevity Diet Based on the Database of Favorite Korean Foods

MEE-SOOK LEE,[a] MEE-KYUNG WOO,[a] CHUNG-SHIL KWAK,[b] SE-IN OH,[b] AND SANG-CHUL PARK[c,d]

[a]*Department of Food and Nutrition, Hannam University, Taejon, Korea*

[b]*Aging and Phsical Culture Research Institute, Seoul National University, Seoul, Korea*

[c]*Department of Biochemistry, Seoul National University College of Medicine, Seoul, Korea*

The traditional Korean diet is reevaluated as the healthy longevity diet, because it is nutritionally balanced and contains less fat and more complex carbohydrates and fiber than the Western diet. In the traditional Korean diet, energy from cereals is 55–60% of total energy, while that from fat energy is 15–20%, and the ratio of the weight of vegetables/meat and fish is over 2. The traditional Korean diet is largely composed of two parts: Joo-sik (staple foods), and Boo-sik (dishes), which in turn is composed of Joo-chan (main dishes) and Boo-chan (side dishes). Joo-sik is boiled rice, the main source of carbohydrates, with some barley, beans, peas, millet, and red beans. Joo-chan consists of meat, fish, eggs, beans, and their products as the sources of protein. Boo-chan contains vegetables, mushrooms, or seaweed as the sources of minerals and vitamins. Besides, soup and Kimchi are always served basically. Soup is made with various vegetables, seaweeds, meat, shellfish, or bone. Especially soybean paste and tofu, which contain saponin, isoflavone, and other active substances, are widely used for soup. The favorite fish are mackerel, soury, and herring, which supply w-3 fatty acids and conjugated linoleic acid. Especially, Kimchi, standing for a group of fermented vegetables enriched with fiber, vitamins, minerals, antioxidants, lactobacillus, and some unknown substances, is reported to have hypolipidemic, anticancer, antimutagenic, microbial, growth inhibitory, and platelet-aggregation inhibitory effects. Garlic, green pepper, ginger, sesame seeds and oil, and the perilla seeds and oil are usually used as seasonings. Based on these data, it is suggested that the traditional Korean diet helps to prevent obesity, cardiovascular disease, cancer, and degenerative diseases, which are the major causes of mortality and morbidity in the elderly.

[d]Corresponding author.

Analysis of Proteins in Aged Rat Kidney: The Effect of Calorie Restriction

HYON-JEEN KIM,[a] HYEON-YOUNG JEONG,[a] BYUNG-PAL YU,[b]
SATARO GOTO,[c] AND HAE-YOUNG CHUNG[a,b]

Vascular Aging Research Group, [a]College of Pharmacy, [b]Research Institute of Genetic Engineering, Pusan National University, Pusan 609-735, Korea

[c]*Department of Biochemistry, School of Pharmaceutical Sciences, Toho University, Miyama, Funabashi, Chiba 274-8510, Japan*

One of characteristic signs of aging is the accumulation of proteins in the cells and tissues. Changes in the protein pattern may be related to the functional decline and pathology of the aging tissue or organs. Because calorie restriction (CR) is the only effective experimental manipulation known to retard aging in rodents, we attempted to document the effect of CR on age-related alteration in protein accumulation. In the study, we quantified the changes in the age-dependent protein pattern and the effect of CR in rat kidney homogenate. Specific pathogen-free male Fischer 344 rats of 6, 12, 18, and 24 months of age were fed *ad libitum* (AL), and CR was used. It is important to note that no evidence of nephrotic lesions were detected in these soy-protein fed rats even at 24 months of age as revealed by histopathological examination. Results showed that the electrophoretic analysis of the protein yielded a major band of albumin with molecular weight of 66.2 kDa that was markedly increased with age in AL rats, whereas CR kept it at low levels throughout at all ages studied. N-terminal amino acid sequencing following eluting confirmed the protein as albumin. Analysis by Western blotting produced additional evidence on the gradual accumulation of albumin with age in AL rats, and its suppression by CR. To test whether renal albumin correlates with serum albumin, we analyzed the age-related changes in serum albumin. The ratio of serum albumin to total serum protein was markedly lower in AL rats than that in CR rats. Decreased serum albumin with age was often taken as a sign of renal dysfunction. However, in view of the absence of nephropathic lesions in these rats, data on the decreased serum protein in AL rats are difficult to explain at present. However, for CR, it may be possible that the antioxidative CR may reduce protein accumulation by reducing glycated proteins. It is known that glycated proteins elicit expression of various proinflammatory genes, which are responsive in changes in renal permeability. The present data suggest that age-related renal protein accumulation needs further clarification as to cause, because oxidatively modified accumulated albumin during aging may be a significant factor contributing to the pathogenic process including inflammation of renal tubules.

This work was supported by Grant PF002201-08 from Plant Diversity Research Center of the 21st Frontier Research Program funded by MSTK.

Analysis of Redox Status in Serum during Aging

JUNG-WON KIM, JAE-KYUNG NO, BYUNG-PAL YU, AND HAE-YOUNG CHUNG

College of Pharmacy, Pusan National University, Pusan, Korea

Aging and age-related diseases are known to be associated with increased oxidative stress. For the protection against the deleterious effects of oxidative stress, a well-coordinated network of both nonenzymatic and enzymatic antioxidant defense systems are essential. Although the redox status of various tissues and organs in the aging process was studied, data concerning serum status are not readily available. In the present study, we investigated the age-related redox status of serum by analyzing hydrogen peroxide, hydroxyl radical, superoxide-scavenging abilities, and other pertinent markers. Blood samples from male Fischer 344 rats of 13 and 31 months of age were drawn and allowed to clot, and the serum was separated and stored at −70°C until analyses were performed. To assess the age-related changes in serum antioxidant status, serum samples were oxidatively challenged with $FeSO_4/H_2O_2$, menadione, or H_2O_2. The extent of the antioxidation of serum was quantified using dichlorofluorescin diacetate (DCFH-DA). Serum peroxide levels were estimated using a PeroXOquant kit. Protein modifications were analyzed by Western blot. Results showed that anti-oxidation abilities were significantly decreased in serum from aged rats that was accompanied with the markedly increased peroxide levels with age. The protein oxidation detected by the OxyBlot kit and subsequent Western blot revealed that oxidized protein levels increased slightly at older ages. Levels of nitrated proteins induced by peroxynitrite treatment were higher in old rats than the young. Our results clearly indicated that balance between pro-oxidant and antioxidant in serum shifted in favor of the oxidation during aging. To confirm further this age-related redox shift, we quantified changes in the major antioxidant, thiol content. It was found that total thiol level significantly decreased (30.6%) in aged group. In this regard, we analyzed the age-related reduction of serum albumin. This reduction of albumin may be responsible in part for the decreased thiol levels, because albumin provides the bulk of total plasma thiols. A similar situation can be explained by low levels of serum GSH in old ages compared to young rats. The significance of the present study is the data showing serum with increased oxidative stress during aging that were caused by decreased major antioxidant components in serum.

This work was supported by Grant PF002201-08 from Plant Diversity Research Center of the 21st Frontier Research Program funded by MSTK.

Animal Model for Alzheimer's Disease by *PS2* Gene Transfer

DAE-YOUN HWANG, KAP-RYONG CHAE, TAE-SURK KANG, DONG-HWAN SHIN, IN-SURK JANG, JIN-HEE HWANG, YEON-JU KIM, JOON-YONG CHO, BUM-JIN KIM, YONG-KYU KIM,[a] AND JUNG-SIK CHO

Division of Laboratory Animal Resources, Korea Food and Drug Administration, National Institue of Toxicological Research, Seoul 122-704, Korea

Alzheimer's disease (AD), the most common cause of dementia occurring in elderly humans, affected 8.3% people over 65 years of age in 1995, and during the next 20 years, the number of persons with AD will exceed 0.62 million in Korea. AD occurs when neurons in the memory and cognition regions of the brain are damaged and ultimately killed. A key step in this process is the polymerization of the Aβ-*peptide* into neurotoxic protein filaments. These filaments are accumulated in the cerebral cortex and hippocampus of AD patients as the extracellular senile *plaques* that are composed of the 40 to 42/3 amino-acid long peptide derived from the amyloid precusor protein (APP) and intracellular neurofibrillary *tangles* that are composed of twisted filament of *tau* protein. The *PS2* gene accounts for about half of all cases of the early onset of AD, leading to the development of AD in patients younger than 60 years. Transgenic mice provide an important advance in the study of how the gene is associated with the human cognitive dysfunction after synaptic transmission between neurons in the brain. To generate transgenic mice, a hybrid gene containing human *PS2 mutant* (*N141I*) coding sequence and tet P consisting of seven copies of the tet O sequence were constructed. Separately, we also prepared another hybrid gene (*pTet-tTAk*) that carries the *Tet-regulated promoter* and *tTAk* coding sequence to generate double transgenic mice by mating with *pTet-PS2* mutant transgenic mice. Prior to microinjection, both of the hybrid genes were tested *in vitro* to see whether Aβ-*peptides* are deposited in transfectant SK-N-MC neuroblastoma cells, and whether TA regulators are induced by tetracycline release in their transfectant cells in a dose-dependent manner. These two hybrid genes were then microinjected into fertilized mouse embryos for study of the *in vivo* function of the *PS2* gene using transgenic mice. Our primary results showed that (1) the level of Aβ-*peptides* was increased in the *PS2*-transfectant cell; (2) expression of the TA genes was enhanced by the release of tetracyline in their TA-transfectants; (3) a total of 11 newborn mice were produced, one of which is identified as a transgenic mouse carrying pNSE-PS2m; and (4) out of 36 founder mice, 7 transgenic mice carrying *pTet-tTAk* were confirmed by PCR analysis.

[a]Corresponding author.

Changes in Growth Factor-induced Signal Transduction during the Aging Process of Human Primary Fibroblasts

EUI-JU YEO[a] AND CHANG-MO KANG[b]

[a]*Department of Biochemistry, Cheju National University Medical School, Cheju, Korea*
[b]*Department of Biochemistry, Seoul National University College of Medicine, Seoul, Korea*

Human primary fibroblasts undergo cellular senescence *in vitro* after a limited number of population doublings. Growth arrest and morphological changes are typical characteristics of the senescent cells. In order to understand further the mechanisms of the aging process, we examined signaling events induced by two mitogenic agonists, platelet-derived growth factor (PDGF) and lysophosphatidic acid (LPA), in young and old cells. PDGF transfer the mitogenic signal via the plasma membrane-bound receptor where the activity of protein tyrosine kinase occurs. LPA acts as an extracellular messenger through pertussis toxin-sensitive guanine nucleotide binding protein (G protein). When [^{3}H]thymidine incorporates into DNA in passages 8–10, cells were compared to those in passage 27 old cells, we observed that there was a reduction of greater than 80% in PDGF-stimulated and about 50% in LPA-stimulated cells. Because changes in intracellular calcium ([Ca^{2+}]$_i$), actin polymerization, and phosphatidyl choline hydrolysis by phospholipase D (PLD) are implicated in many cellular responses such as cell proliferation, differentiation, migration, and secretion, we compared those changes in young and old cells. Both PDGF and LPA generated a rhythmic increase in [Ca^{2+}]$_i$ in young cells. The frequency of the calcium response was reduced, and the response was desensitized in the PDGF-stimulated senescent cells. The frequency of the LPA-induced calcium signal was also reduced, but the magnitude of each was not altered in the senescent cells. Basal level of F-actin content was higher in the old cells than in the young cells. PDGF treatment increased the F-actin level in the young cells but not in the old cells. The effect of PDGF on PLD activation was also reduced significantly. About an 80% reduction of PLD activity was observed in PDGF-stimulated cells, but only about a 20% reduction was seen in LPA-induced cells. The differential effects of aging on PDGF- and LPA-induced signaling events demonstrate that some of events upstream in the PDGF-induced mitogenic process might be altered during the aging process. We examined here the content of PDGF receptor protein extracted by IGEPAL CA630 non-ionic detergent. We suggest that the reduced content of the PDGF receptor protein might be responsible for the reduced response to PDGF.

Contribution of Cyclooxygenase to Age-related Oxidative Stress

HYON-JEEN KIM,[a] BYUNG-PAL YU,[b] MI-AE YU,[b] KYU-WON KIM,[b] JAE-SUK WOO,[c] AND HAE-YOUNG CHUNG[a]

Vascular Aging Research Group, [a]College of Pharmacy, [b]College of Natural Science, and [c]College of Medicine, Pusan National University, Pusan 609-735, Korea

The oxidative stress hypothesis of aging proposes that age-dependent progressive deteriorations are elicited by various reactive species (RS). RS are produced by various metabolic processes under normal and pathologic conditions. A less-documented source of RS generation is the cyclooxygenase (COX)-catalyzed prostaglandin pathway. Recent evidence indicates that COX may be one of the major metabolic sources of superoxide and hydroperoxides through the arachidonic acid cascade pathway. COX is the rate-limiting enzyme in this process generating prostaglandin E_2 (PGE_2), prostacyclin (PGI_2), and thromboxane A_2 (TXA_2). COX exists in two distinct isoforms: COX-1, a constitutive isoform that is detected in most tissues and contributes to the production of physiological levels of prostanoid, and inducible COX-2, produced in response to many proinflammatory stimuli, including several cytokines. In the present study, we attempted to assess the contribution of RS generation of the COX pathway contributing to overall oxidative status. Fischer 344 rats of 6, 12, 18, and 24 months of age were used in this study. We quantified RS generation, the activities and gene expression of COX in aged kidney. Results show that COX-derived RS generation was markedly increased with age in parallel to total RS. This increased RS generation was accompanied by increased COX activity. Data on gene expression of COX-2 corroborated with the changes in the protein and mRNA level of COX-2. It was concluded that a substantial amount of total RS was contributed by the age-related COX-dependent process, which was accompanied by the increased gene expression of COX-2 mRNA and protein levels with age. These results suggest that the upregulation of COX-2 during aging can be a major contributor to oxidative status in the aging process. The significance of our finding is that increased COX activity during aging may be the major cause underlying the inflammation process under oxidative stress.

This work was supported by Korea Research Foundation Grant KRF-99-0005-F00030.

Control of Mitochondrial Redox Balance by the Mitochondrial NADP+-dependent Isocitrate Dehydrogenase

TAE-LIN HUH,[a] SEUNG-HEE JO,[a] MI-KYUNG SOHN,[a] SU-MIN LEE,[b] IN-HWANG SONG,[c] HO-JIN KOH,[a] YONG-OU KIM,[a] AND JEEN-WOO PARK[b]

[a]*Department of Genetic Engineering,* [b]*Department of Biochemistry, Kyungpook National University, Taegu, Korea*

[c]*Department of Anatomy, School of Medicine, Catholic University of Taegu-Hyosung, Taegu, Korea*

The reactive oxygen species (ROS) include superoxide anion, the hydroxyl radical, and the singlet oxygen. The mitochondria are not only a major site where a large amount of cellular ROS is generated, but also they are a main target of ROS; thus, various pathological states including aging have been reported to involve the mitochondrial dysfunctions and ROS generation. However, a catalase, a major enzyme that removes hydrogen peroxide, has been reported to be absent in most mitochondria of mammalian cells. Therefore, mitochondrial GSH is important to the mitochondrial defenses against ROS because it is a prerequisite to the roles of mitochondrial GPx and phospholipid hydrogenperoxide glutathione peroxidase (PHGPx), which play key roles in removing the peroxides in mitochondria. In addition to the role of reducing agent for the regeneration of GSH, NADPH is also necessary to the antioxidant function of the peroxiredoxin family in mitochondria. We have previously reported the isolation and molecular characterization of bovine mitochondrial NADP+-dependent isocitrate dehydrogenase (IDPm). Here, we first report that expression of cloned mouse IDPm cDNA reduces oxidative stress. Conversely, reduction of IDPm in mitochondria by the expression of antisense mouse IDPm cDNA increases spontaneous generation of ROS by stimulating mitochondrial injury. Our findings further support that IDPm is a major producer of mitochondrial NADPH by which the mitochondrial GSH pool required in defense against cellular oxidative stress is replenished.

The Pro- and Antioxidant Role of Glutathione in Selenite-induced Oxidative Stress and Apoptosis

HAN-MING SHEN, CHENG-FENG YANG, JIN LIU, AND CHOON-NAM ONG

Department of Community, Occupational and Family Medicine, Faculty of Medicine (MD3), National University of Singapore, 16 Medical Drive, Singapore 117597

It is well known that glutathione, a major intracellular antioxidant, is closely involved in the metabolism and bioactivity of selenium. One of the unique features of GSH involvement in selenite metabolism is the formation of reactive oxygen species (ROS) from the reaction of selenite with GSH. The elevated level of ROS is believed to be an important mechanism in selenite-induced cytotoxicity. In the present study, glutathione was further demonstrated to play a dual role on selenite-induced oxidative stress and apoptosis in human hepatoma $HepG_2$ cells. The experiment was carried out in two different modes of treatment. In mode A, cells were pretreated with N-acetylcysteine (NAC, 5 mM), buthionine sulfoximine (BSO, 2.5 mM), or reduced glutathione (GSH, 0.25 mM) prior to selenite exposure (10 µM × 24 h). In mode B, cells were treated with selenite and NAC, BSO or GSH simultaneously. Selenite-induced apoptosis was determined by (i) TdT-mediated dUTP nick end labeling (TUNEL) assay and (ii) cell cycle/DNA content analysis. Pretreatment with NAC increased the intracellular GSH level by about 70%, whereas pretreatment with BSO reduced the intracellular GSH by more than 80%. The addition of exogenous GSH failed to alter the intracellular GSH content. It is interesting to note that in mode A, both the increase and depletion of GSH content significantly enhanced selenite-induced oxidative stress and apoptosis in $HepG_2$ cells, whereas NAC was found to protect against selenite-induced oxidative stress and apoptosis when administrated simultaneously with selenite (mode B). On the other hand, the simultaneous addition of exogenous GSH (mode B) significantly magnified the toxic effects of selenite, while GSH pretreatment evidently failed to change selenite toxicity (mode A). Therefore, results from this study clearly demonstrated that GSH has a dual role in the effects of selenite on cancer cells: (i) as a prooxidant facilitating the formation of ROS and promoting oxidative damage and apoptosis, and (ii) as an antioxidant protecting against selenite-induced oxidative stress. Understanding such a unique association between GSH and selenite may help to explain the controversy in the literature on the complex relationship between selenium and glutathione, and to gain a better knowledge of the antioxidant property of selenium related to its application in the prevention of degenerative diseases and aging.

Effects of Aging on Aldosterone Secretion in Rat Zona Glomerulosa Cells

MEI-MEI KAU, JIANN-JONG CHEN, AND PAULUS S. WANG[a]

Department of Physiology, School of Life Science, National Yang-Ming University, and National Taipei College of Nursing, Taipei, Taiwan, Republic of China

Clinical reports have revealed an impaired sodium and water balance in elderly persons. The present studies were designed to investigate the effects and mechanisms of aging involved in aldosterone secretion in zona glomerulosa (ZG) cells of young and old ovariectomized rats. Young (3 months) and old (24 months) female rats were ovariectomized four days before decapitation. ZG cells of young and old rats were incubated with angiotensin II (Ang II), tetrandrine, nifedipine, adrenocorticotropic hormone (ACTH), forskolin, 8-bromo-3':5'-cyclic adenosine monophosphate (8-Br-cAMP), and steroidogenic precursors at 37°C for 30 min. Aldosterone concentrations in plasma and cell media, as well as 3':5'-cyclic adenosine monophosphate (cAMP) production in ZG cells, were determined by radioimmunoassay. The effects of aging on the activity of aldosterone synthase and the expression of cytochrome P450 side-chain cleavage enzyme (P450scc) in ZG cells were determined by thin-layer chromatography and Western blot analysis, respectively. Old rats had a lower plasma aldosterone level and a reduced basal aldosterone release from ZG cells than those in young rats. The conversions of steroidogenic precursors to aldosterone and the activity of aldosterone synthase, as well as the expression of P450scc in ZG cells, were lower in the group of old rats than in the young group. Ang II-, ACTH-, forkolin- or 8-Br-cAMP-stimulated aldosterone secretion was attenuated in the group of old rats as compared with the young group. Nifedipine decreased the aldosterone secretion in the group of young rats, but not in the group of old rats. The basal and forkolin-stimulated cAMP accumulations were lower in the old group than in the young group. These results suggest that the age-related decline in aldosterone secretion is in part due to the reduced activities of biosynthetic enzymes, adenylyl cyclase and L-type calcium channel, as well as the expression of P450scc protein in ZG cells.

[a]Corresponding author.

Evidence for Differential Structure and Function of Hsp70 Family Members, Mot-1 and Mot-2, in Control of Cellular Senescence

YOUJI MITSUI, RENU WADHWA, SYUICHI TAKANO, AND SUNIL C. KAUL

National Institute of Advanced Industrial Scuence and Technology,
1-1 Higashi Tsukuba Ibaraki, 305-8566, Japan

Chugai Research Institute for Molecular Medicine,
153-2 Nagai Niihari Ibaraki, 300-41, Japan

The mortalin genes, mot-1 and mot-2, are hsp70 family members that were originally cloned from normal and immortal murine cells, respectively. Their proteins differ by only two amino acid residues in their carboxy-terminus. Mot-1 harbors valine (V618) at 618 amino acid residue (a.a.) and arginine (R624) at 624 a.a. Mot-2 has M618 and G624. According to secondary structure predictions, the change at the 614 residue (R624G) can potentially introduce a turn in the α-helix. We present evidence that the two proteins indeed differ in their structure and function. Two amino acid differences result in their differential mobility on SDS-polyacrylamide gels confirming their different structures. Mot-1 and mot-2 exhibit different subcellular localization and biological activities. Mot-1 is pancytosolically distributed in normal cells, whereas mot-2 is found in the perinuclear region in immortal cells. Whereas expression of mot-1 induces cellular senescence in NIH 3T3 cells, an overexpression of mot-2 induces a malignant transformation. The pancytosolic mot-1 protein in normal cells did not show colocalization with tumor suppressor protein p53, but the nonpancytosolic mot-2 overlapped significantly with p53 in immortal cells. Transfection of mot-2, but not of mot-1, abrogated nuclear translocation and transactivation function of p53 demonstrating that a novel mechanism of p53 inactivation by mot-2 operates in tumors with wild type p53.

Expression of Growth-Related Genes in the Tissues of Aged Rat Brain

DEOK-KYU AN, SEON-GIL DO, JUN-GYO SUH, JAE-BONG PARK, AND JAE-YONG LEE[a]

Department of Biochemistry, Experimental Animal Center, College of Medicine, Hallym University, Chunchon, 200-702, Korea

Although molecular analyses have identified the changes in gene expression and the activity of gene products during aging, the involvement and the expression of cell-growth-related genes in the various tissues of brain during brain aging have not been established sufficiently. We attempted to analyze the mRNA expression of $p21^{WAF1/CIP1}$, $p27^{KIP1}$, c-*fos*, c-*jun*, and c-*myc* by RT-PCR and in various tissues (medulla, cerebellum, cerebral cortex, olfactory, and hippocampus) of young (7 month), adult (20 month), and old (25 month) rat brain. The results showed that mRNA expression of *p21* and *p27*, *KIP*-family cyclin-dependent kinase-inhibitor genes, was gradually elevated during brain aging in all tissues of the brain, except olfactory. mRNA expression of *p21* and *p27* was too low to be detected in 7-month-old rat brain. mRNA expression of c-*fos,* one of immediately early genes, was decreased gradually in all tissues of old rat brain, as reported previously. However, mRNA expression of c-*myc*, another immediately early gene, was unexpectedly elevated in old rat brain. Interestingly, mRNA expression of these genes is not detected in olfactory tissue for both young and old brain. Protein expression of these genes was also measured in the cortex of young and old rat brain by Western analysis. The result showed a similar pattern, as seen in mRNA expression.

[a]Corresponding author.

Expression of Peroxiredoxin in the Skin and Change of Peroxiredoxin by Ultraviolet B Irradiation

A Possible Antioxidant Role against Oxidative Stress in the Skin

SEUNG-CHUL LEE, JUNG EUN LEE, JEE-BUM LEE, YOUNG PIO KIM, AND HO ZOON CHAE[a]

Department of Dermatology, Chonnam University Medical School, Chonnam, Kwangju, Korea

[a]*Department of Biology, Chonnam National University, College of Natural Sciences, Kwangju, Korea*

Peroxiredoxin (Prx) is a peroxidase family that includes thioredoxin peroxidase, which functions to remove hydrogen peroxide by using the thioredoxin system. Thioredoxin peroxidases are ubiquitous and abundant in mammalian tissue, but very limited data are available on their expression in the skin. In this study, we examined the expression of five isotopes of Prx (I–IV, VI) in the skin. The change of Prx expression by ultraviolet B irradiation was also evaluated. In Western immunoblot with rat skin, three isotypes (except Prx IV and Prx VI) were expressed in the epidermal and dermal extracts. Prx IV expression was barely identified only in the dermal extract. Prx VI was not detected in either epidermal and dermal extracts. Prx IV expression was barely identified only in the dermal extract. Prx VI was not detected in either epidermal and dermal extracts. The same expression patterns of Prx isotypes were identified by Western immunoblot with the cell extracts from primary cells of rat keratinocytes and fibroblasts. In Western immunoblot with human skin, all five isotypes were expressed in the epidermal and dermal extracts. In human cells (primary cells of human keratinocytes and fibroblasts, HaCaT and A431 cells), similar expression patterns of Prx isotypes were found, except in the HaCaT cell: Prx IV was not expressed in the HaCaT cell. Immunofluorescence study showed that Prx expression was mainly localized to the epidermis, hair follicles, and the sebaceous glands. In the epidermis, Prx I–III was expressed in all the layers with isotype-specific patterns, with the stronger expression of basal cell layer for Prx I and III, and the stronger expression of granular layer for Prx II. Prx IV and Prx VI did not show differential expression among epidermal cell layers. In the dermis, however, all isotypes were expressed without isotype-specific variations. The five isotypes of Prx were expressed in all the layers of hair follicles including the outer root sheath, inner root sheath, and the matrix. *In situ* hybridization showed that localization of Prx mRNA was commensurate with Prx protein. Ultraviolet B irradiation with 150 mJ/cm^2 upregulated Prx II expression of the rat skin at an early stage after irradiation (15 min postirradiation). Our study shows that Prx is ubiquitously expressed in mammalian skin with species-specific patterns, which might function as an important antioxidant to remove hydrogen peroxide originating from ultraviolet B irradiation in addition to that of intrinsic origin. Further studies are warranted to elucidate the roles of Prx in photodamaged skin including photoaging.

Genetic Polymorphism of Presenilin-1 Gene and Apolipoprotein E in Korean Elderly with Dementia

JUNG-EUN PARK AND KYUNG-HEA CHO

Department of Biology, Seoul Women's University, Seoul, Korea

Alzheimer's disease (AD) is a progressive neurological illness in the aged population. Genetic studies have led to the identification of two AD-related genes, in which mutations can be risk factors for AD: the presenilin-1 (PS-1) and the apolipoprotein E (apo E) gene. The transmembrane protein gene PS-1, localized at chromosome 14q24.3, has been thought to cause an autosomal dominant form of familial early-onset Alzheimer's disease. Yet a recent observation has lent support to the idea that an intronic polymorphism of PS-1 is a factor for AD: the homozygosity of allele *1* of PS-1 was associated with a doubling of risk for late-onset AD. The gene for apo E locates at chromosome 19q13.2, within the previously associated familial late-onset AD genomic region; the apo E epsilon 4 allele was shown to be a risk factor of AD. To investigate whether the polymorphism of the two genes is related to dementia in the Korean elderly, the distributions of PS-1 and apo E genotypes in demented cases and nondemented controls were analyzed by PCR amplification. As for the PCR products, restriction isotyping was used to rapidly examine PS-1 allele types (allele *1*, allele *2*) with *Bam*HI and apo E isoforms (2, 3, and 4) with *Hha*I. Then the 2 test was finally used to examine the significant differences in genotype and allele frequencies between demented patients and nondemented controls. We found that the frequencies of PS-1 gene allele *1* and apo E 4 were significantly increased in patients with dementia compared with those of nondemented controls. These results were statistically significant at $p < 0.05$.

Impact of Growth Hormone Suppression in the Aging Process and Preliminary Longevity Analysis

ISAO SHIMOKAWA, YOSHIKAZU HIGAMI, KURUMI YANAGIHARA-OUTA, KENJI TANAKA, TOMOSHI TUCHIYA, TAKAHITO KONDO, SHINJI GOTO

Department of Pathology and Department of Biochemistry, Atomic Bomb Disease Institute, Nagasaki University School of Medicine, Nagasaki, Japan

Administration of growth hormone (GH) or its analogs has been considered as a way to prevent physical frailty in elderly persons. Another line of evidence, however, has demonstrated that excessive GH shortens the life span, while congenital deficiency of the pituitary hormones, including GH, is associated with prolonged life span in mice. Lifelong dietary restriction, a powerful antiaging intervention of laboratory rodents, also suppresses the GH-IGF-1 axis. Using a transgenic strain of rats, in which GH-gene expression is suppressed by antisense RNA transgene, we have started a research project to explore the impact of isolated GH suppression on the aging process and longevity. Experimental groups included control Wistar rats, the transgenic rats (Mini), and F1 hybrid rats. Plasma GH and IGF-1, body size, and the amount of daily food intake, were less in the following order: Mini rats, F1 rats, control Wistar rats. At 21 months of age, only 80% of Mini rats were alive, as compared with 90% and 96.7% survival for Wistar rats and F1 rats, respectively. Most rats have died of neoplastic diseases. We also measured the enzyme activity of MnSOD, CuZn-SOD, catalase, and glutathione S-transferase (GST) in the liver, as the enhanced defense system for free radicals may contribute to slowing of the aging process and to extension of the life span. Catalase activity was significantly reduced in Mini rats; the other enzyme activities did not differ among the rat groups. The preliminary results suggested that moderate suppression of GH might be associated with retardation of the aging process and extension of the life span in rats, although severe GH deficiency could accelerate the aging process.

Increased Expression of Calsenilin in the Brains of Scrapie-infected Mice

JIN-KYU CHOI,[a] HYUN-PIL LEE,[a] EUN-KYOUNG CHOI,[b] JAE-KWANG JIN,[a] HYOUNG-GON LEE,[a] WILMA WASCO,[b] JOSEPH D. BUXBAUM,[c] RICHARD I. CARP,[d] AND YONG-SUN KIM[a,e]

[a]*Institute of Environment and Life Science, Hallym Academy of Sciences and* [e]*Department of Microbiology, College of Medicine, Hallym University, Chuncheon, Korea*

[b]*Genetics and Aging Unit, Department of Neurology, Massachusetts General Hospital, Harvard Medical School, Cambridge, Massachusetts, USA*

[c]*Department of Psychiatry and Neurobiology, Mount Sinai School of Medicine, New York, New York, USA*

[d]*New York State Institute for Basic Research in Developmental Disabilities, New York, New York, USA*

Calsenilin, a member of the calcium-binding protein family identified recently, is known to contain four EF-hand motifs and interacts with both calcium and presenilin. The interaction between calsenilin and presenilin has been reported in cell culture, and it is known to modulate intracellular Ca^{2+} homeostasis and processing of presenilin, and thereby affects neuronal apoptosis in Alzheimer's disease (AD). Scrapie, one of the prion diseases, is a transmissible neurodegenerative disease of sheep and goats, and the pathogenesis of neurodegeneration showed a similar pattern with AD. PrP^{Sc}, abnormal prion protein, is the major candidate for the infectious agents in this disease, and can induce neuronal degeneration and glial cell activation. PrP 106–126, a neurotoxic fragment of prion peptide, can also induce an increase in intracellular Ca^{2+} concentration. In the present study, to study the expression of calsenilin in prion disease, we investigated the histochemical localization of the protein and its mRNA level in the brains of control and scrapie-infected mice. In the immunohistochemical study, the localization of calsenilin was observed in neurons of cerebral cortex, striatum, brain stem, and cerebellum of both the control and scrapie-infected groups; their intensity, however, was markedly increased in the brains of scrapie-infected mice. In addition, calsenilin immunoreactivity was observed in the activated astrocytes of the scrapie-infected group, but not in the control groups. Using *in situ* hybridization in the control and scrapie-infected group, calsenilin mRNA is expressed in neuronal cells and activated astrocytes in cerebral cortex and hippocampus in the scrapie infected; however, the expression of calsenilin was detected exclusively in neuronal cells in control brains. These results suggest that increased expression of calsenilin in neuronal cells and activated astrocytes in scrapie-infected brains plays an important role in neurodegenerative mechanisms in prion disease.

Induction of Cellular Senescence in Cervical Cancer Cells by Inhibition of HPV Oncogene Expression

CHAN JAE LEE AND EUN SEONG HWANG[a]

Department of Life Science, University of Seoul, Seoul, Korea

HPV E6 and E7 proteins are continuously expressed in HPV-positive cervical cancer cells, and together induce immortalization of normal keratinocytes, *in vitro*, and are therefore believed to be major etiological agents for human cervical cancer. E6 is not only able to inactivate *p53*, but has been shown to induce telomerase activity and extend the life span of normal keratinocytes and mammary epithelial cells. E7 inactivates Rb, and thereby causes disruption in cell cycle control and helps cells overcome cellular crisis and to become immortale. Previously, it was shown that acute expression of BPV E2 inhibits E6/E7 expression from HPV DNA in certain cervical cancer cell lines, including HeLa, and this is accompanied by an increase in the steady-state level of the *p53* protein, induction of p21WAF1, and the concomitant accumulation of hypophosphorylated Rb protein, resulting in a dramatic growth arrest at the G1 phase. Using this system, it was asked if the depletion of E6/E7 proteins could induce a state of cellular senescence in these HPV-positive cancer cells. In the E2-transduced HeLa cell population, cells positive for senescence-associated β-galactosidase (SA-β-Gal) activity, a marker for cellular senescence, increased dramatically, reaching up to 62% in 3 days post-E2 transduction, while only 5% of cells were positive in the untreated population. Most SA-β-Gal-positive cells also had extended morphology. Treatment of BPV E2 on other HPV-positive cervical cancer cell lines, HT-3 (HPV30), Caski (HPV16), and two keratinocyte lines immortalized by HPV16 DNA, also inhibits E6 and E7 expression and cell proliferation, and induces SA-β-Gal positivity, albeit to a lesser degree. These results strongly indicate that these cells are induced to cellular senescence upon depletion of E6 and E7 oncoproteins, and suggest that HPV-infected cells acquire the immortal phenotype by the activities of the E6 and E7 proteins, while in the absence of them, they somehow sense that they have passed their normal life span and determine to undergo cellular senescence.

[a]Corresponding author.

Induction of Senescence-like Phenotype by an Alkylating Agent, Methyl Methanesulfonante, in Human Diploid Fibroblast

YOUSIN SUH, DEOK-IN KIM, JEONG-SOO PARK, WOONG-YANG PARK, AND SANG CHUL PARK

Department of Biochemistry and Molecular Biology, Seoul National University College of Medicine, Seoul, 110-799, Korea

Alkylating agents represent one of the most abundant chemical DNA-damaging agents in our environment, and consequently cells in every evolutionary spectrum of life are unavoidably exposed to these agents. Because damage to DNA, if left unrepaired and accumulated, has been linked to cellular and organismal aging, we studied the ability of a simple alkylating agent, methyl methanesulfonate (MMS), to induce a senescence-like phenotype in human diploid fibroblast. We showed that MMS induces a growth arrest accompanied by morphological changes and expression of senescence associated β-galactosidase activity, when treated in G1 arrested as well as dividing cells. These arrest responses are irreversible and correlate with persistent induction of p53 and Cdk inhibitors, $p21^{WAF1/CIP1}$ and $p16^{ink4a}$. MMS-induced growth-arrested cells show a marked increase in *p21* and *p53* mRNA and a decrease in *c-fos* mRNA, similar to the level of senescent cells. Furthermore, activation of ERK in response to EGF is abolished or severely delayed in MMS-induced growth-arrested cells as in senescent cells. Taken together, these findings suggest that MMS is able to accelerate the program of cellular aging in human diploid fibroblast, implicating a role of environmental alkylating agents in organismal aging.

Investigation on Natural Peroxynitrite Scavengers

JI-SUNG YOON, BYUNG-PAL YU, AND HAE-YOUNG CHUNG

College of Pharmacy, The Research Institute of Drug Development, Pusan National University, Pusan, Korea

Recent evidence strongly implicates peroxynitrite ($ONOO^-$) as a major culprit in the deleterious action of NO. $ONOO^-$ can induce oxidation of thiol groups, nitration of tyrosine, and lipid peroxidation reactions, altering various cellular functions including signal transduction. Its uncontrolled status may also be involved in several major diseases such as Alzheimer's disease, rheumatoid arthritis, cancer, and atherosclerosis. Because there are no known defense enzymes against $ONOO^-$ in the body, it is important to search for some exogenous sources of scavengers. Our study was launched to find peroxynitrite scavengers in natural products by screening 94 European herbal extracts. The crude samples were extracted with methanol and dried at room temperature for three days. Collected residues were then dissolved in water containing 10% ethanol and further diluted with water to obtain desired concentrations. For the measurement of the antioxidant efficacy, dihydrorhodamine 123 (DHR123) was used. Nonfluorescent dihydrorhodamine is oxidized to rhodamine 123 with fluorescences. $ONOO^-$ scavenging activity was monitored by the oxidation of DHR 123 on a microplate fluorescence spectrophotometry with excitation and emission wavelengths of 485 nm and 530 nm, respectively. The scavenging activity was expressed by IC_{50} values (µg/ml) denoting required concentrations that exert 50% inhibition of the oxidation of DHR123. Results showed that 13 out of 94 herbal extracts (5 µg/ml) exhibited a strong peroxynitrite scavenging effect with more than 70% inhibition. The highest scavenging activity was weeping ash (IC_{50}, 0.028 ± 0.003), witch hazel (IC_{50}, 0.280 ± 0.030), lemon verbena (IC_{50}, 0.399 ± 0.050), elm bark (IC_{50}, 0.549 ± 0.024), and majoram herb (IC_{50}, 0.674 ± 0.034). Interestingly, the superoxide scavenging activities were also detected in these extracts (5 µg/ml) with 60% inhibition. Thus, our data warrant further systematic analysis and characterization on the isolated antioxidants. These endeavors lead to the development of specific peroxynitrite scavengers for new approaches on the effective prevention of peroxynitrite-induced damage.

This work was supported by KOSEF Grant 2000-2-20800-003-5.

Involvement of Caspases in Cell Death Induced by Selenium Compounds in HL-60 Cells

UHEE JUNG, TAE-HO KIM, AND AN-SIK CHUNG

Department of Biological Sciences, Korea Advanced Institute of Science and Technology, Taejon, Korea

Recent studies suggest that the chemopreventive effects of selenium compounds might be related to their ability to induce apoptosis. In this study, we investigated the cellular events that occurred during the apoptosis induced by selenium compounds. It was observed that selenite and Se-methylselenocysteine (MSC) induced apoptosis in HL-60 cells. Filter elution assay showed that MSC induced DNA double-strand breaks only, whereas selenite induced both single- and double-strand breaks. Incubation of cells with MSC induced ROS formation detected by DCFH-DA fluorescence and ROS formation was inhibited by antioxidant N-acetylcysteine, while selenite did not induce ROS formation. MSC and selenite both increased PARP activity, but the activation of caspase-3 and PARP cleavage was observed only in the cells treated with MSC. Several inhibitors of caspases were treated to see which caspases are involved in cell death induced by selenium compounds. z-VAD-fmk, z-DEVD-fmk, z-IETD-fmk, and z-LEHD-fmk inhibited MSC-induced cell death. And they also reduced DNA strand breaks and PARP cleavage in MSC-treated cells. Similar effects were shown by serine protease inhibitor and PARP inhibitor. On the other hand, these inhibitors showed few effects in selenite-treated cells. These results suggested that MSC induces ROS formation, and caspases seems to be crucial for the execution of apoptosis in MSC-treated cells. On the other hand, selenite can induce cell death via caspase-independent pathways.

Lowered 8-Hydroxyguanine Glycosylase Activity in Senescence-accelerated Mice due to a Single-base Mutation

JEONG-YUN CHOI,[a] HUN-SIK KIM,[b,d] DONG-WOOK LEE,[c] AND MYUNG-HEE CHUNG[a]

[a]Department of Pharmacology, Seoul National University Medical College, Seoul, Korea

[b]Department of Pharmacology, Chungbuk National University Medical College, Cheongju, Korea

[c]Laboratory of Biochemistry, Korea Ginseng and Tobacco Research Institute, Taejon, Korea

Senescence-accelerated mouse (SAM), a murine model of accelerated senescence, consists of the senescence-accelerated-prone mouse (SAMP) and senescence-accelerated-resistant mouse (SAMR). SAMP shows aging signs earlier and has a shorter life span than SAMR, whereas SAMR shows characteristics of normal aging. In this animal model of aging, OH^8Gua content in DNA from SAMP was observed to be significantly elevated by 20–40% as compared to the normal SAMR strain. We also discovered that the activity of repair enzyme for OH^8Gua, 8-oxoguanine glycosylase (OGG), was much lower in SAMP than in SAMR in all organs and at all ages tested. In contrast, O^6-methylguanine-DNA methyltransferase, which repairs alkylated DNA, showed no difference in its activity. We also attempted to reveal the molecular basis of these findings in SAMP mice—increased OH^8Gua content in DNA and decreased enzymatic activity for its repair. First, we compared the mRNA expression level of *ogg1*, the gene for OGG, between SAMP1, P8, and SAMR1 mice by Northern blot analysis. The results showed no significant difference between three strains, indicating that the lowered enzymatic activity in SAMP did not result from decreased *ogg1* gene expression. Next, to explore the possibility of structural abnormality in SAMP OGG protein, we determined the nucleotide sequence of cDNA of SAMP *ogg1* mRNA amplified by RT-PCR. From SAMP1 and P8, we found a point mutation at codon 304, with change from Arg (CGG) in SAMR1 to Trp (TGG) in SAMPs. Recombinant OGG proteins were constructed from mRNA of SAMP1 and SAMR1. Purified recombinant OGG protein from SAMP1 showed noticeable impairment in its thermal stability as compared to the recombinant protein of SAMR1 strain. The impairment of OH^8Gua repair activity caused by the 304 mutation in OGG1 may be one of the factors contributing to the high somatic mutation rate and the accelerated senescence observed in SAMP strains.

[d]Corresponding author.

Melatonin-related Compounds Have High Free Radical Scavenging Activity

RYUNG YANG, HAE-YOUNG CHUNG, DONG-BUM SHIN, TAE-YEON CHO, AND SEUNG-HYUN YANG

Department of Biotechnology, Yonsei University, Seoul, Korea

It is known that melatonin has outstanding free radical scavenging activity. We have focused on the physiological roles of melatonin-related compounds in anabolic and catabolic pathways especially by evaluating their free radical scavenging activity. We aimed to elucidate the mechanistic events and molecular insights on oxidative stress. As a main pineal neurohormone, melatonin functions as a mediator; it conveys the influence of light-dark cycle to the body. However, melatonin has received a lot of attention since the 1990s because of its free radical scavenging activity. We have determined test compounds based on the melatonin metabolic pathway. They are tryptophan, 5-hydroxy-tryptophan, serotonin, N-acetyl-serotonin, melatonin, 6-hydroxy-melatonin, 6-hydroxy-melatonin-sulfate, 5-hydroxy-indole-3-acetate, 5-methoxy-indole-3-acetate, and 5-methoxy-tryptamine. We deduce that not only melatonin but also melatonin metabolites have considerable scavenging activity on free radicals because they have both a similar molecular structure and functional groups. We selected some radicals for study: superoxide radical, hydrogen peroxide, hydroxyl radical, peroxinitrite radical, and hypochlorous acid. Melatonin-related compounds have low activity on the superoxide radical, whereas melatonin, N-acetylserotonin, serotonin, and 5-hydroxytryptophan have outstanding scavenging activity on hydrogen peroxide. With respect to lipid peroxidation, serotonin and N-acetylserotonin have high inhibition activity. And melatonin, 5-methoxytryptamin, and 6-hydroxymelatonin have strong activity in hydroxyl radical scavenging. We conclude that melatonin metabolites including melatonin and serotonin have strong radical scavenging activity and a lipid peroxidation inhibition effect. Furthermore, they have potential use as natural and physiological antioxidant materials.

Metabolic Modulation of Cellular Redox Potential Can Improve Cardiac Recovery from Ischemia-Reperfusion Injury

HEUN-SOO KANG,[a] JONG-WAN PARK,[b] YANG-SOOK CHUN,[b] MYUNG-SUK KIM,[b] AND SANG CHUL PARK[a]

Departments of [a]Biochemistry and Molecular Biology, and [b]Pharmacology, Heart Research Institute, Seoul National University College of Medicine, Seoul, 110-799, Korea

Ischemia-reperfusion heart injury is an important pathologic condition against which many strategies, mainly involving antioxidants or radical scavengers, have been developed, but without satisfactory results. In the present experiment, modulation of the cytosolic NADH/NAD ratio by pyruvate and aspartate was tested in order to protect the heart from ischemia-reperfusion injury. The effects of pyruvate and aspartate on cardiac function recovery and redox potential were analyzed in the isolated heart of male Sprague-Dawley rats. Hearts were made globally ischemic for 20 min and then reperfused for 30 min. Pyruvate and aspartate protected against tissue injury and improved contractile function after reperfusion of ischemic hearts; these substances effectively decreased the tissue and cytosolic NADH/NAD ratio of the myocardium in a dose-dependent manner. Postischemic cardiac functions were negatively related to tissue and cytosolic NADH/NAD ratios. Increased NADH selectively inhibited myocardial xanthine dehydrogenase *in vitro*. It was thus expected that a decrease of NADH might limit the production of reactive oxygen species through the recovery of xanthine dehydrogenase activity. These results indicate that a decrease of NADH is related to pyruvate and aspartate-induced protection of ischemic myocardium.

New Directions in Communicating Better Nutrition to Older Adults

GEORGIA SUE GULDAN[a] AND WENDY WAI-HING HUI[b]

[a]Food and Nutritional Sciences Programme, Department of Biochemistry, The Chinese University of Hong Kong, Hong Kong

[b]Dietetic Information Centre, Hospital Authority, Hong Kong

Nutrition education should be an important component of ongoing health promotion for older adults and their caregivers. This is because prevention through sound nutrition and food hygiene practices and regular exercise is the most cost-effective way to deal with their major health problems. Nutrition education services should effectively promote optimum intake and successful self-care. Unfortunately, however, relative to other vulnerable groups, nutrition education for older adults has not been systematically developed or evaluated. Usually older adults care a lot about their health, so this should be a relatively easy group to teach—but their increasing numbers, longevity, and great diversity with respect to health, physical, and economic status and educational level present challenges. Some older adults may not perceive they would benefit from nutrition education, so therefore interesting and motivating them is a challenge. Knowledge of food and nutrition of older people has been acquired through a lifetime of experience. For most older adults in the Asian region, their sources are limited by their limited education, so that their major sources of information have been informal ones, such as television, radio, friends, family, and perhaps newspapers and magazines if they are literate. Nonetheless, dietary advice for older people should build on their existing knowledge and ingrained values. It should provide information useful in daily food selection, and focus on food groups, not nutrients—the same foods and groups considered appropriate for younger people—with messages consistent with those given throughout the population. Attention must also be paid to discovering learning styles in older people. When we teach in schools, the young students are a captive audience resigned to their role of learning. Learning by an older adult, however, reflects an effort to meet his or her perceived needs. Therefore, nutrition education should be a positive experience in a nonthreatening, relaxed, and noncompetitive environment, and perhaps even a social one. The messages also need to be practical and achievable. A needs assessment is essential because our ability to provide the most effective nutrition education will depend on our success in matching the needs—both perceived and unperceived—of this vulnerable group. Therefore, we must go to the potential older learners to assess their interests and preferences. Nutrition education activities for older adults are widespread, but few have been evaluated. Evaluation is therefore also recommended, particularly when new methods are used. Tips from other countries for presenting successful nutrition education will be given, including some examples of applications as attempted in Hong Kong. Research needs will also be described. In conclusion, successful nutrition education for older adults depends on positive needs-based messages. This may be hard to do, because few good examples are available to illustrate these principles.

Nitric Oxide Is Implicated in Apoptotic Cell Death Induced by H_2O_2 in C6 Cells

YOUNG IL LEE, JUNGSOON PARK, YOUNG HEE LEE, AND BOK-GHEE HAN[a]

Laboratory of Degenerative Disease, Department of Biomedical Sciences,
Korean National Institute of Health, Seoul 122-701, Korea

The purpose of this study was to determine NO (nitric oxide) production during the process of lethal oxidative cell injury following exposure of glioma C6 cells to hydrogen peroxide (H_2O_2). NOS activity was determined by immunocytochemical staining and NO_2 measurement with Griess reagent. Cell death was assessed by Tunel staining. Moreover, cell death and changes in succinate dehydrogenase were analyzed simultaneously with histochemistry. Treatment with H_2O_2 increased nitric oxide (NO) production and apoptotic cell death, which seem to be closely related to mitochondrial dysfunction. H_2O_2 caused cell death in a concentration-dependent manner, accompanied by weakened activities of mitochondrial enzymes. In the combined experiment of succinate dehydrogenase (SDH) enzyme histochemistry and apoptosis staining (TUNEL), only the SDH-depleted cells were TUNEL positive. In the enzyme assay with spectrophotometer, the activities of SDH and cytochrome-c oxidase (COX), marker enzymes for mitochondrial function, were also decreased according to the dose of H_2O_2. Taken together, the observed increase of NO production during the H_2O_2-induced apoptotic cell death seems to be also closely related to dysfunction of mitochondria, which leads to a consecutive formation of reactive oxygen species (ROS). These results suggest that NO is implicated in the process of H_2O_2-induced mitochondrial dysfunction and apoptotic cell death.

[a]Corresponding author.

Overexpression of Calsenilin in Sporadic Alzheimer's Disease Brain

JAE KWANG JIN,[a] JIN KYU CHOI,[a] JAE IL KIM,[a] HYOUNG GON LEE,[a] WILMA WASCO,[b] JOSEPH D. BUXBAUM,[c] RICHARD I. CARP,[d] YONG-SUN KIM,[a,e] AND EUN KYOUNG CHOI[b]

[a]*Institute of Environment and Life Science, Hallym Academy of Sciences and* [e]*Department of Microbiology, College of Medicine, Hallym University, Chuncheon, Korea*

[b]*Genetics and Aging Unit, Department of Neurology, Massachusetts General Hospital, Harvard Medical School, Cambridge, Massachusetts, USA*

[c]*Department of Psychiatry, Mount Sinai School of Medicine, New York, USA*

[d]*New York State Institute for Basic Research in Developmental Disabilities, New York, USA*

Familial Alzheimer's disease (FAD) is caused by mutations in the genes encoding presenilin-1 (PS-1), presenilin-2 (PS-2), and amyloid precursor protein (APP). PS-1 mutations induce an apoptosis by disrupting intracellular calcium levels. In sporadic AD brain, abnormal presenilin processing plays an important role in calcium homeostasis. However, the mechanisms by which abnormal processing of presenilin and APP causes AD have not been fully elucidated. The interaction of presenilin with calsenilin may have an important role in abnormal presenilin processing and APP processing. Calsenilin, a recently identified member of calcium-binding protein, is known to contain a four EF-hand motif and interact with both calcium and presenilin. The interaction between calsenilin and presenilin has been reported in cell culture, and it is known to modulate intracellular Ca^{2+} homeostasis and processing of presenilin. In the present study, to determine whether calsenilin and presenilin are colocalized in the brains of patients with sporadic AD, we investigated the histochemical localization of the protein. Immunohistochemically, calsenilin immunoreactivity was observed in neurons of the cerebral cortex and hippocampus of both control and AD brains. In general, immunoreactivity for calsenilin was more intense in neurons from AD brains compared with those of controls. In AD brain, calsenilin immunoreactivity was observed in senile plaques and neurofibrillary tangles, which are typical hallmarks of the disease. In addition, calsenilin immunoreactivity was observed in reactive astrocytes of both frontal cortex and hippocampal formation of the AD brain, but not in the control brain. To determine whether overexpressed calsenilin is involved in neuronal apoptosis, we examined by double staining for terminal deoxynucleotide transferase nick end labeling (TUNEL) and calsenilin expression. In AD brain, apoptotic neurons were present in neurons that express calsenilin. Thus, these findings demonstrated that calsenilin contributes to neuronal apoptosis in AD brain. Taken together, our results suggest that calsenilin may play an important role in neurodegeneration in AD.

Oxidative Stress Associated Antioxidant Enzyme and Neuroendocrine Markers in Dementia

HEUI OG KIM,[a] HYE WON SEO,[a] JUNG EUN PARK,[a,c] KYUNG HEA CHO,[a] AND IN SUNG KIM[b]

[a]*Department of Biology, Seoul Women's University, Seoul, Korea*
[b]*Kongju National Mental Hospital, Kongju, Korea*

Neuroendocrine markers. This study examined the changes in the contents of cortisol, free T4, free T3, red blood cell folate (RBC folate), ferritin, and vitamin B12 from Korean Alzheimer's disease (AD) patients and age-matched controls. The levels of cortisol, free T4, free T3, RBC folate, ferritin, and vitamin B12 in the blood of 25 patients with AD and 25 age-matched controls were measured. According to the MMSE (Mini Mental Status Examination), the subjects were classified into dementia (MMSE ≤ 23) and control (MMSE ≥ 24) groups. All AD patients who met NINCDS-ADRDA and MMSE-K criteria were admitted to the Kongiu National Mental Hospital. A significant decrease in RBC folate ($p < 0.01$) and vitamin B12 ($p < 0.05$) levels was found in AD patients. The levels of ferritin in patients with AD showed an increased tendency, but were not statistically significant. No significant changes were found in free T3 and free T4 between AD patients and controls. It was reported that hypothalamic-pituitary-adrenal (HPA) axis hyperactivity accelerates cognitive impairment and neuronal loss and that the raised cortisol levels associated with prolonged activation of the HPA axis cause neuronal loss in the hippocampus, with consequent impairment of memory and cognition (Sapolsky *et al.* 1990). The main cause of folate and vitamin B12 deficiency in patients was reported to be nutritional deficiencies and neuronal death caused by the process of AD. Our results suggest that RBC folate and vitamin B12 may be involved in the severity of cognitive impariment of AD.

Antioxidant enzymes. Our study examined the changes in the activities of antioxidant enzymes superoxide dismutase (SOD), catalase, glutathione peroxidase (GSH-Px), glutathione reductase (GSSG-R), glutathione S-transferase (GST), glucose-6-phosphate dehydrogenase (G6PDH), and lactate dehydrogenase (LDH). We assayed the activities of these antioxidant enzymes in blood of 25 patients with AD and 25 age-matched controls. According to the MMSE, the subjects were classified into dementia (MMSE ≤ 23) and control (MMSE ≥ 24) groups. All AD patients who met NINCDS-ADRDA and MMSE-K criteria were admitted to the Kongju National Mental Hospital. The activities of total SOD ($p < 0.001$), Mn-SOD ($p < 0.001$), catalase ($p < 0.001$), GSH-Px ($p < 0.01$), GSSG-R ($p < 0.01$), G6PDH ($p < 0.000$), and LDH ($p < 0.001$) were significantly increased in AD patients. These results showed that significant association exists between variables of the antioxidant system, mea-

[c]*Corresponding author.*

sured in blood samples, and AD. The present data suggest that AD patients may be affected by increased oxidative stress including hydroxy radical and superoxide anion.

p38 Mitogen-activated Protein Kinase Is Involved in H_2O_2-induced Phospholipase D Activation in Vascular Smooth Muscle Cells

EUNG-GOOK KIM, EUN-YOUNG SHIN, DO SIK MIN, BYOUNG-HEE PARK, KYUNG-SUN SHIN, MIN-SOO HYUN, JI-CHEOL SHIN, HEE-YUL AHN, ROGER J. DAVIS, AND SEUNG-RYUL KIM

Department of Biochemistry, College of Medicine, Chungbuk National University, Cheongju, Korea

Reactive oxygen species (ROS) are implicated as mediators of vascular disorders. To examine the role of ROS in this process, we investigated the effect of hydrogen peroxide on the activation of phospholipase D (PLD) in vascular smooth muscle cells (VSMCs). Exposure to H_2O_2 resulted in the accumulation of [^{3}H]phosphatidylbutanol in VSMCs in a concentration- and time-dependent manner. We also found that H_2O_2 treatment activated p38 mitogen-activated protein kinase (p38MAPK) in a time-dependent manner. Interestingly, specific inhibition of p38MAPK with SB203580 attenuated H_2O_2-induced PLD activation. Furthermore, transient expression of the dominant negative forms of MKK3/6 also inhibited H_2O_2-induced PLD activation. In a previous report, we showed that tyrosine kinase(s) and PKC are involved in PLD activation in Swiss 3T3 cells. We therefore examined the possible involvement of these kinases in the activation of p38MAPK in H_2O_2-stimulated VSMCs. Genistein dose-dependently suppressed H_2O_2-induced p38MAPK activation and PLD activation in VSMCs. Calphostin C also partially prevented activation of both p38MAPK and PLD by H_2O_2. However, treatment with a combination of SB203580, genistein, and calphostin C did not completely obliterate H_2O_2-induced PLD activity. These results suggest that PLD activation may be mediated in part via a sequence of tyrosine kinase/PKC → p38MAPK, in response to oxidative stress (H_2O_2).

Photoaging in Asian Skin: New Grading System and the Influence of Environmental Factors

JIN HO CHUNG, SEONG HUN LEE, CHOON SHIK YOON, AND HEE CHUL EUN

Department of Dermatology, Seoul National University College of Medicine, Seoul, 110-744, Korea

Clinical assessment of photoaging can be evaluated by various characteristic features presented in the photodamaged skin such as fine and coarse wrinkling, pigmented lesions, roughness of the skin, telangiectasia, and laxity. In evaluating these parameters of photodamaged skin, the conventional assessments primarily resorted to the documented grading scales, which have limitations on objective assessment and, furthermore, tend to cause intra- and interobserver differences. The characteristics of photodamaged skin in the Asian population may be different from those of Caucasians. In Asian skin, pigmentary changes, in addition to wrinkling, are a hallmark of photodamaged skin. Therefore, we developed a new photographic scale to assess the degree of photoaging in the Asian skin. This new scale may be useful in selecting the photoaged patients and in evaluating the efficacy of anti-aging agents for clinical trials for Asian skin. In order to investigate the influences of various environmental factors on photoaging in Korean skin, a questionnaire was administered to quantify cigarette smoking, sun exposure, age, and sex in a total of 407 volunteers. The severity of wrinkling and dyspigmentation in volunteers was assessed using our new photographic scale. After controlling for age and sex, we demonstrated premature wrinkling increased with increased pack-years of smoking, and heavy smokers (>50 pack/year) were 4.7 times more likely than nonsmokers to have premature wrinkling. When smoking and sun exposure coexisted, the effects on wrinkling were synergistic.

Plasma Concentrations of an Endogenous Nitric Oxide Synthase Inhibitor, N^G,N^G-Dimethylarginine

A Novel Risk Factor for Cerebral Infarction in the Elderly

JUN-HYUN YOO[a] AND SUNG-CHANG LEE[b]

[a]*Department of Family Medicine, Samsung Medical Center, Center for Clinical Research, Samsung Biomedical Research Institute, Seoul, Korea*

[b]*Samsung Biomedical Research Institute, Seoul, Korea*

Risk factors associated with stroke, such as hypercholesterolemia, hypertension, diabetes mellitus, smoking, aging, and hyperhomocyst(e)inemia are linked to endothelial dysfunction. Endothelial-derived nitric oxide (NO) has inhibitory effects on key processes in atherothrombogenesis. Asymmetric dimethylarginine (ADMA) is an endogenous inhibitor of NO synthase, of which concentration in a pathophysiological range potently reduces vascular NO synthesis. The aim of this study is to examine whether plasma ADMA concentration is associated with cerebral infarction in the elderly. In a hospital-based setting, 25 patients with recurrent stroke, 27 patients with first stroke, and 35 control subjects matched for age and sex were examined. Plasma ADMA and homocyst(e)ine concentration were determined using high-performance liquid chromatography and fluorescence detection. Patients with first or recurrent cerebral infarction had significantly higher concentrations of plasma ADMA than did controls without stroke (2.28 ± 1.63, 1.46 ± 0.77, 0.93 ± 0.32 mmol/L, respectively, p = 0.0001). After adjustment for hypertension, hypercholesterolemia, smoking, diabetes, and old age, upper median ADMA level (≥ 1.26 mmol/L) was associated with cerebral infarction (OR = 5.10, 95% CI; 2.46–10.59, p = 0.03), and odds ratio for recurrent cerebral infarction was 7.03 (95% CI: 3.42–14.4, p = 0.007). In addition, old age, diabetes mellitus, and hyperhomocyst(e)inemia were significant determinants of elevated plasma ADMA concentration. This finding indicates that elevated ADMA concentrations are associated with increased risk for cerebral infarction in the elderly, with a pronounced magnitude in recurrent stroke. Increased plasma ADMA concentrations may account for increased risk for stroke in elderly subjects with diabetes mellitus or hyperhomocyst(e)inemia.

Protection of Mitochondria Permeability Transition by Dihydroxybenzaldehyde against Hydroxyl Radicals

HAE YOUNG CHUNG,[a] HYON JEEN KIM,[a] YOUNG HWAN YANG,[a] WON CHUL CHOI,[b] HYE JIN PARK,[c] JAE SUE CHOI,[c] CHANG MO KANG,[d] AND SANG CHUL PARK[d]

[a]*College of Pharmacy,* [b]*College of Natural Science, Pusan National University, Pusan, Korea*

[c]*Department of Food and Life Science, Pukyung National University, Pusan, Korea*

[d]*College of Medicine, Seoul National University, Seoul, Korea*

Accumulated evidence strongly implicates the role of mitochondria in cell death that is often accompanied by a release of its components such as cytochrome c and apoptosis-inducing factor. The release of cytochrome c from the mitochondrial electron transport chain can cause the impairment of ATP generation, resulting in eventual cell death. Mitochondrial integrity and its Ca^{2+} homeostasis are tightly regulated by Ca^{2+} channels coupled with other ion permeability movements. Under increased oxidative stress, cells may undergo death because of dysregulation of $[Ca^{2+}]_i$. A mitochondrial Ca^{2+} megachannel, located in the inner membrane, may play a crucial role in the maintenance of Ca^{2+} homeostasis through a mitochondria permeability transition (MPT) process. Because hydroxyl radicals are the most destructive oxidants, in the present study, we investigated the protection of 3,4-dihydroxybenzaldehyde (3,4-DB), isolated from *Salvia miltiorrhiza* and red algae, and its derivatives against hydroxyl radical attack on MPT. To monitor the cell viability by the protective effect of DB against hydroxyl radical-induced cell lysis, trypan blue exclusion was used. MPT activity was monitored by changes in optical density of suspended mitochondria in an appropriate media by spectrophotometry. Results found that treatment of mitochondria with 3,4-DB showed protection with increased cell viability in a dose-dependent manner. Mitochondrial ROS generation by hydroxyl radicals was also suppressed by 3,4-DB. It was found that hydroxyl radical challenge caused high $[Ca^{2+}]_i$ levels that were suppressed by 3,4-DB. Hydroxyl radicals caused the opening of the megachannel, allowing swelling of mitochondria. It was found that this structural alteration resulted in the release of cytochrome c from the inner membrane of mitochondria into the incubating media. Data showed that 3,4- and 2,3-DB effectively suppressed MPT, and consequently prevented cytochrome c release. Since hydroxyl radicals deplete mitochondrial GSH levels, mitochondrial GSH content was measured. When mitochondria were treated with 3,4- and 2,3-DB, the GSH depletion was prevented, thus showing their sparing action of GSH. We conclude that DB protects mitochondria against hydroxyl radical attack by at least two processes: protection of the megachannel and sparing the mitochondrial GSH level. Further investigation on the precise mechanisms underlying the nature of protection of MPT, cytochrome c release, and sparing of GSH provides a better understanding of mitochondrial Ca^{2+} homeostasis.

Risk Factors for Total Mortality in Centenarians in Aichi Prefecture, Japan

KIYOKO YAGYU,[a] SHOGO KIKUCHI,[a] AND HISASHI TAUCHI[b]

[a]*Department of Public Health, Aichi Medical University, Aichi, Japan*
[b]*Institute for Medical Science of Aging, Aichi Medical University, Aichi, Japan*

In order to investigate risk factors for total mortality and survival in centenarians, we analyzed the data of 299 centenarians (60 male and 239 female) in Aichi Prefecture, Japan. The data was collected from 1992–1996 by a questionnaire administered in a direct interview or by mail. Informed consent was obtained, and subjects were followed thereafter. Information on gender, age, living environment, family members, occupational and educational history, smoking and drinking habits, lifestyle and dietary habits, physical functions and conditions, present and past illness, activities of daily living, personality traits and others was collected. Participants were followed until the end of December 1996, and death certificates were checked by governmental permission. Cox's Proportional Hazard Model was applied. Of the 299 centenarians, 175 were deceased by December 31, 1996. Cause of death included circulatory diseases in 69 (30.4%) subjects, senility in 48 (27.4%), respiratory diseases in 34 (19.4%), cancer in 9 (5.1%), and other causes in 15 subjects (17.7%). Statistically significant hazard ratios adjusted by age were as follows: gender (HR: 1.21, 95%CI: 1.00–1.56), smoking (HR: 1.05, 95%CI: 1.01–1.08), health status (HR: 0.93, 95%CI: 0.90–0.99), physically weakened (HR: 1.04, 95%CI: 1.01–1.08), episode of heart disease (HR: 1.25, 95%CI: 1.02–1.62), unable to feed oneself (HR: 1.59, 95%CI: 1.19–2.14), unable to change clothes independently (HR: 1.98, 95%CI: 1.48–2.64), visual difficulty in daily life (HR: 1.48, 95%CI: 1.12–1.96), and adherence (personality traits) (HR: 1.12, 95%CI: 1.01–1.25.) When mutually adjusted, significant prognosis-related factors were (1) unable to change clothes independently (HR: 1.23, 95%CI: 1.05–1.44) and (2) visual difficulty in daily life (HR: 1.07, 95%CI: 1.01–1.14). Alcohol, green tea, meat, fish and vegetable intake and sleep disturbance were not associated by risk.

The Activation Mechanisms of NF-κB and Inflammatory Enzymes during Aging

HYUN JOO KWON,[a] HYON JEEN KIM,[a] MIN JU KANG,[a] RYOYA TAKAHASHI,[b] SATARO GOTO,[b] BYUNG PAL YU,[c] AND HAE YOUNG CHUNG[a,c]

[a]*Vascular Aging Research Group, College of Pharmacy, Pusan National University, Pusan 609-735, Korea*

[b]*Faculty of Pharmacy, Toho University, Chiba 274-8510, Japan*

[c]*Research Institute of Genetic Engineering, Pusan National University, Pusan 609-735, Korea*

Evidence indicates that increased oxidative stress is a common characteristic found in the aged organism. Age-related oxidative stress is thought to be a causative factor responsible for a wide variety of damaged cellular constituents, leading to age-related dysfunction and various pathological conditions, such as the inflammatory process. Inflammation, a pathogenic expression of immunologically related responses, is often exacerbated under increased oxidative stress as in the case of aging. Many factors have been implicated as modulators in the inflammatory process. At the molecular level, for instance, the redox-sensitive transcription factor, NF-κB, plays the most important key role in the regulation of the inflammatory process, along with inducible nitric oxide synthase (iNOS), heme oxygenase-1 (HO-1), and cyclooxygenase-2 (COX-2). In the present study, we studied the mechanism underlying the modulation of the inflammatory reaction with age by investigating NF-κB activation and gene expression of the aforementioned factors in hepatic tissues isolated from young and old rats. We further expanded the investigation of these factors in rats that were injected with inflammatory activator, lipopolysaccharide (LPS, 5 mg/kg, i.p.). Data showed that NF-κB activity was upregulated with age, and this age-related activation was further enhanced by LPS injection, indicating the increased susceptibility and sensitivity to the inflammatory stimulus with age. To explore further the molecular events leading to the NF-κB activation, the inhibitory component of the NF-κB complex, IκB, was investigated. The cytosolic IκBα, but not IκBβ, was significantly decreased in both old and LPS-treated rats, signifying the enhanced migration of cytosolic NF-κB complex into the nucleus following dissociation from the inhibitor. The appearance of p65, as determined in the nucleus, corresponded with the change in IκBα, further provided supporting evidence of the molecular process involved the NF-κB activation. Our investigation on three proinflammation-related enzymes, COX-2, iNOS, and HO-1, clearly showed an age-related increase, in corroboration with the NF-κB activation. It was noteworthy that LPS injection caused the enhanced gene expression of these enzymes. Thus, it was concluded that under oxidatively stressed conditions during aging, the inflammatory status of the aged organism would be more sensitized because of the enhanced responses by NF-κB and other proinflammatory enzyme activities. More importantly, at the molecular level, the increased dissociation of IκBα that occurred in cytosol facilitates the increased NF-κB translocation.

Vitamin and Mineral Supplement Use among Independent-living Korean and American Older Adults

SEUNG-YOUN HONG

Gerontology Program, University of South Carolina, Columbia, South Carolina, USA

Malnutrition is one of the greatest nutritional problems in the older population. Although many dietary recommendations for the elderly were already available such as RDAs, research shows evidence of inadequate nutrient consumption from food alone. The data from the Nationwide Food Consumption survey indicated that the consumption of diets providing at least 61% of the RDA of nine selected nutrients (vitamins A, C, B_6, B_{12}, thiamin, riboflavin, calcium, iron, and magnesium) was reported by only 31% of persons 65 to 84 years old and by 21% of those 85 years and older. Based on the literature review, the following survey was performed to investigate factors associated with vitamin and mineral supplements used by noninstitutionalized American and Korean adults aged 60 years and older. The purpose of this was to investigate (1) the prevalence of vitamin/mineral supplementation among independent-living elderly people in South Carolina, (2) racial differences in the use of supplements, (3) the relationship between supplement use and contributing factors (e.g., gender, age, marital status, living arrangement, level of education), and (4) cultural differences among environmental factors, attitude, and knowledge about vitamin use. The survey was administered in the form of an in-person interview. The final samples consisted of 34 noninstitutionalized adults over 60 years of age: 17 Koreans and 17 Americans. All subjects met the criterion of independent living. The survey questions can be divided into six categories: (1) Demographic assessment (e.g., race, gender, age, marital status, living arrangement, level of education, and current carrier), (2) prevalence of use of vitamin/mineral supplements, (3) knowledge of vitamins, (4) attitude toward supplementation, (5) environmental factors, and (6) perceived health status/behaviors. Data obtained from completed interviews were manually coded and entered into the computer database system Excel. The data was exported into PC-SPPS, version 8.01, for analysis of the survey. The main dependent variable was defined as current use versus nonuse of any type of vitamin/mineral supplements. Result: In former research, approximately 30 to 40% of older adult used vitamin and mineral supplements. However, in this survey, 76% of older adults consumed them, and no difference by race was found in the use of vitamin/mineral supplements. Studies report that the most commonly used vitamin/mineral supplements among the older population are single supplements vitamins C, E, and B-complex, and multiple-nutrient supplements containing a combination of vitamins and minerals. However, in this study, the most commonly used single vitamins were vitamins C and E. Moreover, Koreans seemed likely to use fewer single vitamin/mineral supplements than did older American adults. Fifty-three percent of participants responded they consumed vitamin/minerals 6–9 times/week. There was no gender or age effect on the use of vitamins; however, marital status, living arrangement, and level of education influenced the use of vitamin/mineral supplements. American seniors seem to use more specific vitamins and minerals than do Koreans, but it was not statistically significant. As for environmental factors affecting use of vitamin and mineral supplements, a difference between races ($p < .05$) was shown. For older Korean adults, family is the strongest influence followed by articles in newspapers and magazines, and friends. However, older American adults are primarily influenced by reading news articles rather than by family or friends. Neither race has enough knowledge of micronutrients (30% of respondents correctly answered questions). Sixty-five percent of the Korean group answered "don't know," whereas 52% of the Americans gave the same response. Likewise, attitude toward supplement use was not different between groups ($p < .05$).

Vitamin D and Estrogen Receptor Gene Polymorphism and Their Interaction Associated with Bone Mineral Density in Korean Postmenopausal Women

IN SOON KWON, TAIWOO YOO, BYUNG JOO PARK, HEUNG SIK KANG, CHANG MO KANG, IN KYU KIM, SANG HOON BAE, HYUN CHAN CHO, HAENG SHIN LEE, AND CHO-IL KIM

The Aging and Physical Culture Research Institute, Medical Research Center, Seoul National University, Seoul, Korea

Osteoporosis is characterized by low bone mineral density and related fractures. The major determinant of bone mineral density is heritability, which is estimated to account for 40–80% of variation from twin and family studies. Association of vitamin D receptor (VDR) and estrogen receptor (ER) gene polymorphism with bone mineral density study results are inconsistent in Korea and countries of other ethnic backgrounds. Suggested reasons for this discrepancy are limited sample size, age, race, ethnic differences, and gene interaction with environmental factors such as age, diet and exercise, and gene by gene interactions that regulate bone mass. The goal of the present study is to evaluate (1) the relationship between VDR and ER gene polymorphism and bone mineral density after adjusting for confounding factors and (2) the possibility of the VDR and ER gene interaction that impacted bone mass in postmenopausal Korean women. The association between bone mineral density and restriction fragment length polymorphism (RFLP) with Bsm I endonuclease at the vitamin D gene and Pvu II and Xba I endonuclease with the ER gene were studied in 132 postmenopausal Korean women aged 45 to 71. Capital letters (B,P,X) signify the absence, and small letters (b, p, x) the presence, of restriction sites. Clinical characteristics, bone-related hormones, biochemical markers, and bone mineral density were also measured. Multiple regression was used to predict variables contributing to bone mineral density. Age, height, weight, years since menopause, and VER B genotype and ER P and X were used as independent variables. Age, body mass index, menarche and years since menopause, diet and exercise habits, biochemical markers, and bone mineral density were not significantly different according to VDR and ER genotypes. After controlling for confounding factors (age, body mass index, menarche, years since menopause), a significant ER X genotype effect on femoral neck bone mineral density and an increased significance with gene by gene interaction (VDR B*ER X) effect on femoral neck bone mineral density was observed by multiple regression analysis. Xba I RFLP of the ER gene is associated with femoral neck bone mineral density in Korean postmenopausal women. A more significant contribution of the VDR B and ER X gene interaction on femoral neck mineral was also observed.

Vitamin-E Dose-Associated Alterations in Mouse Immune Function

HYUN-SOOK KIM, JI-HYE LEE, AND YOU-SOOK LEE
Department of Food and Nutrition, Sookmyung Women's University, Chungpa-dong 2-ka, Yongsan-ku Seoul 140-742, Republic of Korea

Evidence from animal and human trials suggest an association between vitamin E and immune function. In this study, we investigated the vitamin-E dose-associated alteration in mouse immunity. Two different doses of vitamin E—20 IU vitamin E/kg b.w. for the optimal supplement group, and 80 IU vitamin E/kg b.w. for the overdose group—were injected daily into the intraperitonial cavity for 14 days in male ICR mice. Mouse splenocyte proliferation against mitogen stimulation, such as Con A, LPS, PWM, of each group was assessed as an index of immune function, and compared with that of a control group injected with the same volume of saline. Serum vitamin-E concentration was analyzed by HPLC to assure that intraperitonially injected vitamin E was appropriately absorbed. The animals in the high dose of vitamin-E supplement group showed significantly lower body weight gain and spleen index compared to those in the optimun level of the vitamin-E supplement group. More importantly, while the splenocyte proliferation of optimal vitamin-E supplement group was significantly enhanced, the overdose of vitamin-E-injected animals represented a much suppressed proliferation capacity compared to that in control animals. Consequently, optimum supplementation of vitamin E would be required for the proper immunity capacity, while overdose of vitamin-E supplementation may rather impair the immunocompetance.

Index of Contributors

Abe, R., 54–64
Ahn, H.-Y., 376
Ahn, J.Y., 346
An, D.-K., 358
Annapurna, V.V., 113–120
Arking, R., 157–167

Bae, S.H., 384
Black, A., 287–295
Buxbaum, J.D., 363, 373

Carmeli, E., 212–225
Carp, R.I., 182–186, 347, 363, 373
Carrillo, M.-C., 248–260
Chae, H.Z., 359–360
Chae, K.-R., 351
Chang, I.-M., 281–286
Chefer, S., 316–326
Chen, J.-J., 356
Cho, H.C., 384
Cho, J.-S., 351
Cho, J.-Y., 351
Cho, K.-A, 79–84
Cho, K.-H., 361, 374–375
Cho, K.-J., 141–156
Cho, S.Y., 261–273
Cho, T.-Y., 369
Chock, P.B., 48–53
Choi, E.-K., 182–186, 347, 363, 373
Choi, J.-K., 363, 373
Choi, J.S., 379
Choi, J.-Y., 368
Choi, S.-I., 182–186
Choi, W.C., 379
Choy, H.E., 65–70
Chun, Y.-S., 370
Chung, A.-S., 141–156, 367
Chung, H.-Y., 39–47, 327–335, 349, 350, 353, 366, 369, 379, 381
Chung, J.H., 377
Chung, M.-H., 368

Davis, R.J., 376
Do, S.-G., 358

Eun, H.C., 377

Franceschi, C., 85–96
Fujiki, H., 274–280
Fukui, K., 168–175
Furuichi, Y., 121–131

Goto, S., 54–64, 345, 349, 362, 381
Guldan, G.S., 371

Han, B.-G., 346, 372
Han, E.H., 346
Handy, A.., 287–295
Hanes, M., 132–140
Harman, D., 1–21
Hayashi, T., 54–64
Herbert, D.C., 132–140
Higami, Y., 362
Hong, K.W., 176–181
Hong, S.-Y., 382–383
Huh, T.-L., 354
Hui, W.W.-H., 371
Hwang, D.-Y., 351
Hwang, E.S., 364
Hwang, J.-H., 351
Hyun, M.-S., 376

Ikeno, Y., 132–140
Imai, K., 274–280
Ingram, D.K., 287–295, 305–315, 316–326
Intano, G., 132–140
Ivy, G.O., 248–260

Jang, I.-S., 351
Jeong, B.-H., 347
Jeong, H.-Y., 349
Ji, L.L., 236–247
Jin, J.-K., 182–186, 347, 363, 373
Jo, S.-H., 354
Jun, H.-S., 200–211
Jung, U., 367

Kanai, S., 248–260
Kang, C.-M., 352, 379, 384
Kang, H.-S., 370, 384
Kang, M.J., 381
Kang, S.-O., 48–53
Kang, T.-S., 351
Kau, M.-M., 356
Kaul, S.C., 357
Kikuchi, S., 380
Kim, B.-J., 351
Kim, C.-I., 384
Kim, D.-I., 79–84, 365
Kim, E.-G., 376
Kim, H.-J., 327–335, 349, 353, 379, 381
Kim, H.O., 374–375
Kim, H.-S., 368, 385
Kim, I.K., 384
Kim, I.S., 374–375
Kim, J.H., 65–70
Kim, J.-I., 182–186, 373
Kim, J.W., 327–335, 350
Kim, K.-W., 353
Kim, M.-S., 370
Kim, N.-H., 182–186
Kim, S.-R., 376
Kim, T.-H., 367
Kim, Y.-J., 351
Kim, Y.-K., 351
Kim, Y.-O., 354
Kim, Y.P., 359–360
Kim, Y.-S., 182–186, 347, 363, 373
Kitani, K., 248–260
Koh, H.-J., 354
Kondo, T., 362
Kozak, C.A., 347
Kumiyama, A., 54–64
Kwak, C.-S., 348
Kwak, I.H., 176–181
Kwon, H.J., 381
Kwon, I.S., 384

Lane, M.A., 287–295, 305–315, 316–326
Lee, C., 48–53
Lee, C.-F., 97–112
Lee, C.J., 364
Lee, D.-W., 368
Lee, H.-C., 97–112
Lee, H.-G., 363, 373
Lee, H.-P., 363

Lee, H.S., 384
Lee, J.-B., 359–360
Lee, J.E., 359–360
Lee, J.-H., 385
Lee, J.-Y., 358
Lee, M.-S., 348
Lee, S.-C., 359–360, 378
Lee, S.H., 261–273, 377
Lee, S.-M., 354
Lee, Y.H., 372
Lee, Y.I., 372
Lee, Y.-S., 261–273, 385
Lim, I.K., 176–181
Lim, S.S., 261–273
Liu, J., 355
London, E.D., 316–326
Lu, C.-Y., 97–112

Ma, Y.-S., 97–112
Manguino, D., 132–140
Maruyama, W., 248–260
Matochik, J., 316–326
Matsuyama, S., 274–280
McMahan, C.A., 132–140
Meeker, H.C., 347
Menashe, O., 212–225
Meydani, M., 226–235
Min, D.S., 376
Minami, C., 248–260
Mitsui, Y., 357
Moscrip, T.D., 316–326

Nakachi,, K., 274–280
Nam, K.H., 65–70
Nelson, J., 132–140
No, J.-K., 350

Oh, S.-I., 348
Okabe, S., 274–280
Ong, C.-N., 355
Onodera, K., 168–175

Packer, L., 141–156
Pang, C.-Y., 97–112
Park, B.-H., 376
Park, B.J., 384
Park, H.J., 379
Park, J., 346, 372

INDEX OF CONTRIBUTORS

Park, J.-B., 358
Park, J.-E., 361, 374–375
Park, J.-S., 79–84, 365
Park, J.-W., 354, 370
Park, S.C., xi–xii, 65–70, 79–84, 176–181, 336–343, 348, 365, 370, 379
Park, W.-Y., 79–84, 365
Perls, T., 85–96

Radak, Z., 54–64
Raji, N.S., 113–120
Rao, K.S., 113–120
Reddick, R., 132–140
Reznick, A.Z., 212–225
Roth, G.S., 287–295, 305–315, 316–326

Seo, H.W., 374–375
Shen, H.-M., 355
Shimokawa, I., 362
Shin, D.-B., 369
Shin, D.-H., 351
Shin, E.-Y., 376
Shin, J.-C., 376
Shin, K.H., 261–273
Shin, K.-S., 376
Shinkai, T., 168–175
Sohn, M.-K., 354
Song, I.-H., 354
Spindler, S.R., 296–304
Stadtman, E.R., 22–38
Stein, H., 212–225
Sueoka, E., 274–280
Sueoka, N., 274–280
Suganuma, M., 274–280
Suh, J.-G., 358
Suh, Y., 365
Suzuki, S., 168–175

Takahashi, R., 54–64, 345, 381
Takano, S., 357
Takenouchi, M., 54–64
Tanaka, K., 362
Tauchi, H., 380
Tilmont, E.M., 287–295

Toda, T., 71–78
Tuchiya, T., 362

Urano, S., 168–175

Van Orsouw, N.J., 85–96
Vijg, J., 85–96

Wadhwa, R., 357
Walter, C.A., 132–140
Wang, C.-W., 97–112
Wang, P.S., 356
Wasco, W., 363, 373
Weed, J., 316–326
Wei, Y.-H., 97–112
Woo, J.-S., 353
Woo, M.-K., 348

Yagyu, K., 380
Yamamoto, T., 248–260
Yanagihara-Outa, K., 362
Yang, C.-F., 355
Yang, R., 369
Yang, S.-H., 369
Yang, Y.H., 379
Yeo, E.-J., 352
Yim, H.-S., 48–53
Yim, M.B., 48–53
Yoo, J.-H., 344, 378
Yoo, T., 384
Yoon, C.S., 377
Yoon, G., 176–181
Yoon, J.-S., 366
Yoon, J.-W., 200–211
Yu, B.-P., 39–47, 327–335, 349, 350, 353, 366, 381
Yu, M.-A., 353
Yun, C.-H., 141–156

Zarzhevsky, N., 212–225
Zhou, Z.-Q., 132–140
Zs.-Nagy, I., 187–199